ORAL AND MAXILLOFACIAL DISEASES

ORAL AND MAXILLOFACIAL DISEASES

An illustrated guide to the diagnosis and management of diseases of the oral mucosa, gingivae, teeth, salivary glands, bones and joints

Third Edition

Crispian Scully
CBE, MD, PhD, MDS, MRCS, FDSRCS, FDSRCPS, FFDRCSI, FDSRCSE, FRCPath, FMedSci
Professor of Special Needs Dentistry, and of Oral Medicine, Pathology and Microbiology
Honorary Consultant
University College London Hospitals, Great Ormond Street
Hospital for Children London and John Radcliffe Hospital, Oxford, and
Dean and Director of Studies and Research
Eastman Dental Institute for Oral Health Care Sciences
University College London, UK

Stephen R Flint
MA, PhD, MBBS, FDSRCS, FFDRCSI, FICD
Senior Lecturer and Consultant in Oral Medicine
Dublin Dental School and Hospital, Trinity College
Dublin, Ireland

Stephen R Porter
FDSRCSEng, FDSRCSEd, PhD, MD
Professor of Oral Medicine
Eastman Dental Institute for Oral Health Care Sciences
University College London, UK

Khursheed F Moos
OBE, FDSRCSEng, MRCS, FDSRCSEd, FDSRCPS, FRCS
Emeritus Professor of Oral and Maxillofacial Surgery
Glasgow Dental Hospital and School, UK

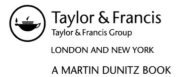

Taylor & Francis
Taylor & Francis Group

LONDON AND NEW YORK

A MARTIN DUNITZ BOOK

First published in the United Kingdom in 1989
by Taylor & Francis, an imprint of the Taylor & Francis Group, 2 Park Square, Milton Park, Abingdon, Oxfordchire
OX14 4RN

Tel.:   +44 (0) 1235 828600
Fax.:   +44 (0) 1235 829000
E-mail: info@dunitz.co.uk
Website: http://www.dunitz.co.uk

Third edition 2004

Although every effort has been made to ensure that all owners of copyright material have been acknowledged in this publication, we would be glad to acknowledge in subsequent reprints or editions any omissions brought to our attention.

Although every effort has been made to ensure that drug doses and other information are presented accurately in this publication, the ultimate responsibility rests with the prescribing physician. Neither the publishers nor the authors can be held responsible for errors or for any consequences arising from the use of information contained herein. For detailed prescribing information or instructions on the use of any product or procedure discussed herein, please consult the prescribing information or instructional material issued by the manufacturer.

This book includes some photographs that predate the recommendations on control of cross-infection: gloves should be worn where appropriate.

A CIP record for this book is available from the British Library.

Library of Congress Cataloging-in-Publication Data
Data available on application

ISBN 1-84184-338-5

Distributed in the United States and Canada by:
Thieme New York
333 Seventh Avenue
New York, NY 10001, USA

Distributed in the rest of the world by:
Thomson Publishing Services
Cheriton House
North Way
Andover, Hampshire SP10 5BE, UK

Composition by Newgen Imaging Systems (P) Ltd, Chennai, India
Printed and bound in Spain by Grafos SA Arte Sobre Papel

CONTENTS

PREFACE TO THE THIRD EDITION   xi

PREFACE TO THE SECOND EDITION   xii

PREFACE TO THE FIRST EDITION   xiii

1 DIFFERENTIAL DIAGNOSES AND MANAGEMENT   **1**
1.1 Differential diagnoses by symptoms or signs   2
1.2 Differential diagnoses by site   14
1.3 Guide to the diagnosis and management of oral diseases   20
1.4 Guide to drugs used in the management of oral diseases   46
1.5 Guide to the oral and perioral side-effects of drug treatment   58

2 VIRAL INFECTIONS   **65**
Hand, foot and mouth disease   66
Herpangina   67
Herpes simplex infections   68
Herpes varicella-zoster   76
Human papillomavirus infections   82
Infectious mononucleosis   85
Measles   87
Molluscum contagiosum   88
Mumps   89
Orf   90
Parvovirus infection   90
Rubella   91
Uvulitis   91
Vaccinia   92
Further reading   92

3 BACTERIAL INFECTIONS   **95**
Actinomycosis   96
Acute necrotizing ulcerative gingivitis   97
Anthrax   98
Cancrum oris (noma)   98
Cat-scratch disease   99
Epithelioid angiomatosis   99
Leprosy   100
Reiter's syndrome   101
Syphilis   102
Tuberculosis   107
Yaws   109
Further reading   110

4 MYCOSES   **111**
Aspergillosis   112
Blastomycoses   113
Candidosis   114
Histoplasmosis   123
Mucormycosis   123
Further reading   123

5 INFESTATIONS AND POSSIBLE INFECTIONS   **125**
Kawasaki's disease   126
Larva migrans   126
Leishmaniasis   127
Myiasis   127
Sarcoidosis   127
Toxoplasmosis   130
Further reading   130

6 NEOPLASMS   **133**
Basal cell carcinoma   134
Granular cell tumour   134
Keratoacanthoma   135
Langerhans' cell histiocytoses   135
Leiomyoma   136
Leukaemias   137
Lipoma   141
Lymphomas   142
Malignant melanoma   146
Melanoacanthoma   147
Metastatic neoplasms   147
Multiple myeloma   149
Mycosis fungoides   151
Myxoma   151
Neuroblastoma   152
Neuroectodermal tumour (congenital epulis)   153
Neuroma   153
Osteoma   155
Plasmacytoma   157
Rhabdomyosarcoma   157
Salivary neoplasms   158
Sarcomas   162
Squamous cell carcinomas   165
Further reading   171

7 HAMARTOMAS   **173**
Haemangioma   174
Lymphangioma   177
Further reading   178

8 ENDOCRINE, NUTRITIONAL AND METABOLIC DISEASES 179

Acrodermatitis enteropathica 180
Acromegaly 181
Addison's disease 183
Carcinoid syndrome 183
Cushing's syndrome 183
Deficiency states 184
Diabetes mellitus 187
Glucagonoma 187
Hyperparathyroidism 188
Hypoparathyroidism 189
Hypophosphatasia 190
Hypothyroidism 191
Lesch–Nyhan syndrome 191
Lipoid proteinosis 192
Mucopolysaccharidoses 192
Multiple endocrine adenoma
    syndrome 194
Further reading 194

9 IMMUNE DISORDERS 197

Amyloidosis 198
Hereditary angioedema 199
Genetically based immune defects 200
Human immunodeficiency virus
    (HIV) disease 203
Further reading 219

10 DISEASES OF THE BLOOD AND BLOOD-FORMING ORGANS 221

Aplastic anaemia 222
Bone-marrow transplantation 222
Chronic granulomatous disease 225
Fanconi's anaemia 225
Folate deficiency 225
Haemoglobinopathies 226
Haemophilias 226
Hypoplasminogenaemia 228
Iron deficiency anaemia 229
Myelodysplastic syndromes 230
Neutropenia 230
Pernicious anaemia 232
Plasmacytosis 233
Plummer–Vinson syndrome 233
Polycythaemia rubra vera 234
Purpura 234
Von Willebrand's disease 236
Further reading 237

11 MENTAL DISORDERS 239

Anorexia nervosa/bulimia 240
Atypical facial pain 241
Learning disability 241
Munchausen's syndrome 242
Oral dysaesthesia 243
Psychogenic oral disease 243
Self-mutilation (oral artefactual disease) 246
Further reading 247

12 DISEASES OF THE NERVOUS SYSTEM 249

Abducent nerve lesion 250
Bell's palsy 250
Cerebral palsy 252
Cerebrovascular accident 252
Congenital pain insensitivity 252
Epilepsy 253
Glossopharyngeal and vagus
    nerve palsy 253
Hypoglossal palsy 254
Lateral medullary syndrome 254
Möbius' syndrome 255
Parkinsonism 255
Riley–Day syndrome 255
Trigeminal neuralgia 256
Trigeminal sensory loss 257
Further reading 258

13 DISEASES OF THE CIRCULATORY SYSTEM 261

Calibre-persistent artery 262
Cardiac transplantation 262
Giant cell arteritis 263
Hereditary haemorrhagic telangiectasia 264
Ischaemic and other heart diseases 265
Midline granuloma 265
Periarteritis nodosa 266
Varices 266
Wegener's granulomatosis 267
Further reading 267

14 DISEASES OF THE RESPIRATORY SYSTEM 269

Antral carcinoma 270
Asthma 271
Cystic fibrosis 271
Fascial space infections 271
Influenza 271
Lung cancer 272

Lymphonodular pharyngitis 272
Maxillary sinusitis 272
Quinsy 273
Tonsillitis 273
Tuberculosis 273
Further reading 274

15 DISORDERS OF TEETH 275

Abrasion 276
Amelogenesis imperfecta 276
Ankylosis 279
Anomalies of tooth shape 280
Attrition 281
Dental caries 282
Dentinogenesis imperfecta 284
Dilaceration 286
Enamel cleft 287
Enamel hypoplasia 287
Enamel nodule 288
Erosion 289
Fluorosis 290
Hypercementosis 290
Hyperdontia 291
Hyperplastic pulpitis 292
Hypodontia 292
Impacted teeth 294
Localized damage 295
Malocclusion 296
Natal teeth 298
Nonvital teeth 299
Odontomes 299
Periapical abscess 301
Periapical cyst 306
Prominent tubercules or cusps 307
Residual cyst 307
Resorption 308
Retained primary tooth 308
Retained root 309
Taurodontism 310
Teratoma 311
Tooth extrinsic staining 311
Tooth intrinsic staining 312
Further reading 314

16 GINGIVAL AND PERIODONTAL DISEASE 317

Abscesses 318
Chronic hyperplastic gingivitis 319
Chronic marginal gingivitis 319
Dental bacterial plaque 320

Dental calculus 320
Desquamative gingivitis 321
Drug-induced swelling 321
Fibrous epulis 322
Giant cell granuloma 322
Gingival cyst 322
Gingival fibromatosis 323
Gingival recession 324
Keratosis 324
Materia alba 325
Pericoronitis 325
Periodontitis 326
Pigmentation 327
Plasma cell gingivitis 328
Pyogenic granuloma 328
Tumours 329
Traumatic occlusion 329
Further reading 330

17 SALIVARY DISORDERS 331

Acute bacterial sialadenitis 332
Adenomatoid hyperplasia 333
Mucoceles 333
Necrotizing sialometaplasia 335
Obstructive sialadenitis 335
Salivary fistula 337
Sialosis 337
Tumours 338
Xerostomia 338
Further reading 339

18 MUCOSAL DISORDERS 341

Aphthae 342
Behçet's syndrome 345
Black hairy tongue 347
Cheek chewing 348
Cheilitis 349
Denture-induced hyperplasia 350
Dermoid cyst 351
Eosinophilic ulcer 351
Ephelis 351
Erythema migrans 352
Erythroplasia 355
Fibrous lump 356
Foliate papillitis 357
Furred tongue 357
Glossitis 357
Glossodynia 358
Keratosis 358
Leukoedema 362

Linea alba   363
Lingual abscess   363
Lingual haematoma   364
Lingual laceration   364
Lingual hemihypertrophy   365
Lip chapping   365
Lip fissure   365
Lip horn   366
Melanotic macules   367
Naevi   367
Oral submucous fibrosis   367
Papillary hyperplasia   368
Papillomatosis   369
Pigmentation   369
Pyogenic granuloma   370
Stomatitis nicotina   370
Tattoos   371
Traumatic ulcers   372
Verrucous hyperplasia   373
Verrucous xanthoma   374
Further reading   374

**19 GASTROINTESTINAL
   DISORDERS   377**
Crohn's disease   378
Gastric regurgitation   381
Gastrointestinal neoplasms   381
Gluten-sensitive enteropathy   382
Melkersson–Rosenthal syndrome   382
Orofacial granulomatosis   383
Peptic ulceration   383
Tylosis   383
Ulcerative colitis   384
Further reading   385

20 DISEASES OF THE LIVER   387
Alcoholic cirrhosis   388
Biliary atresia   388
Chronic active hepatitis   388
Liver transplantation   389
Primary biliary cirrhosis   389
Viral hepatitis   390
Further reading   390

**21 DISEASES OF THE GENITO-
   URINARY SYSTEM   393**
Chronic renal failure   394
Hypophosphataemia   395
Renal transplantation   396
Further reading   396

**22 COMPLICATIONS OF PREGNANCY,
   CHILDBIRTH, PUERPERIUM AND
   THE MENOPAUSE   399**
Chloasma   400
Gingivitis during menstruation   400
Menopause   400
Pregnancy epulis   400
Pregnancy gingivitis   401
Further reading   401

**23 DISEASES OF THE SKIN
   AND SUBCUTANEOUS TISSUES   403**
Acanthosis nigricans   404
Acute lymphadenitis   405
Carbuncle   406
Dermatitis herpetiformis   407
Discoid lupus erythematosus   408
Epidermolysis bullosa acquisita   409
Erythema multiforme   409
Impetigo   412
Lichen planus   413
Lichen sclerosis   422
Linear IgA disease   422
Localized oral purpura   423
Necrotizing fasciitis   423
Pemphigoid   424
Pemphigus   427
Pigmented purpuric stomatitis   431
Psoriasis   431
Stevens–Johnson syndrome   433
Toxic epidermal necrolysis   434
Vitiligo   434
Further reading   434

24 DISEASES OF CONNECTIVE TISSUE   437
Dermatomyositis   438
Felty's syndrome   439
Mixed connective-tissue disease   439
Raynaud's phenomenon   440
Rheumatoid arthritis   440
Scleroderma   442
Sjögren's syndrome   445
Systemic lupus erythematosus   448
Further reading   451

**25 ODONTOGENIC CYSTS AND
   NEOPLASMS   453**
Adenomatoid odontogenic tumour   454
Ameloblastoma   454

Calcifying odontogenic cyst   456
Calcifying odontogenic tumour   456
Dentigerous cyst   457
Eruption cyst   458
Globulomaxillary cyst   459
Lateral periodontal cyst   459
Nasopalatine duct cyst   460
Odontogenic fibromyxoma   461
Odontogenic keratocyst   461
Further reading   462

26 DISORDERS OF BONE   465
Albright's syndrome   466
Alveolar atrophy   467
Aneurysmal bone cyst   467
Cemento-ossifying fibroma   468
Cherubism   469
Dry socket   470
Exostoses   471
Fibrous dysplasia   471
Giant cell granuloma
    (central giant cell granuloma)   474
Haemorrhagic bone cyst   475
Ossifying fibroma   475
Osteomyelitis   476
Paget's disease   479
Stafne bone cavity   483
Torus mandibularis   483
Torus palatinus   484
Further reading   484

27 JOINT DISORDERS   487
Condylar ankylosis   488
Polyvinyl chloride acro-osteolysis   488
Temporomandibular joint arthritides   489
Temporomandibular joint subluxation   489
Temporomandibular joint pain-dysfunction
    syndrome   490
Further reading   490

**28 CONGENITAL AND DEVELOPMENTAL
DISORDERS   491**
Abnormal labial fraenum   492
Absent uvula   492
Ankyloglossia   492
Apert's syndrome   493
Ascher's syndrome   494
Bifid uvula   494
Blue rubber-bleb naevus syndrome   495
Branchial cyst   495
Caffey's disease   495

Carney's syndrome   496
Chievitz's organ   497
Chondroectodermal dysplasia   497
Cleft lip and palate   498
Cleidocranial dysplasia   498
Cowden's syndrome   501
Craniofacial microsomia   502
Craniometaphyseal dysplasia   504
Cri du chat syndrome   505
Crouzon's syndrome   505
Cystic hygroma   507
Darier's disease   507
De Lange's syndrome   508
Down's syndrome   509
Dyskeratosis congenita   512
Ectodermal dysplasia   512
Ehlers–Danlos syndrome   514
Epidermolysis bullosa   516
Epiloia   517
Familial gingival fibromatosis   519
Fissured tongue   519
Fordyce's spots   520
Fragile X syndrome   520
Gardner's syndrome   521
Gorlin's syndrome   523
Hallermann–Streiff syndrome   525
Hemifacial hypertrophy   525
Hereditary haemorrhagic telangiectasia   525
Hereditary palmoplantar keratoses   525
Ichthyosis   526
Incontinentia pigmenti   527
Klippel–Trenaunay–Weber syndrome   528
Laband's syndrome   529
Leukoedema   530
Lip pit   531
Maffucci's syndrome   531
Marfan's syndrome   532
Mucinosis   533
Myotonic dystrophy   533
Naevi   534
Olmsted's syndrome   535
Orofaciodigital syndrome   536
Osteogenesis imperfecta   537
Osteopetrosis   538
Pachyonychia congenita   538
Patau's syndrome   539
Peutz–Jegher's syndrome   540
Pierre Robin sequence syndrome   540
Racial pigmentation   540
Romberg's syndrome   541
Smith–Lemli–Opitz syndrome   541
Sturge–Weber syndrome   542

Tetralogy of Fallot	543
Thyroid (lingual)	543
Tori	544
Treacher Collins' syndrome	544
Van der Woude syndrome	545
Von Recklinghausen's disease	545
White sponge naevus	547
Further reading	548

29 CHEMICAL AGENTS **549**

Acrodynia	550
Allergic reactions	550
Amalgam tattoo	551
Angioedema	552
Betel nut staining	552
Body art	553
Burns	553
Candidosis	555
Cheilitis	555
Drug-induced gingival swelling	556
Drug-induced hyperpigmentation	557
Drug-induced mucositis and ulceration	562
Drug-induced xerostomia	563
Erosions	563
Facial palsy	564
Herpesvirus infections	564
Human papillomavirus infections	564
Leukoplakia	564
Lichenoid lesions	564
Neoplasms and potentially malignant lesions	565
Orofacial granulomatosis	565
Osteonecrosis	565
Stomatitis nicotina	566

Tooth erosion	566
Tooth staining	566
Further reading	567

30 PHYSICAL AGENTS **569**

Body art	570
Burns	571
Cicatrization	572
Foreign bodies	573
Frey's syndrome	574
Frictional keratosis	574
Grafts	575
Iatrogenic injury	575
Oroantral fistula	577
Oronasal fistula	577
Surgical emphysema	578
Trauma to dentition	578
Traumatic hyperplasia	578
Traumatic ulcers and haematomas	579
Further reading	581

31 RADIATION EFFECTS **583**

Actinic cheilitis	584
Actinic prurigo	584
Ionizing radiation-induced epithelial changes	584
Ionizing radiation-induced hard-tissue damage	586
Ionizing radiation-induced xerostomia	588
Radiation accidents	589
Further reading	589

INDEX **591**

PREFACE TO THE THIRD EDITION

Many atlases of clinical oral pathology focus on a specific area such as mucosal disease. This atlas, *The Atlas of Oral and Maxillofacial Pathology*, differs significantly from most others, by the inclusion of clinical detail on diseases of the oral mucosa, gingivae, teeth, salivary glands, bones and joints, and of a wide range of the more obvious extraoral manifestations. This third edition has been enhanced by the contribution from an eminent oral and maxillofacial surgeon, and therefore provides one of the most comprehensive illustrated coverages of oral and maxillofacial diseases of which we are aware worldwide. It is intended primarily as a pictorial diagnostic aid for dentists, surgeons and physicians, with text that provides a concise synopsis of stomatology.

The previous editions of this atlas were extremely successful; it has become increasingly popular because of the very wide coverage of oral and maxillofacial diseases and the depth of information contained. Translations have been published in French, German and Portuguese and have been agreed for Spanish and Arabic.

The atlas has been thoroughly revised and updated, further extended and improved to include better examples of many conditions, as well as more examples of the common orofacial conditions or where clinical diagnosis can be difficult because of varied presentations. There is now much more material on hard tissue pathology and the format has been improved.

There are many new illustrations and conditions appearing in this edition, including several drug reactions (such as to bisphosphates, nicorandil and minocycline), a range of lesions seen in HIV/AIDS, organ transplantation, acrodermatitis enteropathica, cholinergic dysautonomia hypoplasminogenaemia, lipoid proteinosis, cat-scratch disease, craniometaphyseal dysplasia, epithelioid angiomatosis, epidermolysis bullosa, dyskeratosis congenita, microsomia, pachyonychia congenita and a number of syndromes (Carney, Gardner, Job, Kawasaki, Klippel–Trenaunay–Weber, Maffucci, Olmsted, von Willebrand).

The section on diagnosis and management has been updated and continues to be presented in a clear and user-friendly format cover: differential diagnoses by symptoms, signs and site, investigations and management of the various conditions covered in the book, the drugs used in the management of oral diseases and the oral and perioral side-effects of drug treatment. The Recommended International Non-proprietary Name (rINN) is used for drugs. The references have been fully updated.

It is impossible to organize the material in a format that will please all and we therefore elected originally to conform fairly closely to the World Health Organization's International Classification of Diseases (ICD). This, like any system, cannot suit all needs but it does have the advantage of having received WHO acceptance.

However, in this edition, we have varied the system where we felt it absolutely necessary to improve ease of use of the atlas. In particular, we have split several chapters and subclassified the original 'Digestive' section into chapters discussing disorders of the teeth, gingiva and mucosa, and disorders of the salivary glands. We have also arranged the material alphabetically for easier reference. Inevitably there is tremendous variation in the lengths of chapters (disorders with pleomorphic presentations, such as lichen planus, almost warrant a chapter on their own) and there is some overlap, especially in the chapters on iatrogenic disease. Also, although many of the genetic disorders appear in the chapter on congenital disease, it should be recognized that there is scarcely a disorder in which some genetic role does not play a part.

We are grateful to our colleagues who have kindly provided illustrations; particular thanks, in addition to those acknowledged in the previous editions, are due to Oslei Paes de Almeida (Piracicaba), Antonio Azul (Lisbon), Jose-Vicente Bagan (Valencia), John Buchanan (London), Noel Claffey (Dublin), Drore Eisen (Cincinnatti), Catherine Flaitz (Houston), Michael Gaukroger (London), Rodney Grahame (London), Aslan Gokbuget (Istanbul), Tim Hodgson (London), Navdeep Kumar (London), Jane Luker (Bristol), Graham Ogden (Dundee), Nick (Roy) Rogers (Rochester), Mary Toner (Dublin), Richard Welbury (Glasgow), and Donald Winstock (London). Thanks also go to our co-authors of *Dermatology of the Lips* (Scully C, Bagan JV, Eisen D, Porter S, Rogers RS) Isis Medical Media (Oxford) 2000; *A Color Atlas of Orofacial Health and Disease in Children and Adolescents* (Scully C, Welbury R, Flaitz C, Almeida ODP) Martin Dunitz (London) 2001; and *Orofacial Disease. An Update for the Dental Team* (Scully C, Porter SR) Elsevier Harcourt, London & Edinburgh, 2002; and to the publishers of the *British Dental Journal*, *British Journal of Dermatology*, *International Journal of Oral and Maxillofacial Surgery*, *Journal of Oral Pathology and Medicine*, *Medicina Oral*, *Oral Diseases*, *Oral Oncology*, and *Oral Surgery, Oral Medicine and Oral Pathology*.

Crispian Scully
Stephen R Flint
Stephen R Porter
Khursheed F Moos
England, Ireland and Scotland

PREFACE TO THE SECOND EDITION

The first edition, *An Atlas of Stomatology*, was extremely successful and it became increasingly popular as readers appreciated that it was more than just an atlas, containing also a textual overview of the subject and covering a wider range of oral diseases than most atlases. Since then, the authors have moved to new positions and have had access to a much wider patient base.

This second edition provides one of the most comprehensive illustrated coverages of oral diseases of which we are aware and has been extended and improved to include more data and tables on diagnosis, management and drug use, as well as several new clinical entities. The references have been fully updated.

There is a new chapter on liver disease, and more than 125 new illustrations, covering a range of recently described new entities such as pigmented purpuric stomatitis, superficial mucoceles, idiopathic plasmacytosis, oral lesions induced by cocaine and other drugs, and oral body art. Other conditions appearing for the first time in this edition include a range of lesions seen in AIDS, organ transplants, myiasis, Laband syndrome, larva migrans, giant-cell arteritis, myotonic dystrophy, Munchausen's syndrome, necrotizing fasciitis, toxoplasmosis,

lichen sclerosus, adenomatoid hyperplasia, mixed connective tissue disease and lingual thyroid.

The expanded section on diagnosis and management is presented in a clear and easy-to-use format and covers differential diagnoses by symptoms, signs and site, investigations and management of the various conditions covered in the book, the drugs used in the management of oral diseases and the oral and perioral side-effects of drug treatment.

We are grateful to our colleagues who have kindly provided some illustrations; particular thanks are due to Dr A Efeoglu (Istanbul, Turkey), Professor O Almeida (Sao Paulo, Brazil), Mr G Bounds (London, UK), Dr R MacLeod (Edinburgh, UK) and Mr A Babejews (Exeter, UK). We are also grateful to Ms Navdeep Singh (London, UK) for her assistance with tables, to Mr Alan Haddock (King's Lynn, UK) and Mr Alex Redhead (Leeds, UK) for help with references, and to Ms Nicci King and Ms Karen Parr (London, UK) for their help with typing.

Crispian Scully
Stephen R Flint
Stephen R Porter
London and Dublin

PREFACE TO THE FIRST EDITION

This atlas gives examples of oral diseases and those lesions in the wide range of systemic disorders that have oral manifestations. It differs from other atlases by the inclusion of a wide range of the more obvious extraoral manifestations and of some disorders of the teeth and hard tissues. It is intended primarily as a pictorial diagnostic aid, both for dentists and physicians, with text that provides a concise synopsis of stomatology. We have added very recent references for most topics, mainly where there are new developments, reviews or points of controversy.

The atlas covers clinical diagnostic features and includes some radiographs, but excludes laboratory tests and does not attempt to discuss management. Neither have we attempted to cover orthodontics, oral surgery or periodontology, as they are dealt with elsewhere.

It is impossible to organize the illustrations in a format that will please all and we have therefore elected to conform fairly closely to the World Health Organization International Classification of Diseases (ICD). This, like any system, cannot suit all needs but it does have the advantage of having received WHO acceptance. We have varied the system where we felt it absolutely necessary.

The illustrations are almost exclusively from our collection in the University Department of Oral Medicine, Surgery and Pathology at Bristol. We are indebted to former and present members of the Department who have contributed to the collection, particularly to the late Professor AI Darling; to

Professors J Fletcher and AK Adatia; to Drs SR Porter and J Luker; and to Mr RG Smith. We are also grateful to Professor DK Mason, under whose care some of the patients were seen in Glasgow. A few slides are from other collections: Dr G Laskaris (Athens) has kindly helped with Figures 2.130, 2.131, 2.140, 14.82, 14.83 and 16.58; our colleagues, O Almeida, D Berry, M Griffiths, S Mutlu, F Nally, S Prime, J Ross, J Shepherd and AS Young have also helped with single contributions.

Most of the illustrations have not previously been published. For those that have, we are indebted to Professor RA Cawson as co-author of some publications; to the editors of the *British Dental Journal*; *Journal of Oral Pathology*; *Oral Surgery, Oral Medicine and Oral Pathology*; *Dental Update and Hospital Update*; and to publishers Churchill Livingstone; Heinemann Medical; Oxford University Press and John Wright for permission to reproduce some of the slides from our collection. We wish to acknowledge any other source whom we may have unwittingly omitted.

We are also grateful to Dr JW Eveson, who joined the Department after this project was started, and who has helped with constructive comments and our further education; to Ni Fathers and Derek Coles, for help with technical aspects related to the illustrations; and to Connie Blake, for typing the manuscript.

CS
SF
Bristol

1 DIFFERENTIAL DIAGNOSES AND MANAGEMENT

1.1 Differential diagnoses by symptoms or signs

1.2 Differential diagnoses by site

1.3 Guide to the diagnosis and management of oral diseases

1.4 Guide to drugs used in the management of oral diseases

1.5 Guide to the oral and perioral side-effects of drug treatment

1.1 DIFFERENTIAL DIAGNOSES BY SYMPTOMS OR SIGNS

Anaesthesia or hypo-aesthesia

Numbness over the chin (numb chin syndrome) may indicate a lesion involving the mental or inferior alveolar nerves or may have more sinister implications.

Traumatic

Jaw fracture. Direct trauma to trigeminal nerve or branches
Iatrogenic (e.g. nerve block anaesthesia, cancer surgery or osteotomy)

Idiopathic

Benign trigeminal sensory neuropathy

Neoplasms

Jaw metastases
Intracranial neoplasia
Pharyngeal neoplasia (Trotter's syndrome)

Disseminated malignancy in the absence of identifiable jaw deposits

Systemic non-malignant disease

Connective tissue disorders
Diabetes mellitus
Sarcoidosis
Amyloidosis
Sickle cell disease
Vasculitides
Infections
Demyelinating diseases

Drugs and poisons

see Section 1.5, page 58

Blisters

(*See* Table 1.1, page 3)

Skin diseases

Pemphigoid (usually mucous membrane pemphigoid)
Pemphigus (usually pemphigus vulgaris)
Intra-epidermal IgA pustulosis
Dermatitis herpetiformis
Linear IgA disease
Erythema multiforme
Epidermolysis bullosa
Lichen planus

Infections

Herpes simplex
Herpes varicella-zoster
Coxsackie viruses
Other enteroviruses

Burns

Angina bullosa haemorrhagica (localized oral purpura)

Drugs (*see* Section 1.5)

Paraneoplastic disorders

Amyloidosis

False blisters

Cysts
Superficial mucoceles
Abscesses

Burning mouth

Deficiency states

Vitamin B_{12} deficiency
Folate deficiency
Iron deficiency
B complex deficiency

Infections

Candidosis

Others

Erythema migrans (geographic tongue)
Diabetes mellitus
Xerostomia

Psychogenic

Cancerophobia
Depression
Anxiety states
Hypochondriasis

Drugs

see Section 1.5, page 58

Table 1.1 DIFFERENTIATION OF THE MORE IMPORTANT ORAL VESICULOBULLOUS DISORDERS*

	Pemphigus	Mucous membrane pemphigoid	Erythema multiforme	Dermatitis herpetiformis	Linear IgA disease	Localized oral purpura
Incidence	Rare	Uncommon	Uncommon	Rare	Rare	Uncommon
Age mainly affected	Middle age	Late/middle age	Young adults	Middle age	Middle age	Middle age/elderly
Sex mainly affected	F	F	M	M	F	M = F
Geographic factors	Italian, Jewish origin	—	—	—	—	—
Predisposing factors	Rarely drugs	Rarely furosemide or other drugs	Drugs, infections	Gluten-sensitive enteropathy	Rarely vancomycin	? Steroid inhalers
Oral manifestations	Erosions; blisters rarely persist; Nikolsky's sign positive	Blisters (sometimes blood-filled), erosions, Nikolsky sign may be positive	Swollen lips, serosanguinous exudate, large erosions anteriorly, occasional blisters	Blisters, ulcers, erythematous patches	Blisters, ulcers	Blood blisters
Cutaneous or other manifestations	Large flaccid skin blisters at some stage. Mucosal lesions common	Rare or minor skin blisters may be mucosal lesions	Target (iris) or other lesions may be present on skin	Pruritic vesicular rash on back and extensor surfaces Gluten-sensitive enteropathy	Crops of plaques in a characteristic annular or polycyclic pattern on upper trunk, shoulders, limbs, face	Rarely, oesophageal blisters
Histopathology	Acantholysis, intraepithelial bullae	Subepithelial bullae	Subepithelial or intraepithelial bullae	Subepithelial bullae	Subepithelial bullae	Subepithelial bullae
Direct immunostaining	Intercellular IgG in epithelium	Subepithelial/BMZ, C3, IgG	Subepithelial IgG†	Subepithelial IgA	Subepithelial IgA	—
Serology	Antibodies to epithelial intercellular cement (desmoglein) in most	Antibodies to epithelial basement membrane in few	—	Antibodies to transglutaminase or endomysium in some	Antibodies to reticulin and endomysium are rare	—
Other investigations	—	—	—	Biopsy of small intestine Tissue transglutaminase	—	Exclude thrombocytopathy

*Lichen planus is rarely bullous; †Non-specific findings; BMZ, basement membrane zone; C3, third component of complement; IgG, immunoglobulin G; IgA, immunoglobulin A.

Cacogeusia

Oral disease

Pericoronitis
Chronic periodontitis
Acute necrotizing ulcerative gingivitis
Chronic dental abscesses
Dry socket
Food impaction
Sialadenitis
Neoplasms

Xerostomia

Drugs
Sjögren's syndrome
Sarcoidosis
Irradiation damage

Psychogenic causes

Depression
Anxiety states
Psychoses
Hypochondriasis

Drugs (*see also* Section 1.5, page 58)

Smoking

Starvation

Nasal or pharyngeal disase

Chronic sinusitis
Oroantral fistula
Neoplasm
Nasal foreign body
Pharyngeal disease
Tonsillitis
Neoplasm

Diabetes

Respiratory disease

Bronchiectasis
Neoplasm

Gastrointestinal disease

Pharyngeal pouch
Gastric regurgitation
Liver disease

Central nervous system disease

Temporal lobe tumours
Temporal lobe epilepsy

Renal disease

Uraemia

Liver failure

Discharges

Dental disease

Chronic dental and parodontal abscesses
Dry socket
Cysts
Oroantral fistula
Osteomyelitis
Osteoradionecrosis
Infection by foreign body

Salivary gland disorders

Sialadenitis
Salivary fistulae

Psychogenic (imagined discharges)

Depression
Hypochondriasis
Psychosis

Dry mouth (xerostomia)

(see also Section 1.5, page 58)

Drugs with anticholinergic or sympathomimetic effects

Dehydration

Uncontrolled diabetes mellitus
Diabetes insipidus
Diarrhoea and vomiting
Severe haemorrhage

Psychogenic

Anxiety states
Depression
Hypochondriasis
Bulimia nervosa

Salivary gland disorders

Sjögren's syndrome
Sarcoidosis
Irradiation or chemotherapy damage
HIV infection
HCV infection
Bone marrow transplantation/graft-versus-
  host disease
Cystic fibrosis
Ectodermal dysplasia
Amyloidosis or other deposits
Salivary gland aplasia

Dysautonomia

Dysarthria

Oral disease

Painful lesions or loss of mobility of the
  tongue or palate
Cleft palate (including submucous cleft)
Oral or oropharyngeal neoplasia
Severe scarring
Tongue piercing

Neurological disorders

Multiple sclerosis
Parkinson's disease
Motor neurone disease
Cerebrovascular accident
Bulbar and pseudo-bulbar palsy
Hypoglossal nerve palsy
Cerebral palsy
Cerebral disease
Myopathies
Dyskinesias

Drugs *(see also* Section 1.5, page 58)

Severe xerostomia

Mechanical

Poorly fitting prostheses
Restricted jaw movement

Dysphagia

Oral or pharyngeal disease

Inflammatory, traumatic, surgical or neoplastic lesions of tongue, palate or pharynx
Xerostomia

Oesophageal disease

Inflammatory, traumatic, surgical or neoplastic lesions
Foreign body
Stricture
Systemic sclerosis (CREST syndrome)
Pharyngeal pouch
Oesophagitis
Extrinsic compressive lesions (e.g. mediastinal lymphadenopathy)

Psychogenic

Hysteria (globus hystericus)

Neurological disorders

Multiple sclerosis
Cerebrovascular accident
Bulbar and pseudo-bulbar palsy
Parkinson's disease
Syringobulbia/syringomyelia
Achalasia of the cardia
Myopathies (e.g. myasthenia gravis)
Lateral medullary syndrome

Facial palsy

Neurological

Bell's palsy
Stroke
Cerebral tumour
Moebius syndrome
Multiple sclerosis
Ramsay–Hunt syndrome
Guillain–Barré syndrome
HSV, HIV or other viral infection
Trauma to facial nerve or its branches
Diabetes mellitus
Leprosy
Kawasaki disease
Lyme disease
Connective tissue disorders
Botulism

Middle ear disease

Cholesteatoma
Malignancy
Mastoiditis

Parotid lesions

Parotid trauma
Parotid malignancy

Others

Melkersson–Rosenthal syndrome
Sarcoidosis (Heerfordt syndrome)
Reiter's syndrome

Myopathies

Facial swelling

Facial swelling is commonly inflammatory in origin, caused by cutaneous or dental infections or trauma.

(Contd)

Inflammatory

Oral infections
Cutaneous infections
Insect bites

Traumatic

Post-operative oedema or haematoma
Traumatic oedema or haematoma
Surgical emphysema

Immunological

Allergic angioedema
C_1 esterase inhibitor deficiency

Facial swelling
(Contd)

Endocrine and metabolic

Systemic corticosteroid therapy
Cushing's syndrome and disease
Myxoedema
Acromegaly
Obesity
Nephrotic syndrome

Superior vena cava syndrome

Cysts

Neoplasms

Congenital (e.g. lymphangioma)
Lymphoma

Foreign bodies

Granulomatous disorders

Crohn's disease (and orofacial
    granulomatosis)
Sarcoidosis
Melkersson–Rosenthal syndrome

Fissured tongue

Fissured tongue is
common and usually
inconsequential,
although erythema
migrans is often
associated.

Isolated

Developmental

With systemic disease

Down's syndrome
Melkersson–Rosenthal syndrome

Halitosis (oral malodour)

Oral sepsis

Food impaction
Dental or periodontal sepsis
Necrotizing ulcerative gingivitis
Dry socket
Pericoronitis
Xerostomia
Ulceration

Oral malignancy

Nasopharyngeal disease

Foreign body
Sinusitis
Tonsillitis
Neoplasm

Volatile foodstuffs

Garlic
Onions
Highly spiced foods
Durian

Drugs (*see also* Section 1.5, page 58)

Systemic disease

Acute febrile illness
Respiratory tract infections
Hepatic failure
Renal failure
Diabetic ketoacidosis
Trimethylaminouria

Psychogenic (delusional)

Neuroses
Psychoses

Hirsutism

Hirsutism is defined as more facial and body hair than is acceptable to a woman living in a particular culture.

ANDROGEN-MEDIATED

Drugs

Androgens
Anabolic steroids
Contraceptive pill

Ovarian

Polycystic ovaries
Ovarian tumours
Insulin resistance

Adrenal

Cushing's syndrome
Congenital adrenal hyperplasia
Androgen-producing tumours

Other

Idiopathic

ANDROGEN-INDEPENDENT

Racial

Pregnancy

Drugs

Minoxidil
Phenytoin
Calcium-channel blockers
Ciclosporin
Corticosteroids
Danazol
Diazoxide

Endocrine

Hypothyroidism
Acromegaly

Hyper-pigmentation

See Pigmentation

Loss of taste

Anosmia

Upper respiratory tract infections
Maxillofacial or head injuries (tearing of olfactory nerves)

Neurological disease

Lesions of chorda tympani
Cerebrovascular disease
Multiple sclerosis
Bell's palsy
Fractured base of skull
Posterior cranial fossa tumours
Cerebral metastases
Trigeminal sensory neuropathy

Psychogenic

Anxiety states
Depression
Psychoses

Drugs (*see also* Section 1.5, page 58)

Others

Irradiation and chemotherapy
Xerostomia
Zinc or copper deficiency

Pain

(*See* Table 1.2, page 10)

Local diseases

Diseases of the teeth
Dentine sensitivity
Pulpitis
Periapical periodontitis

Diseases of the periodontium
Lateral (periodontal) abscess
Necrotizing ulcerative gingivitis
Pericoronitis
Necrotizing periodontitis

Diseases of the jaws
Dry socket
Fractures
Osteomyelitis
Infected cysts
Malignant neoplasms
Neuralgia-inducing cavitational
   osteonecrosis (NICO)

Diseases of the maxillary antrum
Acute sinusitis
Malignant neoplasms

Diseases of the salivary glands
Acute sialadentitis
Calculi or other obstruction to duct
Severe Sjögren's syndrome
HIV disease
Malignant neoplasms

Diseases of the temporomandibular joint
Arthritis
Temporomandibular joint dysfunction
   (facial arthromyalgia)

Vascular disorders
Migraine
Migrainous neuralgia
Giant-cell arteritis

Neurological disorders
Trigeminal neuralgia
Malignant neoplasms involving the
   trigeminal nerve
Multiple sclerosis
HIV disease
Bell's palsy (rarely)
Herpes zoster (including post-herpetic
   neuralgia)
Severe unilateral neuralgia with
   conjunctival tearing (SUNCT syndrome)

Psychogenic pain
Atypical facial pain and other oral
   symptoms associated with anxiety or
   depression

Referred pain
Angina, nasopharyngeal, ocular and aural
   disease
Chest disease (rarely)

Others
Drugs (e.g. vinca alkaloids)

Table 1.2 DIFFERENTIATION OF IMPORTANT TYPES OF OROFACIAL PAIN*

	Idiopathic trigeminal neuralgia	Temporomandibular joint dysfunction	Atypical facial pain	Migraine	Migrainous neuralgia
Age (years)	> 50	Any (mainly 15–30)	30–50	Any	30–50
Sex	F > M	F > M	F > M	F > M	M > F
Site	Unilateral, mandible or maxilla	Unilateral or bilateral mandible, temple	± Bilateral, maxilla usually	Any	Retro-orbital
Associated features	—	± Anxiety ± Life events ± Depression	± Depression	± Photophobia, ± Nausea, ± Vomiting	± Conjunctival injection, ± Lacrimation ± Nasal congestion
Character	Lancinating	Dull	Dull	Throbbing	Boring
Duration of episode	Brief (seconds)	Hours	Continual	Many hours (usually during day)	Few hours (usually during night, often at same time)
Precipitating factors	± Trigger areas	None	None	± Foods ± Stress	± Alcohol, ± Stress
Relieving factors	Carbamazepine Gabapentin Baclofen	Analgesics, antidepressants, anxiolytics, others	Antidepressants	Triptans, ergot derivatives, β-blockers, H$_3$-blockers	Triptans, oxygen, ergot derivatives, β-blockers, H$_3$-blockers, pizotifen

*Most oral pain is caused by local disease.

Pigmentation

(*see* Table 1.3, page 11)

Racial

Pregnancy

Chloasma

Food/drugs (*see* Section 1.5, page 58)

Endocrinopathies

Addison's disease
Nelson's syndrome
Ectopic ACTH production

Others

Pigmentary incontinence
Albright's syndrome
Haemochromatosis/haemosiderosis
β-thalassaemia
Biliary atresia
Permanganate or silver poisoning

Ecchymoses
Ephelis
Melanoma
Melanoacanthoma
Melanotic macule
Naevus
Peutz–Jeghers syndrome
Kaposi's sarcoma
Epithelioid angiomatosis
Smoker's melanosis
Acanthosis nigricans
Heavy-metal poisoning (lead, bismuth and arsenic)
Laugier–Hunziker syndrome
von Recklinghausen's neurofibromatosis
Spotty pigmentation, myxoma, endocrine overactivity syndrome
Tattoos (amalgam, lead pencils, ink, dyes, carbon)

Table 1.3 COMMON BENIGN ISOLATED PIGMENTED LESIONS

Lesion	Main sites	Age affected	Size	Other features
Naevi	Palate	3rd–4th decade	<1 cm	Mostly raised and pigmented blue or brown
Melanotic macules	Lips; gingivae	Any	<1 cm	Macular Mostly in Caucasians Brown or black
Amalgam tattoos	Floor of mouth; mandibular gingivae	Usually after 5 years	<1 cm	Macular Greyish or black

Purpura

Trauma (including suction)

Platelet and vascular disorders

Thrombocytopenia (especially drugs and leukaemias)
Thrombasthenia
Von Willebrand's disease
Scurvy
Ehlers–Danlos syndrome
Chronic renal failure
'Senile' purpura
Marfan syndrome

Infections

Infectious mononucleosis
Rubella
HIV infection

Localized oral purpura (angina bullosa haemorrhagica)

Amyloidosis

Mixed connective tissue disease

Red areas

Generalized redness

Candidosis
Avitaminosis B complex (rarely)
Mucositis
Mucosal atrophy (e.g. avitaminosis B)
Polycythaemia

Localized red patches

Candidosis
Denture-related stomatitis
Erythroplasia
Purpura
Telangiectases

Angiomas (purple)
Kaposi's sarcoma
Epithelioid angiomatosis
Burns
Lichen planus
Lupus erythematosus
Avitaminosis B_{12}
Sarcoidosis
Psoriasis
Mucoepithelial dysplasia syndrome
Geographic tongue
Drug allergies
Wegener's granulomatosis
Deep mycoses

Sialorrhoea (hypersalivation)

Psychogenic (usually)

Painful lesions in the mouth

Foreign bodies in the mouth

Drugs (*see also* Section 1.5, page 58)

Poor neuromuscular coordination

Parkinson's disease
Facial palsy
Other physical disability

Poisoning

Heavy metals
Mercury
Copper sulphate
Insecticides
Nerve agents

Others

Rabies (rarely)
Oesophageal or pharyngeal
obstructions
Learning disability

Telangiectasia

Hereditary haemorrhagic telangiectasia
Chronic liver disease
Scleroderma
Carcinoid

Pregnancy
Oestrogens
Post-irradiation

Trismus

Limited opening of
the jaw may have
several causes,
including the
following:

Extra-articular causes

Infection, haematoma or inflammation in or
   near masticatory muscles or joint
Temporomandibular joint dysfunction
   syndrome (facial arthromyalgia)
Fractured condylar neck
Fibrosis (including scars, systemic sclerosis,
   radiotherapy and submucous fibrosis)
Tetanus
Tetany
Invading neoplasm
Myositis ossificans
Coronoid hypertrophy or fusion to
   zygomatic arch
Hysteria
Lipoid proteinosis

Intra-articular causes

Dislocation or subluxation
Intracapsular fracture
Arthritides
Ankylosis

In contrast, some drugs such as
metoclopramide and phenothiazines may
cause facial muscle spasm inhibiting the
patient from *closing* his or her mouth.

Ulcers

Local causes

Traumatic (may be artefactual)
Chemical, electrical, thermal, radiation burns

Neoplastic

Carcinoma and other malignant tumours

Recurrent aphthous stomatitis

(including Behçet's syndrome/MAGIC syndrome, Sweet's syndrome and acute febrile illness of childhood (PFAPA: periodic fever, aphthae, pharyngitis, adenitis))

Systemic disease

Cutaneous disease: Erosive lichen planus, pemphigus, pemphigoid, erythema multiforme, dermatitis herpetiformis and linear IgA disease, epidermolysis bullosa, epidermolysis bullosa acquisita, IgA intraepithelial pustular dermatosis, chronic ulcerative stomatitis, graft-versus-host disease

Blood or vascular disorders: Anaemia, sideropenia, neutropenias, leukaemias, myelofibrosis, myelodysplasia, multiple myeloma, giant-cell arteritis, periarteritis nodosa

Gastrointestinal: Coeliac disease, Crohn's disease, orofacial granulomatosis ulcerative colitis

Connective tissue disease: Lupus erythematosus, Reiter's disease, mixed connective tissue disease, Felty's syndrome

Infective: Herpes simplex, chickenpox, herpes zoster, hand, foot and mouth disease, herpangina, infectious mononucleosis, cytomegalovirus infection, necrotizing ulcerative gingivitis, tuberculosis, atypical mycobacterial infections, syphilis, aspergillosis, cryptococcosis, leishmaniasis, tularaemia, lepromatous leprosy, mucormycosis, paracoccidioidomycosis, histoplasmosis, coccidioidomycosis, blastomycosis, HIV infection, Gram-negative bacteria

Drugs: Cytotoxics, many others (*see* Section 1.5, page 58)

Others: Wegener's granulomatosis, midline lethal granuloma, Langerhan's cell histiocytoses, angiolymphoid hyperplasia with eosinophilia, necrotizing sialometaplasia, noma, hypereosinophilic syndrome

White lesions

Congenital

White sponge naevus
Dyskeratosis congenita
Pachyonychia congenita
Tylosis
Darier's disease

Acquired

Inflammatory

Infective: Candidosis, hairy leukoplakia, syphilitic leukoplakia, Koplik's spots, papillomas

Non-infective: Lichen planus, lichen sclerosis, lupus erythematosus, pyostomatitis vegetans, xanthomatosis, dermatomyositis

Neoplastic and possibly pre-neoplastic

Keratoses (leukoplakias)
Carcinoma

Others

Drug burns
Grafts

1.2 DIFFERENTIAL DIAGNOSES BY SITE

The lips

Angular stomatitis (cheilitis, cheilosis)

Candidosis (denture-related stomatitis or other types)
Staphylococcal, streptococcal or mixed infections
Ariboflavinosis (rarely), iron, folate or B_{12} deficiency
Crohn's disease and orofacial granulomatosis
Anaemia
Acrodermatitis enteropathica
HIV infection
Diabetes

Bleeding

Trauma
Cracked lips
Erythema multiforme
Angiomas
Underlying haemorrhagic disease aggravates tendency to bleed

Blisters

Herpes labialis
Burns
Herpes zoster
Erythema multiforme
Pemphigus vulgaris
Paraneoplastic pemphigus
Epidermolysis bullosa
Mucoceles
Impetigo
Allergic cheilitis

Desquamation and crusting

Dehydration
Exposure to hot dry winds
Acute febrile illness
Chemical or allergic cheilitis
Mouth-breathing
Actinic cheilitis
Candidal cheilitis
Erythema multiforme
Psychogenic (self-induced)
Drugs
Exfoliative cheilitis

Swellings

There is a wide individual and racial variation in the size of the lips

Diffuse swellings

Oedema (trauma or infection or insect bite)
Angioedema: allergic or C_1 esterase inhibitor deficiency
Crohn's disease and orofacial granulomatosis

Cheilitis granulomatosa
Cheilitis glandularis
Melkersson–Rosenthal syndrome
Lymphangioma
Haemangioma
Macrocheilia
Ascher's syndrome
Sarcoidosis

Localized swellings

Crohn's disease and orofacial granulomatosis
Mucoceles
Chancre
Salivary adenoma
Squamous cell carcinoma
Basal cell carcinoma
Other tumours
Keratoacanthoma
Cysts
Abscesses
Insect bites
Haematomas
Tuberculosis
Warts
Leprosy
Rhinoscleroma
Anthrax
Trichiniasis
Sarcoidosis

Ulceration

Infective

Herpes labialis
Herpes zoster
Syphilis
Leishmaniasis
Mycoses
Impetigo

Tumours

Squamous cell carcinoma
Basal cell carcinoma
Keratoacanthoma
Others

Burns

Mucocutaneous disease

Erythema multiforme
Lichen planus
Lupus erythematosus
Pemphigus
Pemphigoid
Trauma

(Contd)

The lips
(Contd)

White lesions

Keratoses
Leukoplakias
Carcinoma
Lichen planus
Lupus erythematosus
Fordyce spots

Actinic keratosis
Scars
White sponge naevus

The gingivae

Red areas

Redness is usually a sign of chronic gingivitis or periodontitis, but is then restricted to the gingival margins. Other red lesions which may affect the gingiva include:

Congenital

Mucoepithelial dysplasia syndrome
Hereditary haemorrhagic telangiectasia
Cyclic neutropenia

Acquired

Trauma: physical, chemical, radiation, thermal

Drugs: e.g. chlorhexidine, cinnamonaldehyde

Infections: candidosis, *Geotrichum candidum*

Desquamative gingivitis: lichen planus, pemphigoid, pemphigus, dermatitis herpetiformis, linear IgA disease, lupus erythematosus, pyostomatitis vegetans, psoriasis

Epithelioid angiomatosis

Wegener's granulomatosis

Sarcoidosis

Dermatomyositis

Primary biliary cirrhosis

Leukaemia(s)

Neutropenias

Premalignancy (e.g. erythroplasia)

Malignancy — Kaposi's sarcoma

Plasma cell gingivitis (gingivostomatitis)

Bleeding

Periodontal disease

Chronic gingivitis
Chronic periodontitis
(Contd) Acute ulcerative gingivitis

HIV gingivitis
HIV periodontitis
Aggressive periodontitis

Haemorrhagic disease

Primary platelet disorders
Lymphoproliferative disorders
Myelodysplastic disorders
Myelofibrosis
Myeloproliferative disorders
Idiopathic thrombocytopenic purpura
Hereditary haemorrhagic telangiectasia
Ehlers–Danlos syndrome
Scurvy
Angiomas
Chronic renal failure (*see* Section 1.5)

Drugs

Anticoagulants
Non-steroidal anti-inflammatory drugs
Cytotoxics
Sodium valproate

Clotting defects

Hepatobiliary disease
Haemophilias
Von Willebrand's disease

Gingival swelling

Generalized and congenital

Gingival fibromatosis
Jones' syndrome
Murray–Puretic–Drescher syndrome
Mucolipidosis (I-cell disease)
Rutherfurd syndrome
Zimmermann–Laband syndrome
Cross syndrome
Ramon syndrome
Gingival fibromatosis with growth hormone deficiency (Byars–Jurkiewicz syndrome)

The gingivae
(Contd)

Mucopolysaccharidosis 1-H
Fucosidosis
Aspartylglucosaminuria
Leprechaunism (Donohue syndrome)
Pfeiffer syndrome
Amyloidosis
Lipoid proteinosis
Infantile systemic hyalinosis
Hypoplasminogenaemia

Generalized and acquired

Acute myeloid leukaemia
Preleukaemic leukaemia
Aplastic anaemia
Drugs (*see also* Section 1.5, page 58)
    Phenytoin
    Ciclosporin
    Calcium-channel blockers
    Others
Vitamin C deficiency

Localized and congenital

Fabry's syndrome (angiokeratoma corporis
    diffusum universale)
Cowden's syndrome (multiple hamartoma
    and neoplasia syndrome)
Tuberous sclerosis
Focal dermal hypoplasia
Sturge–Weber angiomatosis
Congenital gingival granular cell
    tumour
Hypoplasminogenaemia
Lipoid proteinosis

Localized and acquired

Heck's disease
Lymphomas
Langerhan's cell tumours
Multiple myeloma
Plasmacytomas
Other primary and secondary neoplasms,
    e.g. papillomas, squamous cell carcinoma,
    Kaposi's sarcoma
Wegener's granulomatosis
Pregnancy epulis
Fibroepithelial epulis
Giant cell epulis
Sarcoidosis
Crohn's disease and orofacial granulomatosis
Epithelioid angiomatosis

Ulcers

Ulcers that affect predominantly the gingivae
are usually traumatic, acute ulcerative
gingivitis or occasionally results of
immunodeficiency, especially acute
leukaemia, neutropenias or HIV disease. The
gingivae can, however, be affected by most
other causes of mouth ulcers (*see* page 13).

Enhanced periodontal destruction

Primary immunodeficiencies

Reduced neutrophil number
    Cyclic neutropenia
    Benign familial neutropenias
    Other
Defective neutrophil function
    Hyperimmunoglobulinaemia E
    Chronic granulomatous disease
    Kartagener's syndrome
    Chediak–Higashi syndrome
    Acatalasia
    Leukocyte adhesion deficiency
Other immunodeficiencies
    Fanconi's anaemia
    Down syndrome
    Severe combined immunodeficiency (SCID)

Other congenital disorders

Papillon–Lefèvre syndrome
Haim–Munk syndrome
Hypophosphatasia
Ehlers–Danlos syndrome type VIII
Acro-osteolysis (Hajdu–Cheney syndrome)
Type 1b glycogen storage disease
Oxalosis
Dyskeratosis benigna intraepithelialis
    mucosae et cutis hereditara

Secondary immunodeficiencies

Malnutrition
HIV disease
Pregnancy
Diabetes mellitus
Crohn's disease
Leukaemias

Other acquired causes

Vitamin C deficiency
Tobacco use

The palate

Lumps

Developmental

Unerupted teeth
Torus palatinus
Cysts
Angiomas

Inflammatory

Abscesses
Cysts
Papillary hyperplasia
Necrotizing sialometaplasia
Adenomatoid hyperplasia
Sarcoidosis
Franklin's heavy chain disease

Neoplasms

Oral or antral carcinoma
Salivary tumours
Fibrous overgrowths
Kaposi's sarcoma
Papillomas and condylomas
Lymphomas
Others

Redness

Redness restricted to the denture-bearing area of the palate is almost invariably denture-related stomatitis (candidosis), although erythematous candidosis of HIV disease can commonly occur as a red patch of the palate. Other red lesions may be erythroplasia, Kaposi's sarcoma or other lesions (*see* page 11).

The tongue

Swellings or lumps

Localized

Congenital: Lingual thyroid, haemangioma, lymphangioma, lingual choristoma

Inflammatory: Infection, abscess, median rhomboid glossitis, granuloma, foliate papillitis, insect bite

Traumatic: Oedema, haematoma

Neoplastic: Fibrous lump, papilloma, neurofibroma, carcinoma, sarcoma, granular cell tumour (granular cell myoblastoma)

Others: Foreign body, cysts, warts, condylomas

Diffuse

Congenital: Down syndrome, cretinism, mucopolysaccharidoses, lymphangioma, haemangioma

Inflammatory: Infection, insect bite, Ludwig's angina

Traumatic: Oedema, haematoma

Others: Multiple endocrine adenomatosis type 3; angioedema; amyloidosis; cyst; acromegaly; muscular (Beckwith–Wiedeman syndrome); deposits (glycogen storage disease, I cell disease, mucopolysaccharidoses)

Sore tongue

With obvious localized lesions

Any cause of oral ulceration (*see* page 13)
Geographic tongue
Median rhomboid glossitis
Foliate papillitis

Glossitis (generalized redness and depapillation)

Anaemias
Candidosis
Avitaminosis B
Post-irradiation or chemotherapy

With no identifiable physical abnormality

Anaemia/sideropenia
Depression or cancerophobia
Glossodynia
Diabetes
Hypothyroidism

The major salivary glands

Swellings

Inflammatory

Mumps
Recurrent parotitis
Sjögren's syndrome
Ascending (acute suppurative) sialadenitis
Recurrent sialadenitis
Lymphadenitis
Sarcoidosis
Actinomycosis
HIV salivary gland disease
HCV infection

Neoplasms

Others

Duct obstruction
Sialosis (sialadenosis)
Mikulicz disease (lymphoepithelial lesion and syndrome)
Amyloidosis
HIV disease
Haemochromatosis

Drug-associated (*see also* Section 1.5, page 58)

Salivary gland pain

Inflammatory

Mumps
Stones or other causes of obstruction
Sjögren's syndrome
Acute sialadenitis
Recurrent sialadenitis
HIV sialadenitis

Neoplastic

Salivary gland malignant tumours

Drug-associated (*see also* Section 1.5, page 58)

The neck

Swellings in the neck

Cervical lymph nodes

Inflammatory: Lymphadenitis (nasopharyngeal, antral, dental, tonsillar, aural, facial or scalp infections), glandular fever syndromes (EBV, CMV, Brucella, *Toxoplasma*, HIV, HHV-6), tuberculosis or other mycobacterial infections, other infections (rubella, cat scratch, syphilis)

Neoplasms: Secondary carcinoma (oral, nasopharyngeal or thyroid primary), lymphoma, leukaemia

Others: Connective tissue disease, drugs (e.g. phenytoin), mucocutaneous lymph node syndrome (Kawasaki syndrome), sarcoidosis

Salivary glands

Mumps
Tumours
Sjögren's syndrome
Sarcoidosis
Sialadenitis
Sialosis

Side of the neck

Actinomycosis
Branchial cyst
Parapharyngeal cellulitis
Pharyngeal pouch
Cystic hygroma
Carotid body tumours or aneurysms

Muscle or other soft tissue neoplasm

Focal myositis
Myositis ossificans
Proliferative myositis
Nodular pseudosarcomatous fasciitis

Midline of the neck

Submental lymphadenopathy
Thyroglossal cyst
Ectopic thyroid
Thyroid tumours or goitre
'Plunging' ranula
Ludwig's angina
Dermoid cyst
Other skin lesions

Oral complaints frequently associated with psychogenic factors*

*Organic causes should first be excluded.

Dry mouth
Sore or burning mouth
Bad or disturbed taste
Atypical facial pain
Atypical odontalgia
Supposed anaesthesias and dysaesthesias

Temporomandibular joint dysfunction
Non-existent discharges
Gripping dentures
Vomiting or nausea caused by dentures
Supposed sialorrhoea
Non-existent lumps or spots

1.3 GUIDE TO THE DIAGNOSIS AND MANAGEMENT OF ORAL DISEASES

Condition	Typical main clinical features	Diagnosis
Abscess (dental)	Pain ± swelling	Clinical mainly
Acanthosis nigricans	Hyperpigmented confluent papillomas mainly in groin/axillae	Clinical plus biopsy
Acquired immune deficiency syndrome (AIDS)	Opportunistic infections (especially fungal and viral), Kaposi's sarcoma, lymphomas, encephalopathy	Confirmed by HIV antibodies or RNA
Acromegaly	Increasing prognathism and hand size, headaches, tunnel vision, lethargy, weight gain	Enlarging pituitary fossa Increased growth hormone
Actinomycosis	Purplish indurated swelling(s) over mandible or neck	Clinical plus microbiology 'Sulphur granules'
Acute bacterial sialadenitis	Painful salivary swellings ± fever and/or trismus	Clinical plus bacteriology
Acute necrotizing ulcerative gingivitis	Interdental papillary ulceration and bleeding, halitosis, pain	Clinical mainly
Addison's disease	Weakness, lassitude, loss of weight, hyperpigmentation	Clinical plus low blood pressure, hyponatraemia, hyperkalaemia, reduced cortisol and increased ACTH
Adenoid cystic carcinoma	Firm salivary swelling	Clinical plus investigations
Agammaglobulinaemia	Recurrent pyogenic infections, especially respiratory and cutaneous	Reduced immunoglobulins
Albright's syndrome	Fibrous dysplasia, precocious puberty, hyperpigmentation, endocrine disease	Clinical plus investigations
Alveolar osteitis (dry socket)	Empty painful extraction socket, halitosis	Clinical
Amalgam tattoo	Grey to black pigmented area(s) usually over the mandible	Clinical
Ameloblastoma	Slow growing swelling, usually in mandible	Clinical plus investigations

Investigations	Management
Radiography ± vitality test	Drain either by incision if pointing, or through tooth. Analgesics ± antimicrobials
Biopsy, gastroscopy, barium studies Exclude diabetes mellitus and malignancy	Treat underlying cause
HIV antibodies and viral load CD4 lymphocyte count	Highly active anti-retroviral therapy (HAART). Prophylaxis/treatment of infections
Lateral skull radiography, growth hormone assays, visual fields, CT/MRI	Treatment of pituitary adenoma
Pus for microscopy and culture	Antimicrobial: penicillin for 4 weeks+
Pus for culture and sensitivity	Antimicrobial: flucloxacillin
Smear may help Consider excluding HIV	Antimicrobial: penicillin or metronidazole. Oral hygiene improvement. Mechanical debridement
Blood pressure, electrolytes, 24 hr cortisol Synacthen test	Corticosteroids
Biopsy and radiography	Surgery
Serum immunoglobulins	Immunoglobulin replacement Antimicrobials
Radiography ± bone biopsy	± Surgery ± calcitonin
Radiography to exclude fracture or foreign body	Debridement, obtundent dressing ± antimicrobial
± Radiography. Biopsy if any doubt	Reassurance
Radiography *and* biopsy	Surgery

Condition	Typical main clinical features	Diagnosis
Angioedema [*see also* **hereditary angioedema**]	Facial swelling	Clinical
Angular cheilitis	*See* Cheilitis	
Aphthae	Recurrent oral ulcers only	Clinical
Atypical facial pain	Persistent dull ache typically in one maxilla in a female	Clinical
Bell's palsy	Lower motor neurone facial palsy only	Clinical
Behçet's syndrome	Recurrent oral and genital ulceration, other systemic features	Clinical
Black hairy tongue	Black hairy tongue	Clinical
Bourneville–Pringle disease	Papules or nodules around nose/mouth, subungual fibromas, ash leaf patches	Clinical plus cerebral radio-opacities
Bruton's syndrome	*See* Agammaglobulinaemia	
Bruxism	Attrition and sometimes masseteric hypertrophy	Clinical
Bulimia nervosa	Recurrent self-induced vomiting	Clinical
Burning mouth syndrome	*See* Glossodynia	
Calculus, salivary	Recurrent salivary swelling ± pain at mealtimes	Clinical ± investigations
Cancrum oris	Chronic ulceration	Clinical ± investigations
Candidosis	White or red persistent lesions	Clinical ± investigations
Carcinoma	Ulcer, lump or red or white lesion	Clinical plus investigations
Central papillary atrophy	*See* Median rhomboid glossitis	
Chancre	Single, painless indurated ulcer usually on lip or tongue	Syphilis serology
Cheek-chewing	Shredded or keratotic lesions around occlusal line and/or on lower labial mucosa	Clinical

Investigations	Management
C1 esterase inhibitor, IgE, C3 and C4 levels	Antihistamines/corticosteroids
Full blood picture. Exclude underlying systemic disease (e.g. coeliac disease)	Corticosteroids topically, Amlexanox, topical tetracycline (doxycycline)
Clinical and radiographic exclusion of organic disease	Reassurance, tricyclic antidepressants, SSRIs
Consider excluding middle ear lesion, Lyme disease, cerebellopontine angle tumour, diabetes, hypertension, HIV	Corticosteroids systemically. Protect cornea. Aciclovir may be indicated
Full blood picture, white cell count and differential	Colchicine, thalidomide or azathioprine may be indicated
—	Reassurance. Brush tongue ± tretinoin
Skull radiography. Biopsy skin lesions	Anticonvulsants
Full blood picture, electrolytes	Reassurance. Psychiatric care Restoration of dental erosions
Radiography/sialography	Surgery ± lithotripsy
Consider biopsy Consider immune defect	Debridement. Antimicrobial Improve nutrition
Smear plus culture Consider immune defect	Antifungal
Biopsy. Chest radiography	Surgery ± radiotherapy
Syphilis serology ± biopsy	Antimicrobial: penicillin
—	Avoid habit
—	Occlusal splint ± botulinum toxoid

Condition	Typical main clinical features	Diagnosis
Cheilitis, actinic	Soreness and/or keratosis on lower lip. Sun exposure	Clinical
angular	Soreness of commissures	Clinical
Cherubism	Slowly enlarging swellings over mandible or maxillae	Clinical plus investigations
Child abuse syndrome	Various injuries inconsistent with history	Clinical ± radiography
Chronic granulomatous disease	Recurrent pyogenic infections, cervical lymphadenopathy	Clinical plus investigations
Chronic mucocutaneous candidosis	Persistent mucocutaneous candidosis	Clinical plus investigations
Cicatricial pemphigoid	*See* Mucous membrane pemphigoid	
Cleidocranial dysplasia	Patent fontanelles, clavicles can approximate	Clinical plus radiographs
Coeliac disease	Loose stool, malabsorption, loss of weight/failure to thrive	Clinical plus jejunal villous atrophy. Tissue transglutaminase
Condyloma acuminata	Warts (condylomas)	Clinical
CREST syndrome	Raynaud's phenomenon, changing facial appearance. Mucosal telangiectases ± Sjögren's syndrome	Clinical plus investigations
Crohn's disease	Loose stool, malabsorption, abdominal pain ± orofacial granulomatosis	Clinical plus investigations
Cyclic neutropenia	Recurrent pyogenic infections	Clinical plus neutropenia
Denture-induced hyperplasia	Hyperplasia close to denture flange	Clinical
Denture-related stomatitis	Erythema in denture-bearing area	Clinical
Dermatitis herpetiformis	Pruritic rash	Clinical plus investigations. Small bowel biopsy
Dermatomyositis	Proximal limb and trunk weakness plus heliotrope rash	Clinical plus investigations

Investigations	Management
—	Avoid exposure. Bland UV protecting creams. ± Laser excision ± Imiquimod ± retinoids
Haematological screen Denture assessment	Denture modification/replacement Oral and denture hygiene Antifungal: miconazole
Radiography + biopsy	Reassurance
Photographs + radiography	Protect child from further abuse
Assay neutrophil phagocytosis and killing of bacteria	Antimicrobials Bone marrow transplantation
Assay T cell function. Biopsy + fungal culture	Antifungals
Radiography of skull and clavicles	Remove supernumary teeth/cysts
Gliadin or endomysial antibodies, transglutaminase + small bowel biopsy	Gluten-free diet
Biopsy	Surgery, podophyllum or interferon or imiquimod
Clinical + anti-centromere antibodies + radiographs	Immunosuppressives
Barium meal and follow-through	Sulfasalazine or corticosteroids or tacrolimus
Serial neutrophil counts	Antimicrobial, colony-stimulating factor
—	Ease denture flange; excise hyperplasia
Fungal culture	Leave denture out at night stored in antifungal
Lesional biopsy + small bowel biopsy + gliadin antibodies	Gluten-free diet Dapsone or sulfapyridine
Serum creatine kinase and aldolase Electromyography Skin/muscle biopsy	Systemic corticosteroids, other systemic immunosuppressants and acetylsalicyclic acid

Condition	Typical main clinical features	Diagnosis
Dermoid cyst	Submental swelling	Clinical plus investigations
Desquamative gingivitis	Erythematous desquamating gingivae	Clinical plus biopsy
Diabetes mellitus	Polyuria, polydipsia	Hyperglycaemia
Discoid lupus erythematosus	*See* Lupus	
Dry mouth	*See* Sjögren's syndrome	
Dry socket	*See* Alveolar osteitis	
Ectodermal dysplasia	Dry thin hair, dry skin, fever, hypodontia	Clinical
Ephelis	*See* Freckles	
Epidermolysis bullosa	Blisters at sites of trauma	Clinical plus histology
Epiloia	*See* Bourneville–Pringle disease	
Epulis		
congenital	Firm nodule on gingiva	Clinical
fibrous	Firm nodule on gingiva	Clinical
fissuratum	Firm leaflike swellings	Clinical
giant cell	Purplish swelling in premolar area	Clinical plus investigations
in pregnancy	Soft swelling typically on anterior gingivae	Clinical
Erythema		
migrans	Desquamating patches on tongue	Clinical
multiforme	Oral ulcers, swollen lips. Target lesions	Clinical
nodosum	Tender red lumps on shins	Clinical plus investigations
Erythroplakia [erythroplasia]	Red velvety patch	Clinical plus histology
Facial arthromyalgia	TMJ pain, click, limitation of movement	Clinical
Familial fibrous dysplasia	*See* Cherubism	
Familial white folded gingivostomatitis	White persistent lesions in mouth, rectum, vagina	Clinical plus family history
Felty's syndrome	Rheumatoid arthritis, splenomegaly, neutropenia	Clinical plus investigations

Investigations	Management
Radiography	Surgery
Biopsy ± immunofluorescence	Topical corticosteroids, improve oral hygiene
Blood sugar (fasting) Glucose tolerance test	Diet or insulin ± oral hypoglycaemic agent
Radiography for hypodontia	Restorative dentistry
Biopsy	Protect against trauma Vitamin E ± phenytoin
— — — Exclude hyperparathyroidism Pregnancy test	Excise if no resolution Excise Change denture. Excise Surgery Leave or excise
— — Biopsy ± serum for immune complexes	Reassurance Corticosteroids, aciclovir if herpes-induced Treat underlying cause
Biopsy	Excise
Radiography ± arthroscopy	Reassurance, occlusal splint, anxiolytics or antidepressants
± Biopsy	Reassurance
Full blood picture, rheumatoid factor, erythrocyte sedimentation rate	Salicylates

Condition	Typical main clinical features	Diagnosis
Fibroepithelial polyp	Firm pink polyp	Clinical
Fibroma, leaf	*See* Fibroepithelial polyp	
Fibromatosis, gingival	Firm pink gingival swellings	Clinical
Fibrous dysplasia	Bony swelling	Clinical plus investigations
Fibrous lump	*See* Fibroepithelial polyp	
Foliate papillitis	Painful swollen foliate papilla	Clinical
Fordyce spots	Yellowish granules in buccal mucosae or lips	Clinical
Fragilitas ossium	Spontaneous fractures, blue sclera	Clinical plus investigations
Freckles [ephelides]	Brown macules	Clinical
Frey's syndrome	Gustatory sweating	Clinical
Gardner's syndrome	Osteomas, desmoid tumours, colonic polyps	Clinical plus investigations
Geographic tongue	*See* Erythema migrans	
German measles	Macular rash, fever, occipital lymphadenopathy	Clinical
Glandular fever	Fever, sore throat, generalized lymphadenopathy	Serology for definitive diagnosis
Glossitis		
atrophic	Depapillated tongue	Clinical plus investigations
benign migratory	*See* Erythema migrans	
in iron deficiency	Depapillated tongue	Clinical plus investigations
median rhomboid	*See* Central papillary atrophy	
Moeller's in vitamin B12 deficiency	Depapillated tongue	Clinical plus investigations
Glossodynia	Burning normal tongue	Clinical plus investigations
Gorlin–Goltz syndrome (Gorlin's syndrome)	Odontogenic keratocysts, basal cell naevi, skeletal anomalies	Clinical plus investigations
Haemangioma	Blush or reddish swelling	Clinical $\pm$ aspiration $\pm$ angiography

Investigations	Management
—	Excision
—	Excision
Radiographs and biopsy	Excision or await resolution
—	Reassurance
—	Reassurance
Radiography	Orthopaedic care
—	Reassurance
Starch-iodine test	Glycopyrrolate
Radiography of jaws, colonoscopy	Excision of colonic polyps
—	Symptomatic
White cell count and differential, Paul Bunnell test, consider HIV and other serology	Symptomatic, corticosteroids systemically if airway threatened
Full blood picture, haematinic assay	Treat underlying cause
Full blood picture, serum ferritin	Treat underlying cause
Full blood picture, serum B12	Treat underlying cause
Full blood picture, haematinic assay, fasting blood glucose	Treat underlying cause where possible ± antidepressants
Radiography skull, jaws, chest	Remove cysts. ± Etretinate
Empties on pressure	Leave or cryoprobe, laser or sclerosant

Condition	Typical main clinical features	Diagnosis
Haemophilia	Haemarthroses, ecchymoses, severe bleeding after trauma	Clinical plus investigations
Hairy leukoplakia	White lesions on tongue	Clinical
Halitosis	Oral malodour	Clinical
Hand, foot and mouth disease	Oral ulcers, mild fever, vesicles on hands and/or feet	Clinical
Heck's disease	Oral papules	Clinical
Heerfordt's syndrome	Uveitis, parotitis, fever, facial palsy	Clinical plus investigations
Hereditary angioedema	Recurrent facial swellings	Clinical plus investigations
Hereditary haemorrhagic telangiectasia	Telangiectasia on lips, mouth, hands	Clinical
Herpangina	Oral ulcers, mild fever	Clinical
Herpetic stomatitis	Oral ulcers, gingivitis, fever	Clinical
Herpes labialis	Vesicles, pustules, scabs at mucocutaneous junction	Clinical
Herpes zoster	*See* Shingles	
Histiocytosis (Langerhan's cell)	Osteolytic lesions	Clinical plus investigations
Histoplasmosis	Cough, fever and weight loss	Histology
Hodgkin's lymphoma	Chronic lymph node swelling ± fever	Histology
Horner's syndrome	Bilateral pupil constriction, ptosis	Clinical
Human immunodeficiency virus (HIV)	*See* AIDS	
Human papillomavirus infections	Warty lesions	Clinical
Hyperparathyroidism	Renal calculi, polyuria, abdominal pain Brown tumour in jaws	Investigations

Investigations	Management
Haemostasis assays	Cover surgery with factor replacement ± antifibrinolytics
HIV serology ± biopsy	HAART
Oral/ENT examination and radiography	Treat underlying cause
—	Symptomatic
—	Observe, interferon or remove
Chest radiography. Biopsy, serum angiotensin-converting enzyme, calcium levels	Corticosteroids
C1 esterase inhibitor, C3 and C4 assays	Danazol or stanazolol or Cierferase inhibitor
Full blood picture and haemoglobin	Laser or cryoprobe to bleeding telangiectases
—	Symptomatic
Sometimes smear or serology	Symptomatic ± aciclovir
—	Penciclovir or aciclovir cream
Biopsy Skeletal survey	Depends on type; from no treatment to chemotherapy and irradiation
Biopsy + chest radiography	Fluconazole
Biopsy ± lymphangiogram ± MRI	Radiotherapy/chemotherapy
—	Identify cause
—	Excise, podophyllum, imiquimod or intralesional interferon
Jaw + skeletal radiography, plasma calcium, phosphate and parathyroid hormone, bone scan	Remove parathyroid adenoma

Condition	Typical main clinical features	Diagnosis
Hypo-adrenocorticism	*See* Addison's disease	
Hypohidrotic ectodermal dysplasia	*See* Ectodermal dysplasia	
Hypoparathyroidism, congenital	Tetany, cataracts, enamel hypoplasia	Investigations (may be part of polyendocrinopathy syndrome)
Hypophosphatasia	Anorexia, bone pain, weakness	Clinical plus investigations
Idiopathic midfacial granuloma syndrome	Ulceration	Histology
Impetigo	Facial rash, blisters, often golden yellow	Microbiology
Infectious mononucleosis	*See* Glandular fever	
Kaposi's sarcoma	Purplish macules or nodules	Histology
Kawasaki disease	Lymphadenopathy, conjunctivitis, dry lips, strawberry tongue, desquamation, cardiomyopathy/myocarditis	Clinical mainly
Keratoconjunctivitis sicca	*See* Sjögren's syndrome	
Keratosis		
frictional	White lesion	Clinical
smoker's	White lesion in palate	Clinical
verrucous	Raised or warty white lesion	Clinical and histology
sublingual	White lesion in floor of mouth and ventrum of tongue	Clinical and histology
Langerhans' cell histiocytoses	*See* Histiocytosis	
Leishmaniasis	Mucocutaneous ulceration, lymphadenopathy	Clinical and histology
Leprosy	Hypo- or hyperpigmented patches, lymphadenopathy, neuropathy	Clinical and histology
Letterer–Siwe disease	*See* Histiocytosis	
Leukaemia	Anaemia, bleeding tendency, infections, lymphadenopathy	Blood picture, biopsy
Leukopenia	Recurrent infections	Blood picture, biopsy

Investigations	Management
Plasma parathormone, calcium phosphate levels	Calcium, vitamin D
Plasma calcium phosphate and alkaline phosphatase levels	Calcium, vitamin D
Biopsy, anti-neutrophil cytoplasmic antibody (ANCA)	Chemotherapy
Culture and sensitivity	Antimicrobial: penicillin
Biopsy, HIV serology	Chemotherapy or radiotherapy, HAART
Full blood picture, erythrocyte sedimentation rate, electrocardiogram	Symptomatic
—	Try to eliminate cause
—	Try to eliminate cause
Biopsy	Excise if dysplastic, stop tobacco use
Biopsy	Excise if dysplastic, stop tobacco use
Biopsy	Pentamidine or stibogluconate
Biopsy	Dapsone or clofazimine
Full blood picture + film, bone marrow biopsy	Chemotherapy
Full blood picture, bone marrow biopsy	Antimicrobial

Condition	Typical main clinical features	Diagnosis
Leukoplakia	*See* Keratosis and *see* Hairy leukoplakia	
Lichen planus	Mucosal white or other lesions. Polygonal purple pruritic papules on skin	Clinical and histology
Lichenoid lesions: drug-induced	Mucosal white lesions. Polygonal purple pruritic papules on skin	Clinical and histology
Linear IgA disease	Mucosal vesicles or desquamative gingivitis	Clinical and histology
Localized oral purpura	Blood blisters only in mouth	Clinical
Ludwig's angina	Tender brawny submandibular swelling, fever	Clinical
Lupus erythematosus	Arthralgia, fever, rash, lymphadenopathy, lichenoid mucosal lesions	Clinical plus investigations
Lyme disease	Acute arthritis — mainly knee, rash ± facial palsy	Clinical plus serology
Lymphadenitis acute	Tender swollen lymph nodes	Clinical plus investigations
chronic	Chronically enlarged lymph nodes	Clinical plus investigations
Lymphangioma	Swelling but empties on pressure	Clinical
Lymphoma	Wide spectrum. Swollen lymph nodes, fever, weight loss	Clinical plus histology
Lymphosarcoma	*See* Lymphomas	
McCune–Albright syndrome	*See* Albright's syndrome	
Maffucci's syndrome	Enchondromatosis plus cavernous haemangiomas	Clinical plus investigations
MAGIC syndrome	*See* Behçet's syndrome	
Masseteric hypertrophy	Masseter enlarged on both or occasionally one side	Clinical

Investigations	Management
Biopsy ± immunofluorescence	Corticosteroids or tacrolimus topically, stop tobacco use
Biopsy	Corticosteroids topically, stop taking drug
Biopsy ± immunofluorescence	Dapsone ± sulfapyridine, gluten free diet
Platelet count, biopsy may be needed to differentiate from pemphigoid	Reassurance ± deflate blisters
Pus for culture and sensitivity	Drainage, antimicrobials: penicillin in high dose ± tracheostomy
Antibodies to double-strand DNA	Corticosteroids, antimalarials
Serology	Antimicrobials
Temperature, examine drainage area White cell count and differential	Depends on cause
Temperature, examine drainage area White cell count and differential chest radiograph. Consider biopsy ± HIV testing	Depends on cause
—	Leave or surgery, cryotherapy, laser therapy or sclerosant
Biopsy. Radiography	Chemotherapy ± radiotherapy
Radiography	Reassurance
—	Symptomatic Rarely surgery ± botulinum toxoid

Condition	Typical main clinical features	Diagnosis
Measles	Fever, lymphadenopathy, conjunctivitis, rhinitis, maculopapular rash	Clinical
Median rhomboid glossitis	Rhomboidal red or nodular and depapillated or white, in midline of dorsum of tongue, just anterior to circumvallate papillae	Clinical and microbiology
Melanoma	Usually hyperpigmented papule in palate	Clinical plus histology
Melanotic macules	Hyperpigmented macule	Clinical
Melkersson–Rosenthal syndrome	Facial swelling, fissured tongue, facial palsy	Clinical plus investigations
Migrainous neuralgia	Nocturnal unilateral retro-ocular pain	Clinical
Molluscum contagiosum	Umbilicated papules	Clinical
Morsicatio buccarum	*See* Cheek chewing	
Mucoceles	Fluctuant swelling with clear or bluish contents	Clinical
Mucoepidermoid tumour	Firm salivary swelling	Clinical plus investigations
Mucormycosis	Sinus pain and discharge plus fever and palatal ulceration	Clinical plus investigations
Mucous membrane pemphigoid	Blisters, mainly in mouth occasionally on conjunctivae, genitals or skin. Scarring	Clinical and histology
Multiple basal cell naevus syndrome	*See* Gorlin–Goltz syndrome	
Multiple myeloma	Bone pain, anaemia, nausea, infections, amyloidosis	Clinical plus investigations
Mumps	Fever, painful swollen salivary gland(s) but no pustular discharge from duct	Clinical mainly
Mycosis fungoides	Variable rash	Clinical plus investigations
Myelodysplastic syndrome	Ulcers, anaemia, neutropenia, thrombocytopenia	Clinical plus investigations
Necrotizing sialometaplasia	Ulceration in palate	Clinical ± investigations

Investigations	Management
—	Symptomatic Avoid aspirin
Smear of lesion	Antifungals if *Candida* present Stop smoking
Biopsy (wide excision)	Surgery
—	Reassurance
Exclude Crohn's disease and sarcoidosis	Reassurance ± salazopyrine ± dapsone ± intralesional steroids
—	H_3 blockers, oxygen, analgesics
Consider HIV infection	Pierce with orangewood stick
—	Surgery or cryotherapy
Biopsy ± radiography	Surgery
Biopsy. Radiography. Full blood picture Exclude diabetes	Surgery. Antifungals
Biopsy + immunostaining	Topical corticosteroids
Radiography. Serum and urine electrophoresis. Bone marrow biopsy	Radiography and chemotherapy
Serology may be helpful	Symptomatic
Biopsy. Full blood picture Bone marrow biopsy	Topical chemotherapy ± radiotherapy
Full blood picture. Bone marrow biopsy	Chemotherapy, Bone marrow transplantation
Biopsy may be indicated	Self-healing

Condition	Typical main clinical features	Diagnosis
Neurofibromatosis	Neurofibromas and skin pigmentation	Clinical usually
Noma	*See* Cancrum oris	
North American blastomycosis	Chronic oral ulceration, pulmonary involvement	Clinical plus investigations
Oral dysaesthesia	*See* Burning mouth	
Oral submucous fibrosis	Firm fibrous bands in cheek and/or palate History of chilli use	Clinical
Orf	Umbilicated nodule	Clinical and history
Orofacial granulomatosis	Facial swelling, mucosa cobblestoned, ulcers, angular stomatitis (*see also* Crohn's disease)	Clinical plus investigations
Osler–Rendu–Weber syndrome	*See* Hereditary haemorrhagic telangiectasia	
Osteogenesis imperfecta	*See* Fragilitis ossium	
Osteomyelitis	Pain, swelling, fever	Clinical plus investigations
Osteopetrosis	Anaemia, cranial neuropathies, hepatosplenomegaly	Clinical plus investigations
Osteoradionecrosis	*See* Osteomyelitis	
Osteosarcoma	Pain, swelling	Clinical plus investigations
Paget's disease	Pain, craniofacial neuropathies, cardiac failure	Clinical plus investigations
Pain dysfunction syndrome	*See* Facial arthromyalgia	
Papillary hyperplasia	Small papillae in palate	Clinical
Paracoccidioidomycosis	Chronic oral ulceration, pulmonary involvement. Time in Latin America	Clinical plus investigations
Parodontal abscess	Painful swelling alongside a periodontally involved tooth	Clinical
Pemphigoid	*See* Mucous membrane pemphigoid	
Pemphigus	Skin vesicles + bullae. Mouth ulcers	Clinical plus histology

Investigations	Management
Radiography and biopsy may help	Excise symptomatic tumours
Biopsy ± chest radiography	Antifungals: fluconazole, ketoconazole or amphotericin
—	Avoid chillis and pan. Corticosteroids intralesionally
Electron microscopy ± biopsy	Spontaneous resolution
Exclude Crohn's disease/sarcoidosis Biopsy ± allergy testing	Avoid allergens. Reassurance Corticosteroids intralesionally. Clofazimine, anti-TNF agents
Radiography. Pus for culture and sensitivity	Drainage. Antimicrobials
Radiography. Biopsy	Bone marrow transplant
Radiography. Biopsy	Surgery ± chemotherapy
Radiography, serum alkaline phosphatase, urinary hydroxyproline	Bisphosphonates, acetylsalicyclic acid, calcitonin
—	Surgery or leave alone
Biopsy ± chest radiography	Antifungals: fluconazole, ketoconazole or amphotericin
Radiography, culture pus	Drain. Antimicrobial: penicillin
Biopsy. Serology Immunostaining	Corticosteroids systemically Consider azathioprine or gold or mycophenolate

Condition	Typical main clinical features	Diagnosis
Periadentitis mucosa necrotica recurrens (Sutton's ulcers)	*See* Aphthae	
Periarteritis nodosa	*See* Polyarteritis nodosa	
Pericoronitis	Painful swelling of operculum of partially erupted tooth ± trismus ± fever	Clinical
Periodontitis (acute apical)	Pain, tenderness on touching tooth	Clinical plus investigations
Perleche	*See* Cheilitis, angular	
Phycomycosis	*See* Mucormycosis	
Pleomorphic salivary ademona	Firm salivary swelling	Clinical plus investigations
Polyarteritis nodosa	Fever, weakness, arthralgia, myalgia, abdominal pain, hypertension	Clinical plus raised ESR Histology
Polycythaemia rubra vera	Headache, thromboses, haemorrhage, splenomegaly	Clinical plus investigations
Polyps – fibroepithelial	*See* Fibroepithelial polyp	
Pulpitis	Toothache	Clinical plus investigations
Pyogenic arthritis	Pain, fever, limited jaw movement, swelling	Clinical mainly
Pyogenic granuloma	Swelling, usually on lip, tongue or gum	Clinical
Pyostomatitis vegetans	Irregular oral ulcers and pustules	Clinical plus investigations
Ranula	*See* Mucocele	
Recurrent aphthous stomatitis	*See* Aphthae	
Recurrent parotitis	Recurrent painful parotid swelling	Clinical
Reiter's syndrome	Arthritis, conjunctivitis, mucocutaneous lesions, urethritis	Clinical mainly

Investigations	Management
Radiography	Debridement ± antimicrobial. Reduce occlusion. Consider extracting offending tooth
Radiography ± vitality test	Open tooth for drainage and relieve occlusion (or extract), analgesics ± antimicrobial
Biopsy ± radiography	Surgery
Full blood picture, erythrocyte sedimentation rate. Biopsy	Systemic corticosteroids
Haemoglobin, full blood picture, marrow biopsy	Phlebotomy ± chemotherapy
Radiography ± vitality test	Open tooth (or extract). Extirpate pulp. Analgesics
Radiography, culture joint aspirate	Antimicrobial, analgesics
Biopsy [excision]	Excise
Biopsy. Exclude Crohn's disease and ulcerative colitis	Treat underlying condition
Sialography. Exclude Sjögren's syndrome	Consider duct dilatation. Antimicrobials
Full blood picture, erythrocyte sedimentation rate. Radiography	Tetracycline. Non-steroidal anti-inflammatory drugs

Condition	Typical main clinical features	Diagnosis
Rheumatoid arthritis	Painful swollen small joints ± deformities Associated with Sjögren's syndrome	Clinical plus investigations Check for xerostomia
Rickets	Skeletal deformities, retarded growth, fractures	Clinical plus investigations
Rubella	*See* German measles	
Rubeola	*See* Measles	
Sarcoidosis	Various — especially hilar lymphadenopathy and rashes	Clinical plus investigations
Scleroderma	Tightening facial and other skin Associated with Sjögren's syndrome	Clinical and serology
Scrotal tongue	Fissured tongue	Clinical
Scurvy	Purplish chronically swollen gingivae	Clinical
Shingles	Painful facial rash and oral ulcers if affecting maxillary or mandibular division of trigeminal nerve	Clinical
Sialolithiasis	*See* Calculus, salivary	
Sialorrhoea	Excess salivation	Clinical
Sialosis	Painless persistent bilateral salivary gland swelling	Clinical plus investigations
Sinusitis (acute)	Pain especially on moving head	Clinical plus radiography
Sjögren's syndrome	Autoimmune exocrinopathy. Dry eyes, dry mouth and often a connective tissue disease	Clinical plus investigations
Smoker's keratosis	*See* Keratosis	
South American blastomycosis	*See* Paracoccidioidomycosis	

Investigations	Management
Rheumatoid factor, full blood picture Radiography	Salicylates. Non-steroidal anti-inflammatory drugs
Blood calcium, phosphate, alkaline phosphatase. Radiography. Renal function tests	Vitamin D. Calcitonin
Chest radiograph + serum angiotensin-converting enzyme	Corticosteroids systemically
Serology Scl-70 antibody	Supportive
—	Reassurance
White blood cell count Vitamin C levels	Vitamin C
Consider underlying immune defect	Analgesics, ± aciclovir, ± protect cornea
Salivary flow rate	Avoid anticholinesterases, otherwise reassurance or consider atropinics
Exclude alcoholism, diabetes, bulimia, sarcoidosis, Sjögren's syndrome, liver disease	Remove underlying cause
Radiography	Decongestants, analgesics and antimicrobial
Serology — SS-A (Ro) and SS-B (La) antibodies. Exclude HCV, HIV. Consider labial gland biopsy ± salivary flow rate ± sialography ± scintiscan	Artificial tears and saliva. Preventive dentistry, pilocarpine, cevimeline

Condition	Typical main clinical features	Diagnosis
Staphylococcus aureus **lymphadenitis**	Painful swollen lymph node(s) ± fever	Clinical mainly
Stevens–Johnson syndrome	*See* Erythema multiforme	
Streptococcal tonsillitis	Sore throat. Tonsillar exudate	Clinical mainly
Stroke	Hemiplegia usually ± facial palsy	Clinical
Subluxation-temporo-mandibular joint	Limited jaw movement ± pain, condyle palpably displaced	Clinical
Surgical emphysema	Swelling which crackles on palpation	Clinical
Tori	Asymptomatic bony lumps	Clinical
Toxoplasmosis	Lymphadenopathy ± chorioretinitis	Clinical plus investigations
Trigeminal neuralgia	Severe lancinating pain often associated with trigger zone	Clinical mainly
Tuberculosis	Cough, cervical, lymphadenopathy, weight loss, oral ulceration	Clinical plus investigations
White sponge naevus	*See* Familial white folded gingivostomatitis	
Zygomycosis	*See* Mucormycosis	

Investigations	Management
Pus for culture and sensitivity	Antimicrobials
Throat swab	Antimicrobials
—	Physiotherapy
—	Reduce. Consider Dautrey operation
—	Reassurance. Antimicrobials
—	Reassurance. Surgery if interfering with denture wear
Serology	Sulfonamide + pyrimethamine
Skull base CT, MRI	Avoid trigger zone. Carbamazepine ± phenytoin, gabapentin, baclofen or clonazepam
Chest radiograph Sputum microscopy and culture Biopsy	Antimicrobials: rifampicin, isoniazid, ethambutol, streptomycin

1.4 GUIDE TO DRUGS USED IN THE MANAGEMENT OF ORAL DISEASES

Always check doses, possible interactions and adverse effects before using a drug, with the British National Formulary, or Physician's Desk Reference or www.bnf.org, www.medsafe.govt.n2/profs/datasheet/dsform. asp, or www.nlm.nih.gov/medlineplus/druginformation.html. While every attempt has been made to include accurate data, the authors and publishers accept no liability for Tables 1 to 15.

Table 1 ANALGESICS (including opioids)

Drug	Comments	Route	Adult dose
Aspirin	Mild analgesic: NSAID Causes gastric irritation Interferes with haemostasis Contraindicated in bleeding disorders, asthma, children, late pregnancy, peptic ulcers, renal disease, aspirin allergy	Oral	300–600 mg up to 6 times a day after meals; maximum 4 g daily (use soluble or dispersible or enteric-coated aspirin)
Mefenamic acid	Mild analgesic: NSAID May be contraindicated in asthma, gastro- intestinal, liver and renal disease and pregnancy May cause diarrhoea or haemolytic anaemia	Oral	250–500 mg up to 3 times a day
Diflunisal	Analgesic for mild to moderate pain: NSAID Long action: twice a day dose only Effective against bone and joint pain Contraindicated in renal and liver disease, peptic ulcer, pregnancy, allergies	Oral	250–500 mg twice a day
Paracetamol (Acetoaminophen)	Mild analgesic: not usually termed an NSAID Hepatotoxic in overdose or prolonged use Contraindicated in liver or renal disease	Oral	500–1000 mg up to 6 times a day
Codeine phosphate*	Analgesic for moderate pain Contraindicated in liver disease and late pregnancy Avoid alcohol May cause sedation and constipation Reduces cough reflex	Oral	10–60 mg up to 6 times a day (or 30 mg IM)
Dextropropoxyphene*	Analgesic for moderate pain Risk of respiratory depression in overdose, especially if taken with alcohol May cause dependence Occasional hepatotoxicity No more effective than paracetamol or aspirin alone	Oral	65 mg up to 4 times a day
Diclofenac	Analgesic for moderate pain: NSAID Contraindicated in peptic ulcer, aspirin sensitivity and pregnancy Caution in elderly, renal, liver or cardiac disease	Oral or IM	25–75 mg up to twice daily
Dihydrocodeine tartrate*	Analgesic for moderate pain May cause nausea, drowsiness and constipation Contraindicated in children, asthma, hypothyroidism and renal disease May increase post-operative dental pain	Oral	30 mg up to 4 times a day (or 50 mg IM)

Table 1 (Contd)

Drug	Comments	Route	Adult dose
Nefopam	Analgesic for moderate pain May cause nausea, dry mouth or urine retention Contraindicated in epilepsy	Oral	60 mg up to 3 times a day

Pentazocine*	Analgesic for moderate pain
	May produce dependence, hallucinations or
	   provoke withdrawal symptoms in narcotic addicts
	Contraindicated in pregnancy, children,
	   hypertension, respiratory depression, head
	   injuries or raised intracranial pressure
	There is a low risk of dependence
		Oral	50 mg up to 4 times a day (or 30 mg IM or IV)

Buprenorphine*	Potent analgesic
	More potent than pentazocine and longer action
	   than morphine
	No hallucinations
	May cause salivation, sweating, dizziness
	   and vomiting
	Respiratory depression in overdose
	Can cause dependence
	Contraindicated in pregnancy, children, with
	MAOIs, liver or respiratory disease
		Sub-lingual	0.2–0.4 mg up to 4 times a day (or 0.3 mg IM)

Meptazinol*	Potent analgesic Claimed to have low incidence of respiratory depression Side-effects as buprenorphine	IM or IV	75–100 mg up to 6 times a day
Phenazocine*	Analgesic for severe pain May cause nausea	Oral or sub-lingual	5 mg up to 4 times a day
Pethidine*	Potent analgesic Less potent than morphine Contraindicated with MAOI Risk of dependence	SC or IM	25–100 mg up to 4 times a day
Morphine*	Potent analgesic Often causes nausea and vomiting Reduces cough reflex, causes pupil constriction	SC or IM or oral	5–10 mg as required
Diamorphine*	Potent analgesic More potent than pethidine and morphine but more dependence	SC or IM or oral	2.5 mg by injection; 5–10 mg orally

*Opioids; NSAID, non-steroidal anti-inflammatory drug; IM, intramuscular; IV, intravenous; SC, subcutaneous; MAOI, monoamine oxidase inhibitor.

Table 2 ANTIFUNGALS FOR THE TREATMENT OF ORAL CANDIDOSIS

Drug	Dose	Comments
Amphotericin	10–100 mg 6-hourly	Dissolve in mouth slowly Active topically Negligible absorption from gastro-intestinal tract
Nystatin	500 000 unit lozenge, 100 000 unit pastille, or 100 000 unit per ml of suspension 6-hourly	Dissolve in mouth slowly Active topically Negligible absorption from gastro-intestinal tract
Miconazole	250 mg tablet 6-hourly or 25 mg/ml gel used as 5 ml 6-hourly	Dissolve in mouth slowly Active topically Also has antibacterial activity Negligible absorption from gastro-intestinal tract Theoretically best antifungal to treat angular cheilitis
Ketoconazole	200–400 mg once daily with meal	Absorbed from gastro-intestinal tract Useful in intractable candidosis Contra-indicated in pregnancy and liver disease May cause nausea, rashes, pruritus and liver damage Enhances nephrotoxicity of ciclosporin
Fluconazole	50–100 mg once daily	Absorbed from gastro-intestinal tract Less toxic than ketoconazole Contraindicated in pregnancy, infants and renal disease May cause nausea and abdominal pain

Table 3 ANTIVIRAL THERAPY OF ORAL HERPETIC INFECTIONS

Virus	Disease	Otherwise healthy patient	Immunocompromised patient
Herpes simplex	Primary herpetic gingivostomatitis	Consider oral aciclovir[a,b] 100–200 mg, five times daily as suspension or tablets	Aciclovir 250 mg/m^2 IV[b] every 8 hours
	Recurrent herpetic infection, e.g. herpes labialis	1% penciclovir or 5% aciclovir cream	Consider systemic aciclovir[b] as above depending on risk to patient of infection
Herpes varicella-zoster	Chickenpox	—	As above
	Zoster (shingles)	Consider oral acyclovir[a] 800 mg, five times daily	

[a]In neonate, treat as if immunocompromised.
[b]Systemic aciclovir: caution in renal disease and pregnancy; occasional increase in liver enzymes and urea, rashes.

Table 4 ANTIBACTERIALS

Drug	Comments*	Route	Dose
PENICILLINS	Most oral bacterial infections respond well to drainage ± penicillin Oral phenoxymethyl penicillin is usually effective and cheap Amoxicillin is often used and is usually effective, but almost four times as expensive		
Amoxicillin	Orally effective (absorption better than ampicillin) Broad-spectrum penicillin derivative *Staphylococcus aureus* often resistant Not resistant to penicillinase Contraindicated in penicillin hypersensitivity Rashes in infectious mononucleosis, cytomegalovirus infection, lymphoid leukaemia, allopurinol May cause diarrhoea	Oral, IM or IV	250–500 mg 8-hourly
Augmentin (Co-amoxiclav)	Mixture of amoxicillin and potassium clavulanate Inhibits some penicillinases and therefore active against *Staphylococcus aureus* Inhibits some lactamases and is therefore active against some Gram-negative and penicillin-resistant bacteria Contraindicated in penicillin hypersensitivity Beware of diarrhoea and hepatobiliary events	Oral	125/250 mg 8-hourly
Ampicillin	Less oral absorption than amoxicillin, otherwise as for amoxicillin (There are many analogues but these have few, if any, advantages) Contraindicated in penicillin hypersensitivity	Oral, IM or IV	250–500 mg 6-hourly
Benzylpenicillin	Not orally active Most effective penicillin where organism sensitive Not resistant to penicillinase Contraindicated in penicillin hypersensitivity Large doses may cause K^+ to fall and Na^+ to rise	Oral or IM	300–600 mg 6-hourly
Flucloxacillin	Orally active penicillin derivative Effective against most, but not all, penicillin-resistant staphylococci Contraindicated in penicillin hypersensitivity	Oral or IM	250 mg 6-hourly
Phenoxymethyl penicillin (Penicillin V)	Orally active Best taken on empty stomach Not resistant to penicillinase Contraindicated in penicillin hypersensitivity	Oral	250–500 mg 6-hourly *Contd*

IM, intramuscular; IV, intravenous; K^+, potassium; Na^+, sodium.
*It should be noted that some antibacterials impair the activity of oral contraceptives.

Table 4 (Contd)

Drug	Comments*	Route	Dose
Procaine penicillin	Depot penicillin Not resistant to penicillinase Contraindicated in penicillin hypersensitivity Rarely psychotic reaction	IM	300 000 units every 12 hours
Benethamine penicillin (Triplopen)	Depot penicillin Contains benzyl (300 mg), procaine (250 mg) and benethamine (475 mg) penicillins Not resistant to penicillinase Contraindicated in penicillin hypersensitivity	IM	1 vial every 2–3 days
SULFONAMIDES	Main indications are in prophylaxis of post-traumatic meningitis but meningococci increasingly resistant Co-trimoxazole may be used to treat sinusitis Contraindicated in pregnancy and in renal disease In other patients, adequate hydration must be ensured to prevent the (rare) occurrence of crystalluria Other adverse reactions include erythema multiforme, rashes and blood dyscrasias		
Co-trimoxazole	Combination of trimethoprim and sulfamethoxazole Orally active Broad spectrum Occasional rashes or blood dyscrasias Contraindicated in pregnancy, liver disease May increase the effect of protein-bound drugs	Oral or IM	960 mg twice daily or 3–4.5 ml IM twice daily
TETRACYCLINES	Broad-spectrum antibacterial but of the many preparations there is little to choose between them. However, doxycycline is useful since a single dose is adequate, and minocycline is effective against meningococci; both are safer for patients with renal failure than most of the tetracyclines, which are nephrotoxic Tetracyclines cause discoloration of developing teeth and have absorption impaired by iron, antacids, milk, etc. Use of tetracyclines may predispose to candidosis, and to nausea and gastro-intestinal disturbance Orally active Broad spectrum Contraindicated in pregnancy and children at least up to 8 years Reduced dose indicated in renal failure, liver disease, elderly Frequent mild gastro-intestinal effects	Oral	250–500 mg 6-hourly
Doxycycline	Orally active Broad spectrum	Oral	100 mg once daily

Table 4 (Contd)

Drug	Comments*	Route	Dose
	Single daily dose Contraindicated in pregnancy and children up 　to at least 8 years Safer than tetracycline in renal failure 　(excreted in faeces) Reduce dose in liver disease and elderly Mild gastro-intestinal effects		
Minocycline	Orally active Broad spectrum: active against meningococci Safer than tetracycline in renal disease 　(excreted in faeces) May cause dizziness and vertigo Absorption not reduced by milk Contraindicated in pregnancy and children up to 　at least 8 years May also cause mild hepatic dysfunction, or oral 　pigmentation in adults	Oral	100 mg twice daily
VANCOMYCIN	Reserved for serious infections Extravenous extravasation causes necrosis and phlebitis May cause nausea, rashes, tinnitus, deafness Rapid injection may cause 'red neck' syndrome Contraindicated in renal disease, deafness Very expensive	Oral or IV	500 mg 6-hourly for pseudomem- branous colitis. 1 g IV by slow injection for prophylaxis of endocarditis

IM, intramuscular; IV, intravenous.
*It should be noted that some antibacterials impair the activity of oral contraceptives.

Table 5 OTHER ANTIBACTERIAL AGENTS USED OCCASIONALLY

Drug	Comments*	Route	Adult dose
CEPHALOSPORINS AND CEPHAMYCINS	Broad spectrum, expensive and bactericidal antibiotics 　with few absolute indications for use in dentistry, 　although they may be effective against *Staphylococcus aureus* They produce false-positive results for glycosuria 　with 'Clinitest' Hypersensitivity is the main side-effect Some cause a bleeding tendency Some are nephrotoxic Cefuroxime is less affected by penicillinases than 　other cephalosporins and is currently the preferred 　drug of the many available		*Contd*

Table 5 (Contd)

Drug	Comments*	Route	Adult dose
Cefotaxime and ceftazidime	Not orally active Broad spectrum; third generation cephalosporins Contraindicated if history of anaphylaxis to penicillin Expensive	IM or IV	1 g 12-hourly
Cefuroxime	Not orally active Broad spectrum; second generation cephalosporin Contraindicated if history of anaphylaxis to penicillin	IM or IV	250–750 mg 8-hourly
Ceftriaxone	Orally active; third generation cephalosporin Longer action than most cephalosporins Contraindicated in liver disease or history of anaphylaxis to penicillin	IM or IV	1 g daily as single dose
ERYTHROMYCIN	Similar antibacterial spectrum to penicillin and is therefore used in penicillin-allergic patients Active against most staphylococci, *Mycoplasma* and *Legionnella*, but not always against oral *Bacteroides* Do not use erythromycin estolate, which may cause liver disease		
Erythromycin stearate	Orally active Useful in those hypersensitive to penicillin Effective against most staphylococci and streptococci May cause nausea Rapid development of resistance Reduced dose indicated in liver disease Can increase ciclosporin absorption and toxicity	Oral	250–500 mg 6-hourly
Erythromycin lactobionate	Used where parenteral erythromycin indicated Give not as a bolus but by infusion Comments as above	IV	2 g daily
GENTAMICIN	Reserved for serious infections Can cause vestibular and renal damage, especially if given with furosemide (frusemide) Contraindicated in pregnancy and myasthenia gravis Reduce dose in renal disease	IM or IV	Up to 5 mg/kg daily
METRONIDAZOLE	Orally active Effective against anaerobes Use only for 7 days (or peripheral neuropathy may develop, particularly in liver-disease patients) Avoid alcohol (disulfiram-type reaction) May increase warfarin effect	Oral or IV	200–400 mg 8-hourly (take with meals) *Contd*

Table 5 (Contd)

Drug	Comments*	Route	Adult dose
	May cause tiredness IV preparation available but expensive Suppositories effective Contraindicated in pregnancy		
RIFAMPICIN	Reserved mainly for treatment of tuberculosis Safe and effective but resistance rapidly occurs Body secretions turn red May interfere with oral contraception Occasional rashes, jaundice or blood dyscrasias	Oral or IV	0.6–1.2 g daily in 2–4 divided doses

IM, intramuscular; IV, intravenous. *It should be noted that some antibacterials impair the activity of oral contraceptives.

Table 6 SOME TOPICAL CORTICOSTEROIDS (many more potent preparations are available)

Drug	Dose 6-hourly	Comments
Hydrocortisone hemisuccinate pellets	2.5 mg	Dissolve in mouth close to lesions Use at early stage
Triamcinolone acetonide in carmellose gelatin paste	Apply thin layer	Adheres best to dry mucosa Affords mechanical protection Of little value on tongue or palate
Betamethasone phosphate tablets	0.5 mg as a mouth wash	More potent than preparations above but may produce adrenal suppression
Beclometasone dipropionate (inhaler)	Spray on lesion, 50–200 µg	More potent than preparations above but may produce adrenal suppression

Table 7 SOME INTRALESIONAL CORTICOSTEROIDS

Drug	Dose	Comments
Prednisolone sodium phosphate	Up to 24 mg	Short acting
Methylprednisolone acetate	4–80 mg every 1 to 5 weeks	Also available with lidocaine (lignocaine)
Triamcinolone acetonide	2–3 mg every 1 to 2 weeks	—
Triamcinolone hexacetonide	Up to 5 mg every 3 to 4 weeks	—

Table 8 SOME INTRA-ARTICULAR CORTICOSTEROIDS*

Drug	Dose	Comments
Dexamethasone sodium phosphate	0.4–5 mg at intervals of 3 to 21 days	More expensive than hydrocortisone acetate
Hydrocortisone acetate	5–50 mg	Usual preparation used

*Also used are those listed in Table 7 under intralesional corticosteroids.

Table 9 SYSTEMIC IMMUNOMODULATORY DRUGS

Drug	Comments	Adult dose
Prednisolone	May be indicated systemically for pemphigus and Bell's palsy, and occasionally other disorders	Initially 40–80 mg orally each day in divided doses, reducing as soon as possible to 10 mg daily Give enteric-coated prednisolone with meals
Dexamethasone	May be used to reduce post-surgical oedema after minor oral surgery	5 mg IV with premedication followed by 0.5–1.0 mg daily for 5 days, orally if possible
Betamethasone	May be useful to reduce post-surgical oedema after minor oral surgery	1 mg orally the night before operation 1 mg orally with premedication 1 mg orally every 6 hours for 2 days post-operatively
Methylprednisolone	May be useful to reduce post-surgical oedema after major surgery	Methylprednisolone succinate 1 g IV at operation, 500 mg on evening of operation followed by 125 mg IV every 6 hours for 24 hours. Then methylprednisolone acetate orally 80 mg every 12 hours for 24 hours
Azathioprine	Steroid-sparing for immuno-suppression Myelosuppressive and hepatotoxic, and long-term may predispose to neoplasms Contraindicated in pregnancy. Use only in patients who are TPMT (thiopurine methyl transferase) positive	Orally 2–2.5 mg/kg daily
Dapsone	May be used in some dermatoses Occasional neuropathy, headache, anaemia, rashes Contraindicated in glucose-6-phosphate dehydrogenase deficiency, pregnancy, anaemia, cardiorespiratory disease	Orally up to 1–2 mg/kg daily
Colchicine	May be used in severe oral ulceration Occasional nausea, abdominal pain, or blood dyscrasia Contraindicated in pregnancy, renal or gastro-intestinal disease	Orally up to 500 μg 4 times daily
Thalidomide	May be used in severe oral ulceration Peripheral neuropathy in prolonged use Contraindicated in women likely to become pregnant	Orally 50–200 mg preferably on alternate days (75 mg usually avoids neuropathy)

IV, intravenous.

Table 10 SOME SEDATIVES AND TRANQUILLIZERS

Drug	Comments	Preparations	Route	Adult dose
Chlorpromazine	Major tranquillizer May cause dyskinesia, photosensitivity, eye defects and jaundice Contraindicated in epilepsy IM use causes pain and may cause postural hypotension	25 mg tablet 25 mg/ml syrup 50 mg/2 ml injection	Oral or IM	25 mg 8-hourly
Chlordiazepoxide	Anxiolytic Reduce dose in elderly	5 mg or 10 mg	Oral	5–1 mg 8-hourly
Diazepam	Anxiolytic Reduce dose in elderly	2 mg, 5 mg or 10 mg	Oral, IM or IV	2–30 mg daily in divided doses
Thioridazine	Major tranquillizer Phenothiazine with fewer adverse effects than chlorpromazine Rare retinopathy	10 mg or 25 mg	Oral	10–50 mg 8-hourly
Propranolol	Useful anxiolytic which does not cause amnesia, but reduces tremor and palpitations Contraindicated in asthma, cardiac failure, pregnancy	10 mg or 40 mg	Oral	80–100 mg daily
Haloperidol	Major tranquillizer Useful in elderly	500 μg	Oral	500 μg 12-hourly

IM, intramuscular; IV, intravenous.

Table 11 SOME OTHER DRUGS USED IN THE MANAGEMENT OF ORAL DISEASES

Drug	Comments	Route	Adult dose
Etretinate	Vitamin A analogue which may be used in treatment of erosive lichen planus Effect begins after 2 to 3 weeks Treat for 6 to 9 months, followed by similar rest period Most patients develop dry, cracked lips May cause epistaxis, pruritus, alopecia Contraindicated in pregnancy/liver disease	Oral	0.5–1.0 mg/kg daily in two divided doses
Carbamazepine	Prophylactic for trigeminal neuralgia — not analgesic Occasional dizziness, diplopia and blood dyscrasia, usually with a rash and usually in the first 3 months of treatment Potentiated by cimetidine, dextropropoxyphene and isoniazid Potentiates lithium Interferes with oral contraceptives	Oral	Initially 100 mg once or twice daily. Many patients need about 200 mg 8-hourly. Do not exceed 1800 mg daily

Table 12 SOME ANTIDEPRESSANTS

Drug	Comments	Route	Adult dose
Amitriptyline	Tricyclic Antidepressant effect may not be seen until up to 30 days after start Sedative effect also When treatment established, use single dose at night	Oral	25–75 mg daily in divided dose
Dosulepin	Tricyclic Anxiolytic effect also useful in atypical facial pain When treatment established, use single dose at night	Oral	25 mg three times a day or 75 mg at night
Clomipramine	Tricyclic Equally effective as amitriptyline but less sedative effect Useful in phobia or obsessional states	Oral	10–100 mg daily in divided doses
Fluoxetine	Selective serotonin re-uptake inhibitor Less sedative or cardiotoxic than tricyclics Contraindicated in cardiovascular, hepatic or renal disease, pregnancy, diabetes and epilepsy	Oral	20 mg daily
Flupentixol	Not a tricyclic or MAOI Fewer side-effects Contraindicated in cardiovascular, hepatic or renal disease, Parkinsonism or overexcitable/over-active patients	Oral	1–3 mg in the morning

MAOI, monoamine oxidase inhibitor.

Table 13 ANTIDEPRESSANTS: INTERACTIONS AND CAUTIONS

Tricyclics and tetracyclics	Monoamine oxidase inhibitors (MAOIs)
USE WITH CAUTION IN: Cardiovascular disease Epilepsy Liver disease Diabetes Hypertension Glaucoma Mania Urinary retention Prostatic hypertrophy	USE WITH CAUTION IN: Cardiovascular disease Epilepsy Liver disease Phaeochromocytoma

Contd

Table 13 (Contd)

Tricyclics and tetracyclics	Monoamine oxidase inhibitors (MAOIs)
MAY INTERACT WITH: Barbiturates MAOIs Antihypertensives General anaesthetics	MAY INTERACT WITH: Barbiturates Some sympathomimetic amines Tricyclics Narcotics Antihypertensives Foods such as some meat or yeast extracts, cheese, wine

Note: Neither group significantly interacts with (lidocaine) prilocaine, articaine or doses of adrenaline (epinephrine) found in dental local analgesic solutions. Either group may worsen xerostomia.

Table 14 SOME HYPNOTICS

Drug	Comments	Preparations	Route	Adult dose
Chlormethiazole	Contraindicated in liver disease Useful in elderly May cause dependence	192 mg capsule 250 mg/5 ml syrup	Oral	500 mg
Diazepam	Useful hypnotic Reduce dose in elderly May cause dependence	5 mg or 10 mg	Oral	5–10 mg
Dichloralphenazone	Derivative of chloral hydrate Contraindicated in porphyria, with oral anticoagulants Useful in elderly	650 mg	Oral	1300 mg
Nitrazepam	No more useful than diazepam Avoid in elderly May cause dependence Hangover effect	5 mg	Oral	5–10 mg
Temazepam	Useful in elderly May cause dependence Less hangover effect than nitrazepam	10 mg	Oral	10–20 mg

Table 15 ANTIFIBRINOLYTIC AGENTS

Drug	Comments	Route	Adult dose

ε-amino
  caproic acid
	Useful in some bleeding tendencies
	May cause nausea, diarrhoea, dizziness, myalgia
	Contraindicated in pregnancy, history of
	    thromboembolism, renal disease
		Oral	3 g, 4–6 times daily

Tranexamic acid	As above, but tranexamic acid is usually the preferred drug	Oral, IV	1–1.5 g, 6 or 12 hourly Slow injection 1 g 8-hourly

IV, intravenous.

1.5 GUIDE TO THE ORAL AND PERIORAL SIDE-EFFECTS OF DRUG TREATMENT

Most oral and perioral side-effects to drug treatment are rare but the more common causes are indicated in **bold** in the following section. For further details the reader is referred to (for example) the Physicians Desk Reference or British National Formulary.

ANGIOEDEMA

Acetylsalicylic acid
Angiotensin-converting enzyme
    (ACE) inhibitors
Asparaginase
Aspirin (acetylsalicylic acid)
Barbiturates
Captopril
Carbamazepine
Cephalosporin derivatives
Clindamycin
Clonidine
Co-trimoxazole
Droperidol
Enalapril
Epoetin alpha
Ibuprofen
Indometacin
Iodine and iodides
Ketoconazole
Local anaesthetic agents
Mianserin
Miconazole
Naproxen
Nitrofurantoin
Penicillamine
Penicillin derivatives
Pyrazolone derivatives
Quinine
Streptomycin
Sulfonamides
Thiouracil

BRUXISM

Amfetamines
Ecstasy

CANDIDOSIS

**Broad spectrum
    antimicrobials**
Corticosteroids
Drugs causing xerostomia
Immunosuppressives

CERVICAL LYMPHADENOPATHY

Phenytoin

Phenylbutazone
Primidone

CHEILITIS

Actinomycin
Atorvastatin
Busulfan
Clofazimine
Clomipramine
Cyancobalamin
Cytotoxic agents
Ethyl alcohol
Etretinate
Gold
Indinavir
Isoniazid
Isotretinoin
Lithium
Menthol
Methyldopa
Penicillamine
Phenothiazines
Psoralens
Selegiline
Streptomycin
Sulfasalazine
Tetracycline
Vitamin A

DRY MOUTH

Alfuzosin
Amiloride
Amitriptyline
Amoxapine
Benzhexol
Benztropine
Biperiden
Bupropion
Buspirone
Cannabis
Cetirizine
Chlormezanone
Chlorpromazine
Citalopram
Clemastine
Clomipramine
Clonidine

Clozapine
Cyclizine
Cyclobenzaprine
Desipramine
Dexamfetamine
Diazepam
Dicyclomine
Dideoxyinosine
Dihydrocodeine
Disopyramide
Donopezil
Dosulepine
Doxepin
Duloxetine
Ecstasy
Elliptinium
Ephedrine
Fenfluramine
Fluoxetine
Furosemide (frusemide)
Guanfacine
Hyoscine
Imipramine
Indoramine
Interferon alpha
Interleukin-2
Ipratropium
Iprindole
Isocarboxazid
Isotretinoin
Ketorolac
Ketotifen
Lansoprazole
L-Dopa
Lithium
Lofepramine
Lofexidine
Loratadine
Maprotiline
Mepenzolate
Methyldopa
Mianserine
Mirtazapine
Monoamine oxidase inhibitors
Morphine
Moxonidine
Nabilone
Nefopam

Nortriptyline
Olanzapine
Omeprazole
Orphenadrine
Oxitropium
Oxybutynin
Paroxetine
Phenelzine
Pipamperone
Pipenzolate
Pirenzipine
Poldine
Pratropium
Procyclidine
Propafenone
Propantheline
Propiverine
Pseudoephedrine
Quetiapine
Reboxetine
Rilmenidine
Risperidone
Rizatriptan
Selegiline
Sertraline
Sibutramine
Sucralfate
Tamsulosin
Terazosin
Thiabendazole
Tiapride
Tiotropium
Tizamidine
Tolterodine
Tramadol
Tranylcypromine
Trazodone
Trepium chloride
Triamterene
Trimipramine
Trospium
Venlafaxine
Viloxazine
Zopiclone

ERYTHEMA MULTIFORME

Acetylsalicylic acid
Allopurinol
Amlodipine
Arsenic
Atropine
Barbiturates
Busulfan
Carbamazepine
Cephalosporins
Chloral hydrate
Chloramphenicol
Chlorpropamide
Clindamycin
Codeine
Co-trimoxazole
Diclofenac
Diflunisal
Digitalis
Diltiazem
Ethambutol
Ethyl alcohol
Fluconazole
Fluorouracil
Furosemide (frusemide)
Gold
Griseofulvin
Hydantoin
Hydrochlorothiazide
Indapamide
Measles/mumps/rubella vaccine
Meclofenamic acid
Mercury
Mesterolone
Minoxidil
Nifedipine
Omeprazole
Oxyphenbutazone
Penicillin derivatives
Phenolphthalein
Phenylbutazone
Phenytoin
Piroxicam
Progesterone
Pyrazolone derivatives
Quinine

Retinol
Rifampicin
Streptomycin
Sulindac
Sulfasalazine
Sulfonamides
Tenoxicam
Tetracyclines
Theophylline
Tocainide
Tolbutamide
Trimethadione
Vancomycin
Verapamil
Zidovudine

FACIAL HIRSUTISM

Ciclosporin
Cyproterone acetate
Formestane
Medroxyprogesterone
Minoxidil
Nandrolone decanoate
Norethisterone
Oxemetholone
Phenytoin
Testosterone
Tibolone

FACIAL FLUSHING

Adenosine
Alprostadil
Buserelin
Calcitonin
Calcium channel blockers
Caroprost
Chlorpropamide
Clomifene
Co-dergocrine
Danazol
L-Dopa
Flumazenil
Formestane
Loxapine
Morphine

Contd

Nicotinic acid
Pentoxifylline (Oxpentifylline)
Pentamidine
Protirelin
Quinine
Rifampicin
Ritodrine
Sermorelin
Tamoxifen
Thymoxamine
Thyroxine
Trilostane

FACIAL MOVEMENTS

Butyrophenones
Carbamazepine
L-Dopa
Lithium
Methyldopa
Metoclopramide
Metirosine
Phenothiazines
Phenytoin
Tetrabenazine
Tricyclic antidepressants
Trifluoroperazine

FACIAL OEDEMA

Cinoxacin
Corticosteroids
Ciclosporin
Trilostane

GINGIVAL SWELLING

Amlodipine
Ciclosporin
Co-trimoxazole
Diltiazem
Diphenoxylate
Erythromycin
Ethosuximide
Felodipine
Interferon-α
Ketoconazole
Lacidipine
Lamotrigine

Lithium
Mephenytoin
Nifedipine
Nitrendipine
Norethisterone + mestranol
Oral contraceptives
Phenobarbital
Phenytoin
Primidone
Sertraline
Topiramate
Valproate
Verapamil
Vigabatrin

GLOSSITIS

Captopril
Chloramphenicol
Cytotoxics
Enalapril
Ergot alkaloids
Flunisolide
Gold
Griseofulvin
Isoniazid
Methyldopa
Metronidazole
Phenelzine
Phenothiazine derivatives
Streptomycin
Sulindac
Tetracycline
Tricyclic antidepressants
Zidovudine

HALITOSIS

Dimethyl sulfoxide (DMSO)
Disulfiram
Isorbide dinitrate

HYPERPIGMENTATION

ACTH
Amodiaquine
Anticonvulsants
Arsenic
Betel

Bismuth
Bromine
Busulfan
Chlorhexidine
Chloroquine
Clofazimine
Coal
Copper
Cyclophosphamide
Doxorubicin
Gold
Heroin
Iron
Lead
Manganese
Mepacrine
Methyldopa
Minocycline
Oral contraceptives
Phenolphthalein
Phenothiazines
Quinacrine
Quinidine
Silver
Thallium
Tin
Vanadium
Zidovudine

HYPERSALIVATION

Alprazolam
Amiodarone
Anticholinesterases
Buprenorphine
Buspirone
Clonazepam
Diazoxide
Ethionamide
Gentamicin
Guanethidine
Haloperidol
Imipenem/cilastatin
Iodides
Kanamycin
Ketamine
Lamotrigine
L-Dopa

Mefenamic acid
Mercurials
Nicardipine
Niridazole
Pentoxifylline
  (Oxpentifylline)
Remoxipride
Risperidone
Rivastigmine
Tacrine
Tobramycin
Triptorelin
Venlafaxine
Zaleplon

LICHENOID REACTIONS

Allopurinol
Amiphenazole
Antimalarials
Barbiturates
BCG vaccine
Beta blockers
Captopril
Carbamazepine
Carbimazole
Chloral hydrate
Chloroquine
Chlorpropamide
Cholera vaccine
Cinnarizine
Clofibrate
Colchicine
Dapsone
Dipyridamole
Ethionamide
Flunarizine
Gaunoclor
Gold
Griseofulvin
Hepatitis B vaccine
Hydroxychloroquine
Interferon-α
Ketoconazole
Labetalol
Levamisole
Lincomycin
Lithium

Lorazepam
Mepacrine
Mercury (amalgam)
Metformin
Methyldopa
Metronidazole
Niridazole
Oral contraceptives
NSAIDs
Oxprenolol
Para-aminosalicylate
Penicillamine
Penicillin derivatives
Phenindione
Phenothiazines
Phenylbutazone
Phenytoin
Piroxicam
Practolol
Prazosin
Procainamide
Propranolol
Propylthiouracil
Prothionamide
Quinidine
Quinine
Rifampicin
Rofecoxib
Streptomycin
Sulfonamides
Tetracycline
Tocainide
Tolbutamide
Triprolidine

LUPOID REACTIONS

Ethosuximide
Gold
Griseofulvin
Hydralazine
Isoniazid
Methyldopa
Para-aminosalicylate
Penicillin
Phenytoin
Phenothiazines
Procainamide

Streptomycin
Sulfonamides
Tetracyclines

OSTEONECROSIS

Bisphosphonates

PAIN

Benztropine
Biperidin
Griseofulvin
Lithium
Penicillins
Phenothiazines
Stilbamidine
Ticarcillin
Vinca alkaloids
Vitamin A

PEMPHIGOID-LIKE REACTIONS

Amoxicillin
Azapropazone
Clonidine
Furosemide (frusemide)
Ibuprofen
Isoniazid
Mefenamic acid
Nadolol
Penicillin v
Penicillamine
Phenacetin
Practolol
Salicylic acid derivatives
Sufasalazine
Sulfonamides

PEMPHIGUS-LIKE REACTIONS

Ampicillin
Arsenic
Benzylpenicillin
Captopril
Cefadroxil
Cefalexin
Diclofenac
Gold   *Contd*

Interferon-β
Interleukin-2
Oxyphenbutazone
Penicillamine
Phenobarbital
Phenylbutazone
Piroxicam
Probenecid
Procaine penicillin
Rifampicin

SALIVA DISCOLORATION

Clofazimine
L-Dopa
Rifabutin
Rifampin

SALIVARY GLAND PAIN OR SWELLING

Bethanidine
Bretylium
Cimetidine
Clonidine
Clozapine
Deoxycycline
Famotidine
Guanethidine
Insulin
Interferon
Isoprenaline
Methyldopa
Naproxen
Nicardipine
Nifedipine
Nitrofurantoin
Oxyphenbutazone
Phenylbutazone
Phenytoin
Ranitidine
Ritodrine
Trimepramine

TASTE DISTURBANCE

Acarbose
Acetazolamide
Alcohol

Allopurinol
Amiloride
Amitryptiline
Amfetamines
Amphotericin
Amrinone
Aspirin
Atorvastatin
Auranofin
Aurothiomalate
Azathioprine
Azelastine
Aztreonam
Baclofen
Biguanides
Bleomycin
Bretylium
Calcitonin
Captopril
Carbamazepine
Carbimazole
Carboplatin
Ceftirizine
Cefamandole
Chlorhexidine
Chlormezanone
Cholestyramine
Choline magnesium trisalicylate
Cilazapril
Cisplatin
Clarithromycin
Clidinium
Clofibrate
Clomipramine
Cocaine
Diazoxide
Dicyclomine
Diltiazem
Dipyridamole
EDTA
Enalapril
Ethambutol
Ethionamide
Etidronate
Flunisolide
Fluoxetine

Flurazepam
5-Fluorouracil
Fluvoxamine
Glycopyrrolate
Griseofulvin
Hexetidine
Hydrochorothiazide
Hydrocortisone
Hyoscyamine
Imipenem
Indometacin
Interferon-γ
Iodine
Isotretinoin
L-Dopa
Levamisole
Levodopa
Lincomycin
Lisinopril
Lithium
Lomefloxacin
Losartan
Lovastatin
Methimazole
Methotrexate
Methyl methacrylate
Methylthiouracil
Metronidazole
Nifedipine
Niridazole
Nitroglycerin
Ofloxacin
Omeprazole
Penicillamine
Pentamidine
Pergolide
Perindopril
Phenformin
Phenindione
Phenylbutazone
Phenytoin
Procaine penicillin
Propafenone
Propantheline
Propranolol
Propylthiouracil

Quinapril
Ramipril
Rifabutin
Rivastigmine
Selegiline
Sodium lauryl sulfate
Spironolactone
Sulfasalazine
Terbinafine
Tetracycline
Thiamazole
Tocainide
Topiramate
Trandolapril
Triazolam
Venlafaxine
Zopiclone

TOOTH DISCOLORATION

Antibiotics
Betel
Chlorhexidine
Clarithromycin
Enalapril
Essential oil
Etidronate
Fluoride
Fosinopril
Imipenem
Iron
Lisinopril
Metronidazole
Penicillin
Pentamidine
Perindopril
Propafenone
Quinapril
Ramipril
Smoking

Terbinafine
Tetracycline
Trandolopril
Zopiclone

TRIGEMINAL PARAESTHESIA OR HYPOAESTHESIA

Acetazolamide
Amitryptiline
Articaine
Chlorpropamide
Colistin
Ergotamine
Gonadotropin-releasing hormone
    analogues
Hydralazine
Interferon-α
Isoniazid
Labetalol
Mefloquine
Methysergide
Monoamine oxidase inhibitors
Nalidixic acid
Nicotinic acid
Nitrofurantoin
Pentamidine
Phenytoin
Prilocaine
Propofol
Propranolol
Prothionamide
Stilbamidine
Streptomycin
Sulfonylureas
Sulthiame
Tolbutamide
Tricyclics
Trilostane
Vincristine

ULCERATION

Alendronate
Allopurinol
Aurothiomalate
Aztreonam
Captopril
Carbamazepine
Clarithromycin
Cytotoxic agents
Diclofenac
Dideoxycytidine
Emepromium
Flunisolide
Gold
Indometacin
Interferons
Interleukin-2
Isoprenaline
Ketorolac
Losartan
Molgramostim
Naproxen
Nicorandil
NSAIDs
Olanzapine
Pancreatin
Penicillamine
Phenindione
Phenylbutazone
Phenytoin
Potassium chloride
Proguanil
Sertraline
Sulindac
Vancomycin

DRUG-RELATED HYPERPIGMENTATION; DIFFERENT COLORS

Blue	Brown (hypermelanosis)	Black	Grey	Green
Amiodarone	Aminophenazone	Amiodiaquine	Amiodiaquine	Copper
Antimalarials	Betel nut	Betel nut	Chloroquine	
Bismuth	Bismuth	Bismuth	Fluoxetine	
Mepacrine	Busulfan	Methyldopa	Hydroxychloroquine	
Minocycline	Clofazimine	Minocycline	Lead	
Phenazopyridine	Contraceptives		Silver	
Quinidine	Cyclophosphamide		Tin/zinc	
Silver	Diethylstilbestrol			
Sulfasalazine	Doxorubicin			
	Doxycycline			
	Fluorouracil			
	Heroin			
	Hormone-replacement therapy			
	Ketoconazole			
	Menthol			
	Methaqualone			
	Minocycline			
	Phenolphthalein			
	Propranolol			
	Smoking			
	Zidovudine			

Further Reading

Scully C, Bagan JV. Adverse drug reactions. Crit Rev Oral Biol Med 2004; 15(4):

2 VIRAL INFECTIONS

- hand, foot and mouth disease (vesicular stomatitis with exanthem)
- herpangina
- herpes simplex infections
- herpes varicella-zoster (chickenpox)
- human papillomavirus infections
- infectious mononucleosis (Paul–Bunnell positive glandular fever)
- measles (rubeola)
- molluscum contagiosum
- mumps
- orf (ecthyma contagiosum)
- parvovirus infection
- rubella (German measles)
- uvulitis
- vaccinia.

HAND, FOOT AND MOUTH DISEASE *(vesicular stomatitis with exanthem)*

This Coxsackie or other enterovirus infection produces small painful vesicles surrounded by an inflammatory halo especially on the dorsum and lateral aspects of the fingers and toes (**Figs 2.1, 2.2**). The infection has an incubation period of up to a week. Coxsackievirus A16 is usually implicated, but A5, A7, A9 and A10 or viruses of the B9 group or other enteroviruses may be responsible.

A rash is not always present or may affect more proximal parts of the limbs or buttocks. The vesicles usually heal spontaneously in about 1 week. Reports of other systemic manifestations such as encephalitis are very rare, except in enterovirus 71 infection.

The oral lesions in this condition are non-specific, usually affecting the tongue or buccal mucosa. Ulcers are shallow, painful and very small, surrounded by an inflammatory halo (**Fig. 2.3**).

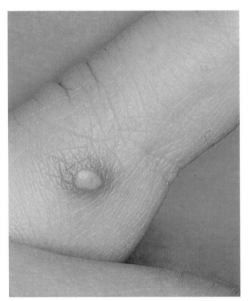

2.1

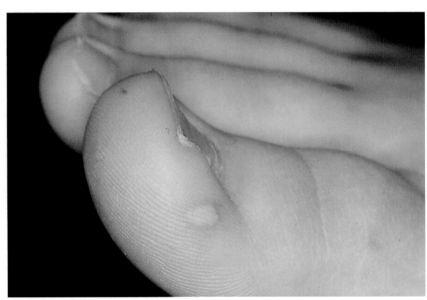

2.2

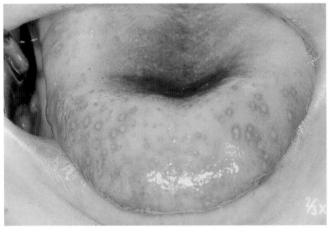

2.3

HERPANGINA

Herpangina, a Coxsackie or enterovirus infection, presents with fever, malaise, headache and a sore throat caused by an ulcerating vesicular eruption in the oropharynx (**Fig. 2.4**).

The vesicles rupture to leave painful, shallow, round ulcers, mainly on the fauces and soft palate (**Fig. 2.5**). Ulcers heal spontaneously in 7–10 days. Herpangina is usually caused by Coxsackieviruses A1–A6, A8, A10, A12 or A22, but similar syndromes can be caused by other viruses, especially Coxsackie B and echoviruses. Most herpangina is seen in schoolchildren and their contacts.

Herpangina Zahorsky, caused by Coxsackievirus A4, particularly affects infants and small children. Lesions resembling Koplik's spots may be seen in echovirus 9 infections, along with a rash and aseptic meningitis. Faucial ulcers, sometimes with a rash and aseptic meningitis, are characteristics of echovirus 16 infection.

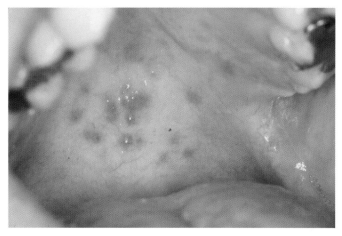

2.4

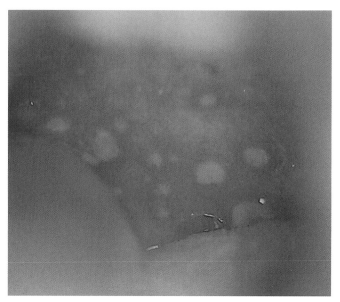

2.5

HERPES SIMPLEX INFECTIONS

After an incubation period of approximately 6–7 days, gingival oedema, erythema and ulceration (**Figs 2.6–2.12**) are prominent features of primary infection with herpes simplex virus (HSV), usually caused by HSV-1. Widespread vesicles break down to leave pinpoint ulcers which enlarge and fuse to produce irregular painful oral ulcers.

Typically a childhood infection between ages 2–4 years, an increasing number of adults are now affected and HSV-2 is sometimes implicated in orofacial infection. HIV-1 can also cause ano-genital infection.

Affected patients, especially adults, can be severely ill, with malaise, fever and cervical lymph node enlargement. The tongue is often coated

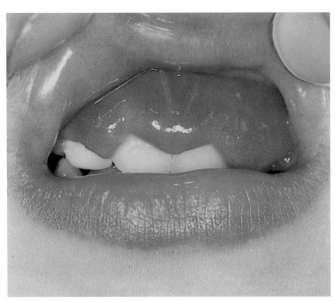

2.6

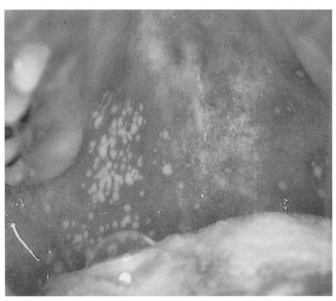

2.7

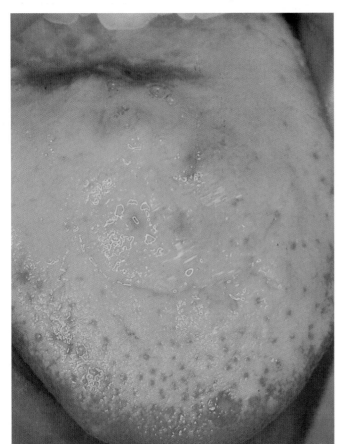

2.8

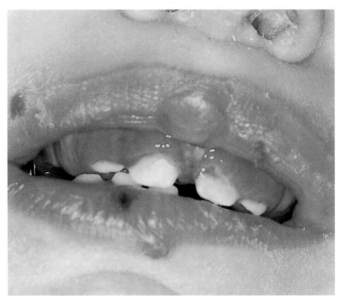

2.9

with oral hygiene difficult to maintain; there is halitosis and, rarely, acute ulcerative gingivitis follows. Additionally, the saliva is heavily infected with HSV which may cause lip and skin lesions (**Figs 2.10, 2.13**) and is a source for cross-infection.

Rare complications of HSV infection include encephalitis and mononeuropathies including Bell's palsy, and erythema multiforme.

Primary infection of the finger by HSV can cause a painful whitlow (**Fig. 2.13**). This is an occupational hazard for nonimmune dental, medical or paramedical personnel if they do not wear protective gloves, and may recur.

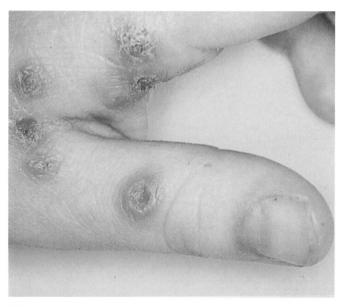

2.10

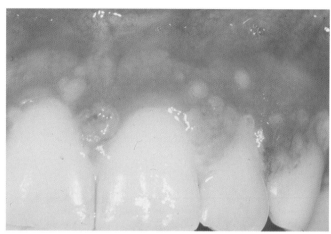

2.11

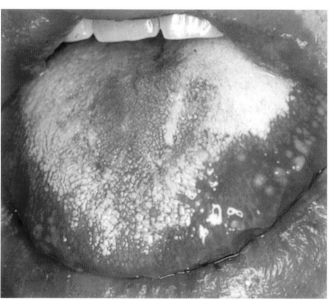

2.12

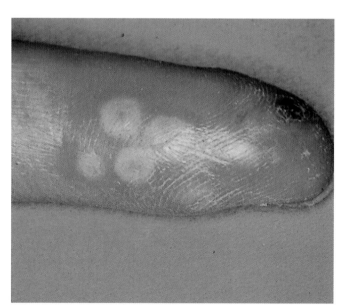

2.13

Recurrent herpes simplex infection

Reactivation of HSV latent in the trigeminal ganglion — for example, by fever, sunlight, trauma or immunosuppression — can produce herpes labialis (**Figs 2.14–2.20**). It presents as macules which rapidly become papular and vesicular, typically at the mucocutaneous junction of the lip. Lesions then become pustular, and scab and heal without scarring (see **Figs 2.18–2.20**).

Some 6–14% of the population have recurrent HSV infections. Any mucocutaneous site can be affected, including the anterior nares (**Figs 2.21–2.23**). At the commissure, HSV can mimic angular cheilitis (**Fig. 2.24**). Occasionally infection can recur at sites other than mucocutaneous junctions and can simulate zoster (**Fig. 2.25**).

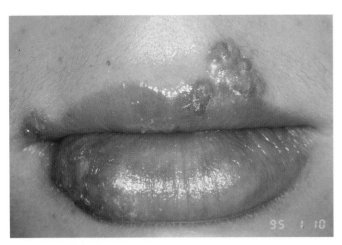

2.14

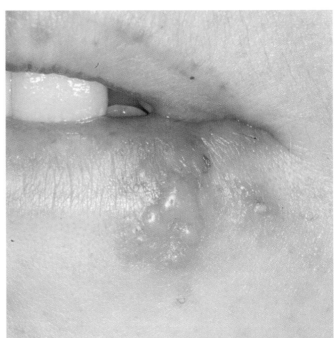

2.15

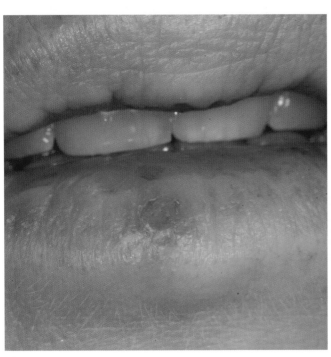

2.16

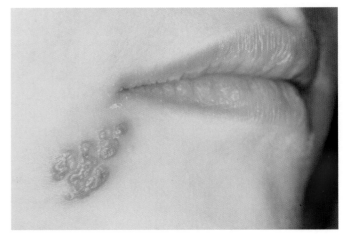

2.17

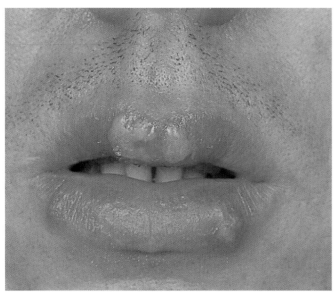

2.18

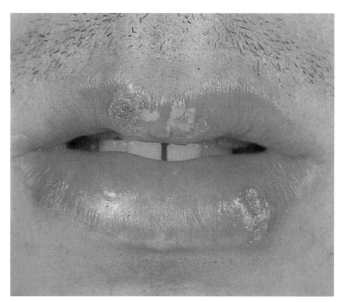

2.19

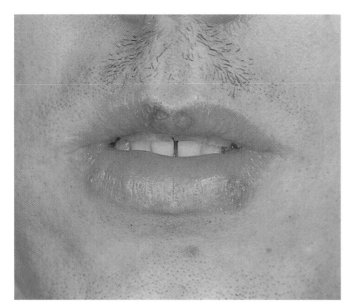

2.20

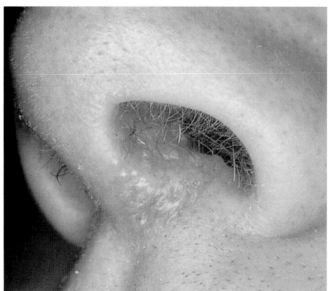

2.21

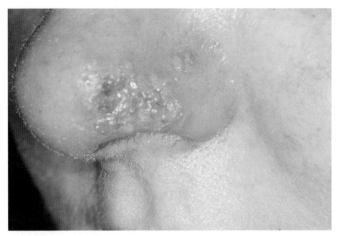

2.22

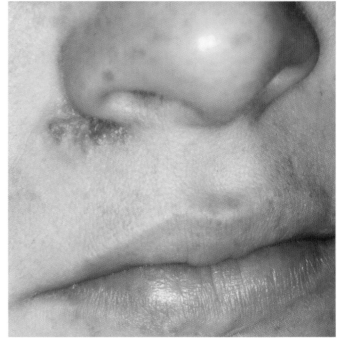

2.23

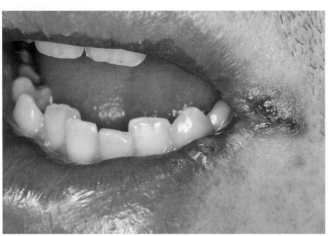

2.24

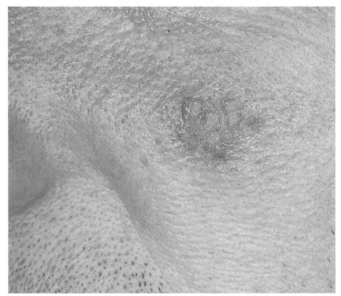

2.25

Intraoral infection may follow trauma (such as that from a local analgesic herpetic injection) or may be seen in immunocompromised persons.

The lesions of herpes labialis eventually heal after crusting. Patients with T-cell immune defects are predisposed to recurrent herpes (Fig. 2.26). Widespread lesions can affect debilitated patients, such as this man recovering from pneumonia (Fig. 2.27).

Haemorrhage into lesions produces a deceptive appearance in a leukaemic or other patient with thrombocytopenia (Fig. 2.28).

Impetigo can mimic or complicate herpes labialis (Figs 2.29–2.31).

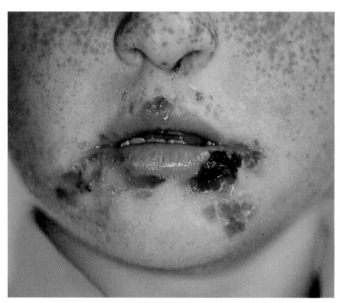

2.26

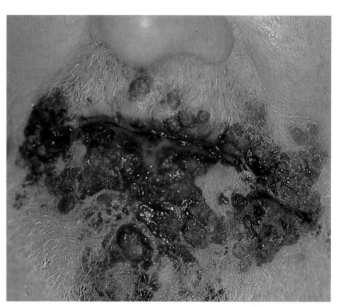

2.27

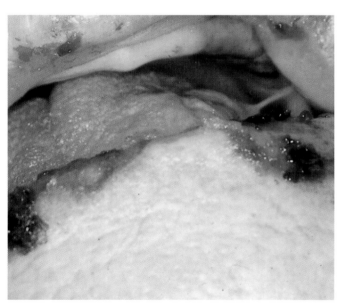

2.28

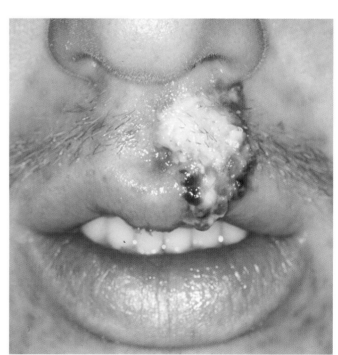

2.29

Eczema herpeticum

Eczema, other diseases of the skin, and the use of topical corticosteroids predispose to disseminated herpetic lesions (eczema herpeticum, Kaposi's varicelliform eruption; **Fig. 2.32**). Skin lesions in otherwise healthy patients are rare but a macular, vesicular or purpuric rash may be seen.

Recurrent intraoral herpes

Herpes simplex infection due to reactivation of latent HSV is rare intraorally, but may follow the trauma of a local anaesthetic injection (**Figs 2.33–2.35**) or may be seen in immunocompromised patients. Recurrent intraoral herpes in normal patients tends to affect the tongue, hard palate or gingiva and heals within 1–2 weeks.

Immunocompromised patients may develop chronic, often dendritic, ulcers from HSV reactivation. So-called 'geometric herpetic stomatitis' may be seen in HIV disease or leukaemia (**Fig. 2.36**). Clinical diagnosis tends to underestimate the frequency of these lesions.

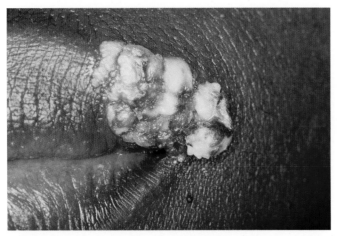

2.30

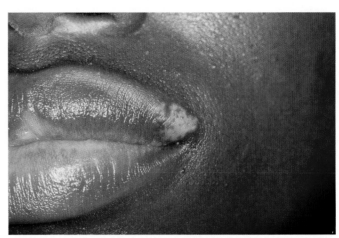

2.31

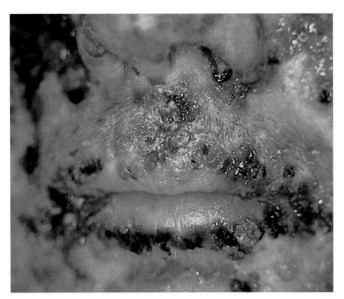

2.32

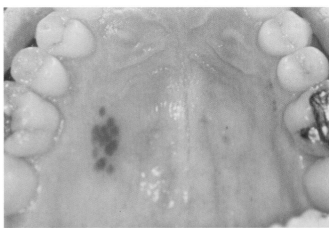

2.33

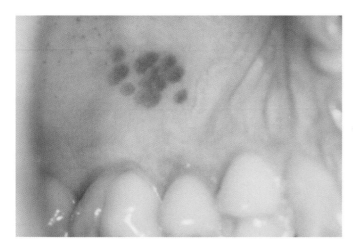

2.34

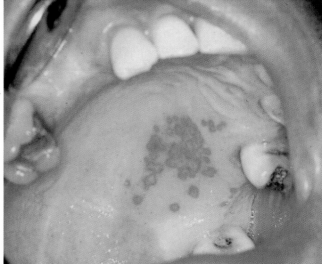

2.35

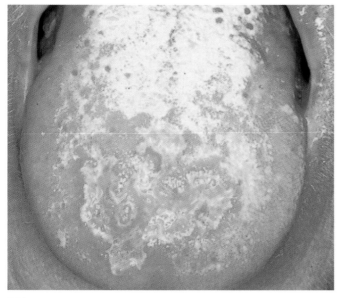

2.36

HERPES VARICELLA-ZOSTER
(chickenpox)

Varicella is a highly contagious infection caused by the varicella-zoster virus (VZV). After an incubation period of 2–3 weeks, a variably dense rash appears, concentrated mainly on the trunk, head and neck (**Fig. 2.37**). The typical rash goes through macular, papular, vesicular and pustular stages before crusting (**Fig. 2.38**). The rash crops in waves over 2–4 days, so that lesions at different stages are typically seen.

The oral mucosa is commonly involved but there may be isolated lesions only. Vesicles appear, especially in the palate, and then rupture (**Figs 2.39–2.43**). Ruptured oral vesicles produce painful round or ovoid ulcers with an inflammatory halo. Diagnosis is typically made on the basis of a widespread rash with oral ulceration.

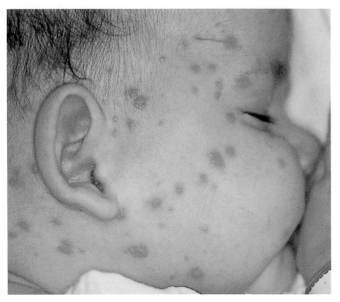

2.37

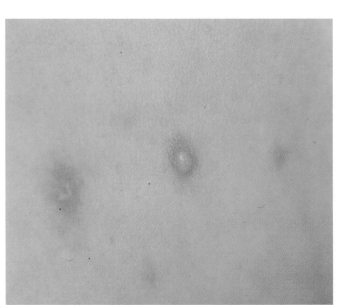

2.38

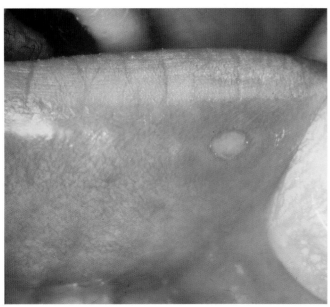

2.39

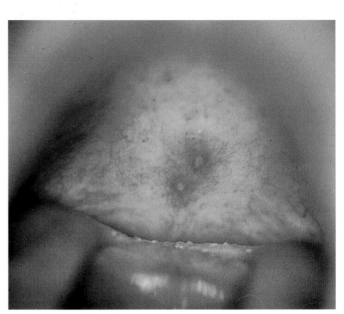

2.40

Herpes zoster *(shingles)*

Herpes zoster is caused by reactivation of VZV latent in dorsal root ganglia and, rarely, by reinfection. It has a bimodal distribution affecting a group of young adults, who appear perfectly healthy otherwise, and the elderly.

Zoster most typically affects the elderly and those with cellular immune defects, especially lymphomas or HIV infection, and causes pain and a rash restricted to a dermatome, usually thoracic or lumbar. Zoster affecting the trigeminal nerve may result in orofacial lesions (the mandibular division of the trigeminal nerve; **Figs 2.44–2.46**).

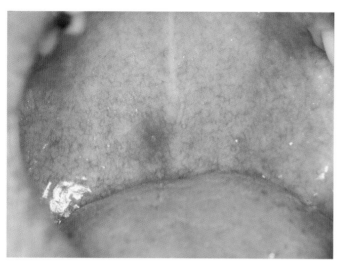

2.41

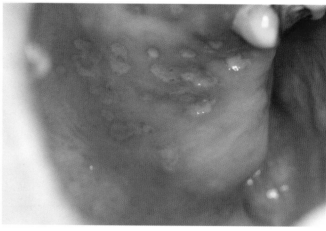

2.42

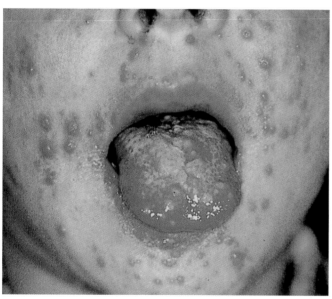

2.43

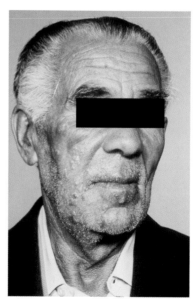

2.44

Mandibular and maxillary zoster may simulate toothache — the pain may precede the rash. Healing is usually uneventful but there may be scarring, bone necrosis, tooth loss or hypoplasia of developing teeth.

Zoster of the maxillary division of the trigeminal nerve causes a rash and periorbital oedema but the eye is not involved (**Fig. 2.47**). Ulceration affects the ipsilateral palate and vestibule mainly (**Fig. 2.48**). The rash of zoster resembles that of varicella and occasionally pocks are

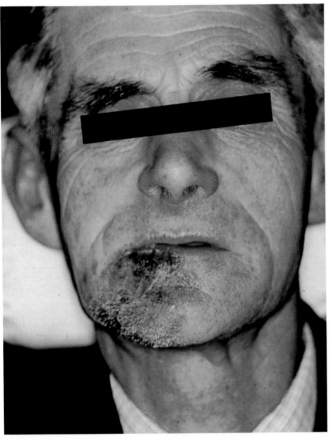

2.45

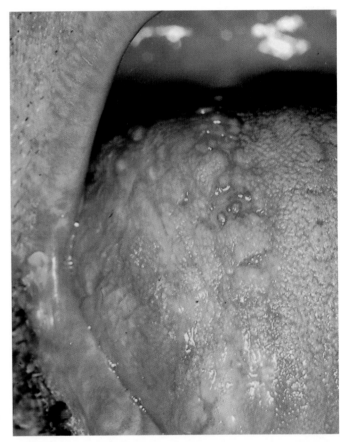

2.46

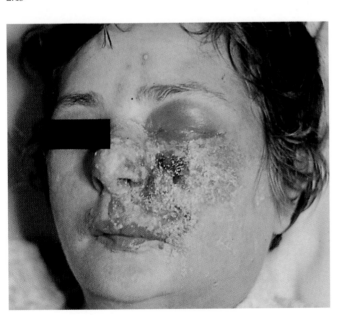

2.47

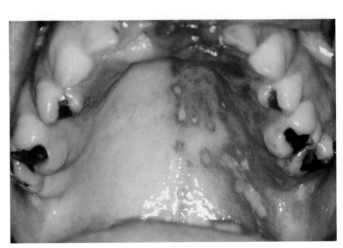

2.48

seen beyond the affected dermatome; note lesions on the forehead in **Fig. 2.47**. Occasionally, oral lesions appear in the absence of a rash.

Occasionally, zoster affects a branch of one of the trigeminal divisions. Zoster of the ophthalmic division of the trigeminal nerve (**Figs 2.49, 2.50**) threatens sight, with the possibility of corneal ulceration or panophthalmitis. Ophthalmic zoster also produces chemosis and

periorbital oedema which may become bilateral (**Fig. 2.50**). Involvement of the central nervous system is common when zoster affects cranial nerves, and meningeal signs and symptoms (headache, neck stiffness, vomiting — meningism) are frequent. Zoster more typically affects thoracic dermatomes or, occasionally, other dermatomes (**Figs 2.51–2.53**).

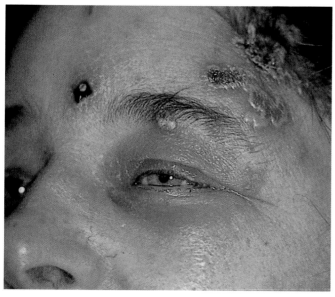

2.49

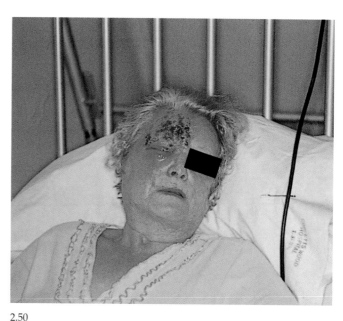

2.50

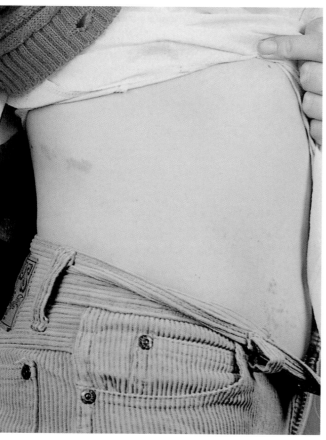

2.51

Occasionally, cervical dermatomes are affected (see **Fig. 2.52**).

There is an increased prevalence of zoster in persons with immuno-compromised cellular immunity, including those with HIV infection (see **Fig. 9.42**), malignancy and following bone-marrow transplantation. This patient, with Hodgkin's lymphoma, has sciatic zoster (see **Fig. 2.53**). Radiotherapy and chemotherapy also reactivate VZV.

Zoster may leave sequelae such as scarring (here, **Fig. 2.54**, from mandibular zoster and **Fig. 2.55** from ophthalmic zoster), sometimes with pigmentation or depigmentation, and post-herpetic neuralgia. Tissue destruction and severe post-herpetic neuralgia are more common in those who are immunocompromised. Infection of zoster lesions with *Staphylococcus aureus* can lead to a form of impetigo with delayed

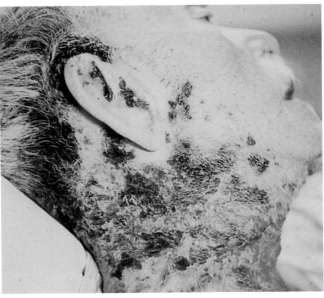

2.52

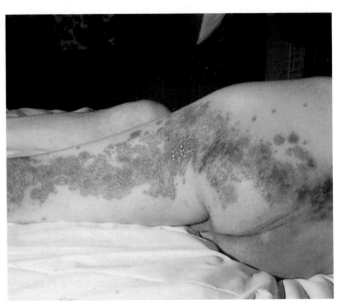

2.53

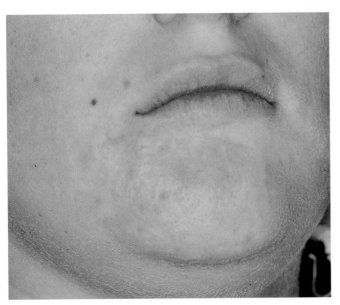

2.54

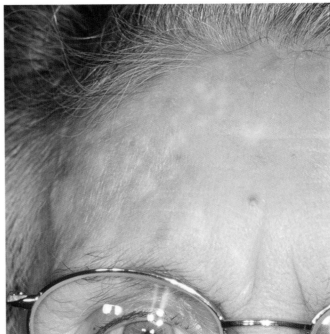

2.55

healing, greater scarring of the zoster lesions and dissemination of the bacterial lesions.

Ramsay Hunt syndrome

Although zoster almost invariably affects sensory nerves, motor nerves may be involved occasionally. In Ramsay Hunt syndrome, zoster of the geniculate ganglion of the facial nerve can cause ipsilateral lower motor neurone facial palsy (**Fig. 2.56**) with ipsilateral pharyngeal ulceration.

A rash may be seen in the external ear, in the distribution of a sensory branch of the facial nerve (**Fig. 2.57**).

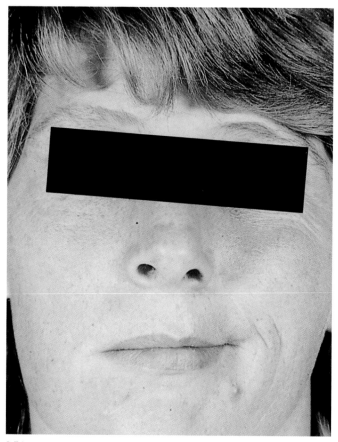

2.56

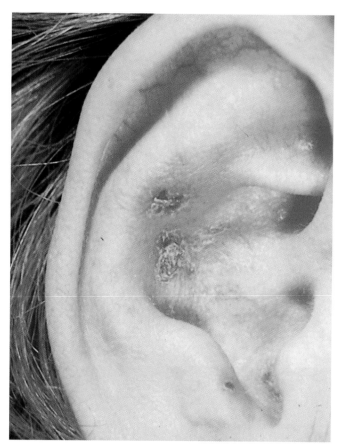

2.57

HUMAN PAPILLOMAVIRUS INFECTIONS

There are around 200 human papillomaviruses (HPV) described. HPV can cause various epithelial lesions, especially verruca vulgaris (common wart) (**Fig. 2.58**), papilloma, condyloma acuminatum (genital wart), and focal epithelial hyperplasia. HPV-16 and other types have been implicated in cervical, anogenital and oropharyngeal carcinoma.

Warts
Infection of the oral regions by contact spread can lead to warts, especially on the skin, lips or tongue (**Figs 2.59, 2.60**).

Papillomas
Papillomas are most common on the palate or gingiva. The cauliflower-like appearance is obvious but indistinguishable from a wart (**Figs 2.61–2.64**).

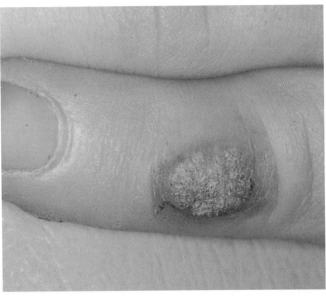

2.58

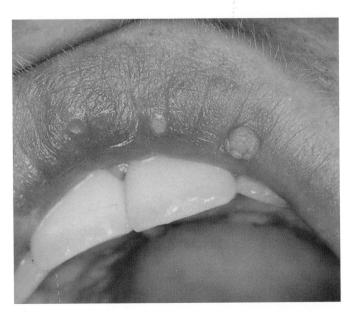

2.59

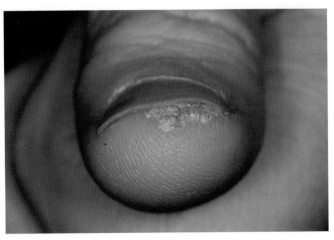

2.60

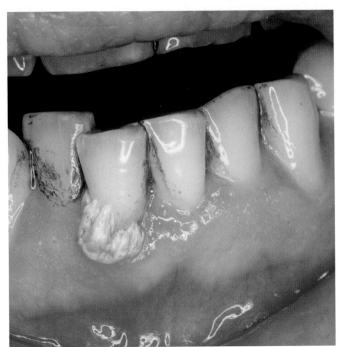

2.61

Condyloma acuminatum

Condyloma acuminatum (genital wart) is caused by HPV. It usually results from orogenital or oroanal contact and appears as a cauliflower-like lump, mainly in the anterior mouth (**Figs 2.65–2.67**). The lesions are increasingly common, especially in sexually active people and as a complication of HIV disease.

Focal epithelial hyperplasia

Focal epithelial hyperplasia (Heck's disease) is an HPV-13 or HPV-32 infection most frequent in Inuits and Native Americans but also reported in many other ethnic groups. Multiple painless, sessile, soft papules, generally whitish in colour, are found, usually in the buccal or lower labial mucosa (**Fig. 2.68**).

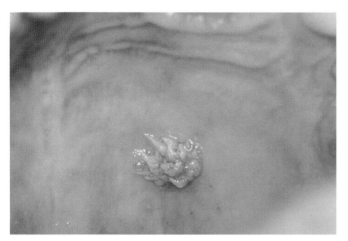

2.62

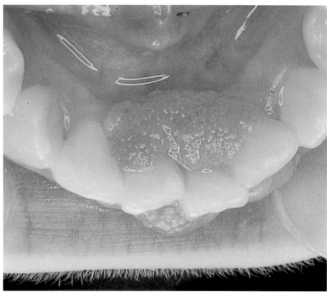

2.63

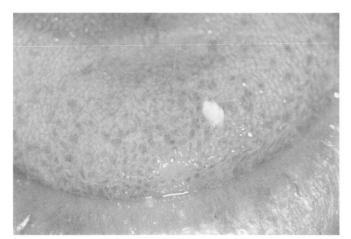

2.64

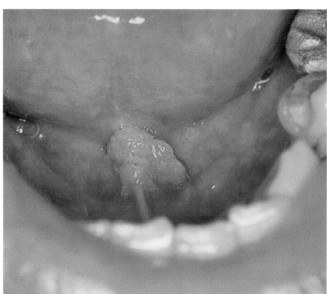

2.65

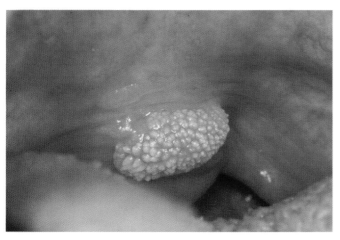

2.66

Proliferative verrucous leukoplakia

HPV are implicated in proliferative verrucous leukoplakia (PVL). This is a multifocal and progressive lesion of the oral mucosa, seen mainly in older females, and characterized by a high recurrence rate and high rate of transformation into verrucous or oral squamous cell carcinoma (**Figs 2.69, 2.70**).

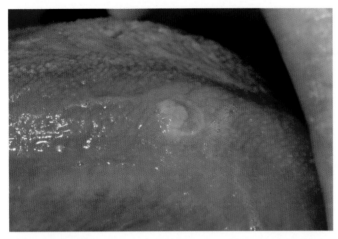

2.67

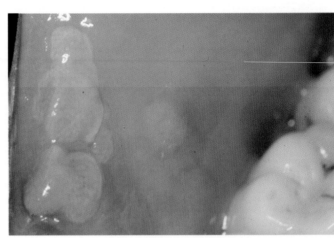

2.68

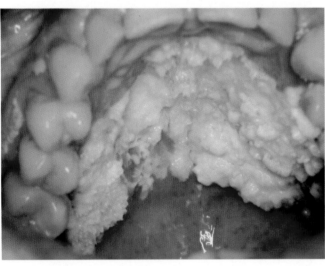

2.69

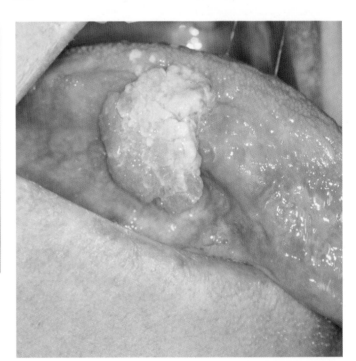

2.70

INFECTIOUS MONONUCLEOSIS *(Paul–Bunnell positive glandular fever)*

Infectious mononucleosis (IM) is caused by Epstein–Barr virus (EBV). More common in teenagers and young adults, the incubation of 30–50 days is followed by fever, sore throat and lymph node enlargement. Mouth ulcers (**Fig. 2.71**) may be seen together with faucial oedema and tonsillar exudate (**Fig. 2.72**: the white lesion on the soft palate is candidosis).

The faucial oedema and a thick yellow to white tonsillar exudate are typical of IM (**Fig. 2.73**) although diphtheria may also produce a tonsillar pseudomembrane. There can be severe dysphagia and on rare occasions the faucial oedema can obstruct the airway (**Fig. 2.74**).

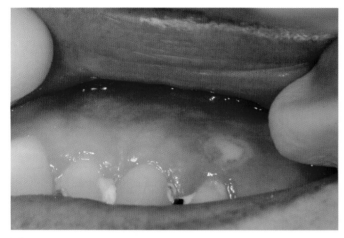

2.71

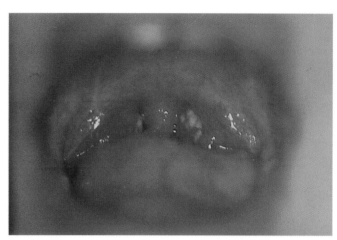

2.72

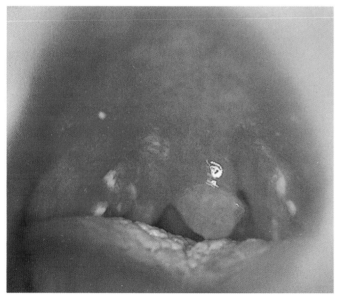

2.73

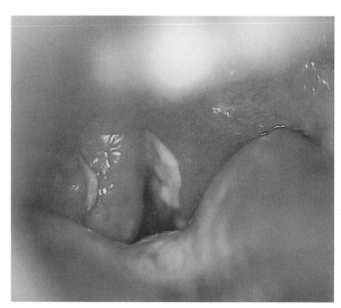

2.74

A glandular fever type of illness in young adults is still usually caused by IM. Generalized lymph node enlargement is present and the degree of cervical lymphadenopathy can be seen in **Fig. 2.75**. Palatal petechiae, especially at the junction of the hard and soft palate, are almost pathognomonic of IM, but can be seen in other viral infections such as HIV (**Fig. 2.76**) or rubella.

A rare presentation of IM is an isolated lower motor neurone facial palsy.

A feature that may suggest IM is the occurrence of a rash if the patient is given ampicillin or amoxicillin; this may also be seen in lymphoid leukaemias (**Fig. 2.77**). A few patients develop a maculopapular rash even if they are not taking synthetic penicillins. This rash is often morbilliform and does not represent penicillin allergy.

EBV may also cause persistent malaise and has associations with Duncan's disease (X-linked lymphoproliferative syndrome), hairy leukoplakia, Burkitt's lymphoma and lymphomas in immunocompromised persons, and other neoplasms.

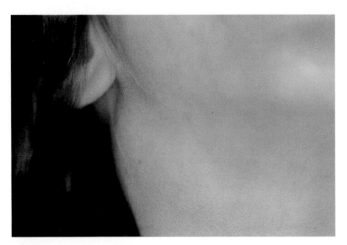

2.75

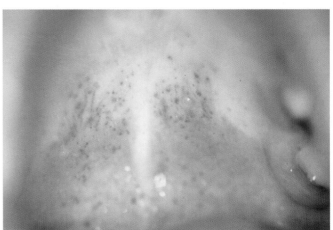

2.76

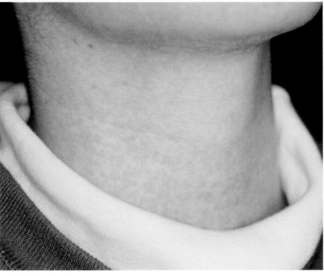

2.77

MEASLES *(rubeola)*

Measles is an acute contagious infection with a paramyxovirus. The incubation of 7–10 days is followed by fever, rhinitis, cough, conjunctivitis (coryza) and then a red maculopapular rash (**Fig. 2.78**). The rash appears initially on the forehead and behind the ears, and spreads over the whole body. It is less immediately obvious in a

dark-skinned patient (**Fig. 2.79**). Mucosal lesions include conjunctivitis (**Fig. 2.80**) and Koplik's spots: small, whitish, necrotic lesions, said to resemble grains of salt (**Fig. 2.81**). These spots are found in the buccal mucosa and occasionally in the conjunctiva or the genitalia. They precede the rash by 1–2 days and are pathognomonic.

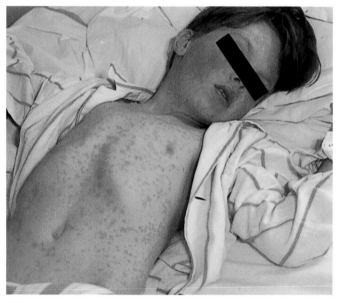

2.78

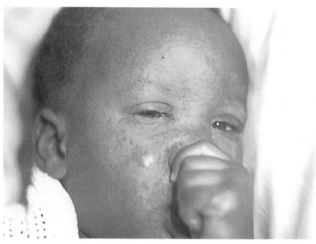

2.79

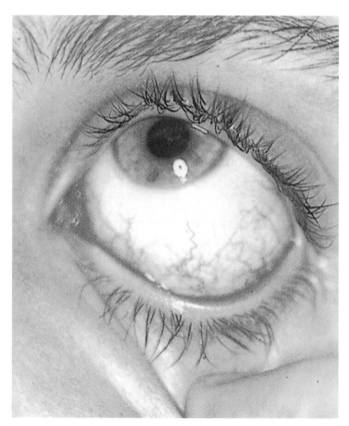

2.80

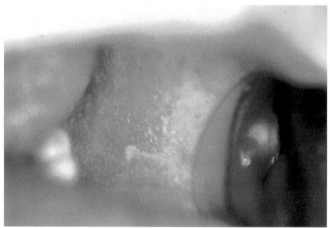

2.81

MOLLUSCUM CONTAGIOSUM

Molluscum contagiosum is a poxvirus infection producing characteristic umbilicated non-tender papules, typically on the skin of male children (**Figs 2.82–2.84**; see also **Fig. 9.53**). Oral lesions are rare.

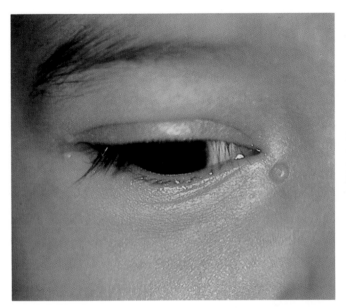

2.82

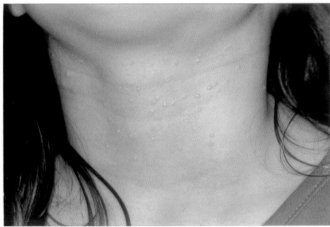

2.83

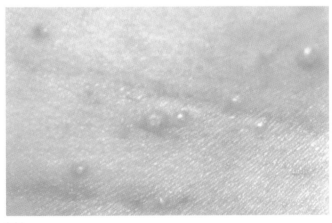

2.84

MUMPS

Mumps is an acute infection with the mumps virus, which predominantly affects the major salivary glands. The parotid glands are usually affected and there is tender swelling with trismus. This may be unilateral (**Fig. 2.85**) but is more frequently bilateral. The usual causal agent is a paramyxovirus but some Coxsackie-, echo-, and other viruses occasionally cause similar features.

The incubation period of 2–3 weeks is followed by fever, malaise and sialadenitis, which can affect not only the parotids but also the submandibular glands (**Fig. 2.86**). Pancreatitis, oophoritis and orchitis are less common features.

The most obvious intraoral feature of mumps is swelling and redness at the duct orifice of the affected gland (papillitis) (**Fig. 2.87**).

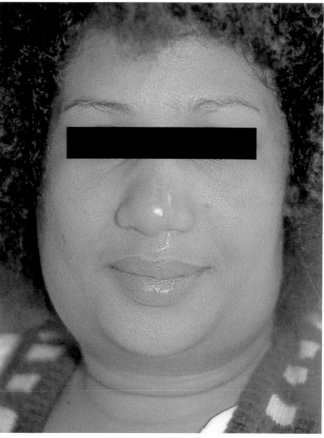

2.86

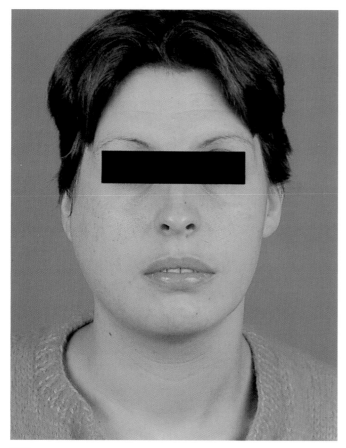

2.85

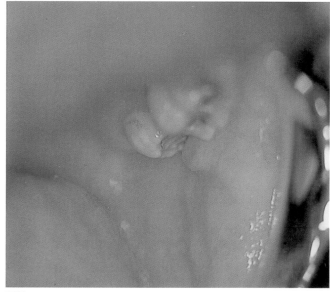

2.87

ORF *(ecthyma contagiosum)*

Orf is a parapoxvirus infection of sheep and goats that rarely affects those in contact with it. It starts as a small, firm, reddish papule which becomes umbilicated. Rare cases affect the lip (**Fig. 2.88**).

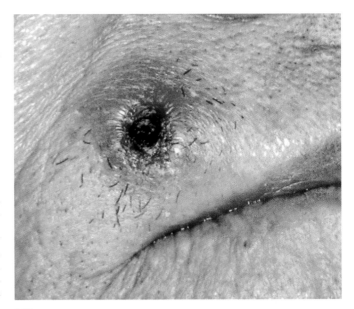

PARVOVIRUS INFECTION

Parvovirus is a DNA virus that may cause an acute febrile illness (fifth disease or erythema infectiosum), with a rash that produces a 'slapped cheek' appearance on the face (**Fig. 2.89**).

Pharyngitis, conjunctivitis, lymph node enlargement, splenomegaly and polyarthritis may occasionally be seen, especially in adults. The exanthem typically evolves into a reticular configuration (**Fig. 2.90**).

Parvovirus infection may occasionally precipitate aplastic crises, especially in those with sickle-cell anaemia. No oral features have been recorded.

2.88

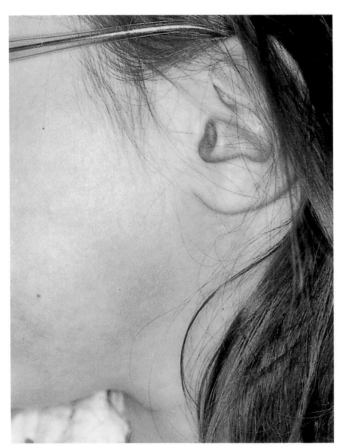

2.89

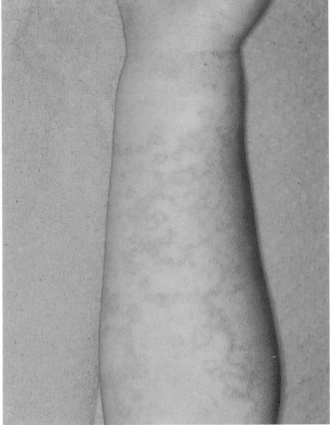

2.90

RUBELLA *(German measles)*

Rubella is a togavirus infection with an incubation period of 2–3 weeks, followed by mild fever, mild conjunctivitis, a diffuse maculopapular rash (**Fig. 2.91**) and lymphadenopathy. Some enteroviruses, especially echovirus type 9, may cause a similar rash. There are no specific oral manifestations but there may be oral petechiae, known as Forchheimer's spots.

Maternal infection during the first trimester of pregnancy may lead to congenital rubella, causing learning disability, deafness, blindness and cardiac defects, depending on the timing of the intrauterine infection.

Congenital rubella may cause hypoplasia of the deciduous dentition (**Fig. 2.92**). Similar defects may be found in other intrauterine infections, such as toxoplasmosis, cytomegalovirus, herpes simplex and Coxsackie B.

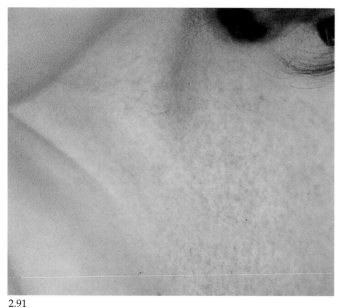

2.91

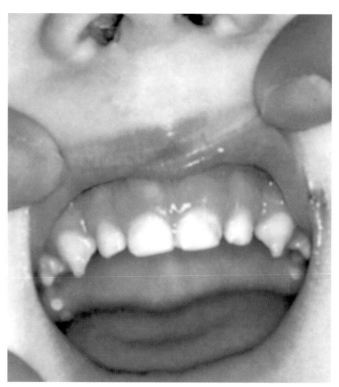

2.92

UVULITIS

Uvulitis is a rare, potentially serious, infection. *Haemophilus influenzae* type b, may cause uvulitis in isolation or is associated with epiglottitis and/or bacteraemia. Group A streptococci may also cause uvulitis. The uvula is often more oedematous than shown here (**Fig. 2.93**) and the airway may be threatened. There may be palatal petechiae.

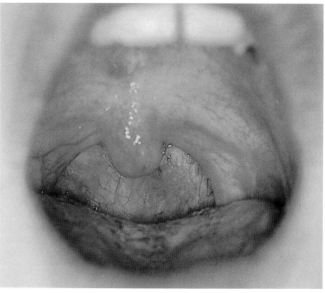

2.93

VACCINIA

Autoinoculation of vaccinia virus from a vaccination site can produce single or multiple vaccinial lesions, with a central scab and pronounced erythema and oedema (**Fig. 2.94**). The vaccination site is shown in **Figure 2.95**.

Occasionally, in young children especially, vaccinial lesions were disseminated widely by autoinoculation. Vaccination is no longer necessary since smallpox has been eradicated but is being considered in view of the potential for biological warfare.

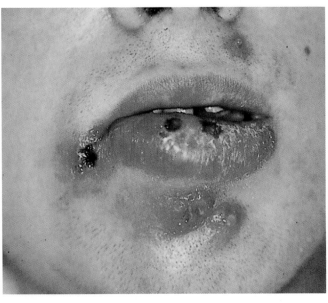

2.94

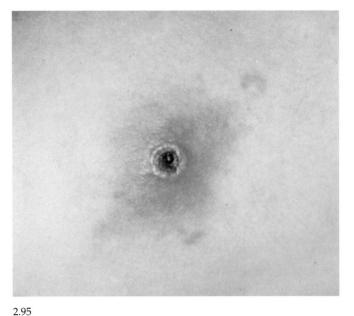

2.95

FURTHER READING

Anderson KM, Perez-Montiel D, Miles L, Allen CM, Nuovo GJ. The histologic differentiation of oral condyloma acuminatum from its mimics. Oral Surg Oral Med Oral Pathol Oral Radiol Endod 2003; 96: 420–8.

Bagg J. Common infectious diseases. Dent Clin North Am 1996; 40: 385–93.

Beyari MM, Hodgson TA, Cook RD, et al. Multiple human herpesvirus-8 infection. J Infect Dis 2003; 188: 678–89.

Bez C, Lodi G, Scully C, Porter SR. Genoprevalence of TT virus among clinical and auxiliary UK dental health care workers: a pilot study. Br Dent J 2000; 189: 554–5.

Blevins JY. Primary herpetic gingivostomatitis in young children. Pediatr Nurs 2003; 29: 199–202.

Cook RD, Hodgson TA, Waugh AC, et al. Mixed patterns of transmission of human herpesvirus-8 (Kaposi's sarcoma-associated herpesvirus) in Malawian families. J Gen Virol 2002; 83: 1613–19.

Di Alberti L, Ngui SL, Porter SR, et al. Presence of human herpesvirus-8 variants in oral tissues of HIV-infected persons. J Infect Dis 1997; 175: 703–7.

Di Alberti L, Piattelli A, Artese L, et al. Human herpes virus 8 variants in sarcoid tissue. Lancet 1997; 350: 1655–61.

Di Alberti L, Porter SR, Speight PM, et al. Detection of human herpesvirus-8 DNA in oral ulcer tissues of HIV-infected individuals. Oral Dis 1997; 3: S133–4.

Eksborg S, Pal N, Kalin M, Palm C, Soderhall S. Pharmacokinetics of acyclovir in immunocompromised children with leukopenia and mucositis after chemotherapy: can intravenous acyclovir be substituted by oral valacyclovir? Med Pediatr Oncol 2002; 38: 240–6.

Femiano F, Gombos S, Scully C. Recurrent herpes labialis; efficacy of topical therapy with penciclovir compared with acyclovir (aciclovir). Oral Diseases 2001; 7: 31–2.

Holmstrup P, Poulsen AH, Andersen L, Skuldbol T, Fiehn NE. Oral infections and systemic diseases. Dent Clin North Am 2003; 47: 575–98.

Hooi PS, Chua BH, Lee CS, Lam SK, Chua KB. Hand, foot and mouth disease: University Malaya Medical Centre experience. Med J Malaysia 2002; 57: 88–91.

Kojima A, Maeda H, Kurahashi N, et al. Human papillomaviruses in the normal oral cavity of children in Japan. Oral Oncol 2003; 39: 821–8.

Laskaris G. Oral manifestations of infectious diseases. Dent Clin N Amer 1996; 40: 395–423.

Leao JC, Porter S, Scully C. Human herpesvirus 8 and oral health care: an update. Oral Surg Oral Med Oral Pathol Oral Radiol Endod 2000; 90: 694–704.

Leao JC, Caterino-De-Araujo A, Porter SR, Scully C. Human herpesvirus 8 (HHV-8) and the etiopathogenesis of Kaposi's sarcoma. Rev Hosp Clin Fac Med Sao Paulo 2002; 57: 175–86.

Lodi G, Porter SR, Scully C, Teo CG. Prevalence of HCV-infection in healthcare workers in a UK dental hospital. Br Dent J 1997; 183: 329–332.

Nomura Y, Kitteringham N, Shiba K, Goseki M, Kimura A, Mineshita S. Use of the highly sensitive PCR method to detect the Herpes simplex virus type 1 genome and its expression in samples from Behcet disease patients. J Med Dent Sci 1998; 45: 51–8.

Phelan JA. Viruses and neoplastic growth. Dent Clin North Am 2003; 47(3): 533–43.

Porter SR, Di Alberti L, Kumar N. Human herpes virus 8 (Kaposi's sarcoma herpesvirus). Oral Oncol 1998; 34: 5–14.

Scott LA, Stone MS. Viral exanthems. Dermatol Online J 2003; 9(3): 4.

Scully C. New aspects of oral viral diseases. Current Topics in Pathology, 90. Berlin: Springer Verlag, 1996, pp. 30–96.

Slots J, Sabeti M, Simon JH. Herpesviruses in periapical pathosis: an etiopathogenic relationship? Oral Surg Oral Med Oral Pathol Oral Radiol Endod 2003; 96: 327–31.

Walling DM, Flaitz CM, Nichols CM. Epstein–Barr virus replication in oral hairy leukoplakia: response, persistence, and resistance to treatment with valacyclovir. J Infect Dis 2003; 188: 883–90.

Whitley RJ. Herpes simplex virus in children. Curr Treat Options Neurol 2002; 4: 231–7.

Whitley RJ. Herpes simplex virus infection. Semin Pediatr Infect Dis 2002; 13: 6–11.

3 BACTERIAL INFECTIONS

- actinomycosis
- acute necrotizing ulcerative gingivitis
- anthrax
- cancrum oris (noma)
- cat-scratch disease
- epithelioid angiomatosis
- leprosy
- Reiter's syndrome
- syphilis
- tuberculosis
- yaws.

ACTINOMYCOSIS

Actinomyces israelii is a common oral commensal but rarely causes disease. Trauma, such as jaw fracture or tooth extraction, appears to initiate infection, which usually presents on the skin of the upper neck, typically just below or over the angle of the mandible (**Figs 3.1, 3.2**). The lesion appears as a purplish firm swelling that enlarges and may eventually discharge through multiple sinuses, although this classical presentation is now rare. The discharge may contain colonies of actinomyces, resembling sulphur granules (**Fig. 3.3**). Rare cases affect bone or salivary glands. Cervicofacial actinomycosis is more common than thoracic or abdominal actinomycosis.

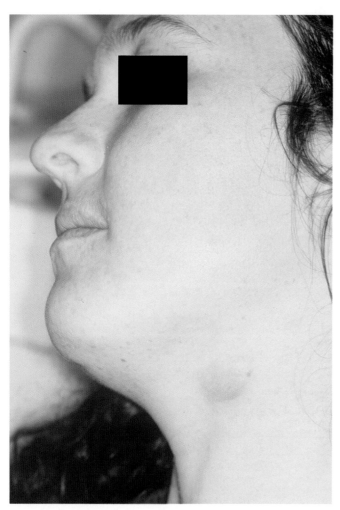

3.1

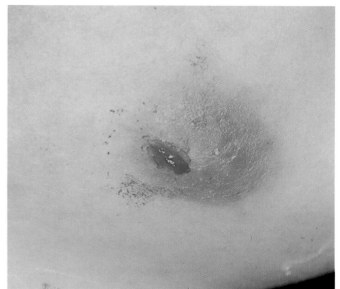

3.2

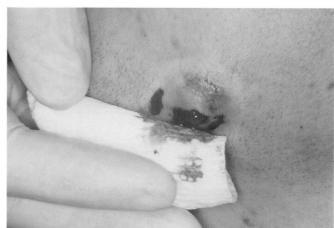

3.3

ACUTE NECROTIZING ULCERATIVE GINGIVITIS *(Vincent's disease)*

Chiefly affecting young adults, acute necrotizing ulcerative gingivitis (ANUG; acute necrotizing gingivitis, ANG; acute ulcerative gingivitis, AUG) is associated with proliferation of *Borrelia vincentii*, fusiform bacilli and other anaerobes. Ulceration of the interdental papillae is the typical feature of this condition (**Fig. 3.4**) which is predisposed by smoking, respiratory infections, poor oral hygiene and immune defects. HIV infection is a recognized predisposing factor in some patients (see **Fig. 3.5 and page 212**).

Painful gingival ulceration occasionally spreads from the papillae to the gingival margins (**Figs 3.6, 3.7**) with sialorrhoea, halitosis and pronounced tendency to gingival bleeding. The gingival bleeding can be profuse and the patient may have malaise, low fever and regional lymph node enlargement. Occasionally patients have primary herpetic stomatitis complicated by ANUG (**Fig. 3.8**; note ulcer in upper vestibule).

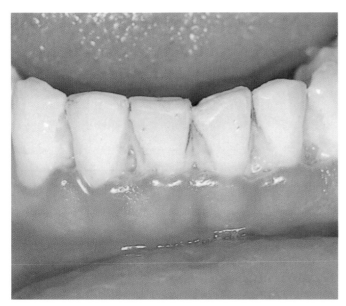

3.4

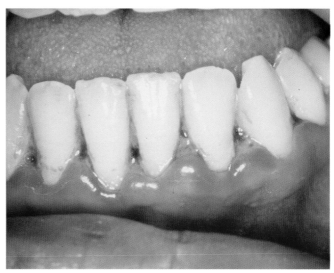

3.5

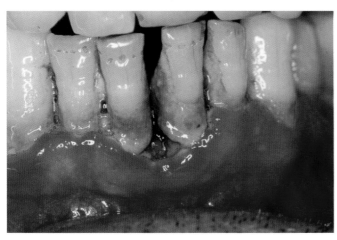

3.6

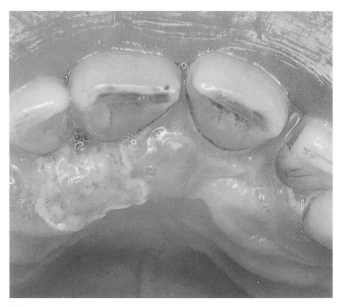

3.7

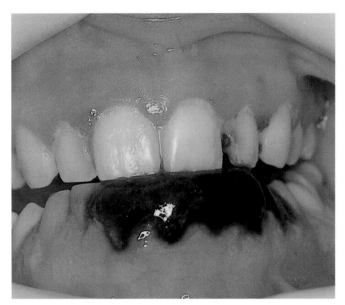

3.8

ANTHRAX

Cutaneous anthrax, a rare infection in workers with cowhides, and caused by *Bacillus anthracis*, presents as a black eschar at the site of inoculation (malignant pustule) (**Fig. 3.9**).

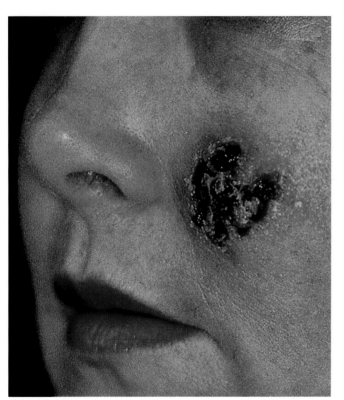

3.9

CANCRUM ORIS *(noma)*

Although usually a trivial illness in healthy persons, ANUG in patients who are malnourished, debilitated, infected with measles, or immunocompromised may extend onto the oral mucosa and skin with gangrenous necrosis (cancrum oris, noma) (**Fig. 3.10**). Anaerobes, particularly Bacteroides (Porphyromonas) species, have been implicated, and the condition is especially seen in malnourished patients from the developing world. Phylotypes unique to noma infections in Africa include those in the genera Eubacterium, Flavobacterium, Kocuria, Microbacterium, and Porphyromonas and the related *Streptococcus salivarius* and genera Sphingomonas and Treponemes.

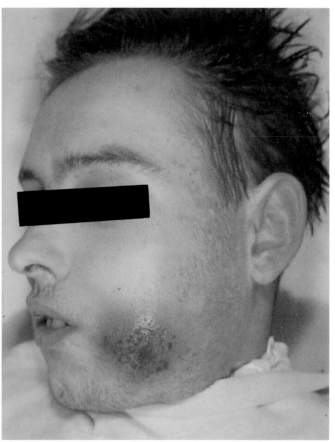

3.10

CAT-SCRATCH DISEASE

Cat-scratch disease is caused by infection with *Bartonella*, usually *B. (Rochilamea) henselae* or *B. quintana*, and has been documented from both immunocompetent and HIV-infected individuals. In immunocompetent individuals cat-scratch disease (**Figs 3.11, 3.12**), bacillary (epithelioid) angiomatosis, bacillary splenitis, bacteraemia and endocarditis may result. In immunocompromised individuals, *B. henselae* can cause bacillary angiomatosis, peliosis hepatitis and bacteraemia. *B. claridgeiae* may also be responsible for human cat-scratch disease.

EPITHELIOID ANGIOMATOSIS

In immunocompromised individuals, *B. henselae* can cause bacillary angiomatosis which clinically and histologically can mimic Kaposi's sarcoma (**Fig. 3.13**).

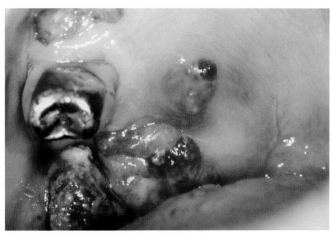

3.13

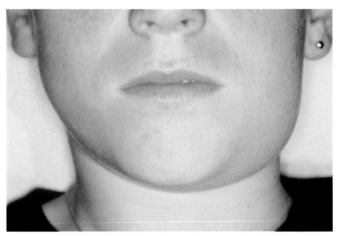

3.11

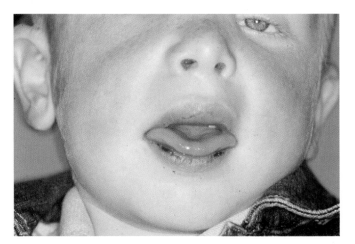

3.12

LEPROSY

Lepromatous leprosy, caused by *Mycobacterium leprae*, can produce widespread lesions, sometimes involving the mouth. Nodules can involve the lips or gingiva and elsewhere (**Figs 3.14–3.16**). The palate may necrose. The classic neural form of leprosy causes thickening of the greater auricular nerve and there may be cranial nerve lesions.

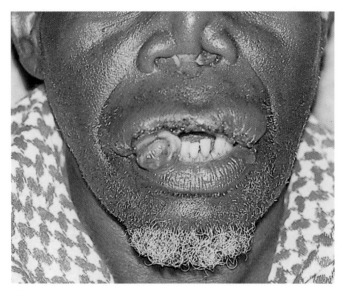

3.14

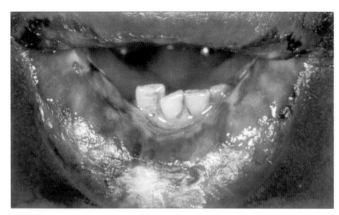

3.15

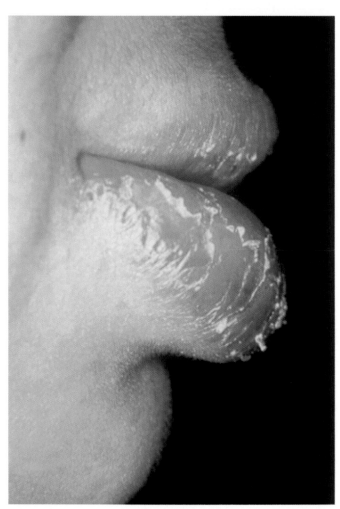

3.16

REITER'S SYNDROME

Reiter's syndrome is a disease predominantly of young males and may follow gonorrhoea, chlamydial or infection with HIV or enteric infection with *Salmonella, Shigella* or *Yersinia*. Features include urethritis, uveitis or conjunctivitis, polyarthritis, and macular or vesicular lesions on the palms and soles (keratoderma blenorrhagica). Mucocutaneous lesions are found in up to half the patients but are typically painless initially. Red lesions, sometimes with a whitish border or superficial painful erosions in the mouth resembling erythema migrans (**Figs 3.17, 3.18**) may be seen. Rarely, the temporomandibular joint is involved in the polyarthritis. Facial palsy may also be seen on rare occasions. Urethritis (**Fig. 3.19**) may follow mouth lesions and there may be circinate balanitis.

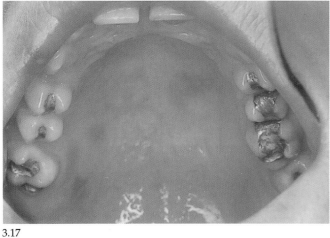

3.17

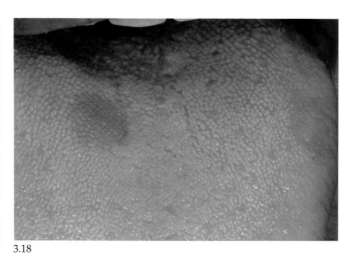

3.18

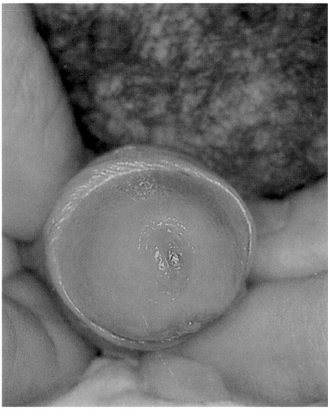

3.19

SYPHILIS

Syphilis is a sexually transmitted disease caused by *Treponema pallidum*.

Primary syphilis

The incubation period of acquired syphilis is 10–90 days and the primary lesion (chancre) is usually seen in the anogenital region (**Figs 3.20–3.24**). Oral chancres (hard or Hunterian chancre) begin as a papule which becomes a painless lump then a hard-based ulcer with regional lymph node enlargement. The chancre, which is usually on the lip, tongue or palate, heals in a few weeks but the patient remains infected and infectious.

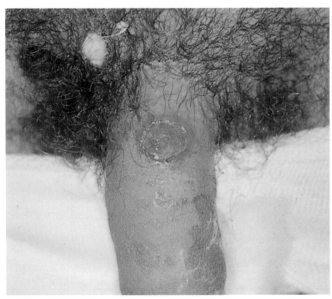

3.20

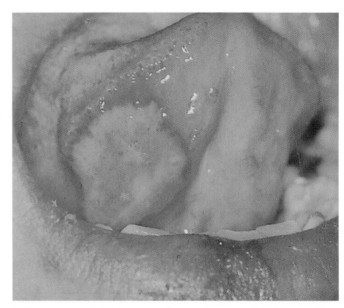

3.21

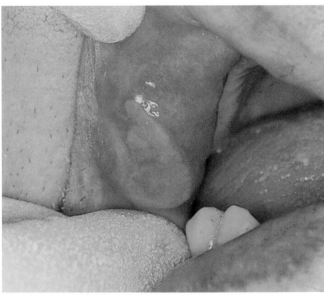

3.22

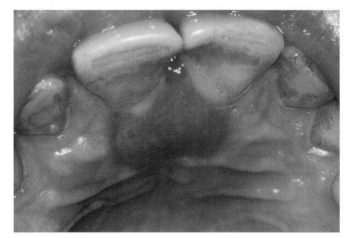

3.23

Occasionally, chancres appear on the breast, nose or other extragenital sites (**Fig. 3.25**).

Secondary syphilis

Some 6–8 weeks after primary infection, the patient develops nonspecific general symptoms, such as fever and malaise, with generalized lymph node enlargement. Rashes are common — typically a macular rash on the palms and soles — but are extremely variable. Papular rashes (papular syphilides) and maculopapular rashes may be seen. Flat, painless, oval or round patches (mucous patches; **Fig. 3.26**) or ulcers (snailtrack ulcers; **Fig. 3.27**) may appear in the mouth or on the genital mucosae. Atypical lesions may be seen in HIV disease (lues maligna).

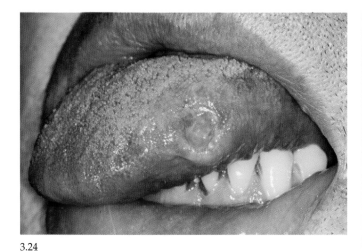

3.24

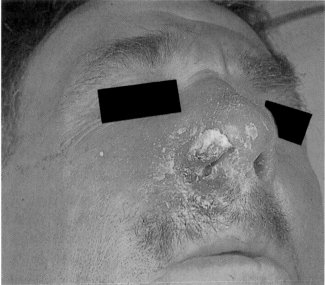

3.25

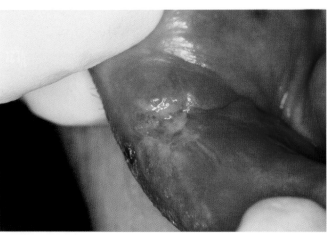

3.26

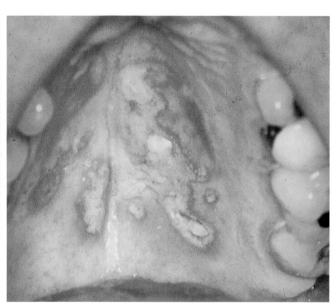

3.27

Lesions at the commissure (split papules; **Fig. 3.28**) or condyloma lata are not uncommon in secondary syphilis. Oral lesions are highly infectious.

Tertiary syphilis

Tertiary or late syphilis appears 4–8 years after infection and may cause mucocutaneous, cardiovascular and/or neurological disease (involvement of the cardiovascular or nervous system has been called quaternary syphilis). Meningovascular syphilis, general paresis and tabes dorsalis are the main syndromes of neurosyphilis. Bilateral ptosis (**Fig. 3.29**) causes the typical compensatory wrinkled brow.

Another feature of tertiary syphilis is a gumma, a painless nodule that undergoes necrosis, forming a punched-out ulcer that eventually heals with scarring. The site of predilection in the mouth is the hard palate but lesions may affect the tongue or other sites (**Fig. 3.30**). Any organ may be affected. Atrophy of the papillae of the dorsum of the tongue produces, with endarteritis, an atrophic glossitis which leads to leukoplakia with a high malignant potential (**Fig. 3.31**).

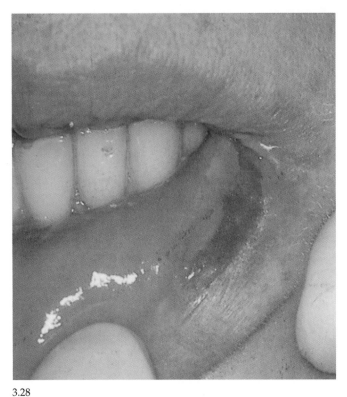

3.28

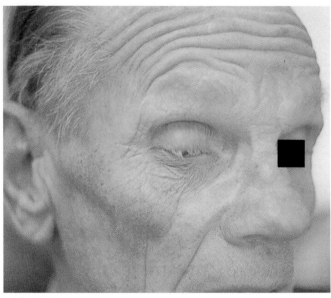

3.29

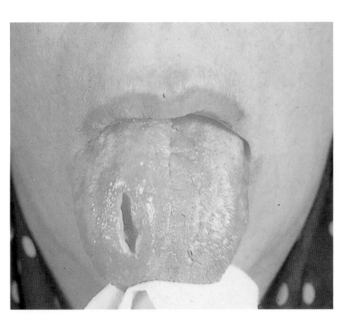

3.30

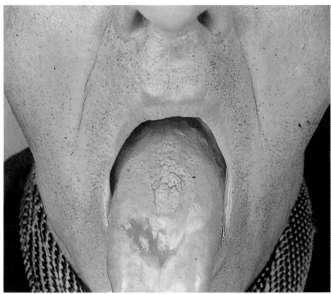

3.31

Syphilitic osteitis is a rare complication of this stage of the disease (**Fig. 3.32**).

Congenital syphilis

Congenital syphilis is rare. *Treponema pallidum*, the causal bacterium of this sexually transmitted disease, crosses the placenta only after the fifth month and can then produce dental defects, typically Hutchinson's incisors (**Fig. 3.33**). The teeth have a barrel shape, often with a notched incisal edge. The molars may be hypoplastic (Moon's molars or mulberry molars; **Figs 3.34, 3.35**). Dysplastic permanent incisors, along with nerve deafness and interstitial keratitis, are combined in Hutchinson's triad (**Fig. 3.36**).

Other stigmata include scarring at the commissures (rhagades or Parrot's furrows), high-arched palate and a saddle-shaped nose (**Fig. 3.37**). Frontal and parietal bossing (nodular focal osteoperiostitis of the frontal and parietal bones called Parrot's nodes) may be seen, and learning disability is common (**Fig. 3.38**).

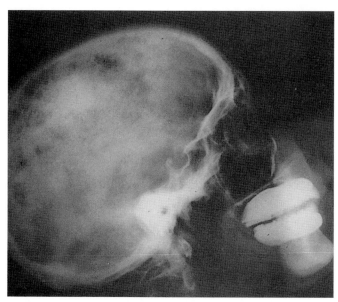

3.32

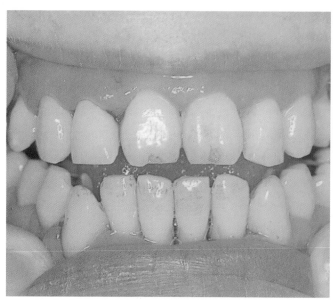

3.33

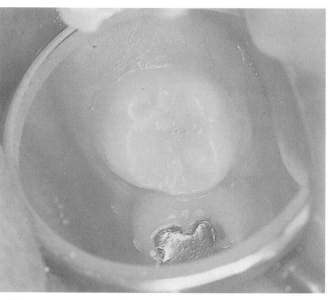

3.34

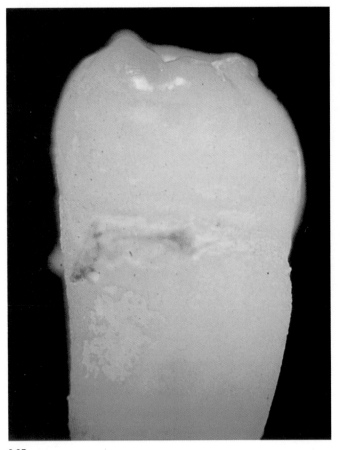

3.35

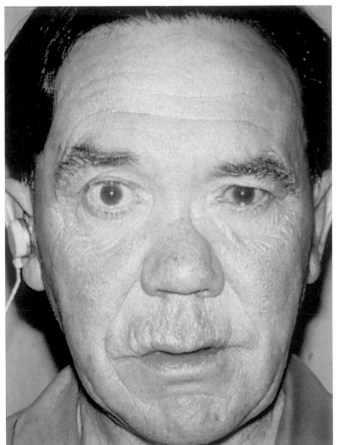

3.36

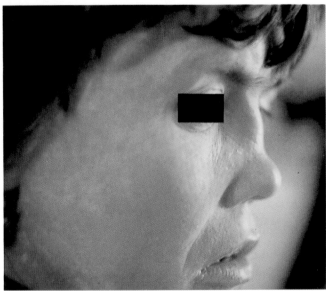

3.37

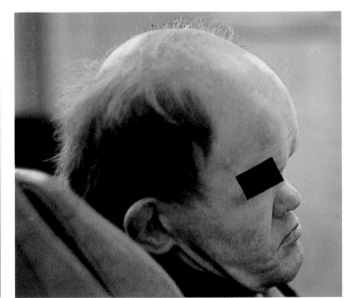

3.38

TUBERCULOSIS

Tuberculosis is usually caused by *Mycobacterium tuberculosis*, although atypical mycobacteria may be implicated, particularly in immunocompromised patients. *M. scrofulaceum, M. avium-intracellulare, M. kansasii* or others may be implicated. Oral lesions of tuberculosis are rare. The most common is a painless, irregular ulcer of the dorsum of the tongue, secondary to pulmonary tuberculosis (**Figs 3.39, 3.40**).

Typically the edge of the ulcer is undermined. Tuberculosis can be spread by the respiratory route.

The most common form of skin tuberculosis is lupus vulgaris. Lesions appear most frequently on the head and neck (**Fig. 3.41**), rarely intraorally. Lupus vulgaris begins as multiple red lesions, from their appearance called 'apple-jelly nodules'. The lesions ulcerate and scar (**Fig. 3.42**).

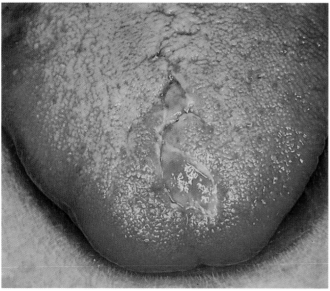

3.39

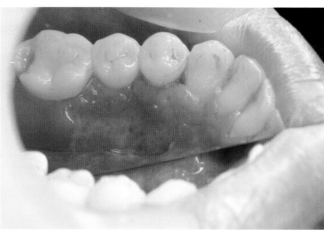

3.40

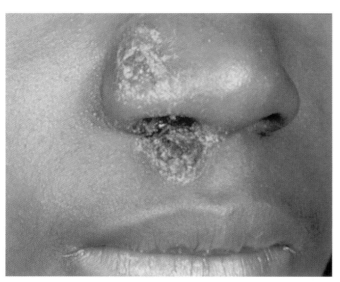

3.41

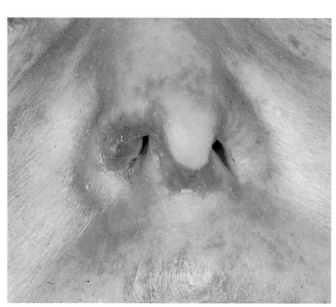

3.42

Tuberculous cervical lymphadenitis (**Fig. 3.43**) is uncommon but may be seen particularly in Asian or African patients and usually caused by *Mycobacterium tuberculosis* or *M. bovis*. The site of entry of the organism is usually the tonsils and, in some cases, *M. scrofulaceum, M. avium-intracellulare* or *M. kansasii* may be implicated. Tuberculous

lymphadenitis caseates and discharges through multiple fistulae (scrofula), with scars on healing (**Fig. 3.44**).

Haematogenous spread of tuberculosis is usually to the vertebrae or long bones, rarely to the jaw (**Fig. 3.45**).

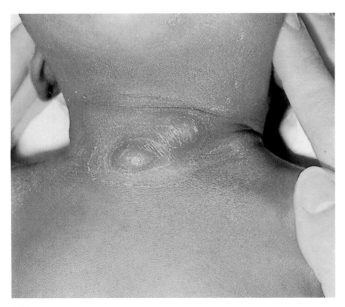

3.43

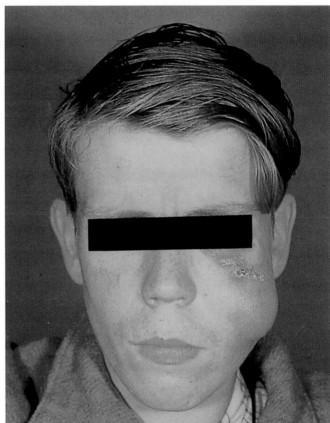

3.45

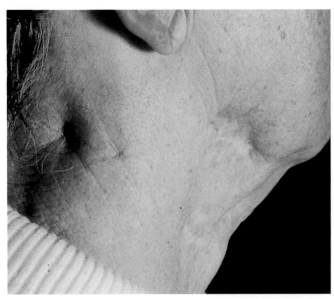

3.44

YAWS

Non-venereal syphilis, yaws and pinta (the 'endemic' treponematoses) follow a course not dissimilar from syphilis, with primary, secondary and tertiary stages. Yaws, caused by *Treponema pertenue* is seen predominantly in equatorial regions. The primary lesion (the mother yaw) is usually a single, painless papule that appears after 3–6 weeks and ulcerates (**Figs 3.46, 3.47**).

After a secondary stage with lesions similar to the primary lesions, late lesions present as gummas (**Fig. 3.48**), especially on the lower extremities. The skin may heal with 'tissue-paper' scarring and depigmentation (**Fig. 3.49**).

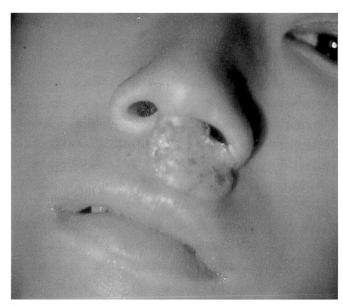

3.46

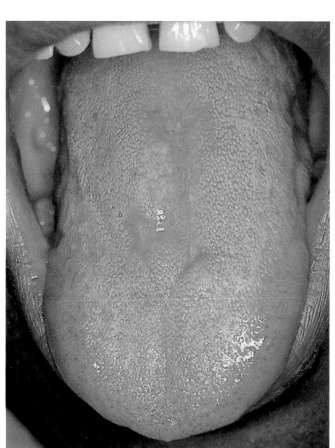

3.47

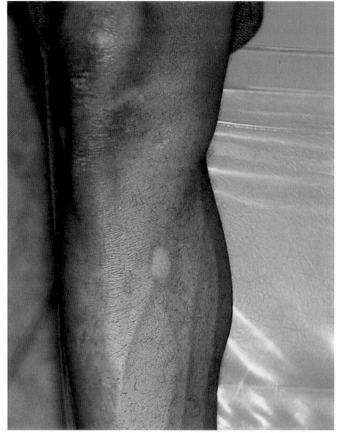

3.48

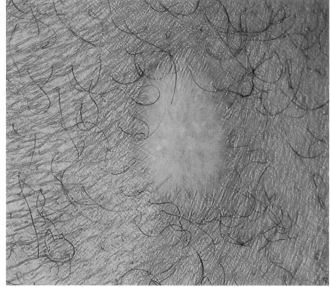

3.49

FURTHER READING

Aguiar AM, Enwonwu CO, Pires FR. Noma (cancrum oris) associated with oral myiasis in an adult. Oral Dis 2003; 9(3): 158–9.

Alam F, Argiriadou AS, Hodgson TA, Kumar N, Porter SR. Primary syphilis remains a cause of oral ulceration. Br Dent J 2000; 189: 352–4.

Baratti-Mayer D, Pittet B, Montandon D, *et al*. Guess What! Localised bacillary angiomatosis of the tongue. Eur J Dermatol 1998; 8(4): 283–4.

Cox HJ, Brightwell AP, Riordan T. Non-tuberculous mycobacterial infections presenting as salivary gland masses in children: investigation and conservative management. J Laryngol Otol 1995; 109: 525–30.

Dixon TC, Meselson M, Guillemin J, Hanna PC. Anthrax. N Engl J Med 1999; 341(11): 815–26.

Enwonwu CO, Sanders C. Nutrition: impact on oral and systemic health. Compend Contin Educ Dent 2001; 22(3 Spec No): 12–18.

Fotiou G, Laskaris G. Reiter's syndrome oral manifestations. Hell Stomatol Chron 1988; 32(2): 148–51.

Golden MR, Marra CM, Holmes KK. Update on syphilis: resurgence of an old problem. JAMA 2003; 290: 1510–14.

Ilyas SE, Chen FF, Hodgson TA, Speight PM, Lacey CJ, Porter SR, Llyas SE. Labial tuberculosis: a unique cause of lip swelling complicating HIV infection. HIV Med 2002; 3: 283–6.

Jaquinet A, Schrenzel J, Pittet D, Geneva Study Group on Noma. Noma: an 'infectious' disease of unknown aetiology. Lancet Infect Dis 2003; 3(7): 419–31.

Levell NJ, Bewley AP, Chopra S, Churchill D, French P, Miller R, Gilkes JJ. Bacillary angiomatosis with cutaneous and oral lesions in an HIV-infected patient from the UK. Br J Dermatol 1995; 132(1): 113–15.

Lopez de Blanc S, Sambuelli R, Femopase F, Luna N, Gravotta M, David D, Bistoni A, Criscuolo MI. Bacillary angiomatosis affecting the oral cavity. Report of two cases and review. J Oral Pathol Med 2000; 29(2): 91–6.

Maurin M, Birtles R, Raoult D. Current knowledge of *Bartonella* species. Eur J Clin Microbiol Dis 1997; 16: 487–506.

Monteil RA, Michiels JF, Hofman P, *et al*. Histological and ultrastructural study of one case of oral bacillary angiomatosis in HIV disease and review of the literature. Eur J Cancer B Oral Oncol 1994; 30B(1): 65–71.

Naidoo S, Chikte UM. Noma (cancrum oris): case report in a 4-year-old HIV-positive South African child. SADJ 2000; 55(12): 683–6.

Nunez-Marti JM, Bagan JV, Scully C, Penariocha M. Leprosy: dental and periodontal status of the anterior maxilla in 76 patients. Oral Dis 2004; 10: 19–21.

Paster BJ, Falkler WA Jr, Enwonwu CO, *et al*. Prevalent bacterial species and novel phylotypes in advanced noma lesions. J Clin Microbiol 2002; 40(6): 2187–91.

Rivera H, Correa MF, Castillo-Castillo S, Nikitakis NG. Primary oral tuberculosis: a report of a case diagnosed by polymerase chain reaction. Oral Dis 2003; 9(1): 46–8.

Tramont EC. Syphilis in adults: from Christopher Columbus to Sir Alexander Fleming to AIDS. Clin Infect Dis 1995; 21: 1361–71.

4 MYCOSES

- aspergillosis
- blastomycoses
- candidosis
- histoplasmosis
- mucormycosis.

ASPERGILLOSIS

Infection with *Aspergillus* species, usually *Aspergillus fumigatus*, but also *A. flavus* and *A. niger*, can present in several ways. The most serious is systemic aspergillosis, or respiratory tract *Aspergillus* infection, in immunocompromised patients. In *Aspergillus* sinusitis, there are normally noninvasive fungus balls, although infection of the antrum (**Fig. 4.1**) may rarely invade the palate, orbit or brain. Antral aspergillosis can be precipitated by overfilling maxillary root canals with endodontic material containing zinc oxide and paraformaldehyde. Oral ulceration may occasionally be caused by aspergilia (**Fig. 4.2**).

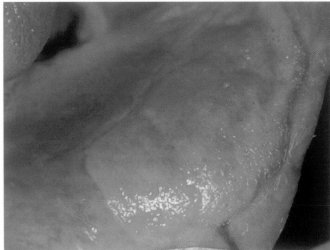

4.2

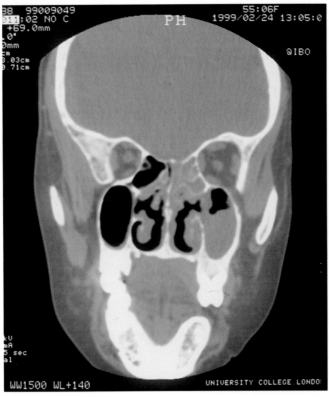

4.1

BLASTOMYCOSES

North American blastomycosis

North American blastomycosis (Gilchrist's disease) is a rare fungal disease. Caused by *Blastomyces dermatitidis*, it mainly affects the lungs and skin. Nearly 25% have oral or nasal lesions, usually an ulcer with a warty surface which may simulate a neoplasm (**Fig. 4.3**).

South American blastomycosis

The oral lesions of South American blastomycosis (paracoccidioidomycosis; Lutz's disease) are similar to those of the North American form of the fungal disease (**Figs 4.4, 4.5**). The causal organism, *Paracoccidioides brasiliensis*, may enter the body through the lungs or periodontium and cause granulomatous or ulcerative lesions and lymphadenopathy. Both the clinical appearance and the pseudoepitheliomatous hyperplasia on histology can mimic carcinoma.

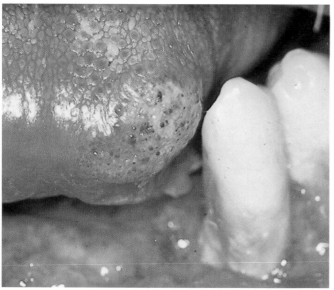

4.3

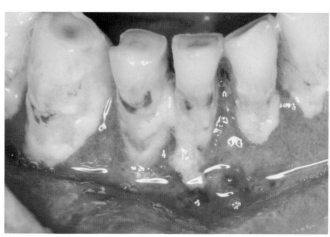

4.4

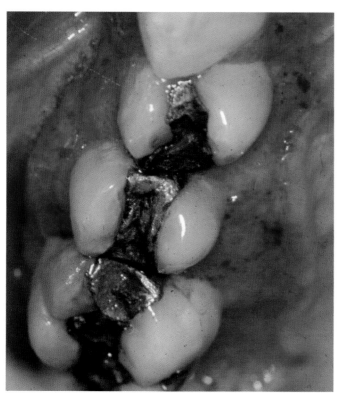

4.5

CANDIDOSIS

Acute candidosis *(thrush; candidiasis; acute pseudomembranous candidosis; moniliasis)*

Candida species are common oral commensals. *Candida albicans* is the most common and virulent species, which can act as an opportunistic pathogen, causing thrush (**Figs 4.6–4.8**) but *C. tropicalis*, *C. parapsilosis*, *C. guilliermondii* and *C. krusei* may also be implicated, especially in immunocompromised persons. *C. glabrata* is commonly seen after radiotherapy. New species such as *C. dubliniensis* are seen in HIV disease.

Thrush appears as white flecks or plaques, which are easily removed with gauze to leave an erythematous base (**Fig. 4.9**). Apart from neonates, who have no immunity to *Candida* species, thrush indicates an immunocompromised patient or a local disturbance in oral flora, such as that caused by xerostomia, antibiotic treatment or corticosteroids.

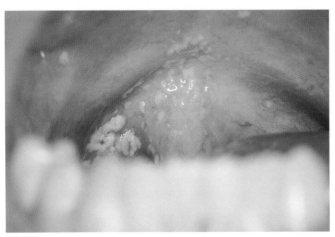

4.6

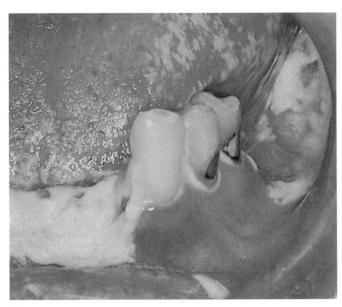

4.7

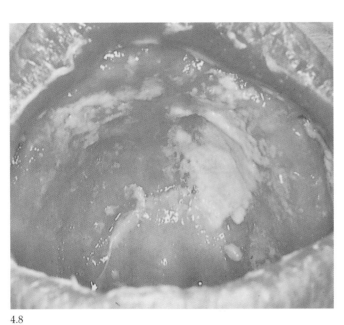

4.8

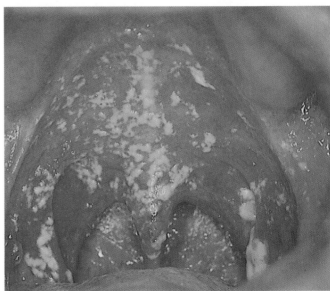

4.9

Thrush can affect any oral site, typically the palate or upper buccal vestibule posteriorly (**Figs 4.10, 4.11**). It is a feature in many immune defects, especially leukaemia, HIV disease and particularly where there has also been radiotherapy affecting the mouth and salivary glands.

In severely immunocompromised patients, there may also be other fungal infections, such as *Aspergillus*, *Mucor* or *Trichosporon* species.

Thrush can be an early feature of HIV (**Fig. 4.11**; see also **Fig. 9.21**) or related disease. Orogenital and anogenital transmission of *Candida* is also possible. Local causes of thrush should always be excluded: the use

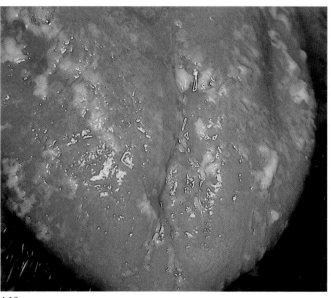

4.10

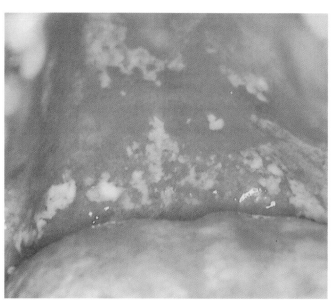

4.11

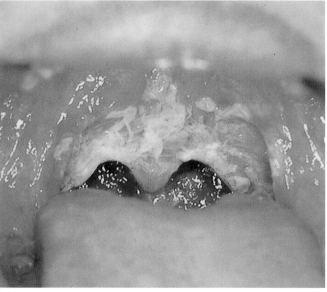

4.12

of corticosteroid inhalers may produce faucial and oropharyngeal thrush (**Fig. 4.12**).

Acute atrophic candidosis *(antibiotic sore tongue)*
Broad-spectrum antimicrobials such as tetracycline or ampicillin, and corticosteroids, predispose to an acute atrophic erythematous candidosis that causes redness, soreness, or a burning sensation, especially of the tongue (**Fig. 4.13**).

Erythematous candidosis
This is also seen in HIV disease (**Figs 9.24–9.27**).

Chronic atrophic candidosis
(denture-related stomatitis)
Chronic atrophic candidosis is common beneath complete upper dentures, especially in the elderly (**Figs 4.14–4.22**). Although termed 'denture sore mouth', it is usually asymptomatic unless complicated by

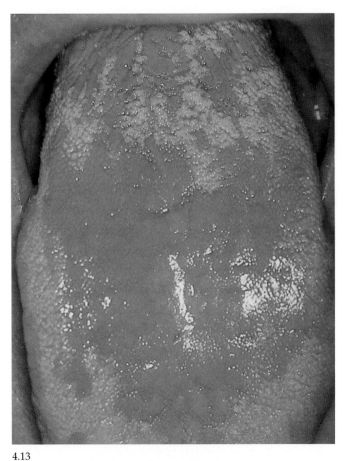

4.13

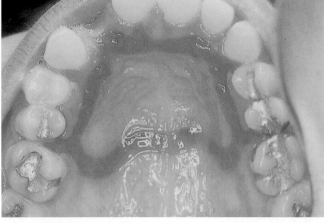

4.14

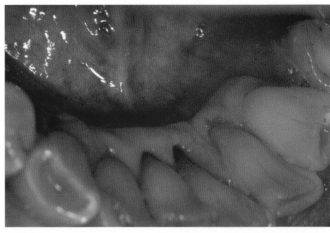

4.16

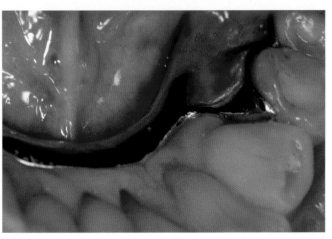

4.15

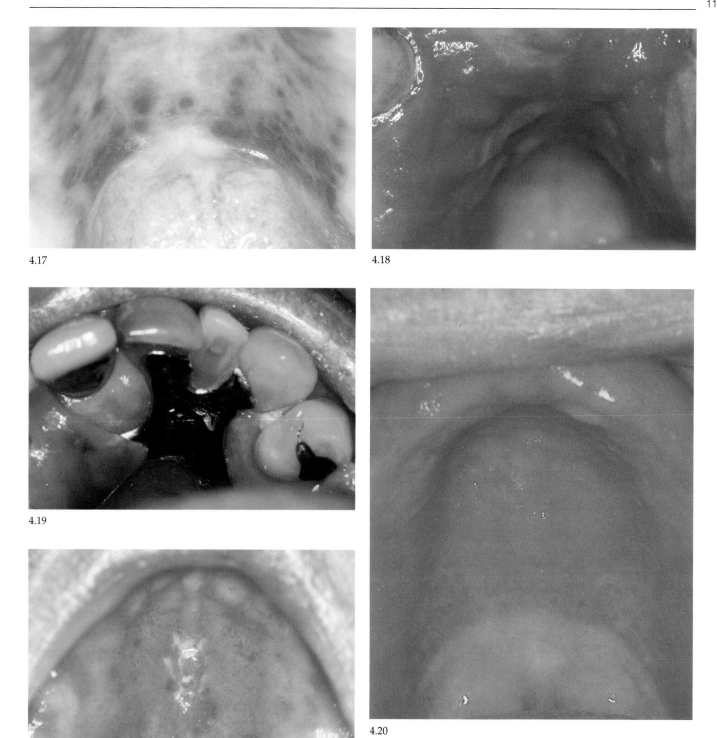

4.17

4.18

4.19

4.20

4.21

thrush (see **Fig. 4.22**). Characteristically there is erythema limited to the denture-bearing area (**Fig. 4.14**). It is rare below lower dentures.

Newton described three types, from punctate erythema (localized simple type; type 1; see **Fig. 4.21**), to complete erythema of the denture-covered area (type 2; see **Fig. 4.20**), to inflammatory papillary hyperplasia (granular type; type 3).

Patients with denture-related stomatitis are usually otherwise healthy. The lesion is caused by *Candida* and bacteria proliferating on the denture surface, especially when it is worn during sleep. Inadequate dentures predispose to the lesion in some patients. Occasionally the lesion is complicated by the development of papillary hyperplasia or angular stomatitis.

Angular stomatitis *(angular cheilitis; cheilosis; perlèche)*
Denture-related stomatitis may predispose to angular stomatitis, which is bilateral and produces erythema, fissuring or ulceration (**Fig. 4.23**; see also **Figs 4.24–4.26**) which can be painful and occasionally very disfiguring (**Fig. 4.25**).

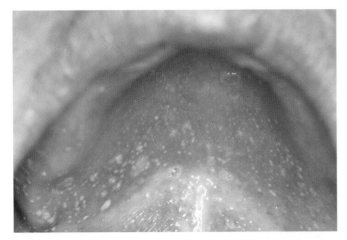

4.22

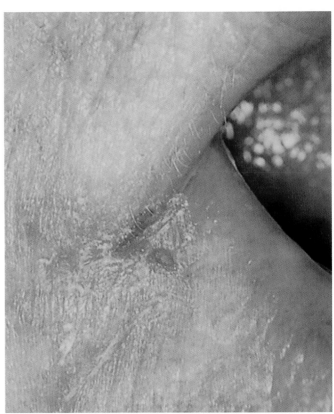

4.23

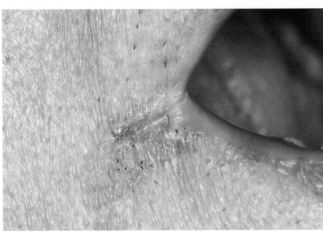

4.24

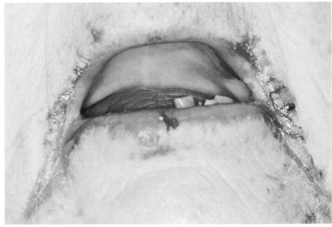

4.25

Rarely, angular stomatitis is a manifestation of iron deficiency (**Fig. 4.26** – there is also glossitis), or of vitamin B deficiency, when there may also be glossitis and mouth ulcers, or of an immune defect (see **Fig. 9.23**). Although *Candida albicans* is the prevalent organism, *Staphylococcus aureus* and other microorganisms may sometimes be isolated.

Median rhomboid glossitis

Median rhomboid glossitis, although originally thought to be a developmental lesion, is rarely seen in children and may be chronic focal candidosis (**Figs 4.27, 4.28**). It is a fairly common lesion and predisposed by diabetes, cigarette smoking, the wearing of dentures and HIV infection (see also Chapter 9).

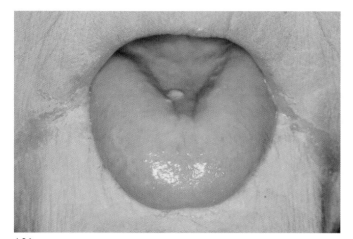

4.26

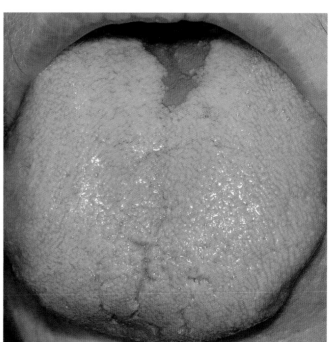

4.27

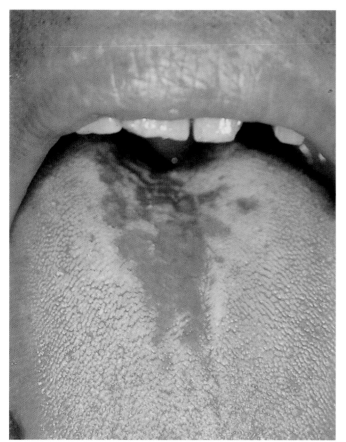

4.28

Multifocal chronic candidosis

Focal chronic candidosis may occur in the palate in apposition to the tongue lesion — the 'kissing lesions' (**Figs 4.29, 4.30**).

Multifocal chronic candidosis may appear as red, white or mixed lesions and is usually seen in smokers.

Candidal leukoplakia

Chronic hyperplastic candidosis, or candidal leukoplakia, is a firm, white, adherent plaque, usually seen inside the commissures (**Fig. 4.31**), or on the tongue. These leukoplakias may have a higher malignant potential than many forms of keratosis.

Candidal leukoplakia may be a speckled red and white lesion (**Fig. 4.32**). HIV infection or deficiencies of haematinics may underlie chronic candidosis.

Chronic mucocutaneous candidosis

Chronic mucocutaneous candidosis (CMC) is a heterogeneous group of syndromes characterized by recurrent or persistent cutaneous, oral and

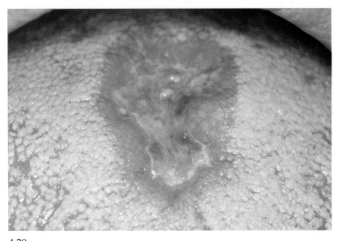

4.29

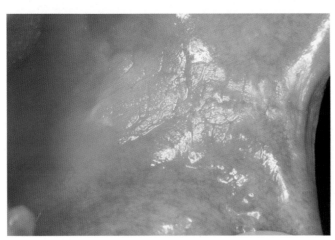

4.31

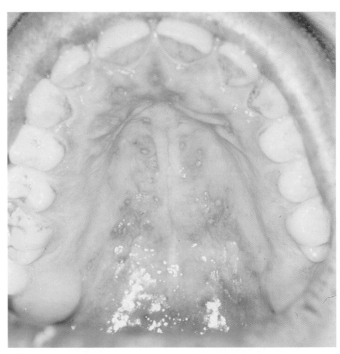

4.30

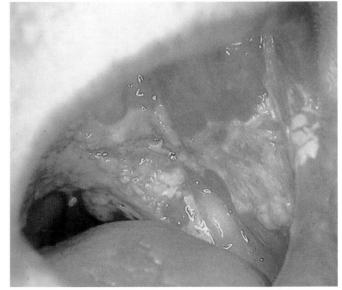

4.32

other mucosal candidosis, usually from early life. Early lesions are white and resemble thrush, as here (**Fig. 4.33**), in one variant (candidosis — endocrinopathy syndrome: Wells' type 3 CMC) that also includes hypoparathyroidism (note dental defects) and often hypoadrenocorticism, hypothyroidism and diabetes mellitus. *Candida*

albicans is the usual cause but *C. tropicalis*, *C. parapsilosis*, *C. guilliermondii* and *C. krusei* may also be implicated.

The white plaques eventually become widespread, thick and adherent, and the tongue fissured (**Figs 4.34 and 4.35**). The CMC extends over the palate and into the oropharynx (**Fig. 4.36**). Antifungal

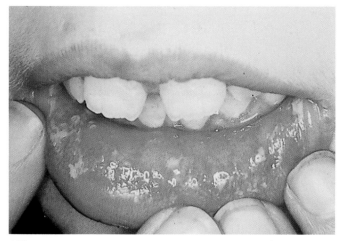

4.33

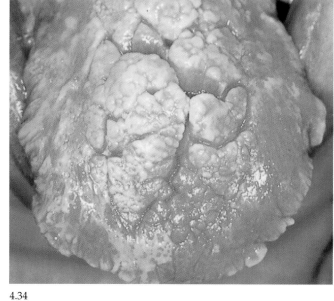

4.34

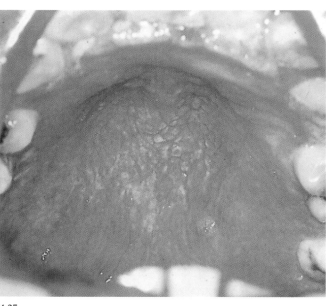

4.35

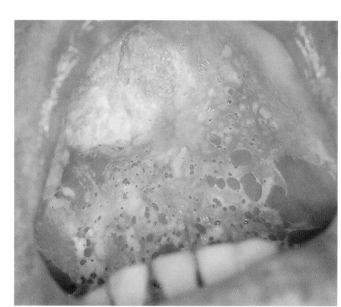

4.36

treatment is at least transiently effective (**Fig. 4.37**, which is the same patient as in **Fig. 4.36**).

Chronic oral candidosis is often associated with malignant thymoma in this type of CMC (Good's syndrome). Enamel hypoplasia may also be seen in candidosis endocrinopathy syndrome (**Fig. 4.38**).

In CMC, the nails are usually involved but both cutaneous and nail involvement vary in severity (**Fig. 4.39**).

Granulomas may be seen in the diffuse variant of CMC (**Fig. 4.40**). These patients also have chronic oral candidosis, which may affect the larynx and eyes. There can be a familial pattern and early onset of disease.

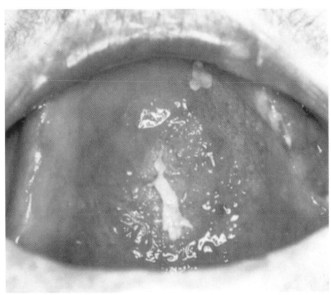

4.37

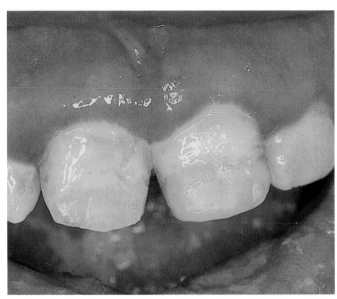

4.38

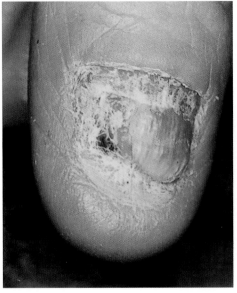

4.39

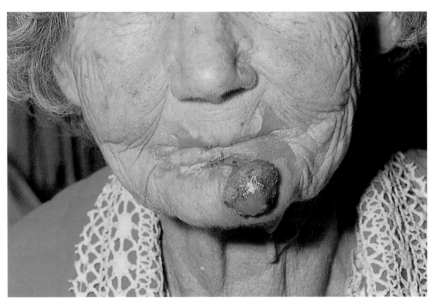

4.40

HISTOPLASMOSIS

Oral histoplasmosis, caused by *Histoplasma capsulatum*, may be seen especially in immunocompromised patients or in endemic areas such as the Ohio and Mississippi valleys in the USA. Oral lesions appear as mucosal nodules or nonspecific indurated ulcers (**Fig. 4.41**). There may be associated low-grade fever, lymphadenopathy and hepatosplenomegaly (see also **Figs 9.67–9.69**).

MUCORMYCOSIS *(phycomycosis; zygomycosis)*

Despite the fact that *Rhizopus*, *Mucor* and *Absidia* are fungi ubiquitous in decaying vegetation and some sugary foods, infection is rare and seen almost exclusively in immunocompromised patients. Nasal and paranasal sinus mucormycosis is seen especially in poorly controlled diabetics, and in particular presents resembling sinusitis. However, it may invade the orbit, frontal lobe, palate (**Fig. 4.42**) and elsewhere.

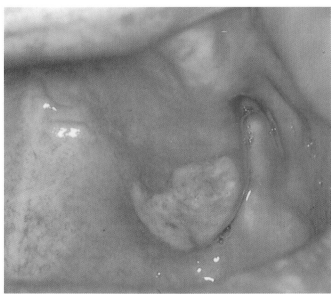

4.41

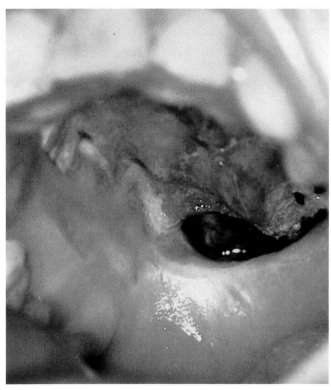

4.42

FURTHER READING

Al-Karaawi ZM, Manfredi M, Waugh AC, *et al*. Molecular characterization of *Candida* spp. isolated from the oral cavities of patients from diverse clinical settings. Oral Microbiol Immunol 2002; 17: 44–9.

Almeida ODP, Scully C. Fungal infections of the mouth. Brazil J Oral Sci 2002; 1: 19–26.

Almeida ODP, Jacks J, Scully C. Paracoccidioidomycosis of the mouth; an emerging deep mycosis. Crit Rev Oral Biol Med 2003; 14: 377–383.

Bartie KL, Williams DW, Wilson MJ, Potts AJ, Lewis MA. PCR fingerprinting of *Candida albicans* associated with chronic hyperplastic candidosis and other oral conditions. J Clin Microbiol 2001; 39: 4066–75.

Bedi R, Scully C. Tropical oral health. In Manson's Tropical Diseases, 21st Edition, edited by Cook GC, Zumla A. WB Saunders; Elsevier, Edinburgh, 2002, 515–531.

Casariego Z, Rey Kelly G, Perez H, *et al*. Disseminated histoplasmosis with orofacial involvement in HIV-1-infected patients with AIDS: manifestations and treatment. Oral Dis 1997; 3: 184–7.

Correa ME, Soares AB, de Souza CA, *et al*. Primary aspergillosis affecting the tongue of a leukemic patient. Oral Dis 2003; 9(1): 49–53.

Epstein JB, Hancock PJ, Nantel S. Oral candidiasis in hematopoietic cell transplantation patients: an outcome-based analysis. Oral Surg Oral Med Oral Pathol Oral Radiol Endod 2003; 96(2): 154–63.

Groll AH. Itraconazole — perspectives for the management of invasive aspergillosis. Mycoses 2002; 45 Suppl 3: 48–55.

Gupta AK, Tomas E. New antifungal agents. Dermatol Clin 2003; 21(3): 565–76.

Hay RJ. Antifungal drugs used for systemic mycoses. Dermatol Clin 2003; 21(3): 577–87.

Hodgson TA, Rachanis CC. Oral fungal and bacterial infections in HIV-infected individuals: an overview in Africa. Oral Dis 2002; 8 Suppl 2: 80–7.

Kauffman CA. Quandary about treatment of aspergilloma persists. Lancet 1996; 347: 1640.

Kretzschmar DP, Kretzschmar JL. Rhinosinusitis: review from a dental perspective. Oral Surg Oral Med Oral Pathol Oral Radiol Endod 2003; 96(2): 128–35.

Lilic D. New perspectives on the immunology of chronic mucocutaneous candidiasis. Curr Opin Infect Dis 2002; 15: 143–7.

Moraru RA, Grossman ME. Palatal necrosis in an AIDS patient: a case of mucormycosis. Cutis 2000 66(1): 15–18.

Myoken Y, Sugata T, Myoken Y, Kyo T, Fujihara M, Mikami Y. Antifungal susceptibility of Aspergillus species isolated from invasive oral infection in neutropenic patients with hematologic malignancies. Oral Surg Oral Med Oral Pathol Oral Radiol Endod 1999; 87(2): 174–9.

Perheentupa J. APS-I/APECED: the clinical disease and therapy. Endocrinol Metab Clin North Am 2002; 31: 295–320.

Preston SL, Briceland LL. Fluconazole for antifungal prophylaxis in chemotherapy-induced neutropenia. Am J Health Syst Pharm 1995; 52(2): 164–73.

Scully C, El-Kabir M, Samaranayake LP. Candida and oral candidosis. Crit Rev Oral Biol Med 1994; 5: 124–58.

Scully C, de Almeida OP, Sposto MR. The deep mycoses in HIV infection. Oral Dis 1997; 3 Suppl 1: S200–7.

Scully C, van Bruggen W, Diz Dios P, Casal B, Porter S, Davison MF. Down syndrome: lip lesions (angular stomatitis and fissures) and Candida albicans. Br J Dermatol 2002; 147: 37–40.

Shams MG, Motamedi MH. Aspergilloma of the maxillary sinus complicating an oroantral fistula. Oral Surg Oral Med Oral Pathol Oral Radiol Endod 2003; 96(1): 3–5.

Silverman S, Scully C. Infectious diseases. In 3rd World Workshop in Oral Medicine, edited by Millard D, Mason DK, University of Michigan Press, 2000.

Sitheeque MA, Samaranayake LP. Chronic hyperplastic candidosis/candidiasis (candidal leukoplakia). Crit Rev Oral Biol Med 2003; 14(4): 253–67.

Vargas PA, Mauad T, Bohm GM, Saldiva PH, Almeida OP. Parotid gland involvement in advanced AIDS. Oral Dis 2003; 9(2): 55–61.

Vazquez JA, Sobel JD. Mucosal candidiasis. Infect Dis Clin North Am 2002; 16: 793–820.

Willard CC, Eusterman VD, Massengil PL. Allergic fungal sinusitis: Report of 3 cases and review of the literature. Oral Surg Oral Med Oral Pathol Oral Radiol Endod 2003; 96(5): 550–60.

Williams DW, Wilson MJ, Potts AJ, Lewis MA. Phenotypic characterisation of Candida albicans isolated from chronic hyperplastic candidosis. J Med Microbiol 2000; 49: 199–202.

5 INFESTATIONS AND POSSIBLE INFECTIONS

- Kawasaki's disease (mucocutaneous lymph node syndrome)
- larva migrans
- leishmaniasis (mucocutaneous leishmaniasis; espundia)
- myiasis
- sarcoidosis (Boeck's sarcoid)
- toxoplasmosis.

KAWASAKI'S DISEASE *(mucocutaneous lymph node syndrome)*

Of uncertain but probably infective origin, this condition can cause cardiac involvement together with lymphadenopathy, a 'strawberry'

tongue, cheilitis and desquamation of the palms and soles (**Figs 5.1, 5.2**). Uvulitis, palatal palsy and facial nerve palsy have also been observed.

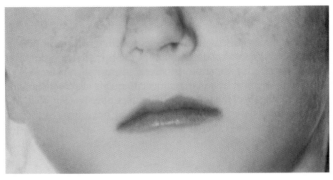

5.1

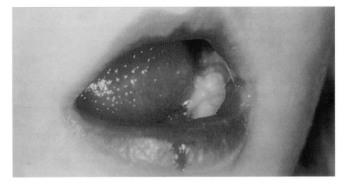

5.2

LARVA MIGRANS

Nematodes that are not normally parasitic to man often fail to develop fully if they infect humans, and may wander, causing one of several forms of 'larva migrans' before they die. The syndrome of visceral larva migrans is synonymous with toxocariasis, i.e. infection by larvae from roundworms of dogs, cats or wild carnivores. The syndrome of cutaneous larva migrans (creeping eruption) is caused by the larvae of hookworms from various animals, mainly dogs and cats.

Cutaneous larva migrans is characterized by itchy serpiginous tracks, affecting mainly the feet, hands or buttocks. It is common in

tropical countries and in Central and South America the nematode *Ancylostoma braziliense* is the main aetiological agent. Cutaneous larva migrans is now being seen increasingly in persons visiting the developing world.

Although common in the skin, larva migrans is rare in the mouth, with very few reports in the literature. As in the skin, the mouth infection probably mainly occurs by direct contact with contaminated sand but ingestion of contaminated food may also be responsible.

Larva migrans in this patient involved the tongue, lips, cheeks, floor of the mouth, palate and oropharynx (**Figs 5.3, 5.4**), but not the skin.

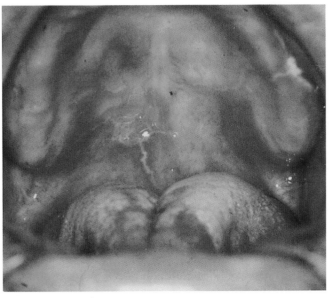

5.3

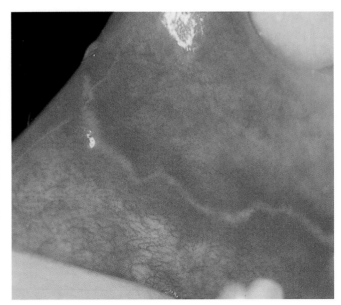

5.4

LEISHMANIASIS *(mucocutaneous leishmaniasis; espundia)*

The protozoa *Leishmania braziliensis* is found mainly in South America. A sandfly bite transmits infection and this usually heals although, in some, there is later metastasis to the mucocutaneous junctions of the mouth or nose (**Fig. 5.5**). The palate is frequently affected and ulcerates. Leishmaniasis may also be found around the Mediterranean (*L. donovani* or *L. tropica*). Chronic ulcers or swellings may be seen on the lips or face and in HIV disease, oral ulceration may be seen.

SARCOIDOSIS *(Boeck's sarcoid)*

Sarcoidosis is a multisystem noncaseating granulomatous condition of unknown aetiology. The semblance to tuberculosis has suggested a microbial aetiology, as yet unproved. Sarcoidosis mainly affects the lungs, lymph nodes and eyes, and though oral minor salivary tissue may contain granulomas, frank oral lesions are seldom seen. Acute sarcoidosis usually manifests as hilar adenopathy with erythema nodosum (HAEN). The salivary glands may be affected (**Fig. 5.7**) with

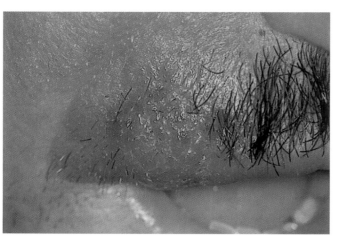

5.5

MYIASIS

Myiasis (from the Greek *myia* for 'flying') is the infestation of body tissues of animals by the larvae, commonly known as maggots, of two-winged flies (the Diptera). Oral myiasis has only rarely been reported in the English-language literature. Flies can affect a tooth-extraction site (**Fig. 5.6**).

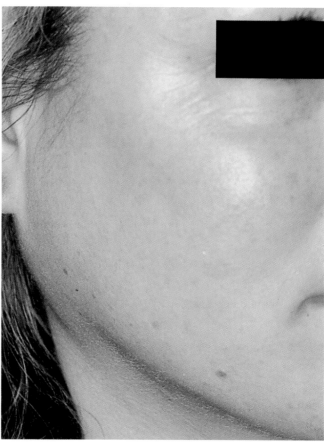

5.7

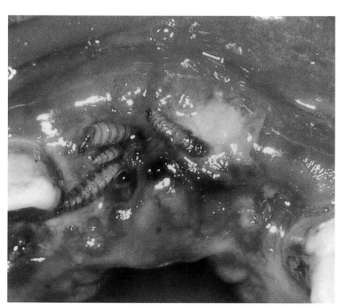

5.6

firm, painless swelling and xerostomia and, rarely, with fever, uveitis and facial palsy (Heerfordt's syndrome, uveoparotid fever).

Chronic swelling of the lip may be a feature of sarcoidosis (**Fig. 5.8**) and difficult to differentiate from oral Crohn's disease, Melkersson–Rosenthal syndrome, orofacial granulomatosis and cheilitis granulomatosa.

Obvious oral lesions are uncommon but include red nodules which may affect any oral site, including the gingiva (**Figs 5.9, 5.10**). The tongue is rarely involved but sarcoid may be seen in the palate (**Figs 5.11, 5.12**). Palatal biopsy, even from an apparently normal palate, may show granulomas.

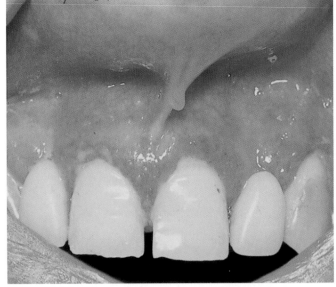

5.9

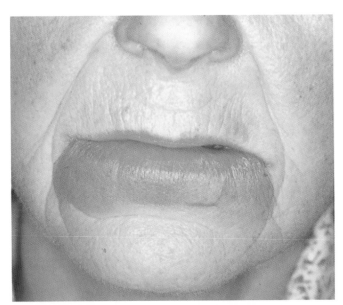

5.8

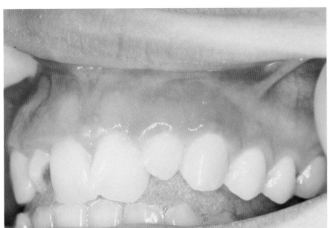

5.10

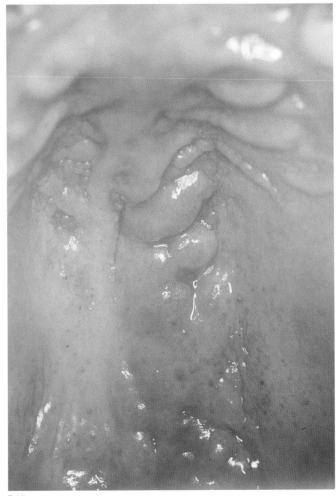

5.11

Multiple small, purple-brown dermal macules, papules or nodules are common in early active sarcoidosis but may be transient (**Fig. 5.13**). Lupus pernio (**Fig. 5.14**) — large, persistent, red or violaceous infiltrations of the skin — is a typical feature of chronic sarcoidosis and may be associated with pulmonary fibrosis.

Arthropathy is a prominent early feature, associated with fever and erythema nodosum. Chronic periarticular swelling affects the fingers and toes especially and there may be bony changes.

Sarcoidosis may be rarely associated with primary biliary cirrhosis, Crohn's disease, coeliac disease or amyloidosis, and some patients develop lymphomas. It is as yet unclear which, if any, of these associations are true overlap syndromes.

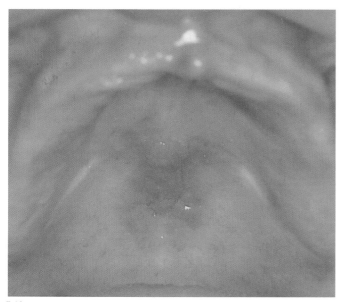

5.12

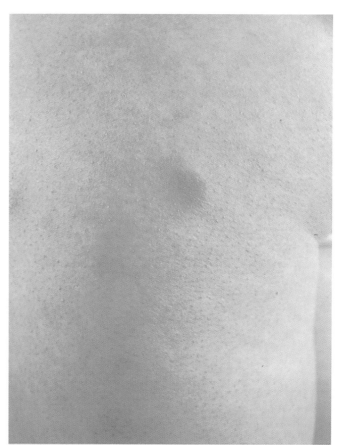

5.13

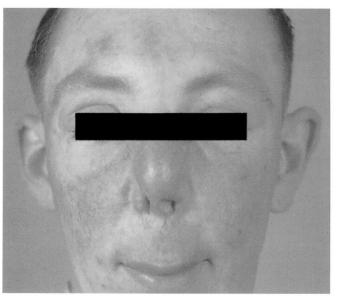

5.14

TOXOPLASMOSIS

Toxoplasmosis is an infection by the protozoan *Toxoplasma gondii*, contracted mainly by the ingestion of the parasite from infected meat (especially pork) or material contaminated with cat faeces. *T. gondii* can also cross the placenta, and can be transmitted in blood, tissues or organs.

Lymphadenopathy is the most common manifestation of toxoplasmosis, typically being seen in the neck. Chorioretinitis is a serious manifestation. Immunocompromised persons are also especially liable to pneumonitis, myocarditis, pericarditis, hepatitis, polymyositis, or encephalitis or meningoencephalitis.

Congenital toxoplasmosis may cause intrauterine death or severe fetal damage, and may present with enamel hypoplasia (**Fig. 5.15**) and deafness (**Fig. 5.16**).

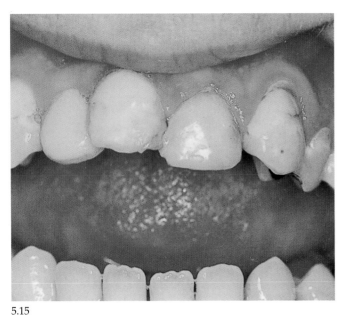

5.15

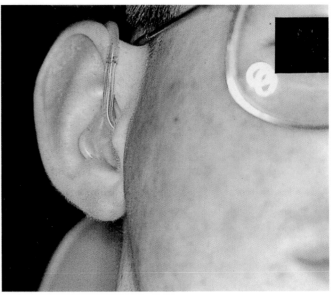

5.16

FURTHER READING

Aliaga L, Cobo F, Mediavilla JD, *et al*. Localized mucosal leishmaniasis due to *Leishmania (Leishmania) infantum*: clinical and microbiologic findings in 31 patients. Medicine (Baltimore) 2003; 82(3): 147–58.

al-Ismaily M, Scully C. Oral myiasis: report of two cases. Int J Paediatr Dent 1995; 5(3): 177–9.

Alrajhi AA, Saleem M, Ibrahim EA, Gramiccia M. Leishmaniasis of the tongue in a renal transplant recipient. Clin Infect Dis 1998; 27(5): 1332–3.

Arvand M, Kazak I, Jovanovic S, Foss HD, Liesenfeld O. Cervical cat scratch disease lymphadenitis in a patient with immunoglobulin M antibodies to *Toxoplasma gondii*. Clin Diagn Lab Immunol 2002; 9(2): 496–8.

Bedi R, Scully C. Tropical oral health. In Manson's Tropical Diseases, 21st edition, edited by Cook GC, Zumla A. WB Saunders; Elsevier, Edinburgh, 2002, 515–31.

Berman J. Current treatment approaches to leishmaniasis. Curr Opin Infect Dis 2003; 16(5): 397–401.

Blinder D, Yahatom R, Taicher S. Oral manifestations of sarcoidosis. Oral Surg Oral Med Oral Pathol Oral Radiol Endod 1997; 83: 458–61.

Cascio A, Antinori S, Campisi G, Mancuso S. Oral leishmaniasis in an HIV-infected patient. Eur J Clin Microbiol Infect Dis 2000; 19(8): 651–3.

Chaudhry Z, Barrett AW, Corbett E, French PD, Zakrzewska JM. Oral mucosal leishmaniasis as a presenting feature of HIV infection and its management. J Oral Pathol Med 1999; 28(1): 43–6.

Ciftcioglu N, Altintas K, Haberal M. A case of human orotracheal myiasis caused by *Wohlfahrtia magnifica*. Parasitol Res 1997; 83(1): 34–6.

Costa JW Jr, Milner DA Jr, Maguire JH. Mucocutaneous leishmaniasis in a US citizen. Oral Surg Oral Med Oral Pathol Oral Radiol Endod 2003; 96(5): 573–7.

Di Alberti L, Piattelli A, Artese L, *et al*. Human herpesvirus 8 variants in sarcoid tissues. Lancet 1997; 350: 1655–61.

Erol B, Unlu G, Balci K, Tanrikulu R. Oral myiasis caused by hypoderma bovis larvae in a child: a case report. J Oral Sci 2000; 42(4): 247–9.

Felices RR, Ogbureke KU. Oral myiasis: report of case and review of management. J Oral Maxillofac Surg 1996; 54(2): 219–20.

Garcia-Pola MJ, Gonzalez-Garcia M, Garcia-Martin JM, Villalain L, De los Heros C. Submaxillary adenopathy as sole manifestation of toxoplasmosis: case report and literature review. J Otolaryngol 2002; 31(2): 122–5.

Henry J. Oral myiasis: a case study. Dent Update 1996; 23(9): 372–3.

Joshi A, Agrawal S, Garg VK, Thakur A, Agarwalla A, Jacob M. Severe mucosal involvement in a patient with cutaneous leishmaniasis from Nepal. Int J Dermatol 2000; 39(4): 317–18.

Lata J, Kapila BK, Aggarwal P. Oral myiasis. A case report. Int J Oral Maxillofac Surg 1996; 25(6): 455–6.

Linss G, Richter C, Janda J, Gantenberg R. Leishmaniasis of the lips mimicking a mycotic infection. Mycoses 1998; 41 Suppl 2: 78–80.

Macey-Dare LV, Kocjan G, Goodman JR. Acquired toxoplasmosis of a submandibular lymph node in a 9-year-old boy diagnosed by fine-needle aspiration cytology. Int J Paediatr Dent 1996; 6: 265–9.

Martin S. Congenital toxoplasmosis. Neonatal Netw 2001; 20(4): 23–30.

Milian MA, Bagan JV, Jimenez Y, Perez A, Scully C. Oral leishmaniasis in an HIV-positive patient. Report of a case involving the palate. Oral Diseases 2002; 8: 59–61.

Ohtsuka S, Yanadori A, Tabata H, Yamakage A, Yamazaki S. Sarcoidosis with giant parotomegaly. Cutis 2001; 68: 199–200.

Tan JS. Human zoonotic infections transmitted by dogs and cats. Arch Intern Med 1997; 157(17): 1933–43.

Thongngarm T, Fratkin JD, Harisdangkul V. Sarcoidosis presenting as Heerfordt's syndrome with myopathy. Clin Exp Rheumatol 2001; 19: 480–1.

6 NEOPLASMS

- basal cell carcinoma
- granular cell tumour (Abrikssoff's tumour; granular cell myoblastoma)
- keratoacanthoma
- Langerhans' cell histiocytoses
- leiomyoma
- leukaemias
- lipoma
- lymphomas
- malignant melanoma
- melanoacanthoma
- metastatic neoplasms
- multiple myeloma (myelomatosis)
- mycosis fungoides
- myxoma
- neuroblastoma
- neuroectodermal tumour (congenital epulis)
- neuroma
- osteoma
- plasmacytoma
- rhabdomyosarcoma
- salivary neoplasms
- sarcomas
- squamous cell carcinomas.

BASAL CELL CARCINOMA

Basal cell carcinoma is the most common malignancy in Caucasians with incidence rates of 300 per 100,000 reported in the USA. Actinic radiation is a major aetiologic factor; greater than 85% occur on the sun-exposed areas of the head and neck. Other significant risk factors for the development of basal cell carcinomas include prior burns, genetic syndromes such as xeroderma pigmentosum, nevoid basal cell carcinoma syndrome, albinism and Bazex's syndrome, and immunosuppression.

On the lip these manifest as pearly, sometimes ulcerated, nodules or papules. Unlike squamous cell carcinomas, basal cell carcinomas only rarely originate on the vermilion but commonly occur periorally (**Figs 6.1, 6.2**). In contrast to squamous cell carcinomas, basal cell carcinomas more commonly arise on the upper than the lower lip.

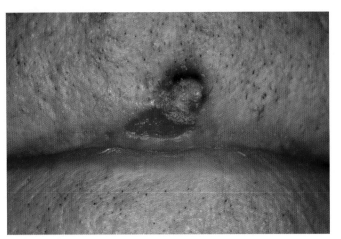

6.1

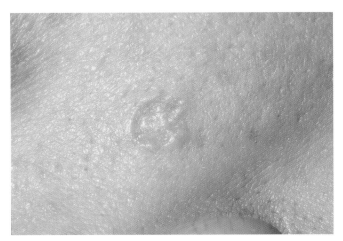

6.2

GRANULAR CELL TUMOUR *(Abrikosov's tumour; granular cell myoblastoma)*

This rare benign lesion of controversial origin may arise in many sites in the body but is most common in the tongue, presenting as a firm, submucosal, painless nodule (**Fig. 6.3**). Some have a whitish surface and occasionally this appearance, with pseudoepitheliomatous hyperplasia on histology, leads to a misdiagnosis of carcinoma.

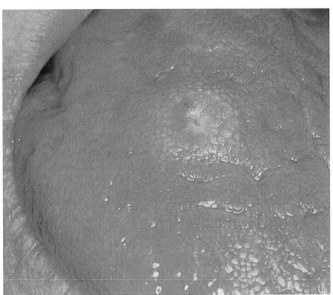

6.3

KERATOACANTHOMA

The keratoacanthoma is a common self-limiting benign tumour that arises most frequently in men after the sixth decade of life. It is a rapidly growing lesion that probably arises from the supraseboglandular part of a sebaceous gland. One variant, the Ferguson–Smith syndrome, is a familial trait.

The lesions mimic squamous cell carcinoma both clinically and microscopically. Keratoacanthomas are rare on the lips but often manifest at the vermilion border, as indurated, dome-shaped, nodules displaying a characteristic central, keratin-filled, crusted and frequently darkened, crater (**Fig. 6.4**). Keratoacanthomas grow rapidly, attaining a size typically greater than 1 cm, may be locally invasive and result in significant tissue damage but, if left untreated, many undergo spontaneous involution after 1–2 months.

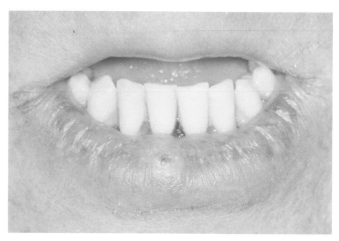

6.4

LANGERHANS' CELL HISTIOCYTOSES

Langerhans' cell histiocytoses are a group of disorders, formerly termed histiocytosis X, arising from Langerhans' cells. Hand–Schüller–Christian disease (**Figs 6.5–6.6**) usually appears at 3–6 years of age with disseminated bone lesions including osteolytic jaw lesions and loosening of teeth (floating teeth), diabetes insipidus and exophthalmos.

Eosinophilic granuloma is a localized benign form of histiocytosis where there are painless osteolytic bone lesions and, sometimes, mouth ulcers (**Fig. 6.6**). The affected teeth may loosen.

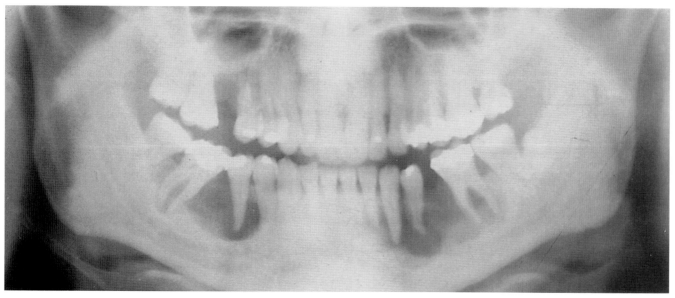

6.5

Letterer–Siwe disease is an acute disseminated and usually lethal form of histiocytosis in children under the age of 3 years. There are destructive bone lesions (**Fig. 6.7**), skin lesions, fever, lymphadenopathy and hepatosplenomegaly.

LEIOMYOMA

This benign tumour of smooth muscle is rare in the oral cavity (**Fig. 6.8**), and usually found on the tongue.

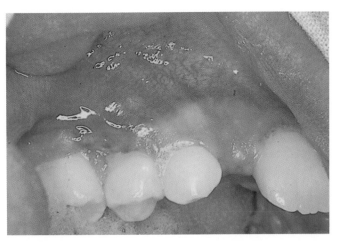

6.6

6.8

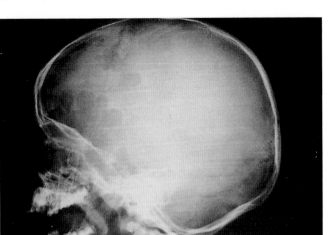

6.7

LEUKAEMIAS

Replacement of bone marrow by leukaemic tissue leads to crowding out of other cellular elements and consequent anaemia and thrombocytopenia. Spontaneous gingival haemorrhage is common (**Fig. 6.9**).

Oral purpura is also common, particularly where there is trauma, such as the suction exerted by an upper denture (**Fig. 6.10**). Chemotherapy may aggravate the bleeding tendency.

Gingival haemorrhage can be so profuse as to dissuade the patient from oral hygiene, but this simply aggravates the problem as the gingivae then become inflamed, more hyperaemic (**Fig. 6.11**) and bleed more profusely.

Leukaemic deposits in the gingivae occasionally cause swelling of variable degree in the gingivae (**Figs 6.15**). This is a feature especially of myelomonocytic leukaemia (a variant of acute myeloid leukaemia).

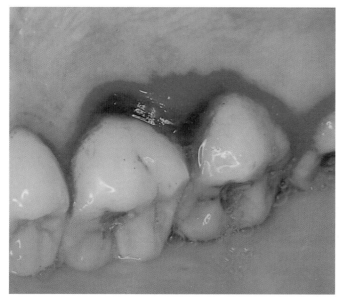

6.9

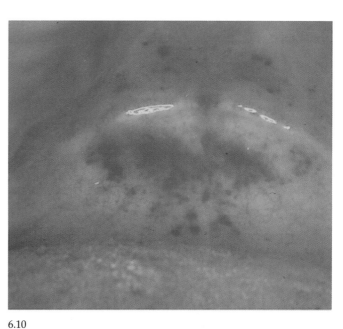

6.10

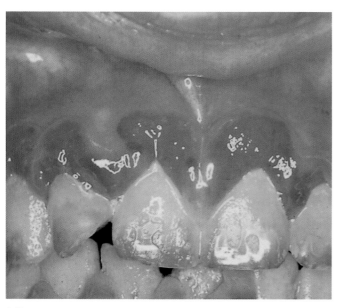

6.11

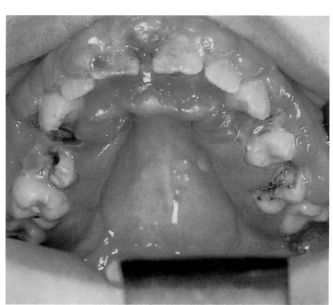

6.12

Simple odontogenic infections can spread widely and be difficult to control (**Fig. 6.16**). Non-odontogenic oral infections are common in leukaemic patients and involve a range of organisms including *Staphylococcus aureus, Pseudomonas aeruginosa, Klebsiella pneumoniae, Staphylococcus epidermidis, Escherichia coli,* enterococci, herpes simplex or varicella-zoster viruses, *Candida* species, *Aspergillus, Mucor* and, occasionally, other opportunists.

Mouth ulcers are common in leukaemia and often lack an inflammatory halo (**Figs 6.17, 6.18**). Some are associated with cytotoxic therapy, some with viral or bacterial infection, and some are non-specific.

Erythroleukaemia or Di Guglielmo's disease is a rare disorder, now recognized as a variant of myeloid leukaemia, characterized by proliferation of erythropoietic cells, with anaemia and hepatosplenomegaly but no lymphadenopathy. Oral ulceration, pallor (**Fig. 6.19**) and purpura are the main features.

Microbial infections in leukaemia are common in the mouth and can be a significant problem. Candidosis is extremely common (**Fig. 6.20**).

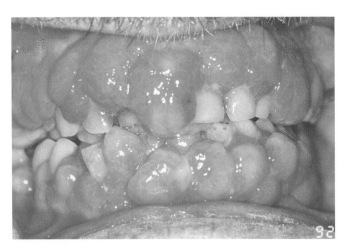

6.13

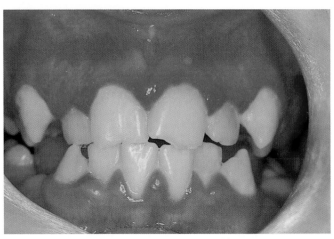

6.14

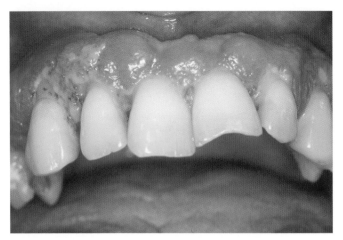

6.15

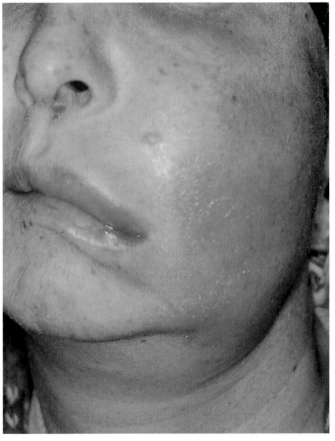

6.16

Of the viral infections, recurrent intraoral herpes simplex is also common. The patient in **Fig. 6.20** also has a dendritic ulcer, caused by herpes simplex virus.

Recurrent herpes labialis is common in leukaemic patients. The lesions can be extensive and, because of the thrombocytopenia, there is often bleeding into the lesion (**Figs 6.21**).

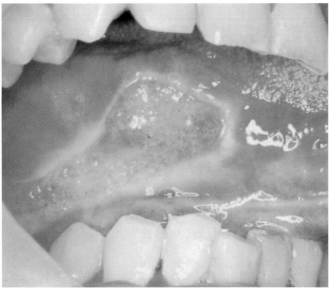

6.17

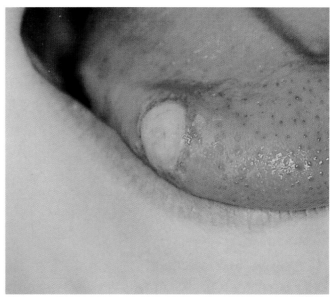

6.18

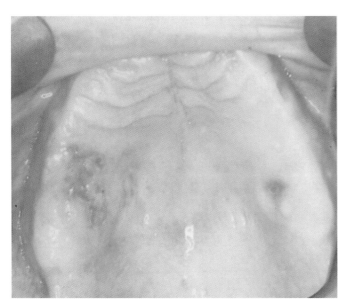

6.19

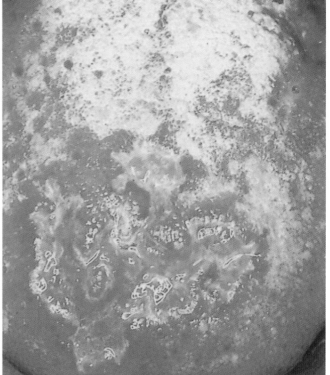

6.20

Zoster is also common in leukaemic patients (**Fig. 6.22**); hairy leukoplakia may rarely be seen.

Bacterial infections, however, are uncommon (**Fig. 6.23**) but a wide range of organisms may be involved, including various enteric organisms such as *Klebsiella* and *Escherichia coli;* septicaemia may originate from oral lesions.

Leukaemic deposits (chloromas) may appear in the mouth (**Fig. 6.24**) or on the face and neck (**Fig. 6.25**) but are uncommon. The most common manifestation in the neck of leukaemic patients is cervical lymph node enlargement.

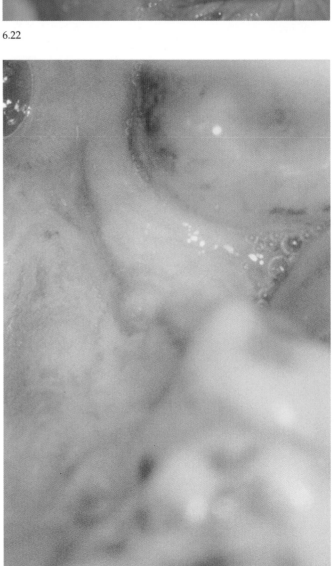

6.22

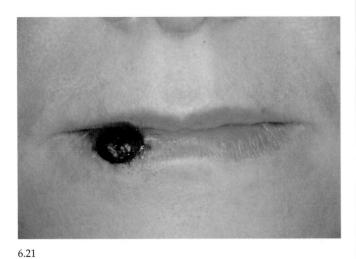

6.21

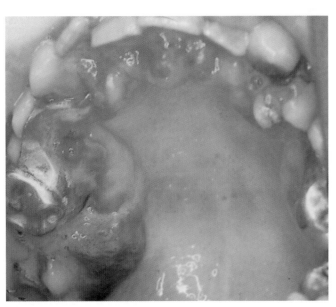

6.23

6.24

Figure 6.26 shows facial pallor and bruising, gingival haemorrhage and herpetic infection in a child with terminal leukaemia. However, the prognosis in childhood leukaemias has now improved. Finally, infiltration of the oral mucosa with leukaemic deposits is most typical of acute myeloid leukaemia although it has been rarely reported in chronic lymphocytic leukaemia.

The precise reason for the variable infiltration of the oral mucosa with different leukaemias is unknown.

LIPOMA

Lipoma is a relatively rare benign intraoral tumour, generally found in adults. The appearance is typical with thin epithelium over the yellowish tumour and prominent superficial blood vessels (**Figs 6.27–6.30**). Lipomas may be very soft on palpation (semi-fluctuant) and mistaken for cysts.

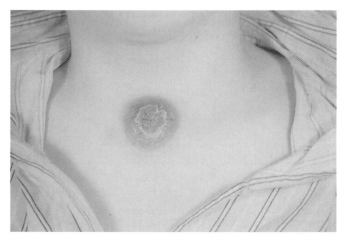

6.25

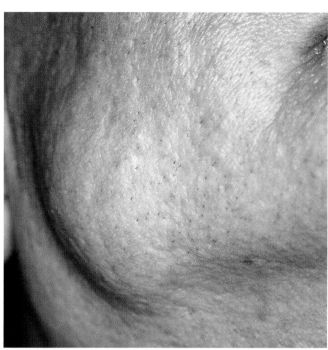

6.27

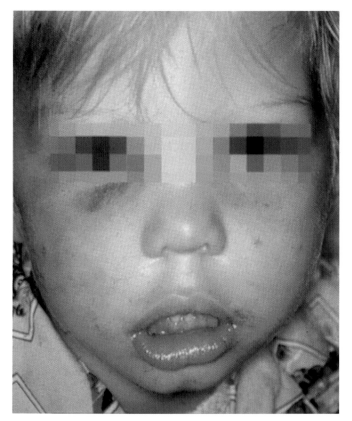

6.26

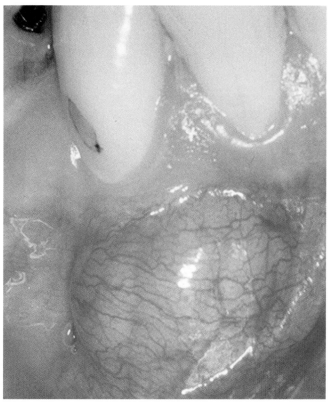

6.28

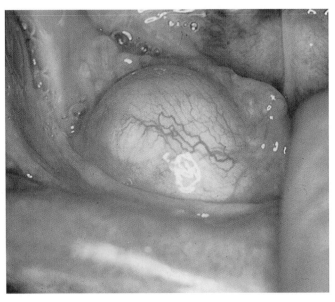

6.29

LYMPHOMAS

Lymphomas are uncommon in the mouth, although cervical lymph node involvement is common. Usually lymphomas present as ulcers or swellings (**Figs 6.30–6.39**). There is an increased prevalence of lymphomas in Sjögren's syndrome and — particularly non-Hodgkin's disease — in HIV infection (see **Fig. 9.54**).

Non-Hodgkin's lymphoma (**Fig. 6.31**) often appears in the tonsillar region, gingiva or palate (see also **Fig. 9.54**). T-cell lymphomas usually

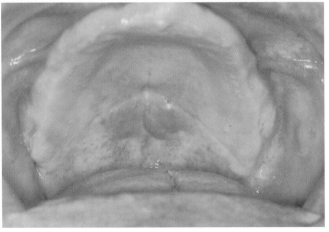

6.30

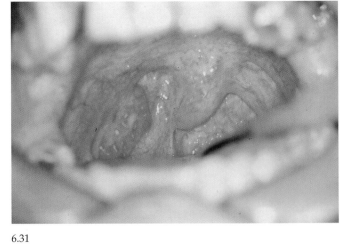

6.31

present as a diffuse painless palatal swelling that eventually ulcerates and may produce considerable destruction (**Figs 6.38, 6.39**).

African Burkitt's lymphoma is associated with Epstein–Barr virus and typically affects children before the age of 12–13 years. The

jaws, particularly the mandible, are common sites of presentation (**Fig. 6.40**). Massive swelling, which ulcerates in the mouth, may be seen. Radiographically, the teeth may appear to be 'floating in the air'.

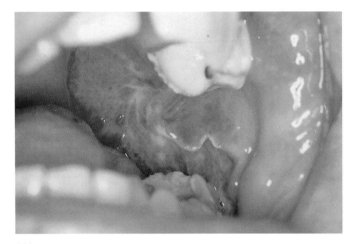

6.32

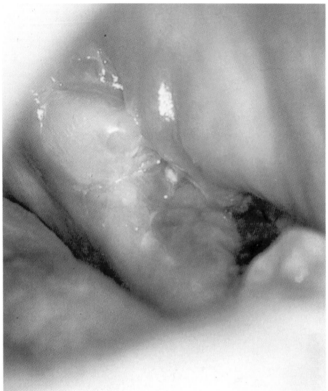

6.33

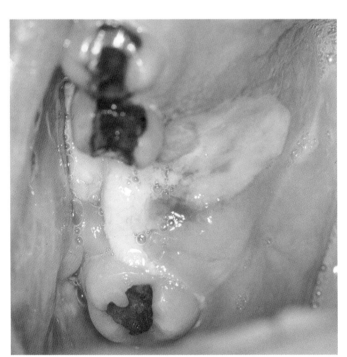

6.34

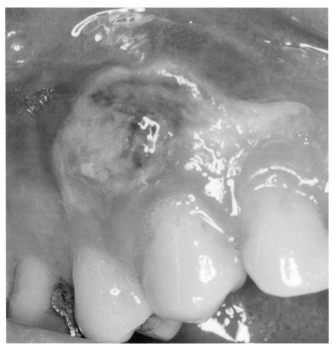

6.35

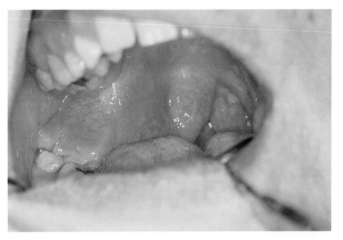

6.36

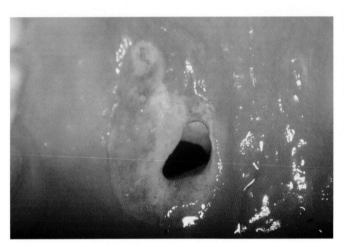

6.38

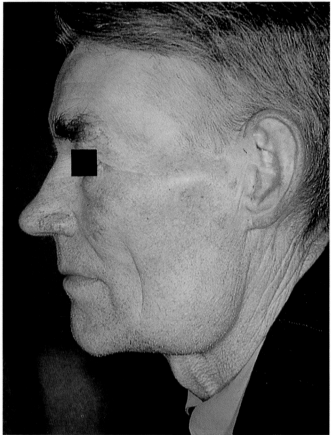

6.37

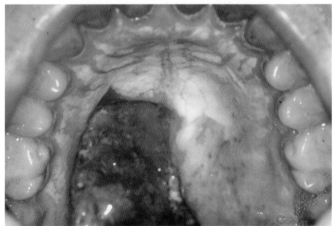

6.39

The jaws are less frequently involved in non-African Burkitt's lymphoma. Discrete radiolucencies in the lower third molar region, destruction of the lamina dura and widening of the periodontal space may be seen on radiography. In **Fig. 6.41** it presents as an ulcerated lump arising from the mandible but the disease may also cause oral pain, paraesthesia or increasing tooth mobility.

The association of non-African Burkitt's lymphoma with Epstein–Barr virus is tenuous and the disease is less common.

Patients with lymphocytic lymphomas are also predisposed to develop squamous carcinomas of the head and neck, possibly owing at least partly to the chemotherapy.

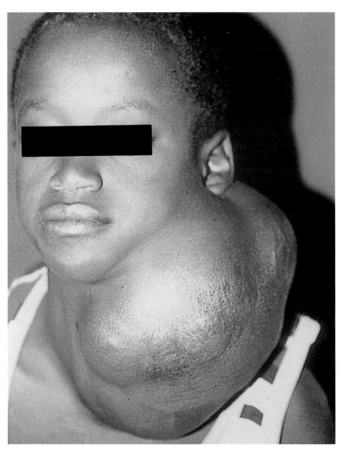

6.40

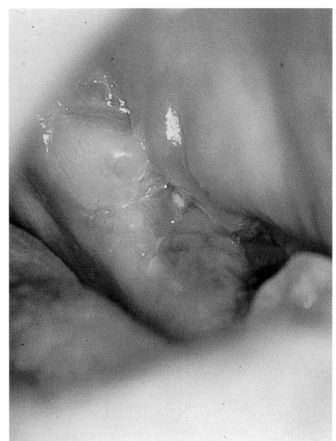

6.41

MALIGNANT MELANOMA

Primary oral melanoma is rare but it affects both sexes equally, is more common in patients of African or Asian derivation, and usually appears in or after middle age. Most malignant melanomas arise in the palate and many are preceded by melanosis (**Figs 6.42, 6.43**). Some vegetate profusely (**Fig. 6.44**, which is a rather extreme example), others remain flattish and spread more deeply. Not all are pigmented. The prognosis is very poor.

It has recently been suggested that patients with melanoma may present with facial erythema.

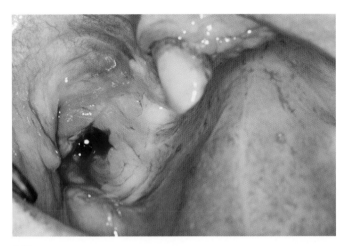

6.42

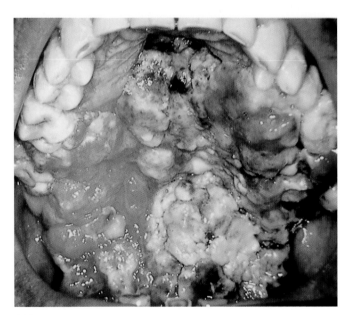

6.44

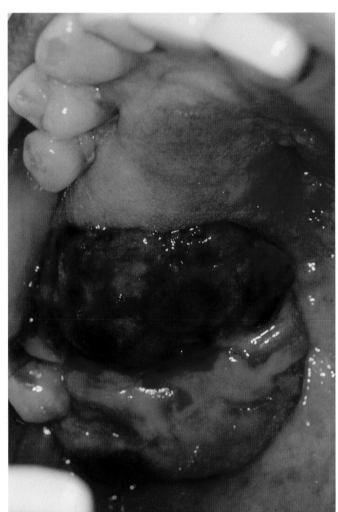

6.43

MELANOACANTHOMA

Melanoacanthoma is a rare condition of the cutaneous and mucosal epithelia, typically in patients of African ancestry, characterized by a proliferation of both melanocytes and keratinocytes, resulting in pigmented macular or plaque-like dark-brown or black lesions (**Fig. 6.45**).

The lesions are generally considered benign. No cases of recurrence or metastasis are reported.

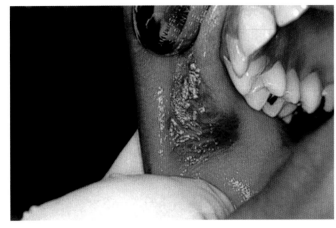

6.45

METASTATIC NEOPLASMS

Metastases are most common in cervical lymph nodes (**Figs 6.46–6.48**). Metastatic lymphatic spread is a particular feature of carcinomas of the oral and perioral regions, and is a poor prognostic finding.

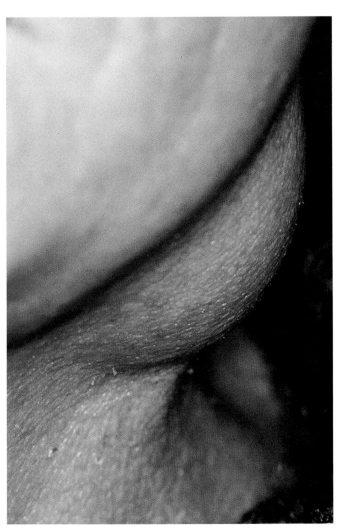

6.46

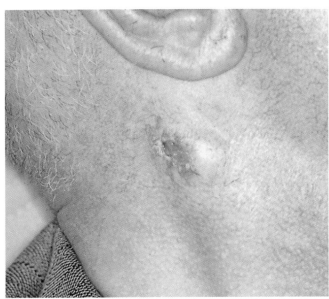

6.47

Blood-borne metastases are rare in the oral soft tissues and most are seen in the mandible, especially the angle and body. They virtually all present with pain or anaesthesia, expansion of the jaw (usually the mandible) or loosening of the teeth. Metastases to the jaw are usually from carcinomas of the breast or bronchus, thyroid, kidney, colorectum, stomach, prostate or uterus (**Figs 6.49–6.51**).

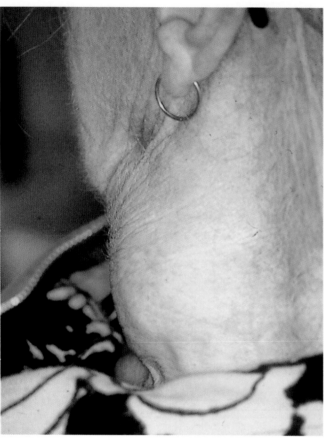

6.48

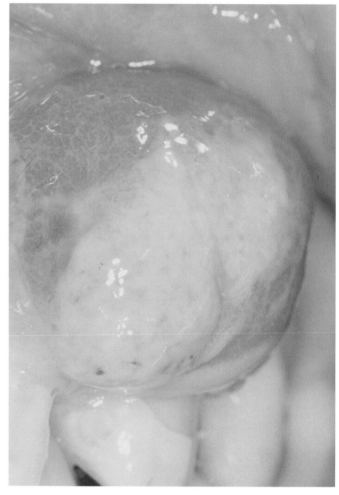

6.49

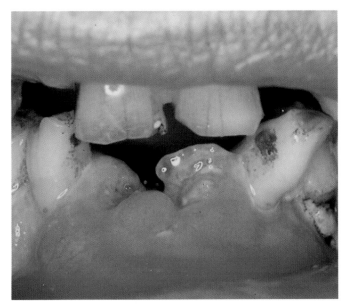

6.50

MULTIPLE MYELOMA *(myelomatosis)*

Myelomatosis is a malignant disorder of plasma cells, predominantly affecting the bone marrow. It is most commonly found in males over 50 years of age and it particularly affects the skull and axial skeleton. The jaws may be involved but soft tissue lesions (**Fig. 6.52**) are rare.

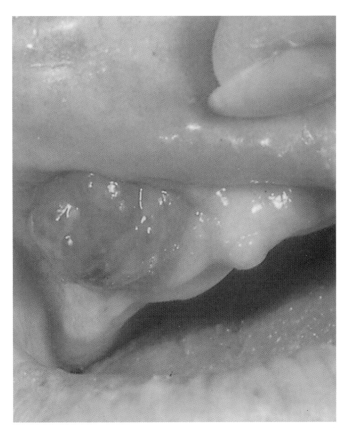

6.52

6.51

The symptomatic stage is preceded by the presence in plasma of an M-type (monoclonal) plasma protein, raised erythrocyte sedimentation rate, and proteinuria. Renal dysfunction may eventually arise. Clinically there may be anaemia, bone pain, swelling, paraesthesia or, occasionally, pathological fractures. Radiography typically shows multiple punched-out radiolucencies (**Figs 6.53–6.55**).

Ultimately, there may be circulatory impairment, Raynaud-type phenomena or a bleeding tendency caused by the paraproteins. Amyloidosis may be seen and there is a predisposition to recurrence of varicella-zoster virus infection.

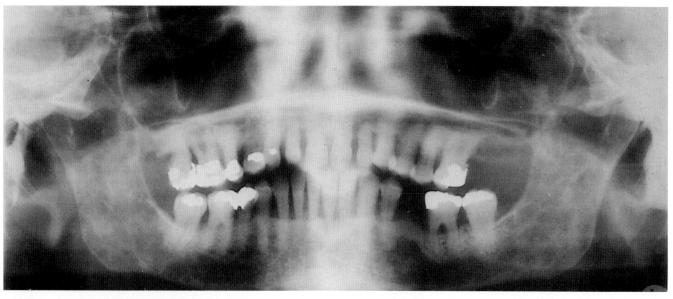

6.53

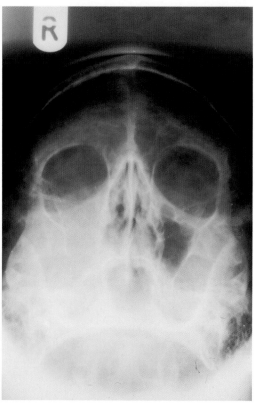

6.54

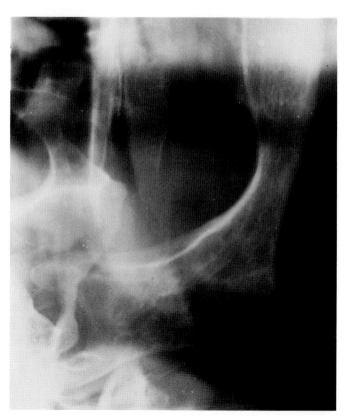

6.55

MYCOSIS FUNGOIDES

Mycosis fungoides is a predominantly cutaneous T-cell neoplasm that may produce oral plaques (**Fig. 6.56**), infiltrates or ulcers, especially on the tongue, vermilion of the lips or buccal mucosa. Incidentally, this patient also has erythema migrans.

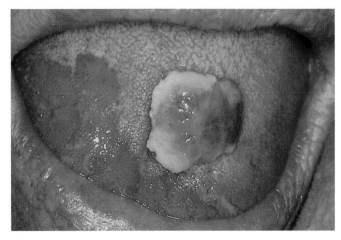

6.56

MYXOMA

Myxomas may have an odontogenic origin (odontogenic myxoma), usually affect the mandible and are most commonly seen in young people (**Figs 6.57, 6.58**). They are slow growing but pain may be a feature.

Bony expansion with cortical destruction, displacement of teeth without root resorption, and a multilocular, or honeycomb appearance, are typical radiographic features (see **Fig. 6.58**).

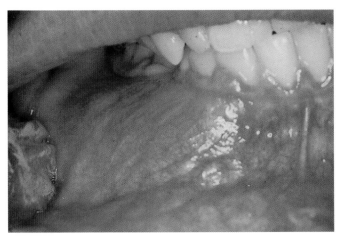

6.57

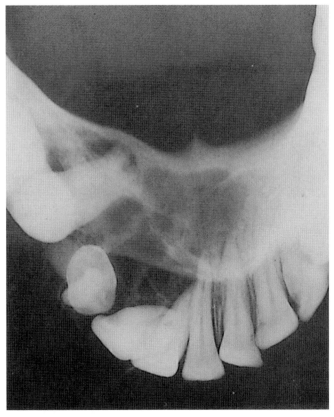

6.58

NEUROBLASTOMA

Neuroblastic tumours include ganglioneuroblastoma (a malignant tumour comprised of mature ganglion cells and nerve fibres, regarded by many to be a fully differentiated neuroblastoma) and ganglio-neuroma (a benign tumour composed of Schwann and ganglion cells). Neuroblastoma is an aggressive malignant tumour derived from primitive neural crest cells; it tends to metastasize rapidly. Survival rates for infants and older children with localized disease have improved but long-term survival for older children with metastatic (widespread) disease at diagnosis is poor (**Figs 6.59, 6.60** – a metastatic tumour).

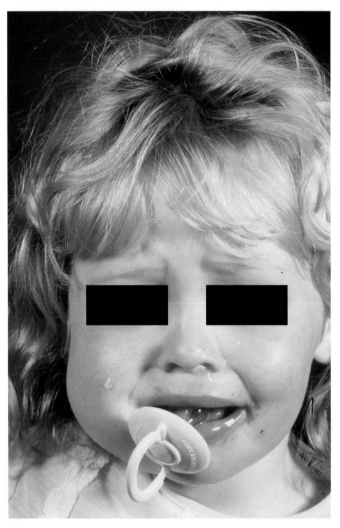

6.59

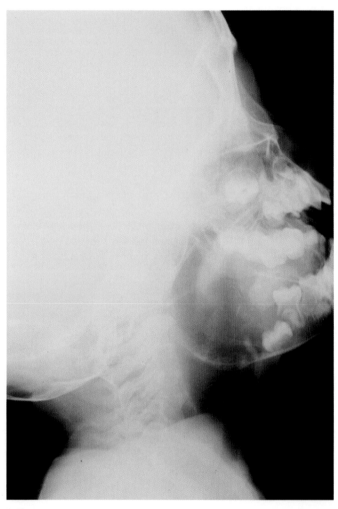

6.60

NEUROECTODERMAL TUMOUR
(congenital epulis)

Congenital epulis of the newborn is a rare lesion seen mostly in females and in the maxilla (**Figs 6.61**) shows an infant with a lump over the anterior mandible. Histologically similar to the granular cell tumour, the congenital epulis is a distinct benign entity, possibly of neural origin. The lesion does not grow after birth and may resolve spontaneously. It may need to be removed if it interferes with feeding.

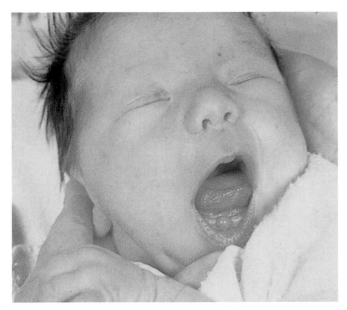

6.61

NEUROMA

Neuroma is usually an isolated benign tumour (**Fig. 6.62**) but may be multiple in MEN (Chapter 8). **Figures 6.63 and 6.64** show a plexiform neurofibroma. Clinically, neurofibromas may present as an isolated lesion, as a nerve sheath tumour, for example in relation to the inferior dental nerve as an expanded radiolucency in bone. They may also present as localised skin lesions and they can present as a widespread lesion affecting all branches of a nerve in a plexiform fashion involving all the soft tissues and invading bone with the loss of muscle function in the area and causing marked changes in the skin which develops a wrinkled brown appearance and then often ulcerates. Treatment is by extensive surgical removal and replacement with a composite free flap, as sarcomatous change may occur in these lesions.

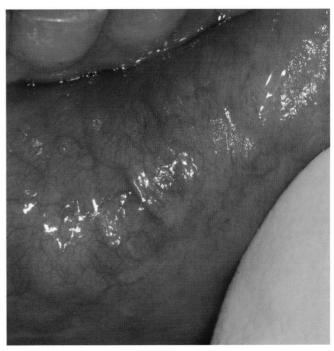

6.62

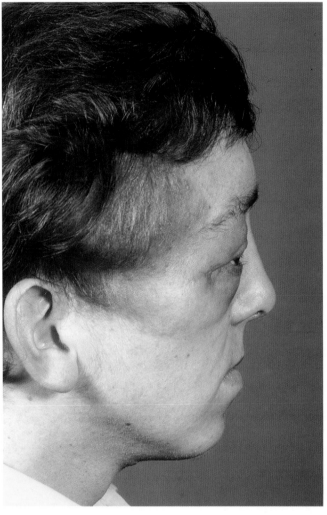

6.63

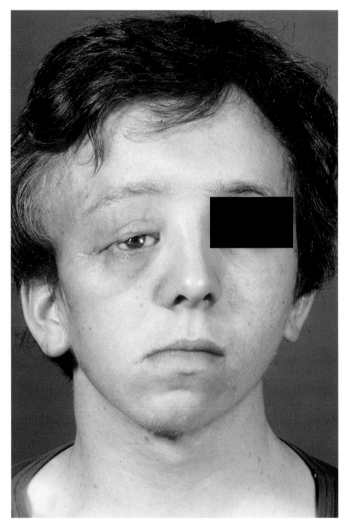

6.64

OSTEOMA

Osteoma is a benign bony outgrowth of membranous bones found mostly on the skull and facial bones. It is seen especially in the inner/outer table of calvarium (usually outer), paranasal sinus (frontal, ethmoid), mandible or nasal bones. Osteomas are well circumscribed, round, extremely dense, structureless and usually less than 2 cm across (**Figs 6.65–6.72**).

Figure 6.66 shows a swelling in the malar region due to a cancellous osteoma of the coronoid process (**Fig. 6.67**). **Figure 6.68** shows the excision specimen. **Figure 6.69** shows a left mandibular osteochondroma, with swelling, deviation of the chin to the right, elongation of the left ramus, and a lateral open bite. Figure 6.70 shows the radiograph.

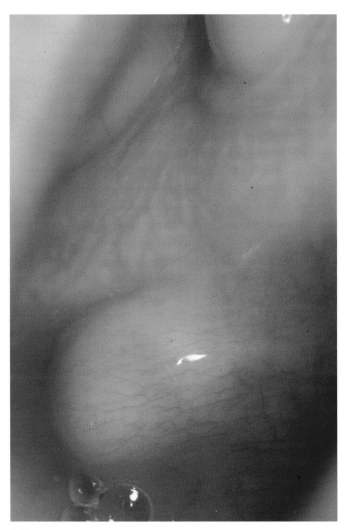

6.65

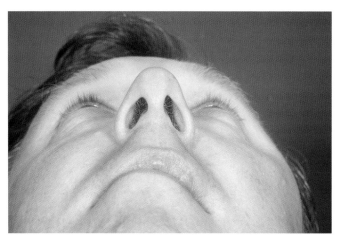

6.66

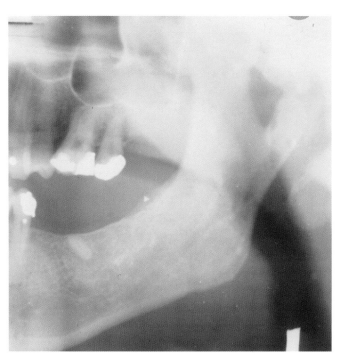

6.67

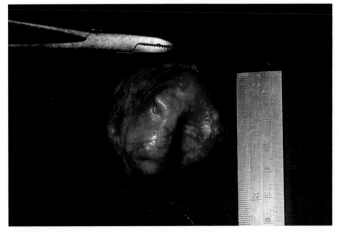

6.68

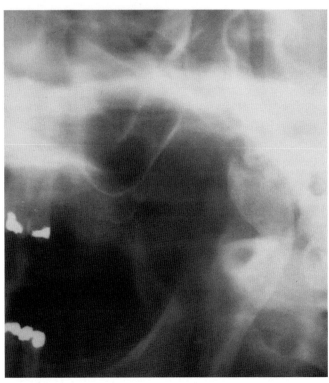

6.70

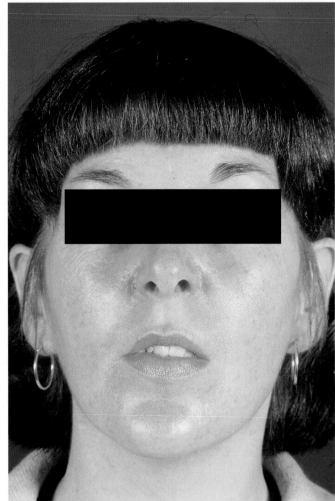

6.69

PLASMACYTOMA

Solitary plasmacytoma (localized myeloma) occasionally forms in the jaws or soft tissues nearby (**Fig. 6.71**) and is more likely than bone lesions to remain localized for a time. There is usually no abnormal immunoglobulin production but, even when present, serum levels are low. Patients should be kept under observation as multiple myeloma can develop in many, even after 20 years.

Local radiotherapy may be useful but cytotoxic chemotherapy is contraindicated.

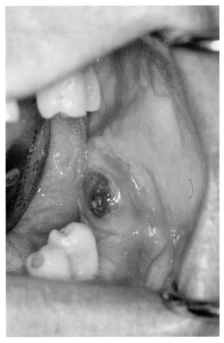

6.71

RHABDOMYOSARCOMA

Rhabdomyosarcoma is a highly malignant sarcoma of striated muscle derived from primitive mesenchymal cells affecting the bone or connective tissue (such as tendon or cartilage). It is the most common soft-tissue tumour in children and can occur anywhere in the body, including the head and neck, where over 25% are located. The brain, cheek, larynx, meninges, neck, oral cavity, parameningeal, parotid, scalp, thyroid and other areas may be affected (**Figs 6.72, 6.73**). Embryonal rhabdomyosarcoma is the most common type, usually found in children under 15 and in the head and neck region and genitourinary tract. The botryoid type is a variant of the embryonal type and arises as a grape-like lesion in mucosal-lined hollow organs such as the vagina and urinary bladder. The alveolar type is a more aggressive tumour, which usually involves the muscles of the extremities or trunk. The pleomorphic type is usually seen in adults and arises in muscles of the extremities. The embryonal rhabdomyosarcoma is considered the most treatable form of the disease.

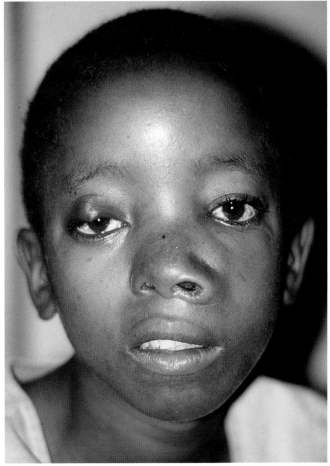

6.73

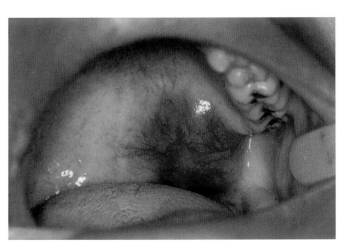

6.72

158

SALIVARY NEOPLASMS

Pleomorphic salivary adenoma *(mixed salivary tumour)*

Salivary gland neoplasms are uncommon and of unknown aetiology, although there is increased incidence in those exposed to atomic or therapeutic irradiation and possibly an association with breast carcinoma. The most common is pleomorphic salivary adenoma (PSA), a benign neoplasm which typically affects middle-aged or elderly persons. There is a slight female predominance and the neoplasm is found mainly in the parotid (**Fig. 6.74**). Sialography may show duct displacement (**Fig. 6.75**).

The majority of salivary neoplasms are benign, most are PSA and most affect the parotid. Swellings of the parotid gland typically appear behind and over the angle of the mandible and evert the lobe of the ear (**Figs 6.76–6.81**).

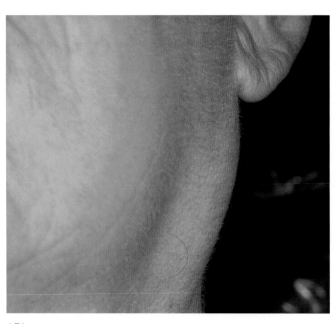

6.74

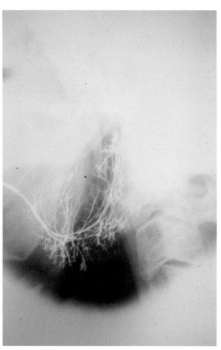

6.75

6.76

PSA is usually painless and has no effect on the facial nerve, despite an often intimate relationship. PSA frequently has a lobulated surface and is slow growing (see **Fig. 6.79**).

Malignant change, although uncommon, is suggested by pain, rapid growth, facial palsy, increased vasculature (see **Fig. 6.77**) or ulceration (**Fig. 6.80**). Metastases are rare. In some cases, the submandibular gland may be the site of PSA (**Fig. 6.81**).

Intraoral salivary gland neoplasms are most common in the palate, usually in the region of the junction of the hard and soft palates (**Figs 6.82–6.83**).

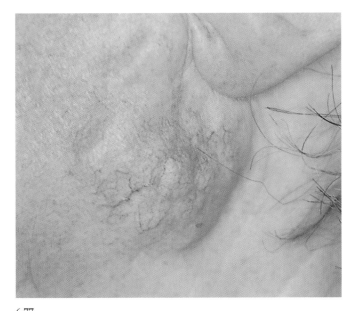

6.77

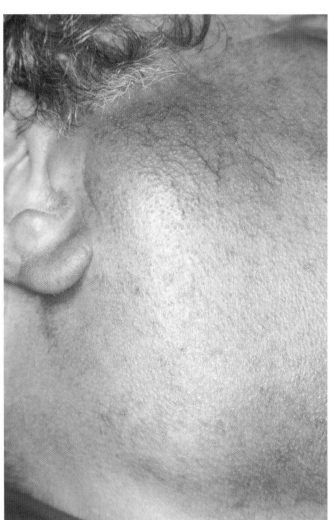

6.78

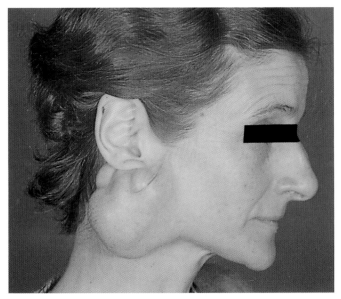

6.79

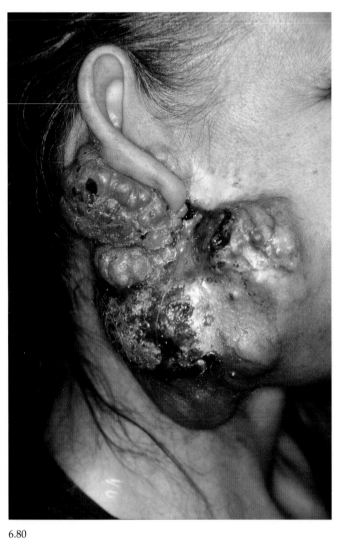

6.80

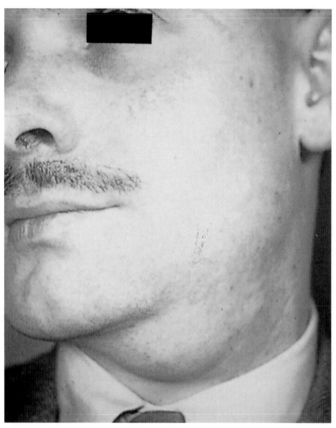

6.81

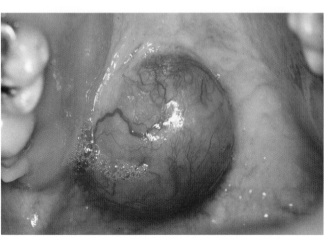

6.82

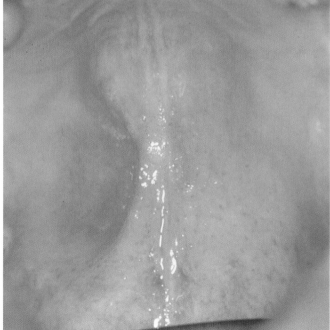

6.83

PSA is not only the most common neoplasm of major salivary glands but also of the minor salivary glands of the lip, palate (**Figs 6.84–6.85**) and elsewhere. A nodule or sometimes a cystic mass, especially in the upper lip, should be considered as a salivary neoplasm until histologically proved otherwise.

Ulceration is uncommon in PSA, even where the lesion has impinged on a denture (**Figs 6.84, 6.85**. Same patient with and without denture.)

Adenoid cystic (adenocystic) carcinoma

Adenoid cystic carcinoma is the most common malignant neoplasm of minor salivary glands and is usually seen in the palate as a fairly slow-growing lump, which eventually ulcerates, or in a major gland (**Fig. 6.86**). Nevertheless, it is invasive, especially perineurally, and has a poor prognosis.

Mucoepidermoid tumour

Mucoepidermoid tumour may be seen in the palate (**Fig. 6.87**). Mucoepidermoid tumour appears to be the most common malignant tumour of salivary glands induced by previous irradiation. Neoplasms are rare in the sublingual gland (**Fig. 6.88**) but are typically malignant, such as acinic cell tumour, mucoepidermoid tumour, adenoid cystic tumour, malignant PSA or adenocarcinoma.

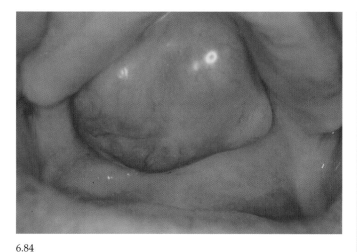

6.84

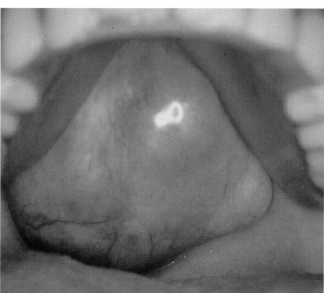

6.85

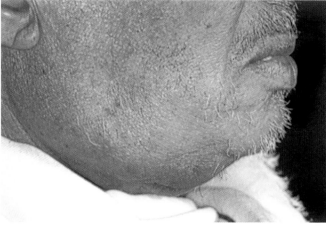

6.86

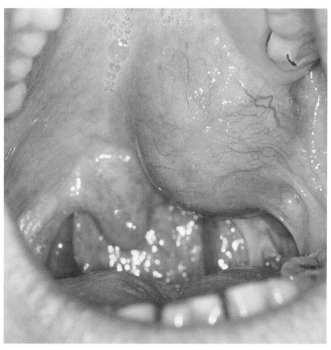

6.87

Monomorphic salivary adenoma

Monomorphic adenomas may occur intraorally (**Fig. 6.89**).

SARCOMAS

Apart from carcinoma, malignant oral lesions are rare. They include melanoma, Kaposi's sarcoma, alveolar soft part sarcoma (**Fig. 6.90**), fibrosarcoma (**Fig. 6.91**), angiosarcoma (**Figs 6.92, 6.93**), osteosarcoma

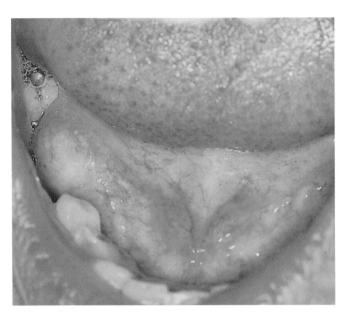

6.88

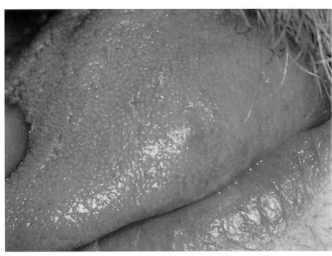

6.90

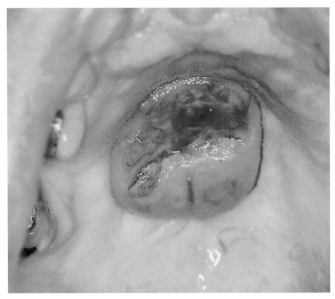

6.89

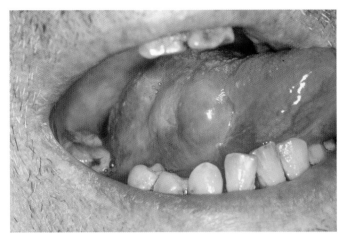

6.91

(Figs 6.94–6.98), malignant fibrous histiocytoma, lymphoproliferative disorders, metastases and others. In most malignant neoplasms, the clinical features are insufficiently specific to give a reliable diagnosis. A young child with osteosarcoma may present with pyrexia and a painful swelling expanding the mandible, it may exhibit a sunray appearance on the postero-anterior radiograph as is seen in **Fig. 6.97**. Treatment is with surgery/radiotherapy and chemotherapy, which appears today to have improved the prognosis.

Figures 6.96–6.98 show an osteogenic carcoma in an adult, which has a more indolent course. This was locally resected followed by radiotherapy with a good result. Biopsy is invariably indicated.

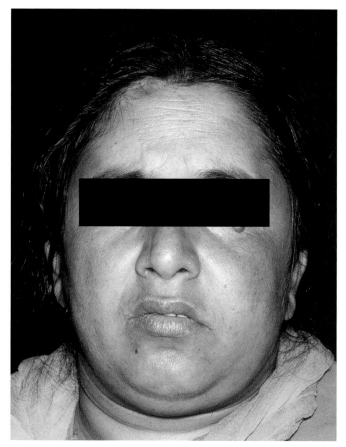

6.92

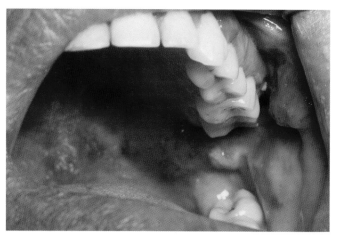

6.93

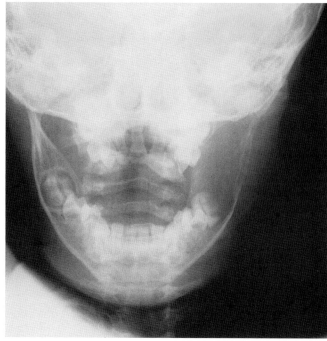

6.94

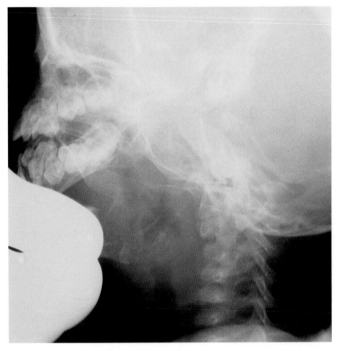

6.95

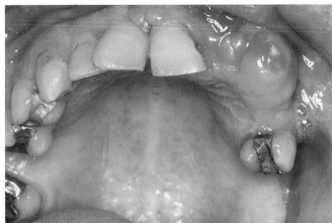

6.96

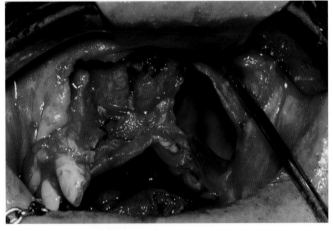

6.97

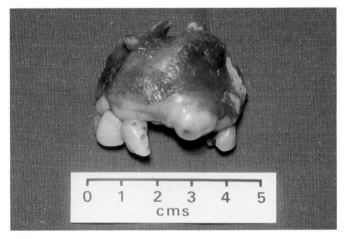

6.98

SQUAMOUS CELL CARCINOMAS

Carcinoma of the lip

Oral carcinoma accounts for less than 3% of cancer deaths in western countries but in some developing countries, particularly parts of India, oral cancer accounts for more than one third of admissions to cancer hospitals. Most oral malignant neoplasms are squamous cell carcinomas, commonly of the lip. Patients with carcinoma of the lip tend to present early and the prognosis is usually good. Oral carcinoma in this site is seen especially in male Caucasians living in sunny climes.

Predisposing factors include chronic sun exposure, possibly smoking, and immunosuppression but the overall incidence is decreasing.

Early carcinoma presents with an asymptomatic red or white lesion, and a small indurated lump or erosion with crusts developing (**Figs 6.99–6.102**). Typically located at the mucocutaneous junction the neoplasm spreads within the vermilion and on to the skin. In extreme examples, a deep ulcer with an irregular surface and rolled edges results. Metastasis is primarily to submental and submandibular lymph nodes.

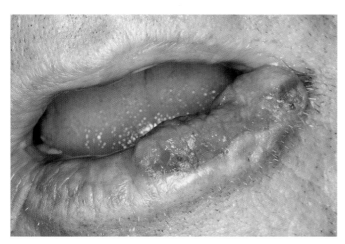

6.99

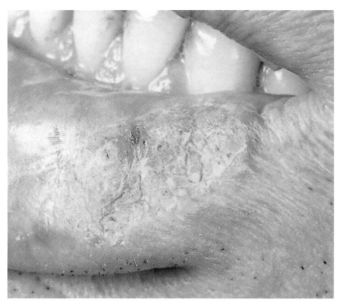

6.101

6.100

Carcinoma of tongue

The tongue is the most common intraoral site of carcinoma. Most tumours are on the lateral margin extending on to the ventrum (**Figs 6.103–6.117**). Tobacco or alcohol use and infections such as tertiary syphilis and chronic candidosis are possible predisposing factors. The incidence of tongue cancer is now increasing.

A lesion predominantly of elderly males, carcinoma presents as a red or white lesion, nodule, erosion or an ulcer. The lesion is indurated, usually sited on the posterolateral margin, and often associated with enlarged submandibular or jugulodigastric lymph nodes, sometimes bilaterally. The tumour tends to metastasize early and the patients present late.

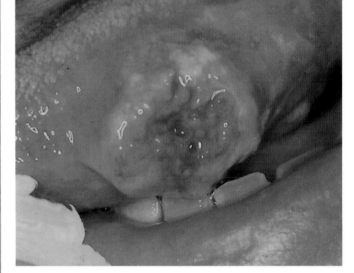

6.103

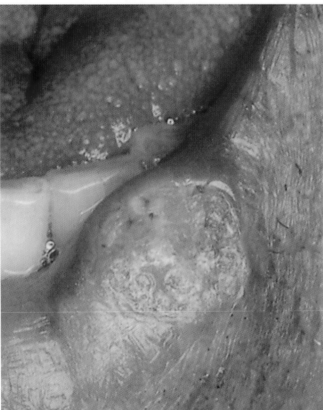

6.102

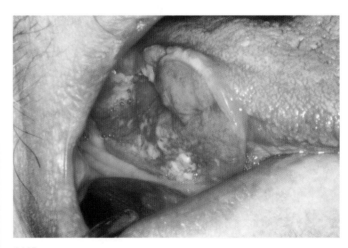

6.105

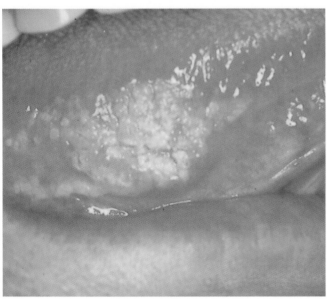

6.104

On rare occasions the carcinoma is exophytic (verrucous carcinoma) and extends on to the dorsum of the tongue (**Fig. 6.107**). Extremely rarely, the carcinoma appears induced by chronic trauma (**Fig. 6.106**)

Carcinoma may present as, or in, a white lesion. Leukoplakia of the floor of the mouth/ventrum of tongue may have a high malignant potential — the so-called 'sublingual keratosis'.

Carcinoma of the gingiva

Carcinoma of the gingiva is rare. It may present as a lump or as a more obvious vegetating mass (**Figs 6.110, 6.111, 6.114**). Tobacco chewing predisposes to carcinoma of the gingiva, buccal mucosa and the floor of the mouth.

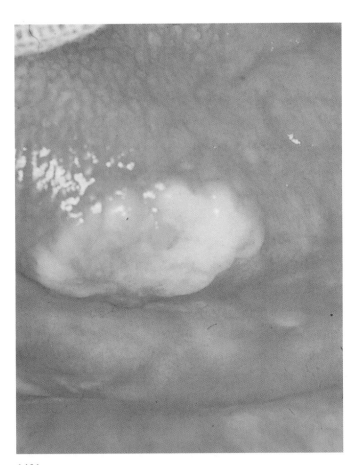

6.106

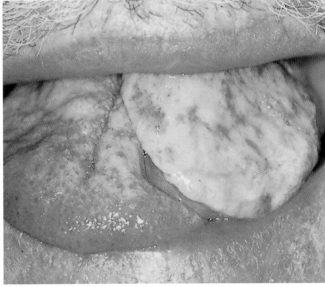

6.107

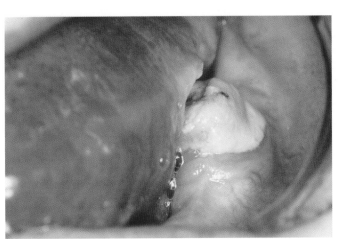

6.108

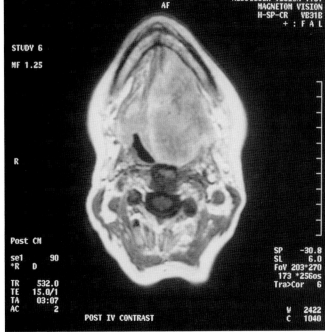

6.109

Suspicious red lesions, white lesions, ulcers or mixed lesions, should be biopsied to exclude carcinoma.

Carcinoma of the alveolar ridge

The variation in the clinical appearance of carcinoma of the alveolus is illustrated in **Figs 6.112–6.114**. In **Fig. 6.113** there is an obvious malignant ulcer with rolled edges and a red base, within an area of keratosis. There is an association between carcinoma in the floor of the mouth and hepatic cirrhosis.

Figure 6.114 is a carcinoma on the alveolus in a person consuming at least a bottle of whisky a day.

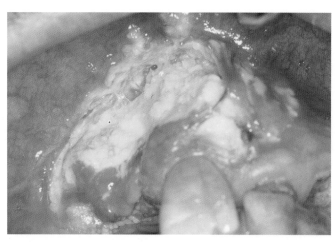

6.110

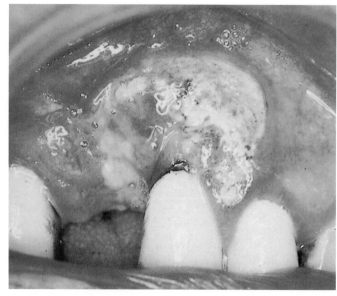

6.111

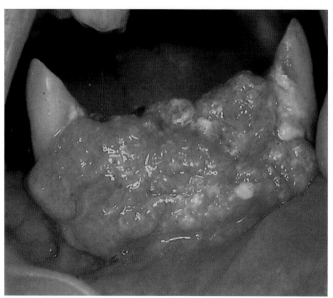

6.112

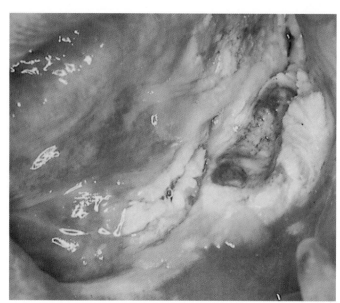

6.113

Carcinoma of the buccal mucosa

Habits such as snuff taking or tobacco chewing (including the use of smokeless tobacco) may predispose to buccal carcinoma. **Figure 6.115** is exophytic. **Figure 6.116** is a carcinoma arising in candidal leukoplakia. The particular example shown in **Fig. 6.117** is diffuse rather than exophytic and has red (erythroplasia) and white (leukoplakia) components. Erythroplasia is often highly dysplastic or malignant.

An ulcerated exophytic malignant ulcer is shown in **Fig. 6.118**. This is a verrucous carcinoma, a variant of squamous cell carcinoma, which is predominantly exophytic, slow-growing and of relatively good

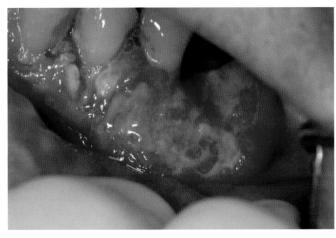

6.114

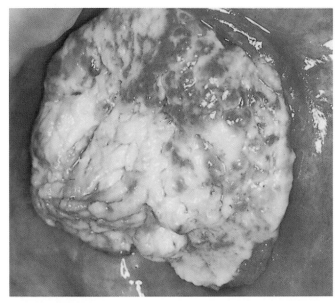

6.115

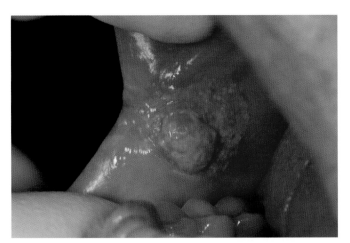

6.116

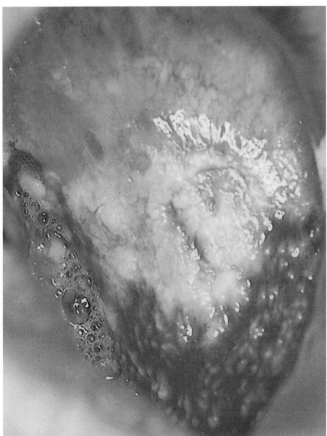

6.117

prognosis. Most common in elderly males, it typically affects the buccal mucosa and has a pebbly surface. A clinically similar condition, verrucous hyperplasia, is probably a variant.

Carcinoma of palate

Palatal carcinoma (**Fig. 6.119**) is very rare in the West but is fairly common in parts of the world where reverse cigarette smoking is practised (e.g. Andrah Pradesh, India; Philippines). Oropharyngeal carcinoma (**Fig. 6.120**) may be associated with human papillomavirus infection.

Carcinoma of antrum

For further information on this, see Chapter 14.

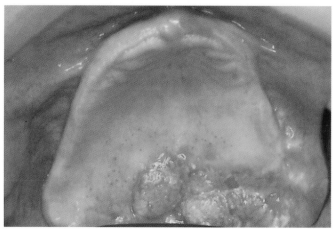

6.119

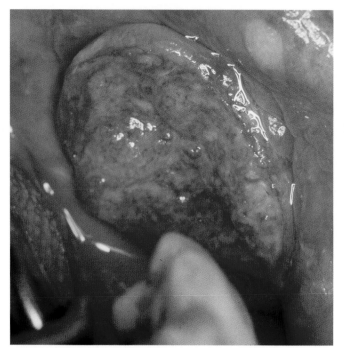

6.118

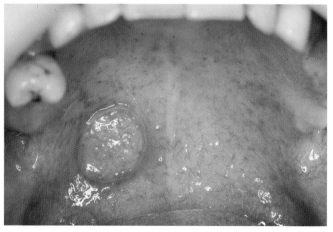

6.120

FURTHER READING

Bagan JV, Murillo J, Poveda R, Gavalda C, Jimenez Y, Scully C. Proliferative verrucous leukoplakia: unusual locations of oral squamous cell carcinomas, and field cancerization as shown by the appearance of multiple OSCCs. Oral Oncol 2004; 40(4): 440–3.

Bagan JV, Jimenez Y, Sanchis JM, et al. Proliferative verrucous leukoplakia; high incidence of gingival squamous cell carcinoma. J Oral Pathol Med 2003; 32: 379–82.

Calabrese L, Tradati N, Nickolas TL, Giugliano G, Zurrida S, Scully C, Boyle P, Chiesa F. Cancer screening in otorhinolaryngology. Oral Oncol 1998; 34: 1–4.

Chetty R, Hlatswayo N, Muc R, Sabaratnam R, Gatter K. Plasmablastic lymphoma in HIV+ patients: an expanding spectrum. Histopathology 2003; 42: 605–9.

Eckardt A, Schultze A. Maxillofacial manifestations of Langerhans cell histiocytosis: a clinical and therapeutic analysis of 10 patients. Oral Oncol 2003; 39(7): 687–94.

Favia G, Lo Muzio L, Serpico R, Maiorano E. Angiosarcoma of the head and neck with intra-oral presentation. A clinico-pathological study of four cases. Oral Oncol 2002; 38(8): 757–62.

Flaitz CM, Nichols CM, Walling DM, Hicks MJ. Plasmablastic lymphoma: an HIV-associated entity with primary oral manifestations. Oral Oncol 2002; 38: 96–102.

Genc A, Atalay T, Gedikoglu G, Zulfikar B, Kullu S. Leukemic children: clinical and histopathological gingival lesions. J Clin Pediatr Dent 1998; 22(3): 253–6.

Genden EM, Ferlito A, Scully C, Shaha AR, Higgins K, Rinaldo A. Current management of tonsillar cancer. Oral Oncol 2003; 39: 337–42.

Genden EM, Ferlito A, Bradley PJ, Rinaldo A, Scully C. Neck disease and distant metastases. Oral Oncol 2003; 39: 207–212.

Gu GM, Epstein JB, Morton TH Jr. Intraoral melanoma: long-term follow-up and implication for dental clinicians. A case report and literature review. Oral Surg Oral Med Oral Pathol Oral Radiol Endod 2003; 96(4): 404–13.

Hoagland HC. Myelodysplastic (preleukaemia) syndromes; the bone marrow factory failure problem. Mayo Clin Proc 1995; 70: 673–7.

Jaber MA, Porter SR, Speight P, Eveson JW, Scully C. Oral epithelial dysplasia: clinical characteristics of western European residents. Oral Oncol 2003; 39(6): 589–96.

Jordan RC, Regezi JA. Oral spindle cell neoplasms: a review of 307 cases. Oral Surg Oral Med Oral Pathol Oral Radiol Endod 2003; 95(6): 717–24.

Junior AT, de Abreu Alves F, Pinto CA, Carvalho AL, Kowalski LP, Lopes MA. Clinicopathological and immunohistochemical analysis of twenty-five head and neck osteosarcomas. Oral Oncol 2003; 39(5): 521–30.

Langdon J. The radiotherapeutic and surgical management of head and neck cancer. In Porter SR and Scully C (eds), Oral Health Care for Those with HIV Infection and Other Special Needs. Northwood, Science Reviews, 1995, pp. 175–87.

Langdon J, Henk J (eds). Malignant Tumours of the Mouth, Jaws and Salivary Glands. London, Edward Arnold; 1995.

Larsson A, Warfvinge G. Malignant transformation of oral lichen planus. Oral Oncol 2003; 39(6): 630–1.

Levy-Polack MP, Sebelli P, Polack NL. Incidence of oral complications and application of a preventive protocol in children with acute leukemia. Spec Care Dentist 1998; 18(5): 189–93.

Li N, Zhu W, Zuo S, Jia M, Sun J. Value of gallium-67 scanning in differentiation of malignant tumors from benign tumors or inflammatory disease in the oral and maxillofacial region. Oral Surg Oral Med Oral Pathol Oral Radiol Endod 2003; 96(3): 361–7.

Luker J. Leukaemias. In Porter SR and Scully C (eds), Oral Health Care for those with HIV Infection and Other Special Needs. Northwood, Science Reviews, 1995, pp. 111–16.

Meurman JH, Pyrhonen S, Teerenhovi L, Lindqvist C. Oral sources of septicaemia in patients with malignancies. Oral Oncol 1997; 33(6): 389–97.

Nikoui M, Lalonde B. Oro-dental manifestations of leukemia in children. J Can Dent Assoc 1996; 62(5): 443–6, 449–50.

Pandey M, Chandramohan K, Thomas G, et al. Soft tissue sarcoma of the head and neck region in adults. Int J Oral Maxillofac Surg 2003; 32(1): 43–8.

Pentenero M, Carrozzo M, Pagano M, Galliano D, Broccoletti R, Scully C, Gandolfo S. Oral mucosal dysplastic lesions and early squamous cell carcinomas: underdiagnosis from incisional biopsy. Oral Dis 2003; 9(2): 68–72.

Philipsen HP, Reichart PA, Takata T, Ogawa I. Verruciform xanthoma — biological profile of 282 oral lesions based on a literature survey with nine new cases from Japan. Oral Oncol 2003; 39(4): 325–36.

Porter SR, Diz Dios P, Kumar N, Stock C, Barrett AW, Scully C. Oral plasmablastic lymphoma in previously undiagnosed HIV disease. Oral Surg Oral Med Oral Pathol Oral Radiol Endod 1999; 87: 730–4.

Porter SR, Scully C. Early detection of oral cancer in the practice. Br Dent J 1998; 185: 72–73.

Rosenthal MA, Mougos S, Wiesenfeld D. High-grade maxillofacial osteosarcoma: evolving strategies for a curable cancer. Oral Oncol 2003; 39(4): 402–4.

Rozman C, Montserrat E. Chronic lymphocytic leukemia. N Engl J Med 1995; 333: 1052–7.

Ruiz-Arguelles GJ, Garces-Eisele J, Ruiz-Arguelles A. ATRA-induced gingival infiltration. Am J Hematol 1995; 49: 364–5.

Salisbury PL 3rd. Diagnosis and patient management of oral cancer. Dent Clin North Am 1997; 41(4): 891–914.

Salisbury PL 3rd, Caloss R Jr, Cruz JM, Powell BL, Cole R, Kohut RI. Mucormycosis of the mandible after dental extractions in a patient with acute myelogenous leukemia. Oral Surg Oral Med Oral Pathol Oral Radiol Endod 1997; 83(3): 340–4.

Schaedel R, Goldberg MH. Chronic lymphocytic leukemia of B-cell origin: oral manifestations and dental treatment planning. J Am Dent Assoc 1997; 128(2): 206–10.

Scully C. Oral malignancy: diagnosis. In Porter SR and Scully C (eds), Oral Health Care for Those with HIV and Other Special Needs. Northwood, Science Reviews, 1995, pp. 167–74.

Scully C. Oral precancer: preventive and medical approaches to management. Oral Oncol: Eur J Cancer 1995; 31B: 16–26.

Scully C. Aetiopathogenesis of intraoral squamous cell oral carcinoma. Contin Prof Develop Dent 2001; 2: 9–13.

Scully C. Oral squamous cell carcinoma; from an hypothesis about a virus, to concern about possible sexual transmission. Oral Oncol 2002; 38: 227–34.

Scully C, Bedi R. Ethnicity and oral cancer. Lancet Oncol 2000; 1: 37–42.

Scully C, Cawson RA. Potentially malignant oral lesions. J Epidemiol Biostat 1996; 1: 3–12.

Scully C, Epstein JB. Oral health care in cancer patients. Oral Oncol 1996; 32B: 281–92.

Scully C, Field J. Genetic aberrations in squamous cell carcinoma of the head and neck (SCCHN) with reference to oral carcinoma. Int J Oncol 1997; 10: 5–21.

Scully C, Ward-Booth P. Detection and treatment of early cancers of the oral cavity. Crit Rev Oncol/Haematol 1995; 21: 63–75.

Scully C, Sudbo J, Speight PM. Progress in determining the malignant potential of oral lesions. J Oral Pathol Med 2003; 32: 251–256.

Sepet E, Aytepe Z, Ozerkan AG, et al. Acute lymphoblastic leukemia: dental health of children in maintenance therapy. J Clin Pediatr Dent 1998; 22(3): 257–60.

Speight PM, Barrett AW. Salivary gland tumours. Oral Dis 2002; 8(5): 229–40.

Whitmyer CC, Esposito SJ, Terezhalmy GT. Radiotherapy for head and neck neoplasms. Gen Dent 1997; 45(4): 363–70; quiz 377–8.

7 HAMARTOMAS

- haemangioma
- lymphangioma.

HAEMANGIOMA

Haemangiomas are fairly common hamartomas in the mouth, especially seen on the lip (**Figs 7.1–7.13**). They are usually symptomless but may cause cosmetic problems if on the tongue and bitten, or because of aesthetics if on the face, if large (**Figs 7.5–7.9**) or because they lie in areas that my be breached during dental or oral surgical care (**Fig. 7.10**).

Some haemangiomas may result in partial enlargement of the soft tissues and underlying bone (Klippel– Trenaunay–Weber or angio-osteohypertrophy syndrome; see Chapter 28) and others may be part of the von Hippel–Lindau syndrome (involving the retina, cerebellum, spinal cord, kidneys, pancreas and liver, but not the mouth), Maffucci's or Sturge–Weber syndromes (see Chapter 28). Facial haemangiomas may rarely be associated with posterior fossa brain abnormalities often of the Dandy–Walker type.

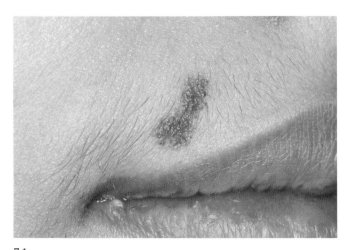

7.1

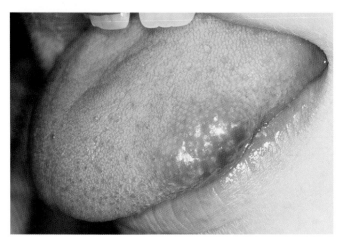

7.3

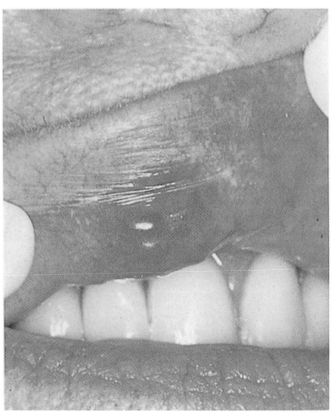

7.2

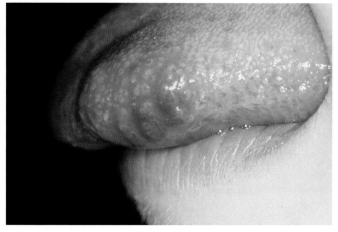

7.4

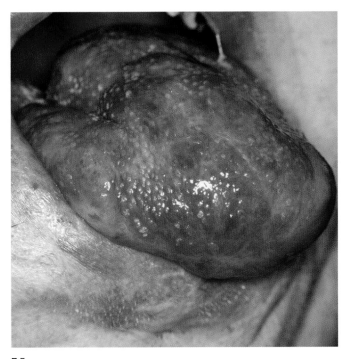

7.5

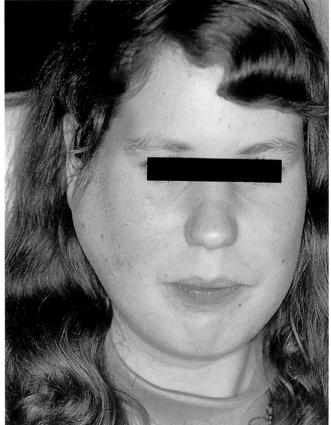

7.6

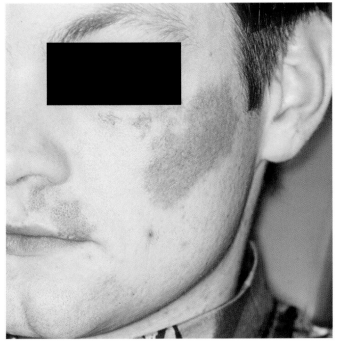

7.7

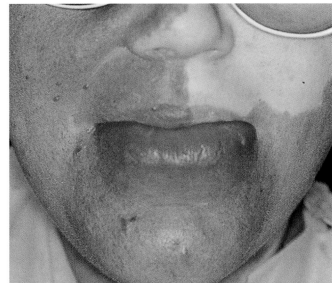

7.8

Figure 7.12 shows an intrabony arterio-venous malformation as opposed to a haemangioma which involved hard and soft tissues. Treatment for the lesion in Figure 7.12 and 7.13 was by selective embolisation followed by surgical removal of the contents of the mandible, which was then bonegrafted without actual resection, again with an excellent result.

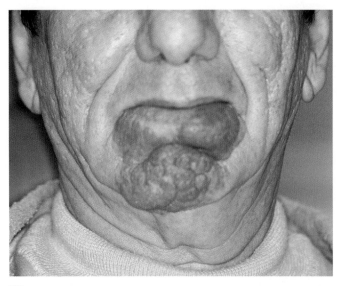

7.9

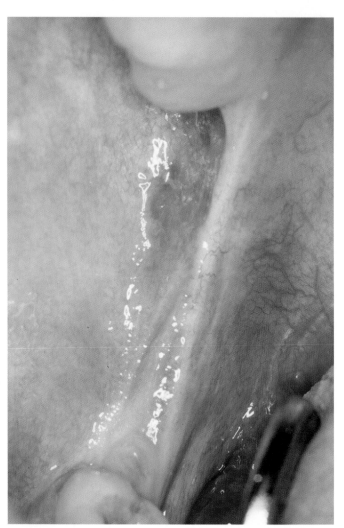

7.10

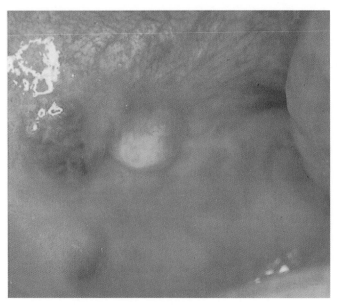

7.11

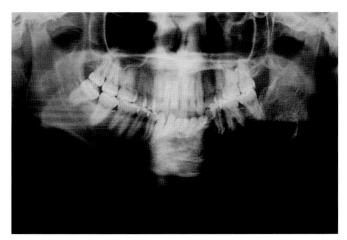

7.12

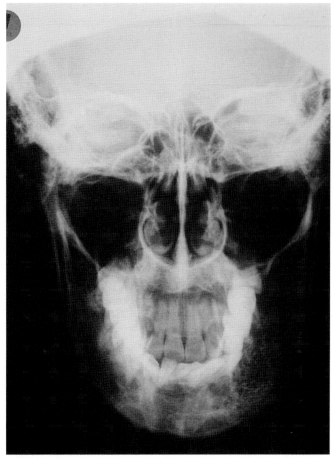

7.13

LYMPHANGIOMA

Lymphangioma is a hamartoma most common in the anterior tongue
(**Figs 7.14–7.16**) or lip (**Fig. 7.17**).

The typical 'frogspawn' appearance of the surface is seen in **Figs 7.15**
and **7.17**. There is often an angiomatous element.

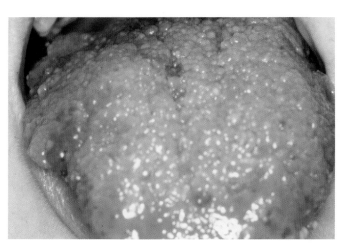

7.14

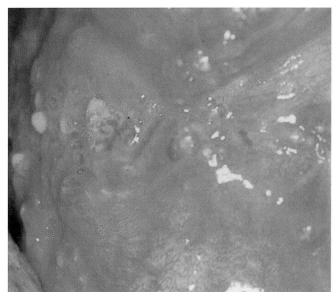

7.15

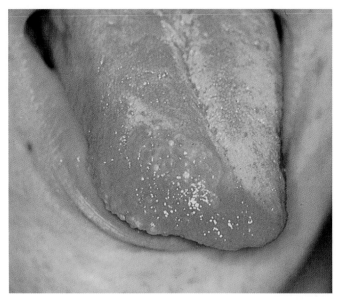

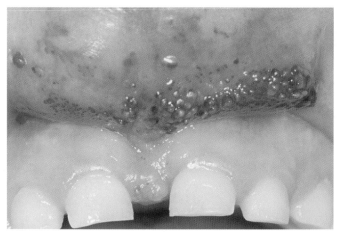

7.17

7.16

FURTHER READING

Andronikou S, McHugh K, Jadwat S, Linward J. MRI features of bilateral parotid haemangiomas of infancy. Eur Radiol 2003; 13(4): 711–16.

Childers EL, Furlong MA, Fanburg-Smith JC. Hemangioma of the salivary gland: a study of ten cases of a rarely biopsied/excised lesion. Ann Diagn Pathol 2002; 6(6): 339–44.

Flaitz CM. Oral and maxillofacial pathology case of the month. Lymphangioma. Tex Dent J 2000; 117: 65, 112–13.

Kaira N, Mahapatra GK, Srivastava D, Vaid L, Taneja HC. Hemangioma of the oral cavity in a seven year old: a case report. J Indian Soc Pedod Prev Dent 2002; 20(2): 49–50.

Orvidas LJ, Kasperbauer JL. Pediatric lymphangiomas of the head and neck. Ann Otol Rhinol Laryngol 2000; 109: 411–21.

Scolozzi P, Laurent F, Lombardi T, Richter M. Intraoral venous malformation presenting with multiple phleboliths. Oral Surg Oral Med Oral Pathol Oral Radiol Endod 2003; 96(2): 197–200.

Toida M, Hasegawa T, Watanabe F, et al. Lobular capillary hemangioma of the oral mucosa: clinicopathological study of 43 cases with a special reference to immunohistochemical characterization of the vascular elements. Pathol Int 2003; 53(1): 1–7.

Van Doorne L, De Maeseneer M, Stricker C, Vanrensbergen R, Stricker M. Diagnosis and treatment of vascular lesions of the lip. Br J Oral Maxillofac Surg 2002; 40(6): 497–503.

8 ENDOCRINE, NUTRITIONAL AND METABOLIC DISEASES

- acrodermatitis enteropathica
- acromegaly
- Addison's disease
- carcinoid syndrome
- Cushing's syndrome
- deficiency states
- diabetes mellitus
- glucagonoma
- hyperparathyroidism
- hypoparathyroidism
- hypophosphatasia
- hypothyroidism
- Lesch–Nyhan syndrome
- lipoid proteinosis
- mucopolysaccharidoses
- multiple endocrine adenoma syndrome type III (MEN type II b, or Schimke's syndrome).

ACRODERMATITIS ENTEROPATHICA

Acrodermatitis enteropathica is an inborn error of metabolism resulting in zinc malabsorption of unknown aetiology, and severe zinc deficiency. A vesiculobullous dermatitis with perioral involvement, often sparing the vermilion may be seen (**Figs 8.1, 8.2**). Angular cheilitis, characterized by erythema, maceration and ulcerations of the lip commissures, is frequently observed. Diarrhoea, mood changes, anorexia, neurological disturbance, growth retardation, alopecia, weight loss and recurrent infections are prevalent in affected children. Skin lesions and poor wound healing are observed in severe forms and the disorder can be lethal.

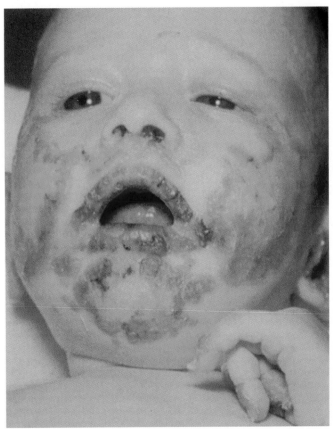

8.1

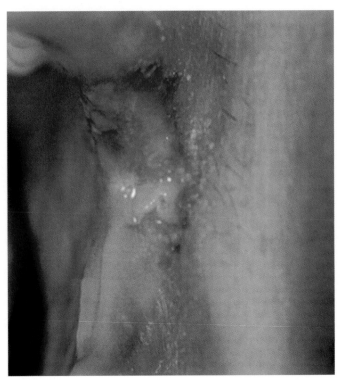

8.2

ACROMEGALY

Acromegaly results from increased growth hormone secretion by a pituitary adenoma. Typical signs are mandibular prognathism (**Figs 8.3–8.5**), generalized thickening of soft tissues, large hands and feet (**Fig. 8.6**), class III malocclusion (**Fig. 8.7**), eventual spacing of the teeth (**Fig. 8.8**) and a large tongue (**Fig. 8.9**).

Enlarged pituitary fossa, as a result of the causal pituitary adenoma, and enlarged supraorbital ridges and mandible may be obvious on radiography (**Fig. 8.10**). Headache and tunnel vision (bitemporal hemianopia) may eventually result as the pituitary neoplasm enlarges.

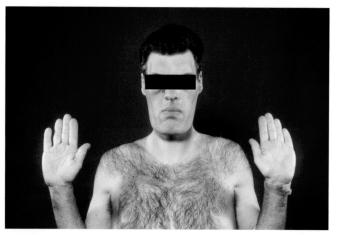

8.4

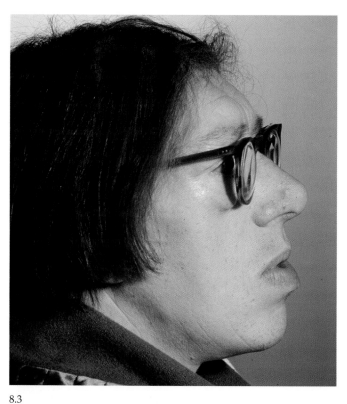

8.3

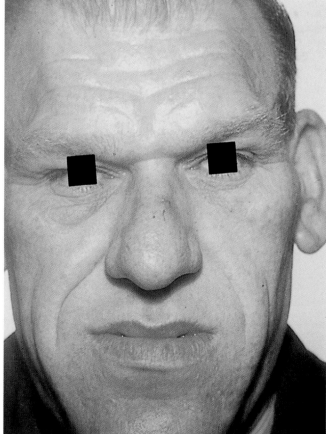

8.5

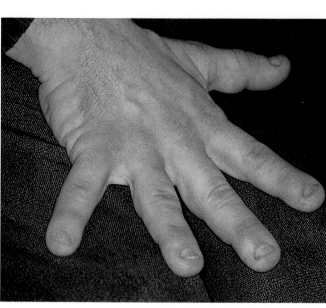

8.6

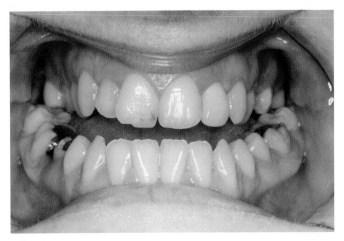

8.7

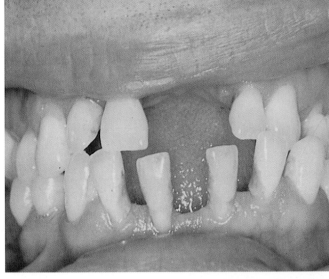

8.8

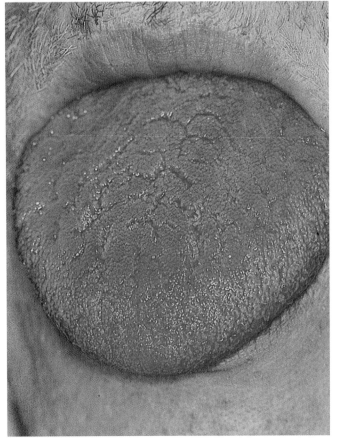

8.9

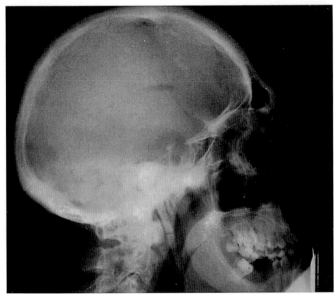

8.10

ADDISON'S DISEASE

Addison's disease is hypoadrenocorticism, often of autoimmune aetiology, but hypoadrenalism may be caused by a tumour, tuberculosis or, rarely, cytomegalovirus or histoplasmosis. Lower plasma cortisol levels result in increased pituitary secretion of adrenocorticotrophic hormone (ACTH) and precursor hormones with MSH-like activity.

Oral hyperpigmentation of a brown, grey or black colour, especially at sites of trauma such as the buccal mucosae or tongue, is typical of Addison's disease (**Fig. 8.11**), although most people with oral hyperpigmentation prove to have other causes.

Generalized skin hyperpigmentation is also seen (**Fig. 8.12**). The skin pigmentation is mainly in sun-exposed or traumatized sites, the areolae and genitalia. Similar hyperpigmentation is also seen in Nelson's syndrome (increased ACTH production after bilateral adrenalectomy).

There are occasional associations of Addison's disease with other diseases, particularly autoimmune diseases, such as the probable TASS syndrome, i.e. thyroiditis, Addison's disease, Sjögren's syndrome and sarcoidosis.

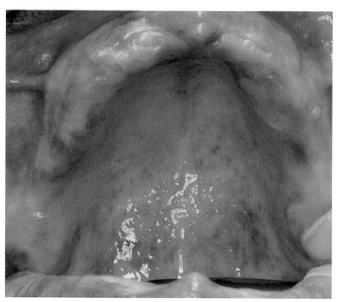

8.11

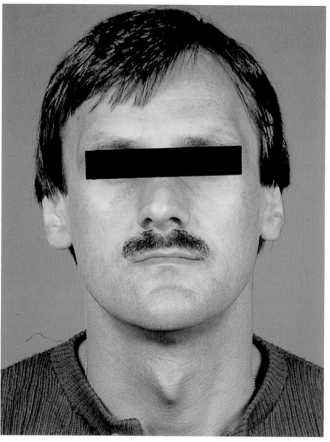

8.12

CARCINOID SYNDROME

Flushing of the face and neck with telangiectasia and sometimes periorbital oedema may be seen in this syndrome.

CUSHING'S SYNDROME

Cushing's *syndrome* arises when glucocorticoid levels are increased from any source, including iatrogenically. (Cushing's *disease* is the consequence of a pituitary adenoma oversecreting ACTH, thus stimulating excess adrenocortical activity.)

The typical features are truncal and facial obesity, hypertension, weakness, hirsutism, purplish abdominal striae, osteoporosis, amenorrhoea and glycosuria. The 'moon face' appearance is typical (**Fig. 8.13**).

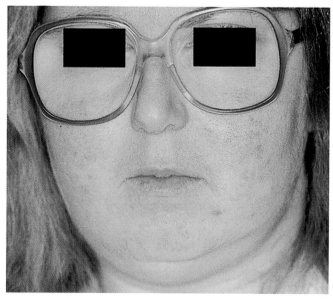

8.13

DEFICIENCY STATES

Deficiency of haematinics (iron, vitamin B_{12}, or folic acid) can manifest with glossitis, angular stomatitis and mouth ulcers. A significant proportion of patients with classical clinical aphthae prove to be deficient in a haematinic.

Vitamin B deficiency

The tongue is completely depapillated and smooth in vitamin B deficiency (**Fig. 8.14**). Oral ulcers and angular stomatitis are also common features. This particular child had coeliac disease, associated with selective IgA deficiency.

Angular stomatitis is seen particularly in vitamin B_{12} deficiency (**Fig. 8.15**) and riboflavin deficiency; it is also seen in iron or folate deficiency. The most common cause of angular stomatitis, however, is candidosis. Vitamin B_{12} deficiency is common in vegans but otherwise is rarely dietary in origin. More usually it is due to pernicious anaemia, gastric or small intestinal disease, or it follows gastrectomy. Gastric bypass surgery for morbid obesity is another surgical cause described.

Atrophic glossitis (**Fig. 8.16**) or red lines or red patches on the tongue (Moeller's glossitis; **Fig. 8.17**), are fairly typical of early vitamin B_{12} deficiency.

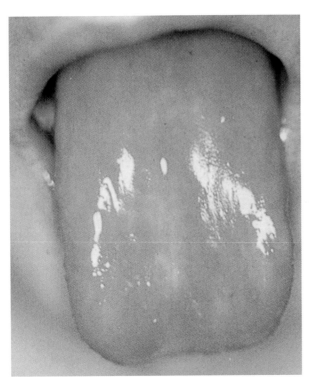

8.14

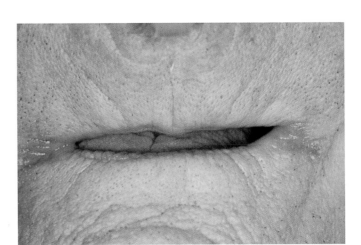

8.15

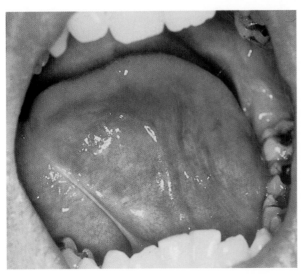

8.17

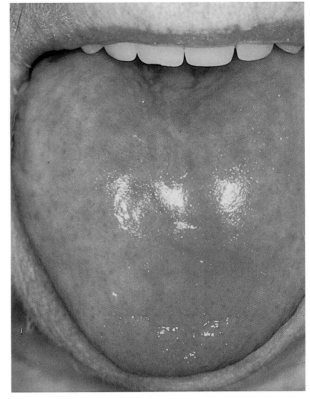

8.16

Pernicious anaemia is often characterized by premature greying of the hair and greying of blue eyes (**Fig. 8.18**). It may progress to neurological damage, especially subacute combined degeneration of the spinal cord. Mouth ulcers may be seen (**Fig. 8.19**).

Scurvy *(vitamin C deficiency)*
Scurvy is a rare cause of gingival swelling (**Figs 8.20, 8.21**) reminiscent of leukaemia. Most patients develop scurvy because they have an abnormal diet, lacking in fresh fruit and vegetables.

Perifollicular haemorrhages are typical of scurvy but occasionally there may be more severe purpura (**Fig. 8.22**). Cutaneous bleeding is most obvious on the legs and buttocks. Small subconjunctival haemorrhages may also be seen (**Fig. 8.23**).

Rickets *(vitamin D deficiency)*
Rickets (**Fig. 8.24**) is uncommon in western countries but has been recorded in Asian patients living in environments where they are exposed to relatively little sunlight and with a diet rich in phytate (found in chupatti flour), which chelates dietary calcium.

Enamel hypoplasia has been seen only in extremely severe rickets (**Fig. 8.25**) where tooth eruption may also be retarded (see also renal rickets).

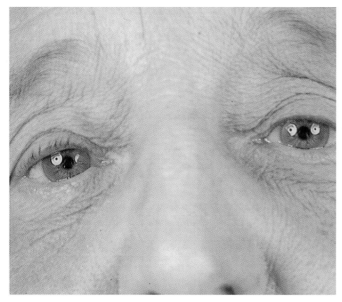

8.18

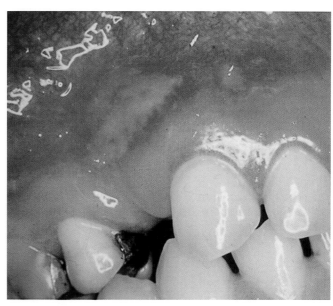

8.19

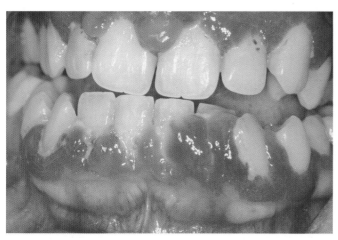

8.20

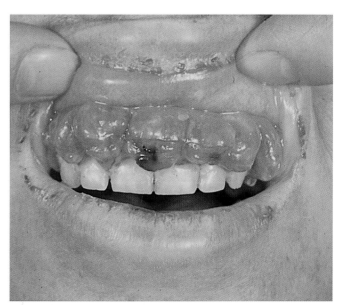

8.21

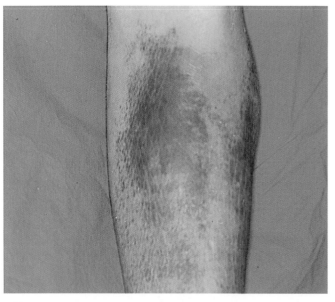

8.22

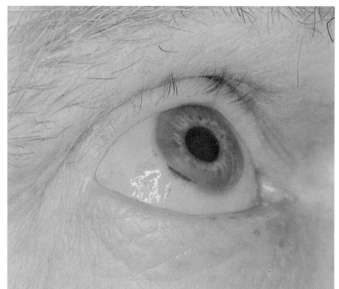

8.23

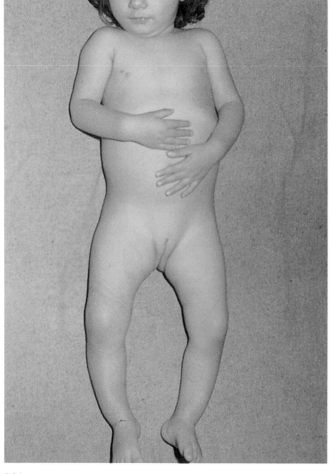

8.24

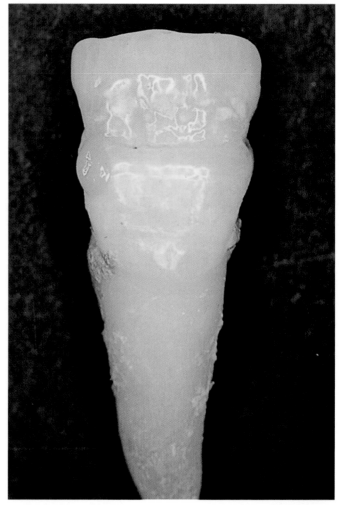

8.25

DIABETES MELLITUS

The oral changes in diabetes are nonspecific and seen mainly in severe insulin-dependent diabetics. Parodontal abscesses, infections and rapid periodontal breakdown are the most obvious features. **Figure 8.26** shows gingivitis mainly in the lower anterior region and an abscess above the upper lateral incisor, which proved to be an abscess related to the nonvital and discoloured central incisor.

Figure 8.27 shows severe periodontal breakdown in a diabetic (there is a healing lesion of herpes labialis on the upper lip).

Hyperglycaemia may result in ketosis and ketone bodies in the breath, which may cause pronounced halitosis. Osmotic diuresis leads to dehydration and often a dry mouth. Other oral lesions in diabetes may include candidosis sometimes with angular stomatitis (**Fig. 8.28**), sialosis, median rhomboid glossitis, glossodynia and lichenoid lesions induced by hypoglycaemic drugs. Autonomic neuropathy may cause xerostomia or gustatory sweating. Mucormycosis is a rare complication of diabetes (Chapter 4). Diabetic angiopathy rarely presents with palatal petechiae and diabetes has rare associations with acanthosis nigricans.

GLUCAGONOMA

Oral ulceration, glossitis and angular stomatitis can be seen in this condition.

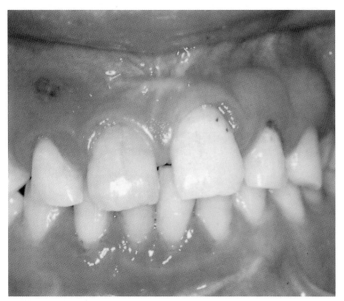

8.26

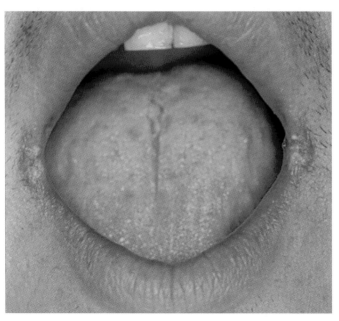

8.28

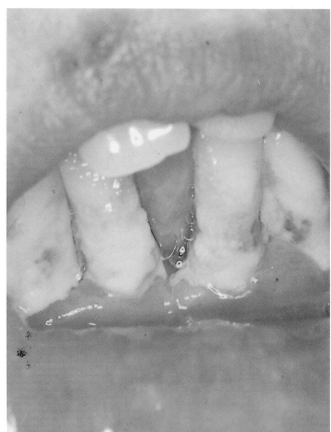

8.27

HYPERPARATHYROIDISM

Giant-cell granulomas are occasionally associated with hyperparathyroidism (**Fig. 8.29**). Skeletal changes in primary hyperparathyroidism typically include generalized rarefaction, and sometimes lytic lesions (osteitis fibrosa cystica), but an almost pathognomonic oral change is the loss of the lamina dura detectable by radiography (**Fig. 8.30**). Almost all patients with primary hyperparathyroidism have skeletal lesions microscopically indistinguishable from the central giant cell granuloma of bone (brown tumours). Skull and jaw involvement is a late complication (**Figs 8.31, 8.32**).

The characteristic radiographic sign of the condition is subperiosteal bone resorption and 'tufting' of the terminal phalanges (**Fig. 8.33**).

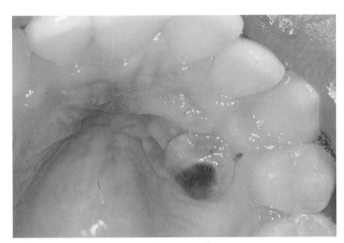

8.29

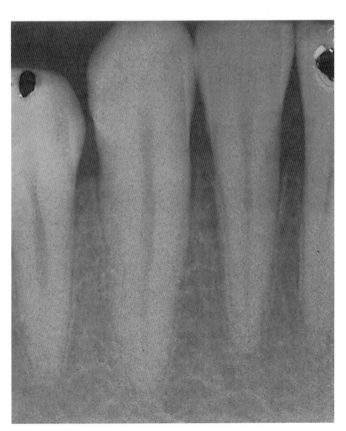

8.30

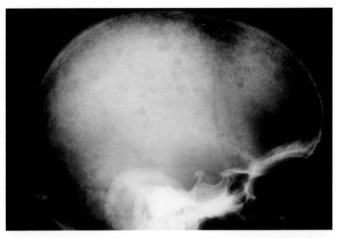

8.31

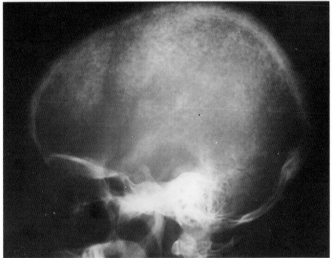

8.32

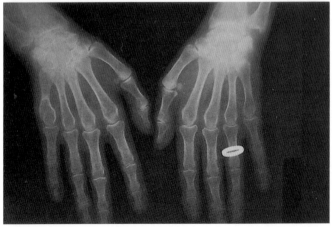

8.33

HYPOPARATHYROIDISM

In congenital hypoparathyroidism, there may be severe hypoplasia of the teeth (**Figs 8.34–8.39**), shortened roots and retarded eruption. Elfin facies (**Fig. 8.35**), short stature, short metatarsals and metacarpals (**Figs 8.36, 8.37**), calcified basal ganglia and enamel hypoplasia are features of the rare, complex, dominant disorder, which is possibly sex linked.

In pseudohypoparathyroidism (**Fig. 8.40**), parathyroid hormone is secreted but the end organs are unresponsive. There is also an association with other endocrine disorders, particularly hypothyroidism.

In rare patients with candidosis–endocrinopathy syndrome and with DiGeorge syndrome there is hypoparathyroidism with chronic mucocutaneous candidosis (Chapter 4).

Acquired hypoparathyroidism in adult life produces facial tetany but no oral manifestations.

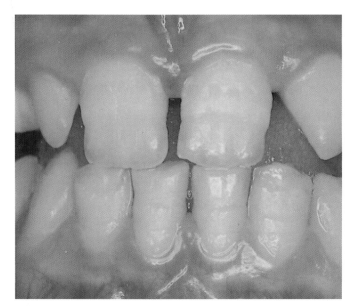

8.34

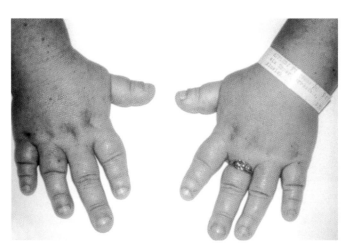

8.36

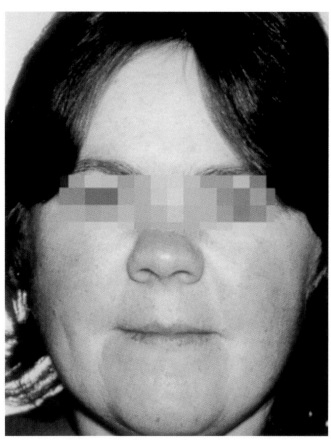

8.35

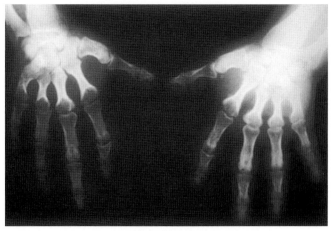

8.37

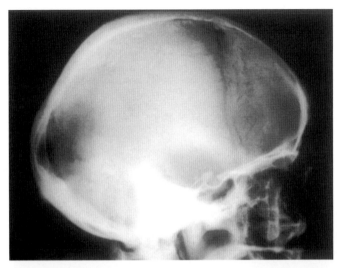

8.38

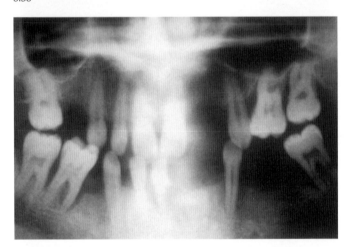

8.39

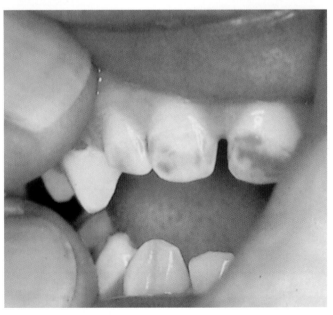

8.40

HYPOPHOSPHATASIA

In hypophosphatasia (vitamin D-resistant rickets; X-linked hypophosphataemia) there is a failure of proximal tubular phosphate reabsorption and defective vitamin D metabolism. Skeletal anomalies are common and the oral manifestations include cemental hypoplasia or aplasia, irregular calcification of the dentine, enlarged pulp chambers, and early loss of deciduous teeth (**Figs 8.41, 8.42**). The deciduous dentition is much more commonly affected than the permanent teeth.

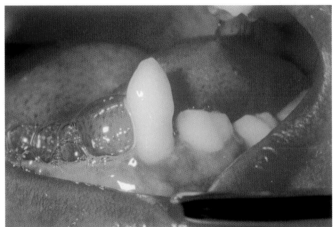

8.41

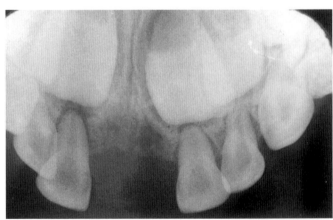

8.42

HYPOTHYROIDISM

Short stature, learning disability and coarse facies (**Fig. 8.43**) are the most obvious features of congenital hypothyroidism (cretinism). Oral changes include macroglossia, delayed eruption and hypoplasia of the teeth.

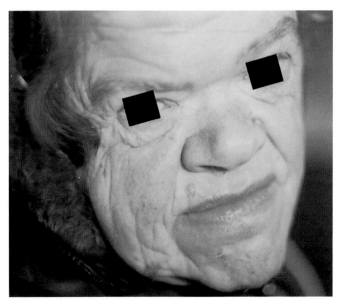

8.43

LESCH–NYHAN SYNDROME

Sex-linked hyperuricaemia, owing to deficiency of the enzyme hypoxanthine guanine phosphoribosyl transferase, is associated with learning disability, choreoathetosis and self-mutilation especially of the tongue and lip (**Fig. 8.44**).

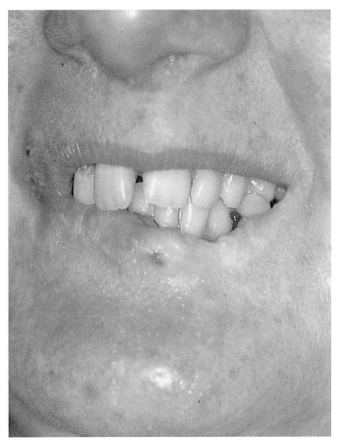

8.44

LIPOID PROTEINOSIS (Haylinosis cutis et mucosae, Urbach–Weithe disease)

Lipoid proteinosis is a rare genetically determined defect of collagen production giving rise to the deposits of hyaline-like material within the mucocutaneous dermis. The lips may be fissured and everted (**Fig. 8.45**) and there may be recurrent enlargement of the major salivary glands (typically the parotids) as a consequence of ductal obstruction. Xerostomia is rare.

The oral mucosa is commonly affected, becoming infiltrated with white elevated pea-size plaques in childhood. The tongue can become infiltrated and firm, with limited mobility, giving rise to dysphagia and dysarthria. Other oral manifestations of lipoid proteinosis may include gingival swelling (**Fig. 8.46**), hypodontia, enamel hypoplasia and yellow pigmentation of the dental crowns.

It has been suggested that penicillamine may be of some therapeutic benefit.

MUCOPOLYSACCHARIDOSES

Deficiency of mucopolysaccharidases leads to the accumulation of mucopolysaccharides (glycosaminoglycans) and to one of a number of syndromes, characterized by dwarfism, hirsutism, coarse features and macroglossia, often with learning diasability, deafness, cardiac failure and corneal clouding. Hurler's syndrome or gargoylism (**Figs 8.47–8.53**) is the most common of these disorders.

Hurler's syndrome manifests in early childhood with deteriorating mental and physical development. Hepatosplenomegaly causes abdominal swelling; umbilical hernia is common (see **Fig. 8.49**).

Characteristic 'claw hand' occurs because the joints cannot be fully extended (see **Fig. 8.50**). There are also flexion contractures in many other joints and talipes is common. There are frequent upper respiratory

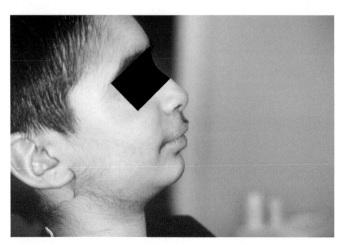

8.45

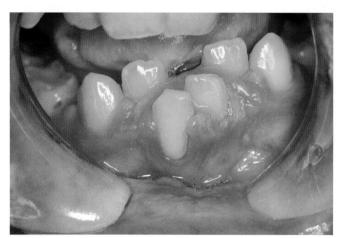

8.46

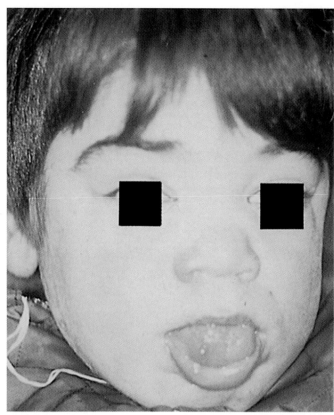

8.47

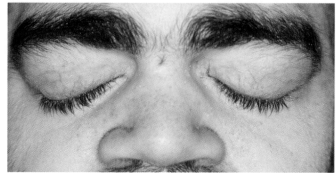

8.48

infections, cardiomegaly and murmurs. The head is large with premature closure of the sagittal and metopic sutures. The pituitary fossa is boot- or slipper-shaped (see **Fig. 8.52**). Delayed or incomplete eruption of teeth (see **Figs 8.51, 8.53**) and radiolucent lesions around the crowns of the lower second molars may be seen, as well as temporomandibular joint anomalies.

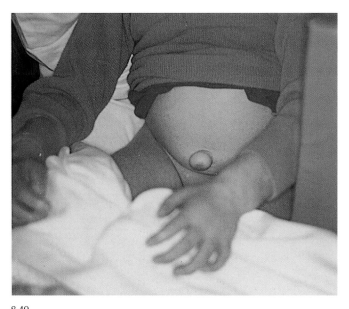

8.49

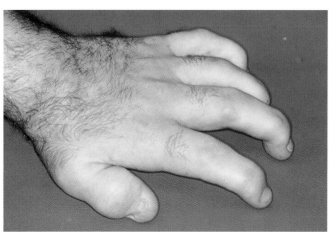

8.50

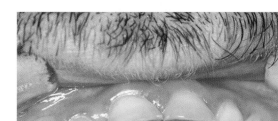

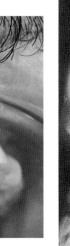

8.51

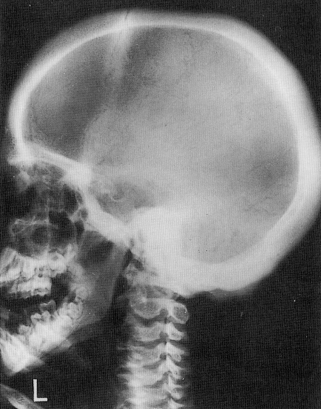

8.52

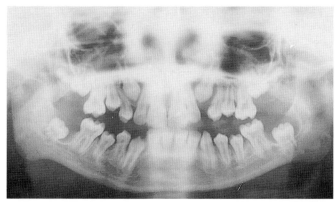

8.53

MULTIPLE ENDOCRINE ADENOMA SYNDROME TYPE III (*MEN Type IIb, or Schimke's syndrome*)

Medullary cell carcinoma of the thyroid, phaeochromocytoma and, occasionally, hyperparathyroidism characterize the type III (IIb)

multiple endocrine adenoma syndrome. Patients may have a marfanoid habitus and macroglossia. Neurofibromas and ganglioneuromatosis coli may also be seen. Mucosal neuromas may be seen on the lips, tongue, nasal and pharyngeal mucosae, conjunctivae and cornea (**Figs 8.54–8.56**).

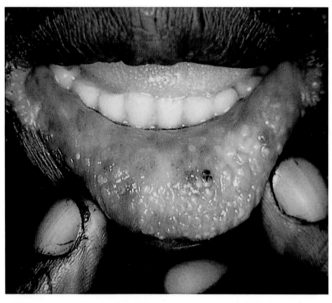

8.54

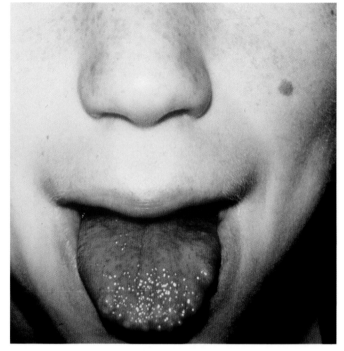

8.56

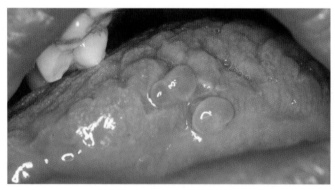

8.55

FURTHER READING

Arvio P, Arvio M, Wolf J, Lukinmaa PL, Saxen L, Pirinen S. Impaired oral health in patients with aspartylglucosaminuria. Oral Surg Oral Med Oral Pathol Oral Radiol Endod 1998; 86(5): 562–8.

Christgau M, Palitzsch KD, Schmalz G, Kreiner U, Frenzel S. Healing response to non-surgical periodontal therapy in patients with diabetes mellitus: clinical, microbiological, and immunologic results. J Clin Periodontol 1998; 25(2): 112–24.

Cleary MA, Francis DEM, Kilpatrick NM. Oral health implications in children with inborn errors of intermediary metabolism. Int J Paed Dent 1997; 7: 133–41.

Diaz-Arias AA, Bickel JT, Loy TS, *et al.* Follicular carcinoma with clear cell change arising in lingual thyroid. Oral Surg Oral Med Oral Pathol 1992; 74: 206–11.

Dougherty N, Gataletto MA. Oral sequelae of chronic neutrophil defects: case report of a child with glycogen storage disease type 1b. Pediatr Dent 1995; 17: 224–9.

Friedlander AH, Marder SR, Pisegna JR, Yagiela JA. Alcohol abuse and dependence: psychopathology, medical management and dental implications. J Am Dent Assoc 2003; 134(6): 731–40.

Haveman CW, Sloan TB, Long RT. Multiple endocrine neoplasia syndrome, type III: review and case report. Spec Care Dentist 1995; 15(3): 102–6.

Huber MA, Drake AJ 3rd. Pharmacology of the endocrine pancreas, adrenal cortex, and female reproductive organ. Dent Clin North Am 1996; 40(3): 753–77.

Kawamura M, Fukuda S, Kawabata K, Iwamoto Y. Comparison of health behaviour and oral/medical conditions in non-insulin-dependent (type II) diabetics and non-diabetics. Aust Dent J 1998; 43(5): 315–20.

Levin JA, Muzyka BC, Glick M. Dental management of patients with diabetes mellitus. Compend Contin Educ Dent 1996; 17(1): 82, 84, 86 passim.

Lingstrom P, Moynihan P. Nutrition, saliva, and oral health. Nutrition 2003; 19(6): 567–9.

Lowe G, Woodward M, Rumley A, Morrison C, Tunstall-Pedoe H, Stephen K. Total tooth loss and prevalent cardiovascular disease in men and women: possible roles of citrus fruit consumption, vitamin C, and inflammatory and thrombotic variables. J Clin Epidemiol 2003; 56(7): 694–700.

Martin W. Oral health and the older diabetic. Clin Geriatr Med 1999; 15(2): 339–50.

Mealey B. Diabetes and periodontal diseases. J Periodontol 1999; 70(8): 935–49.

Mealey BL. Impact of advances in diabetes care on dental treatment of the diabetic patient. Compend Contin Educ Dent 1998; 19(1): 41–4, 46–8, 50 passim; quiz 60.

Orth DN. Cushing's syndrome. N Engl J Med 1995; 332: 791–803.

Pinto A, Glick M. Management of patients with thyroid disease: oral health considerations. J Am Dent Assoc 2002; 133(7): 849–58.

Romito LM. Introduction to nutrition and oral health. Dent Clin North Am 2003; 47(2): 187–207.

Rose LF, Steinberg BJ, Atlas SL. Periodontal management of the medically compromised patient. Periodontol 2000 1995; 9: 165–75.

Sherman RG, Lasseter DH. Pharmacologic management of patients with diseases of the endocrine system. Dent Clin North Am 1996; 40(3): 727–52.

Slavkin HC. Diabetes, clinical dentistry and changing paradigms. J Am Dent Assoc 1997; 128(5): 638–44.

Stephenson E Jr, Haug RH, Murphy TA. Management of the diabetic oral and maxillofacial surgery patient. J Oral Maxillofac Surg 1995; 53(2): 175–82.

Taylor GW. Periodontal treatment and its effects on glycemic control: a review of the evidence. Oral Surg Oral Med Oral Pathol Oral Radiol Endod 1999; 87(3): 311–16.

Thomas G, Hoilat R, Daniels JS, Kalagie W. Ectopic lingual thyroid: a case report. Int J Oral Maxillofac Surg 2003; 32(2): 219–21.

Thomason JM, Girdler NM, Kendall-Taylor P, Wastell H, Weddel A, Seymour RA. An investigation into the need for supplementary steroids in organ transplant patients undergoing gingival surgery. A double-blind, split-mouth, cross-over study. J Clin Periodontol 1999; 26(9): 577–82.

Tinanoff N, Palmer CA. Dietary determinants of dental caries and dietary recommendations for preschool children. Refuat Hapeh Vehashinayim 2003; 20(2): 8–23, 78.

Touger-Decker R. Clinical and laboratory assessment of nutrition status in dental practice. Dent Clin North Am 2003; 47(2): 259–78.

Touger-Decker R, Mobley CC; American Dietetic Association. Position of the American Dietetic Association: Oral health and nutrition. J Am Diet Assoc 2003; 103(5): 615–25.

Williams JD, Slupchinsku O, Sclafani AP, et al. Evaluation and management of the lingual thyroid gland. Ann Otol Rhinol Laryngol 1996; 105: 312–16.

9 IMMUNE DISORDERS

- amyloidosis
- hereditary angioedema
- genetically based immune defects
- human immunodeficiency virus (HIV) disease.

AMYLOIDOSIS

Amyloidosis is a group of diseases in which one of a range of materials is deposited in tissues. Deposits are sufficiently large in size to give a characteristically fibrillar structure on electron microscopy, and green birefringence on polarization microscopy after Congo red staining. Amyloid L arises from immunoglobulin light chains, amyloid A from amyloid A protein, and others are from prealbumin, gamma-trace protein or β_2-microglobulin.

Primary amyloidosis — that associated with plasma cell dyscrasias — particularly affects males over the age of 50 years and is the type of amyloid most commonly associated with deposits in the oral mucosa and sub-endocardium. Macroglossia is typical. The tongue is large, firm and indurated and may show red nodules and/or petechiae, especially at the lateral margins (**Figs 9.1–9.3**); rarely there may be gingival (**Fig. 9.4**) or labial enlargement. Petechiae, ecchymoses or blood-filled blisters may be seen (**Figs 9.5, 9.6**), as there is an acquired deficiency of blood coagulation factor X in patients with the light chain type of amyloid found in plasma cell dyscrasias.

Figure 9.7 shows subconjunctival haemorrhage in the patient shown in **Fig. 9.1**, who subsequently died from amyloid nephropathy, detected through his heavy proteinuria and glycosuria.

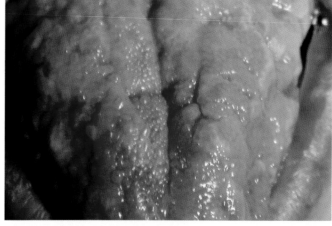

9.3

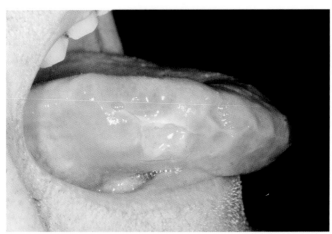

9.1

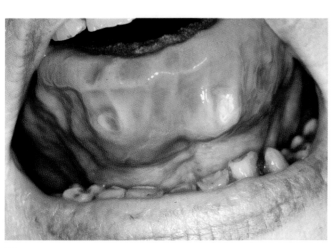

9.2

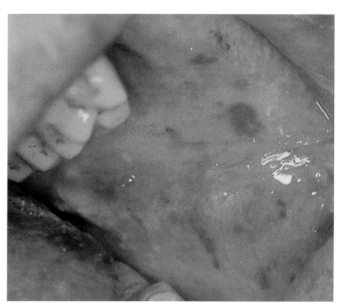

9.4

9.5

Secondary types of amyloidosis — most of those associated with deposits other than of light chains — rarely affect the mouth.

The tongue may be involved in β_2-microglobulin amyloidosis in patients on long-term haemodialysis.

HEREDITARY ANGIOEDEMA

Hereditary angioedema (HANE) is a familial condition transmitted as an autosomal dominant trait, which is not an immune defect as such but is due to a decreased or defective inhibitor of the activated first component of complement (C1). The episodes of angioedema are often precipitated by mild trauma, such as that associated with dental treatment.

Immune diseases occasionally associated with HANE are a lupus-like syndrome, coronary arteritis and autoimmune conditions, including Sjögren's syndrome, rheumatoid arthritis and thyroiditis, possibly because of disturbed immunoregulation.

C1-esterase deficiency is occasionally acquired, especially in lymphoproliferative disorders.

Swelling of the face, mouth and neck (**Fig. 9.8**) in angioedema may embarrass the airway. **Figure 9.9** is the same patient as in **Fig. 9.8** but seen between episodes. There may also be swelling of the abdominal viscera and extremities.

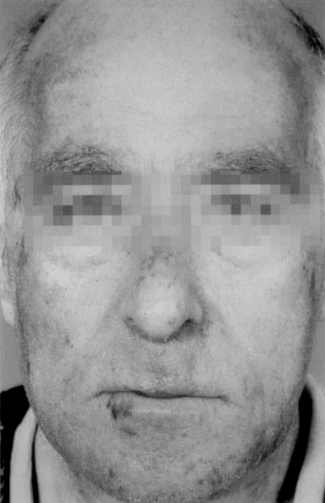

9.6

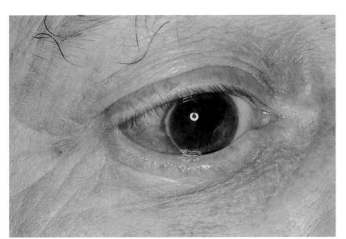

9.7

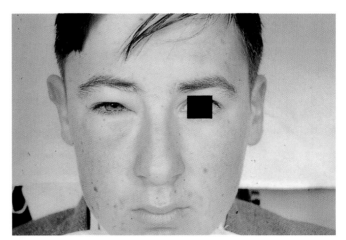

9.8

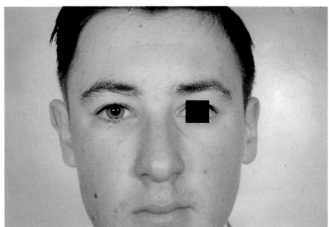

9.9

GENETICALLY BASED IMMUNE DEFECTS

Agammaglobulinaemia *(Bruton's syndrome)*

Panhypoimmunoglobulin aemia affects males almost exclusively and presents mainly with recurrent pyogenic respiratory infections. Several patients with mouth ulcers have been recorded (**Fig. 9.10**).

Severe infections in the neonate can disturb odontogenesis causing enamel hypoplasia (**Fig 9.11**). In the past, tetracycline treatment caused tooth discoloration.

Cell-mediated immunodeficiency

Chronic oral candidosis, which may present with angular stomatitis, is an early and prominent feature in any cell-mediated immune defect (**Fig. 9.12**), and there is a predisposition to recurrent lesions of herpes simplex and varicella-zoster virus.

Oral thrush (**Fig. 9.13**) is an early feature of many T-lymphocyte defects. Herpes labialis is often reactivated during immunosuppression of the cellular response, as in this patient (**Fig. 9.14**) on systemic corticosteroids (see below for discussion of HIV disease).

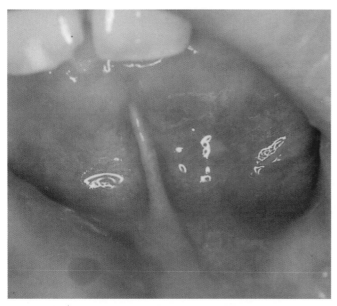

9.10

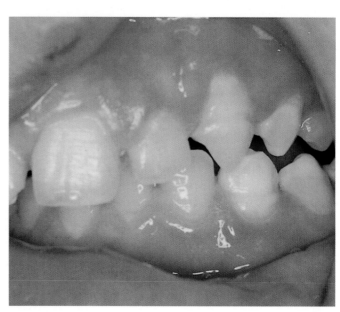

9.11

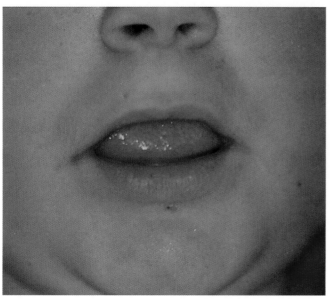

9.12

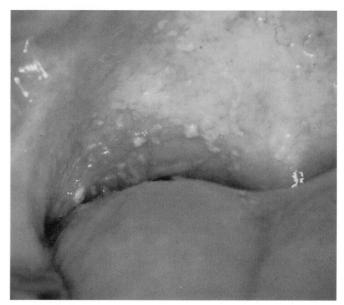

9.13

Job syndrome *(hyper-IgE syndrome)*
Job syndrome is a rare primary immunodeficiency disorder characterized by extremely high levels of serum immunoglobulin E (IgE) and recurrent serious staphylococcal infections of the skin, lungs and joints. Associated features include coarse facies, cold cutaneous abscesses, eczematous rashes and osteopenia. The oral manifestations of Job syndrome include enhanced gingivitis, accelerated periodontitis and oral ulceration (**Figs 9.15–9.18**).

Selective IgA deficiency
Selective IgA deficiency is the most common primary (genetically determined) immune defect. Some patients are healthy but those who

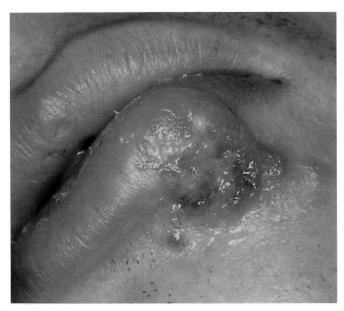

9.14

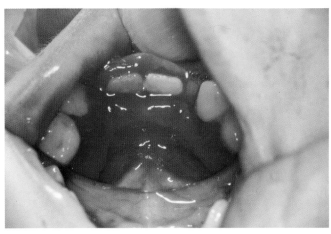

9.15

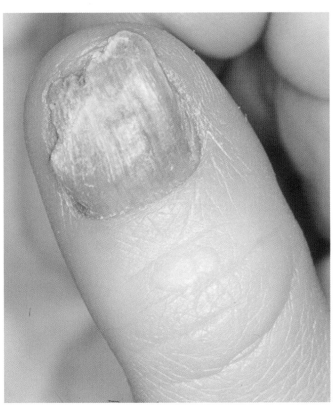

9.16

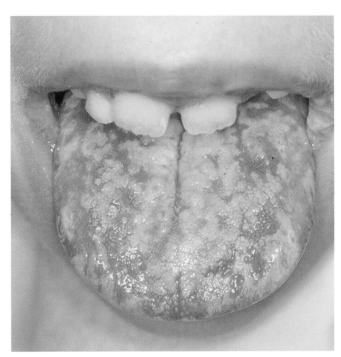

9.17

also lack IgG$_2$ suffer recurrent respiratory infection, autoimmune disorders and atopy. Many have mouth ulcers (**Fig. 9.19**) and there may be a reduced protection against dental caries.

Wiskott–Aldrich syndrome

Wiskott–Aldrich syndrome is the association of thrombocytopenia with immunodeficiency and eczema (TIE syndrome), which may manifest with oral purpura (**Fig. 9.20**).

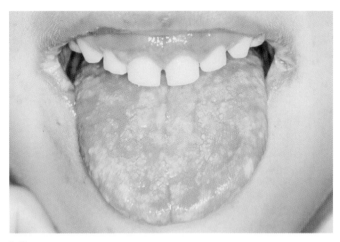

9.18

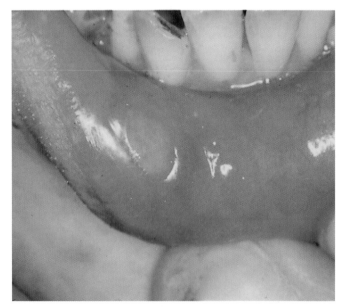

9.19

9.20

HUMAN IMMUNODEFICIENCY VIRUS (HIV) DISEASE

The orofacial manifestations of HIV disease have been significantly influenced by Highly Active Antiretroviral Therapy (HAART) such that many of the lesions discussed below may not arise in treated persons, or may resolve or manifest less profoundly. Nevertheless the majority of HIV-infected persons do not have ready access to such therapies, and indeed HAART can itself give rise to a wide range of oral features: for example, zoster and warts are more common in patients on HAART.

Infection with HIV may cause an initial glandular fever-like illness but this may be asymptomatic. The incubation period (i.e. the time from infection to AIDS) may extend over very many years, depending upon the patient's degree of deprivation and the ability to receive and tolerate HAART.

Infections are common in HIV disease. Oral candidosis, especially thrush, is the most common oral feature of HIV disease and is seen in over 90% of HIV-infected patients (**Fig. 9.21**). It may be a predictor of other opportunistic infections and of oesophageal thrush. Extensive and chronic oral candidosis in HIV disease (**Fig. 9.22**) may become resistant to fluconazole. Other types of oral candidosis may be seen, including angular stomatitis (**Fig. 9.23**), which in non-HIV-infected persons is usually a local infection, emanating from a reservoir of *Candida* beneath an upper denture.

Erythematous candidosis is another common feature, and is seen especially in the palate (**Fig. 9.24**) where it may produce a thumb-print-

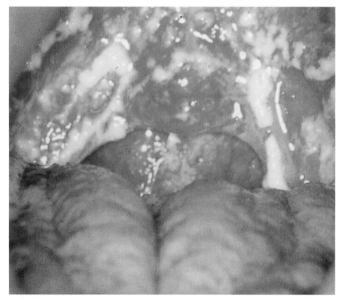

9.21

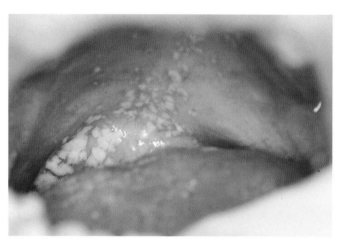

9.22

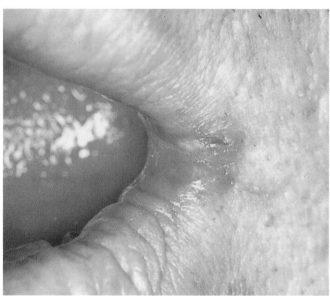

9.23

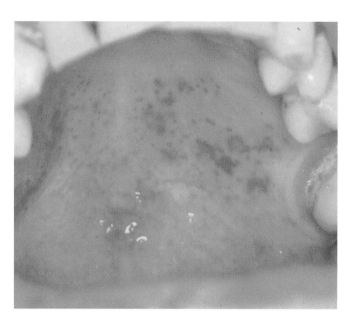

9.24

type pattern (**Figs 9.25, 9.26**). Red lesions of candidosis, such as erythematous candidosis on the tongue, may be multifocal (**Fig. 9.27**), median rhomboid glossitis or others (**Fig. 9.28**) and may be overlooked by the uninitiated.

Viral infections are also common; unusual infections or combinations of lesions may be seen in HIV disease, such as candidosis plus herpes labialis (**Fig. 9.29**). Recurrent herpes simplex infection may be intraoral in HIV/AIDS (**Fig. 9.30**), often as a dendritic ulcer in the midline dorsum

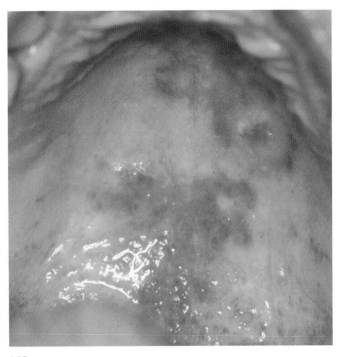

9.25

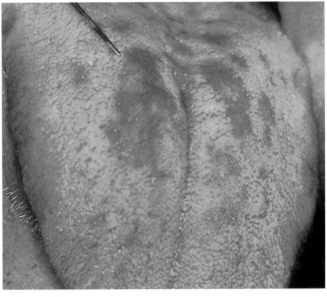

9.27

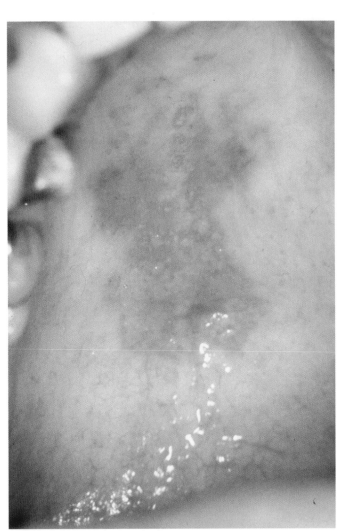

9.26

of the tongue (**Fig. 9.31**). Chronic herpetic lesions in HIV disease (**Fig. 9.32**) can occasionally become resistant to aciclovir, in which cases foscarnet may be required.

Ulcers may also be caused by cytomegalovirus (CMV), alone or in association with herpes simplex virus (**Figs 9.33, 9.34**). In HIV disease, chronic oral ulcers associated with CMV infection typically occur when the infection is disseminated.

Hairy leukoplakia of the tongue is a common feature of HIV disease (**Figs 9.35–9.39**) caused by Epstein–Barr virus (EBV). This lesion is not known to be premalignant although in patients who do not receive HAART it may be a predictor of bad prognosis and of lymphoma elsewhere. Flat white lesions may be seen on the tongue in about one-third of cases. Mild hairy leukoplakia may be overlooked (see **Fig. 9.39**) and hairy leukoplakia is typically more corrugated than it is hairy.

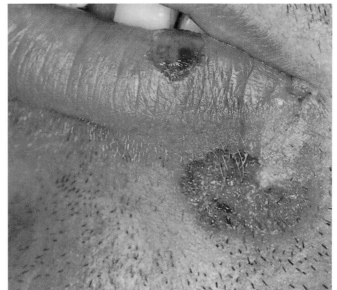

9.29

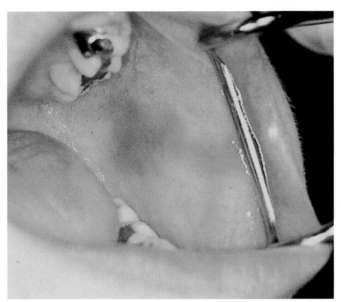

9.28

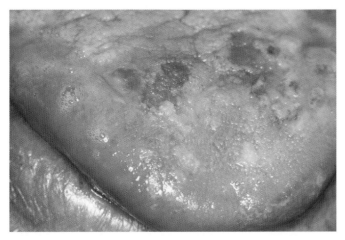

9.30

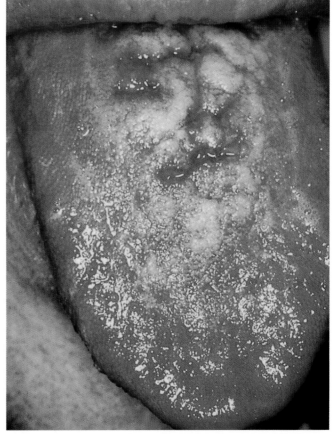

9.31

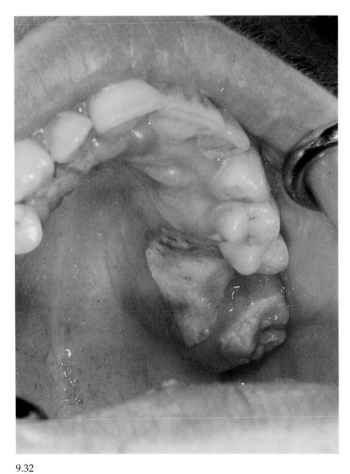

9.32

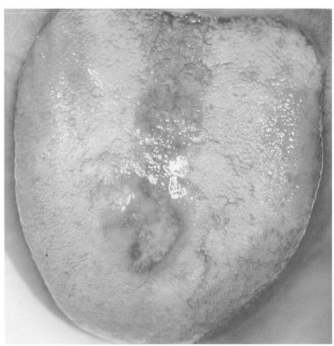

9.33

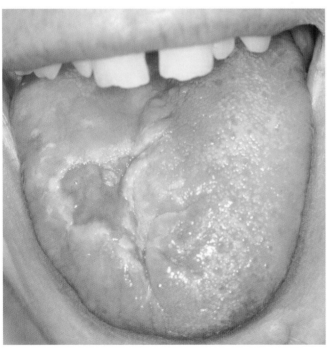

9.34

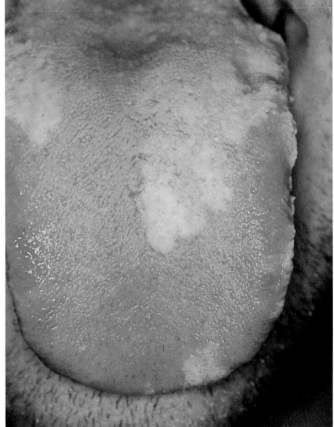

9.35

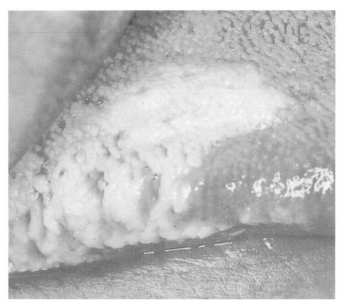

9.36

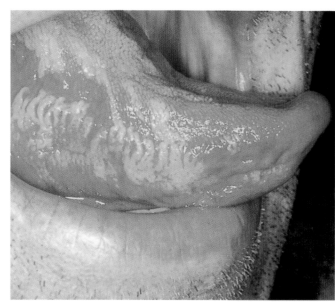

9.37

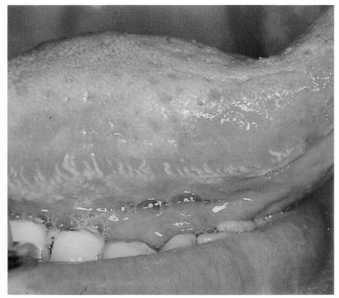

9.38

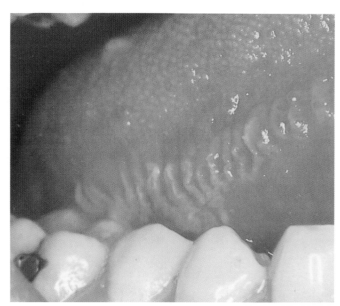

9.39

Hairy leukoplakia is usually bilateral on the lateral margins and the ventrum of the tongue and can simulate candidosis. It may resolve with HAART, aciclovir or ganciclovir.

Other viral infections — including human papillomavirus (HPV) infections and types of papillomavirus which are uncommonly associated with oral lesions — can cause oral lesions in HIV-infected persons, in particular genital warts (condyloma accuminata; **Figs 9.40, 9.41**).

Varicella-zoster virus infection may supervene in AIDS (**Fig. 9.42**) and even in the absence of ophthalmic zoster, may cause retinal damage.

Kaposi's sarcoma (KS), caused by human herpesvirus type 8 (HHV-8), is a late feature of sexually transmitted infection with HIV, especially in men who have sex with men, but may be seen occasionally in other groups of immunocompromised patients. **Figure 9.43** is KS in an African patient with diabetes mellitus following renal transplantation whose HIV status was uncertain.

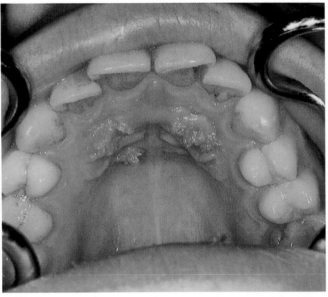

9.40

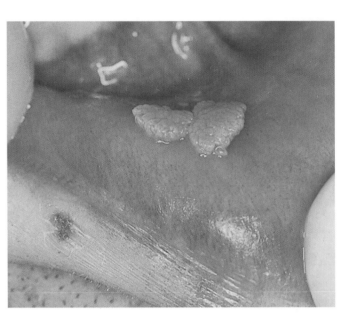

9.41

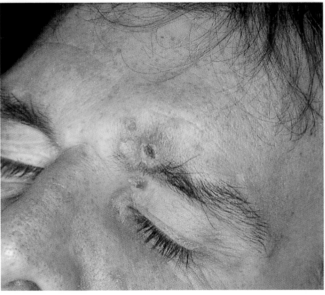

9.42

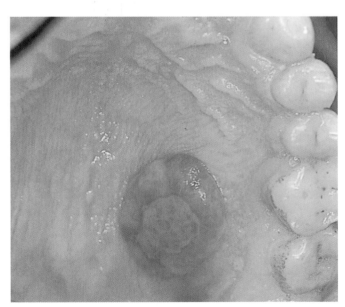

9.43

Oral lesions of KS are macules or nodules, red to purple in colour, and most common on the palate. Multiple KS are common (**Figs 9.44–9.51**). Kaposi's sarcoma is not uncommon extraorally, especially on the nose (**Fig. 9.48**). Epithelioid angiomatosis, a bacterial infection with *Bartonella henselae* or *B. quintana*, is the main differential diagnosis (**Fig. 9.52**).

Molluscum contagiosum is another viral infection that may complicate HIV disease (**Fig. 9.53**).

Lymphomas (typically non-Hodgkin's lymphomas) may be seen in the oropharynx or fauces, and are often associated with EBV (**Figs 9.54, 9.55**). Of note, plasmablastic lymphoma (**Fig. 9.54**) occurs almost exclusively in the mouths of patients with HIV disease.

Squamous carcinomas have also occurred, albeit rarely (**Fig. 9.56**), and may be associated with HPV. Basal cell carcinomas may be seen rarely (**Fig. 9.47**; note also the KS).

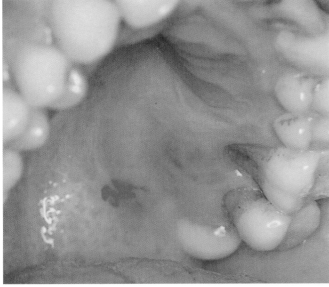

9.44

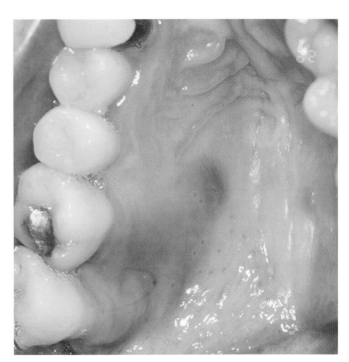

9.45

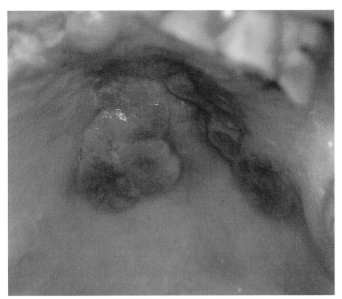

9.46

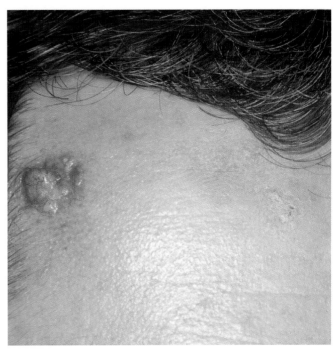

9.47

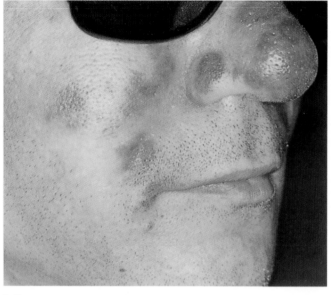

9.48

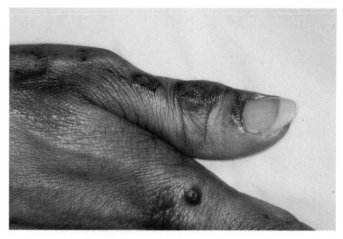

9.49

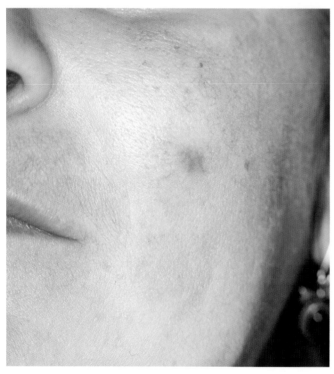

9.50

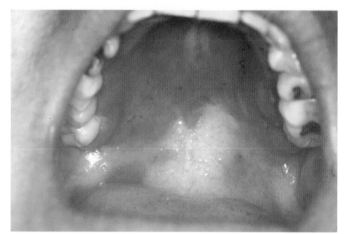

9.51

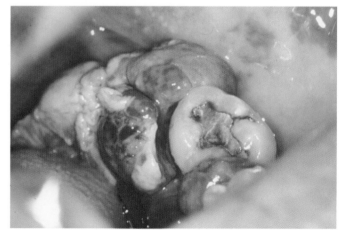

9.52

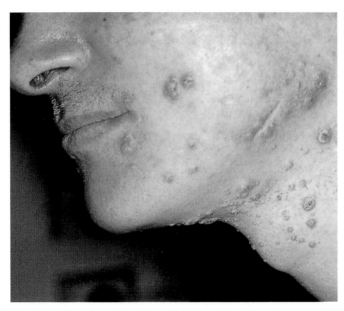

9.53

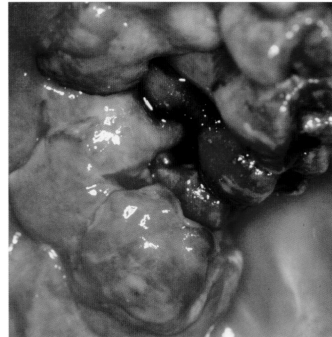

9.54

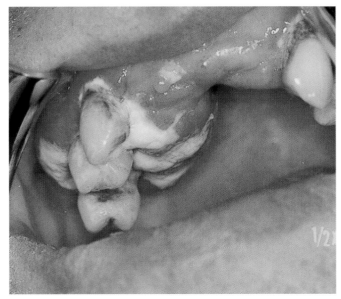

9.55

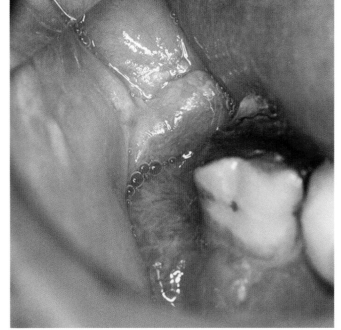

9.56

Periodontal features of HIV infection include mainly ulcerative gingivitis and destructive periodontitis (**Figs 9.57–9.65**). The ulcerative or necrotizing lesions may be widespread and chronic (see **Fig. 9.61**), although localized necrotic periodontal lesions may arise. Periodontal necrosis may result not only from periodontitis but also from viral or fungal infections, or KS. Localized destructive periodontal lesions are not uncommon and alveolar sequestration may follow (see **Fig. 9.64**).

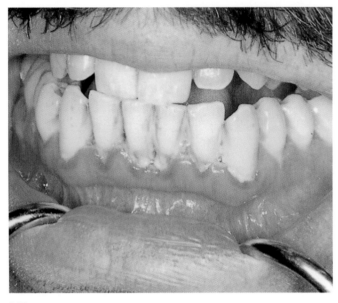

9.57

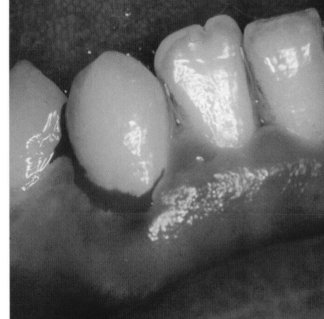

9.58

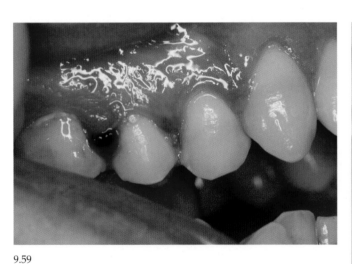

9.59

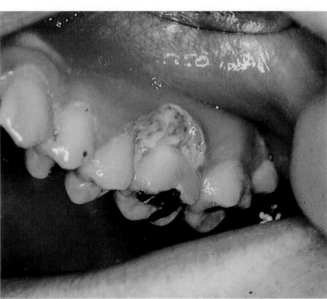

9.60

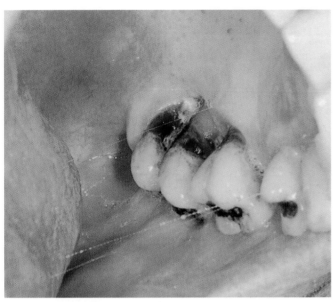

9.61

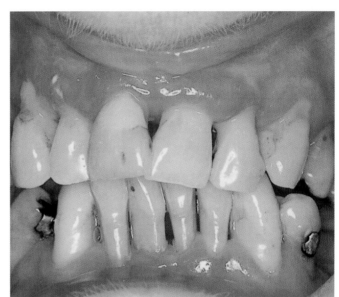

9.62

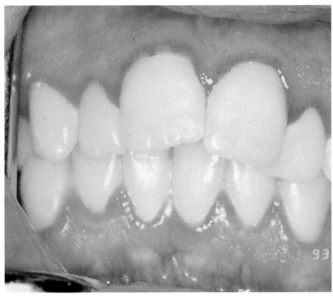

9.63

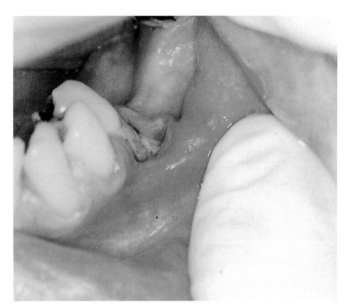

9.64

Finally, linear gingival erythema is sometimes seen in HIV disease (see **Fig. 9.65**) but necrotic lesions are more sinister. Other bacterial infections in HIV disease include syphilis (**Fig. 9.66**) and tuberculosis (chapter 3).

Oral or cutaneous lesions of deep mycoses are uncommon in many areas of the world, although increasingly common in patients with severe HIV disease. *Histoplasma capsulatum*, the causal organism of histoplasmosis — the most common deep mycosis — is found particularly in north-eastern and central USA. It is found especially in bird and bat faeces and in the endemic areas as it is a soil saprophyte. In these areas, over 70% of all adults appear to be infected, typically subclinically. Clinical presentations include acute and chronic pulmonary, cutaneous and disseminated histoplasmosis, the latter of which can affect the reticuloendothelial system, lungs, kidneys and gastrointestinal tract and is typically seen in HIV infection (**Figs 9.66–9.69**) and in other immunocompromised persons.

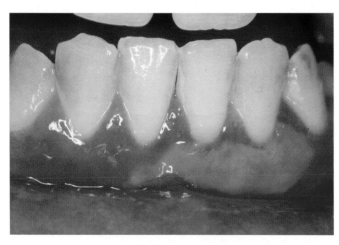

9.65

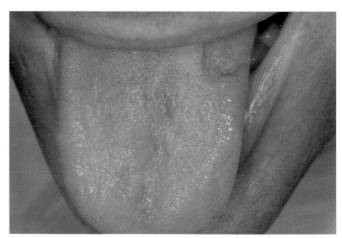

9.66

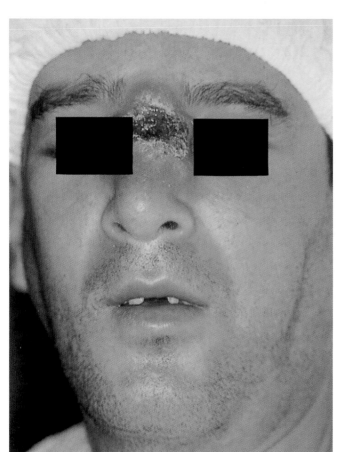

9.67

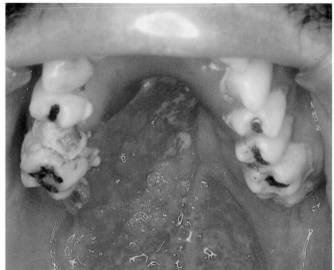

9.68

Oral lesions of *H. capsulatum* infection have been recorded in persons with pulmonary or disseminated histoplasmosis. The oral lesions are usually ulcerative or nodular, have been found on the tongue, palate, buccal mucosa or gingiva, and, rarely, have invaded the jaws. Less common are oral lesions of cryptococcosis, blastomycosis or paracoccidioidomycosis (**Fig. 9.70**).

Oral ulceration seen in HIV disease can have a range of causes. Aphthous-type ulcers, especially of the major type (**Figs 9.71–9.74**), may appear in HIV disease. Mouth ulcers are also occasionally caused by opportunistic pathogens such as herpes viruses, CMV (sometimes in combination), mycobacteria and, rarely, by *Histoplasma Cryptococcus* or *Leishmaniasis*.

Rarely HAART may give rise to erythema multiforme, and HIV-infected patients may be liable to toxic epidermal necrolysis (TEN). Necrotizing stomatitis can be a complication, and syphilis may present atypically (**Fig. 9.75**). Localized osteitis (**Fig. 9.76**), osteomyelitis and other severe oral infections may supervene in AIDS (**Fig. 9.77**). Intrauterine infection with HIV may rarely cause facial dysmorphogenesis and a fetal AIDS syndrome.

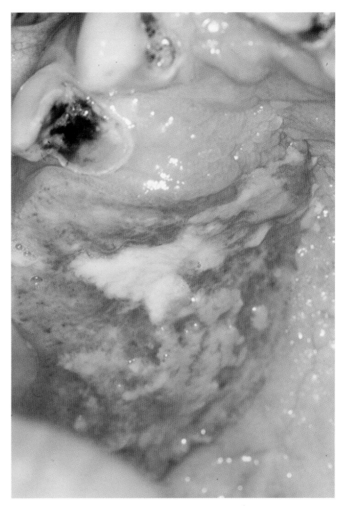

9.70

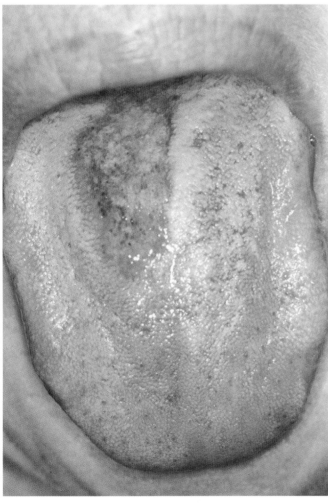

9.69

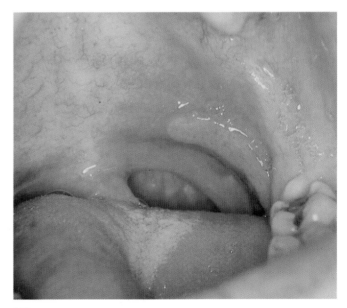

9.71

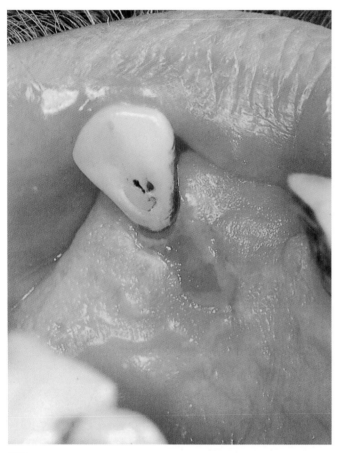

9.72

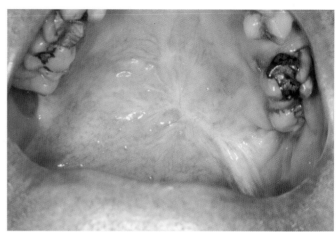

9.73

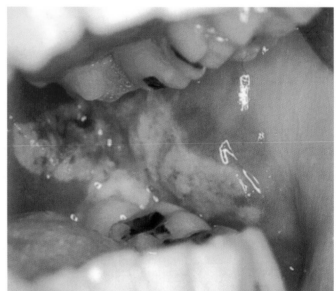

9.74

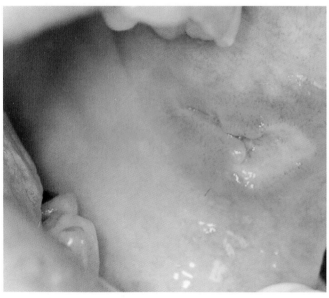

9.75

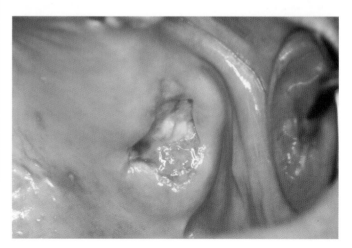

9.76

Other oral and perioral lesions in HIV infection include cervical lymph node enlargement, cheilitis (**Fig. 9.78**), petechiae (**Fig. 9.79**), cranial neuropathies and parotitis. Salivary gland swelling and xerostomia may arise in about 6% of patients with HIV infection (**Figs 9.80, 9.81**) mainly in children, and as part of diffuse lymphocytosis syndrome (DILS). Xerostomia can also arise from drug use, especially didanosine and some protease inhibitor drugs and can lead to caries (**Fig. 9.81**). Lichenoid lesions may rarely occur (**Fig. 9.82**; note that the

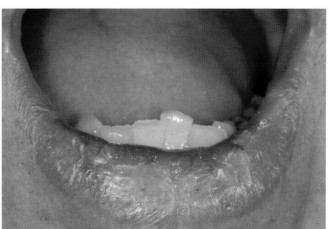

9.78

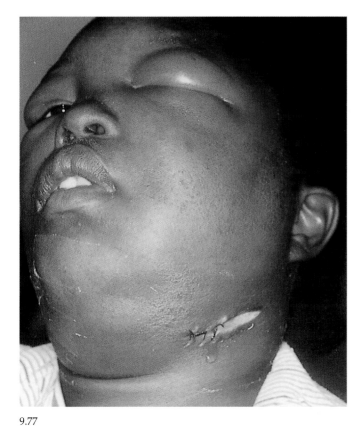

9.77

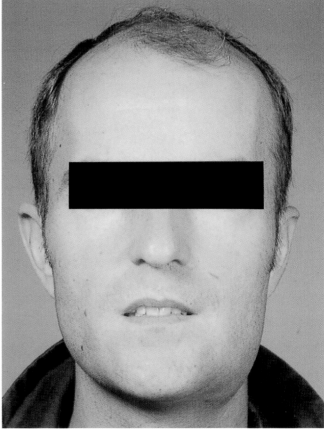

9.80

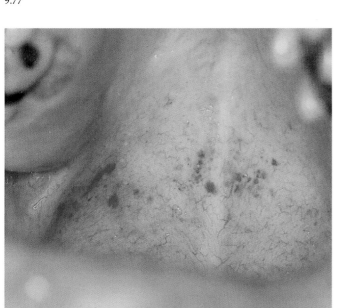

9.79

palatal lesions in this patient are candidosis). Oral hyperpigmentation may also be seen and this may arise from several causes, especially as a drug side-effect (e.g. clofazimine or zidovudine) or as a consequence of adrenocortical damage (**Fig. 9.83**). Some protease inhibitors may give rise to dysgeusia.

Autoimmune disorders may be seen. Spontaneous oral bleeding is sometimes seen in HIV infection often as a consequence of autoimmune thrombocytopenia which can also cause petechiae. Vitiligo may be seen on the face (**Fig. 9.84**).

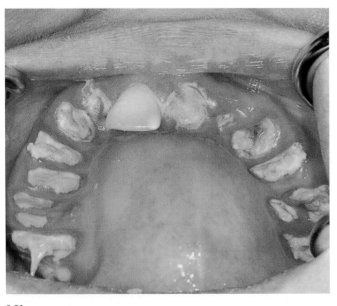

9.81

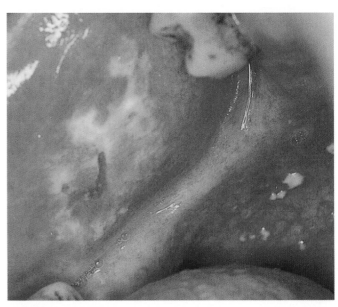

9.82

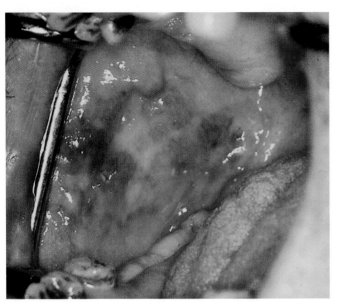

9.83

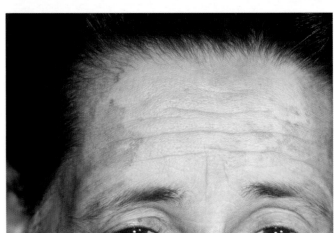

9.84

FURTHER READING

Basak PY, Ergin S, Sezer MT, Sari A. Amyloidosis of the tongue with kappa light chain disease. Australas J Dermatol 2001; 42(1): 55–7.

Coates E, Slade GD, Goss AN, Gorkic E. Oral conditions and their social impact among HIV dental patients. Aust Dent J 1996; 41(1): 33–6.

Cruz GD, Lamster IB, Begg MD, Phelan JA, Gorman JM, el-Sadr W. The accurate diagnosis of oral lesions in human immunodeficiency virus infection. Impact on medical staging. Arch Otolaryngol Head Neck Surg 1996; 122(1): 68–73.

Diz Dios P, Scully C. Adverse effects of antiretroviral therapy: focus on orofacial effects. Expert Opin Drug Saf 2002; 1: 307–17.

Ferguson FS, Nachman S, Berentsen B. Implications and management of oral diseases in children and adolescents with HIV infection. NY State Dent J 1997; 63(2): 46–50.

Filho FJS, Lopes M, Almeida OPD, Scully C. Mucocutaneous histoplasmosis in AIDS. Br J Dermatol 1995; 133: 472–4.

Fukui N, Amano A, Akiyama S, Daikoku H, Wakisaka S, Morisaki I. Oral findings in DiGeorge syndrome: clinical features and histologic study of primary teeth. Oral Surg Oral Med Oral Pathol Oral Radiol Endod 2000; 89(2): 208–15.

Greene VA, Chu SY, Diaz T, Schable B. Oral health problems and use of dental services among HIV-infected adults. Supplement to HIV/AIDS Surveillance Project Group. J Am Dent Assoc 1997; 128(10): 1417–22.

Guyot L, Dubuc M, Pujol J, Dutour O, Philip N. Craniofacial anthropometric analysis in patients with 22q11 microdeletion. Am J Med Genet 2001 15; 100(1): 1–8.

Hoefert S, Schilling E, Philippou S, Eufinger H. Amyloidosis of the tongue as a possible diagnostic manifestation of plasmacytoma. Mund Kiefer Gesichtschir 1999; 3(1): 46–9.

Johnson EM, Warnock DW, Luker J, Porter SR, Scully C. Emergence of azole drug resistance in Candida species among HIV-infected patients receiving prolonged fluconazole therapy for oral candidosis. Antimicrob Agents Chemother 1995; 35: 103–14.

Leao JC, Ferreira AM, Martins S, et al. Cheilitis glandularis: An unusual presentation in a patient with HIV infection. Oral Surg Oral Med Oral Pathol Oral Radiol Endod 2003; 95: 142–4.

Li MC, Chou G, Chen JT, Wong YK, Ho WL. Amyloidosis of medium-sized arteries presenting as perioral mass: a case report. Oral Surg Oral Med Oral Pathol Oral Radiol Endod 2003; 95(4): 463–6.

Madigan A, Murray PA, Houpt M, Catalanotto F, Feuerman M. Caries experience and cariogenic markers in HIV-positive children and their siblings. Pediatr Dent 1996; 18(2): 129–36.

Majorana A, Notarangelo LD, Savoldi E, Gastaldi G, Lozada-Nur F. Leukocyte adhesion deficiency in a child with severe oral involvement. Oral Surg Oral Med Oral Pathol Oral Radiol Endod 1999; 87(6): 691–4.

Mandel L, Hong J. HIV-associated parotid lymphoepithelial cysts. J Am Dent Assoc 1999; 130(4): 528–32.

Marcenes W, Pankhurst CL, Lewis DA. Oral health behaviour and the prevalence of oral manifestations of HIV infection in a group of HIV positive adults. Int Dent J 1998; 48(6): 557–62.

Mateo Arias J, Molina Martinez M, Borrego A, Mayorga F. Amyloidosis of the submaxillary gland. Med Oral 2003; 8(1): 66–70.

Meiller TF, Jabra-Rizk MA, Baqui Aa, Kelley JI, Meeks VI, Merz WG, Falkler WA. Oral Candida dubliniensis as a clinically important species in HIV-seropositive patients in the United States. Oral Surg Oral Med Oral Pathol Oral Radiol Endod 1999; 88(5): 573–80.

Messner AH, Mitchell DP, Roifman CM. Mucosal lesions in severe combined immunodeficiency syndrome. J Otolaryngol 1996; 25(3): 200–2.

Milian MA, Bagan JV, Jimenez Y, Perez A, Scully C. Oral leishmaniasis in a HIV-positive patient. Report of a case involving the palate. Oral Dis 2002; 8: 59–61.

Moroni AM, Benavides A, Retamal Y. Macroglossia and occult amyloidosis. Rev Med Child 2002; 130(2): 215–18.

Patton LL. HIV disease. Dent Clin North Am 2003; 47(3): 467–92.

Patton LL, Phelan JA, Ramos-Gomez FJ, Nittayananta W, Shiboski CH, Mbuguye TL. Prevalence and classification of HIV-associated oral lesions. Oral Dis 2002; 8 (Suppl 2): 98–109.

Porter SR, Scully C. Orofacial manifestations in primary immuno-deficiencies involving IgA deficiency. J Oral Pathol Med 1993; 22: 117–19.

Porter SR, Scully C. Orofacial manifestations in primary immuno-deficiencies: T lymphocyte defects. J Oral Pathol Med 1993; 22: 308–9.

Porter SR, Scully C (eds) Oral Healthcare For Those With HIV and Other Special Needs. Science Reviews (Northwood), 1995.

Porter SR, Luker J, Scully C, Kumar N. Oral lesions in UK patients with or liable to HIV disease – ten years experience. Med Oral 1999; 4: 455–69.

Ramos-Gomez FJ, Flaitz C, Catapano P, Murray P, Milnes AR, Dorenbaum A. Classification, diagnostic criteria, and treatment recommendations for orofacial manifestations in HIV-infected pediatric patients. Collaborative Workgroup on Oral Manifestations of Pediatric HIV Infection. J Clin Pediatr Dent 1999; 23(2): 85–96.

Reichart PA. Oral pathology of acquired immune deficiency syndrome and oro-facial Kaposi's sarcoma. Curr Topics Pathol 1996; 90: 98–121.

Schuman P, Ohmit SE, Sobel JD, Mayer KH, Greene V, Rompalo A, Klein RS. Oral lesions among women living with or at risk for HIV infection. HIV Epidemiology Research Study (HERS) Group. Am J Med 1998; 104(6): 559–64.

Scully C. HIV: Viral infections. In Porter SR and Scully C (eds) Oral Health Care for Those with HIV and Other Special Needs. Northwood, Science Reviews, 1995; pp. 31–42.

Scully C. The dental profession. In Collins J and Kennedy DA (eds) Occupational Blood-Borne Infections. CAB International, 1997; pp. 133–58.

Scully C. The HIV global pandemic: the development and emerging implications. Oral Dis 1997; 3 (Suppl 1): S1–S6.

Scully C. Oral manifestations associated with human immuno-deficiency virus (HIV) infection in developing countries — are there differences from developed countries? Oral Dis 2000; 6: 395.

Scully C, Dios PD. HIV topic update; orofacial effects of antiretroviral therapies. Oral Diseases 2001; 7: 205–210.

Scully C, Porter SR. Orofacial manifestations in primary immunodeficiencies: common variable immunodeficiency. J Oral Pathol Med 1993; 22: 157–8.

Scully C, Porter SR. Orofacial manifestations in primary immuno-deficiencies: polymorphonuclear leukocyte defects. J Oral Pathol Med 1993; 22: 310–11.

Scully C, Spittle M. Malignant tumours of the oral cavity in HIV disease. In Langdon J and Henk JM (eds) Malignant Tumours of the Mouth, Jaws and Salivary Glands, 2nd edn. London, Edward Arnold, 1995, pp. 246–57.

Scully C, Almeida OPD, Sposto MR. Deep mycoses in HIV infection. Oral Dis 1997; 3 (Suppl 1): 200–7.

Scully C, Almeida OPD, Warnakulasuriya KAAS, Johnson NW. Orofacial involvement by systemic mycoses in HIV infection. Oral Dis 1995; 1: 61–2.

Stoopler ET, Sollecito TP, Chen SY. Amyloid deposition in the oral cavity: a retrospective study and review of the literature. Oral Surg Oral Med Oral Pathol Oral Radiol Endod 2003; 95(6): 674–80. Review.

Triantos D, Porter SR, Scully C, Teo CG. Oral hairy leukoplakia: clinicopathologic features, pathogenesis, diagnosis, and clinical significance. Clin Infect Dis 1997; 25: 1392–6.

Tsang PCS, Samaranayake LP, Philipsen HP, *et al*. Biotypes of oral *Candida albicans* isolates in human immunodeficiency virus-infected patients from diverse geographic locations. J Oral Pathol Med 1995; 24: 32–6.

Vargas PA, Mauad T, Bohm GM, Saldiva PH, Almeida OP. Parotid gland involvement in advanced AIDS. Oral Dis 2003; 9(2): 55–61.

Weinert M, Grimes RM, Lynch DP. Oral manifestations of HIV infection. Ann Intern Med 1996; 125: 485–96.

WHO. Primary immunodeficiency diseases. Clin Exp Immunol 1997; 109 (Suppl 1): 1–28.

10 DISEASES OF THE BLOOD AND BLOOD-FORMING ORGANS

- aplastic anaemia
- bone-marrow transplantation (haemopoietic stem cell transplantation)
- chronic granulomatous disease (CGD)
- Fanconi's anaemia
- folate deficiency
- haemoglobinopathies
- haemophilias
- hypoplasminogenaemia
- iron deficiency anaemia
- myelodysplastic syndrome
- neutropenia
- pernicious anaemia
- plasmacytosis
- Plummer–Vinson syndrome (Paterson–Kelly syndrome)
- polycythaemia rubra vera
- purpura
- von Willebrand's disease.

APLASTIC ANAEMIA

Clinical features of aplastic anaemia depend on the predominant cell type affected and aplastic anaemia may therefore present with signs and symptoms of thrombocytopenia, leukopenia, anaemia or a combination of all three (pancytopenia). Profound and spontaneous purpuric or ecchymotic haemorrhages or infection of the skin and mucous membrane, and pallor, can be the presenting features (**Fig. 10.1**).

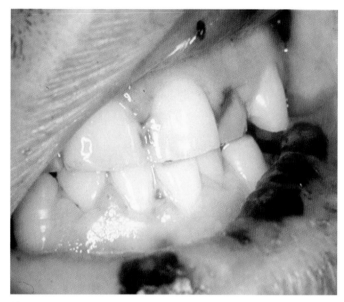

10.1

BONE-MARROW TRANSPLANTATION
(haemopoietic stem cell transplantation)

Bone-marrow transplantation (BMT) is often the treatment for aplastic anaemia. Oral complications include mucositis, candidosis, parotitis, graft-versus-host disease (GVHD) with lichenoid or sclerodermatous reactions, and infections with herpes viruses or fungi such as *Aspergillus*. Xerostomia predisposes to caries.

Oral complications are common and can be a major cause of morbidity following BMT. Mucositis (**Fig. 10.2**), infections (**Fig. 10.2** also shows candidosis), petechiae, bleeding, xerostomia and loss of taste result from the effects of the underlying disease, chemo- and/or radiotherapy, and GVHD. GVHD affects the ventrum of the tongue,

buccal and labial mucosae, palate (**Figs 10.3–10.11**) and gingiva. Acute GVHD manifests with painful mucosal desquamation and ulceration, and/or cheilitis, and lichenoid plaques or striae. Small white lesions affect the buccal and lingual mucosa early on but these clear by day 14. Erythema and ulceration are most pronounced at 7–11 days after BMT. Oral candidosis and herpes simplex stomatitis are common (occasionally zoster) and there may be oral purpura.

The oral lesions in chronic GVHD are coincident with skin lesions, and include generalized mucosal erythema, lichenoid lesions (mainly in the buccal mucosa) and xerostomia with depressed salivary IgA levels in minor gland saliva. Xerostomia is most significant in the first 14 days after transplantation and is a consequence of drug treatment, irradiation and/or GVHD.

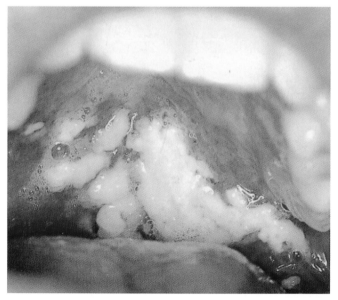

10.2

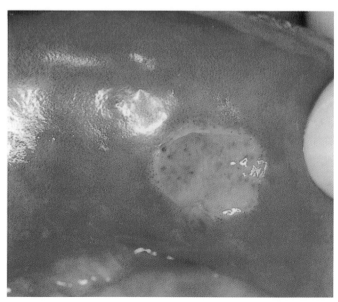

10.3

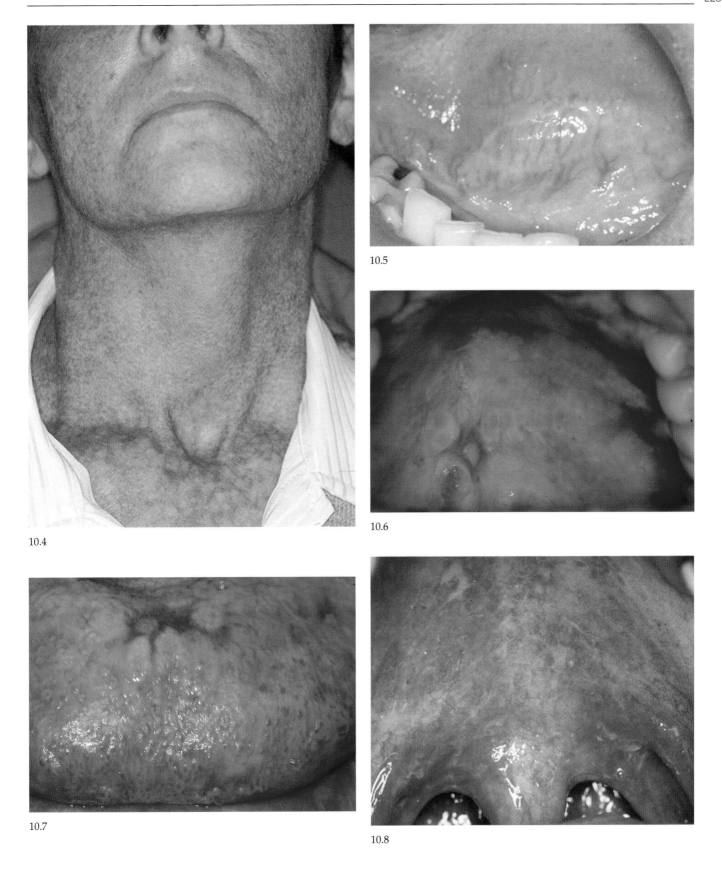

10.4

10.5

10.6

10.7

10.8

Conjunctival lesions may be seen (**Fig. 10.12**) and the face may be swollen from corticosteroid use (**Fig. 10.13**). The chronic immunosuppression needed following organ transplantation predisposes to candidosis, other mycoses and viral infections. Some patients develop white lesions (keratoses) or hairy leukoplakia. Ciclosporin may induce gingival hyperplasia although tacrolimus does not. Rarely, oral malignant neoplasms have been recorded.

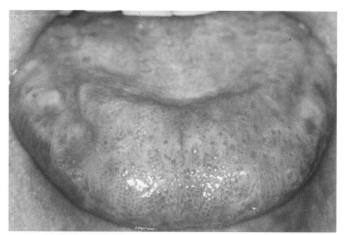

10.10

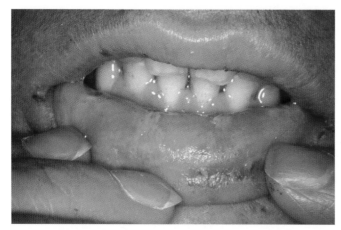

10.9

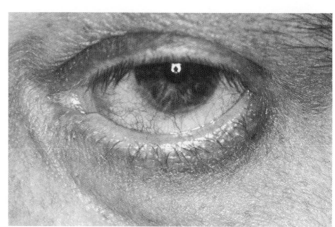

10.12

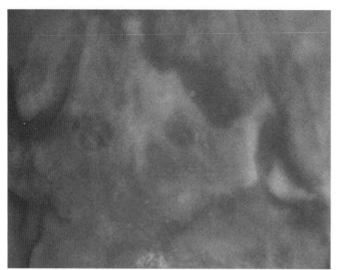

10.11

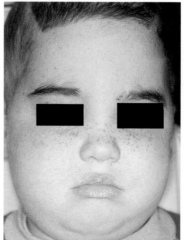

10.13

CHRONIC GRANULOMATOUS DISEASE (CGD)

This predominantly sex-linked leukocyte defect (in which neutrophils and monocytes are defective at killing catalase-positive micro-organisms) typically presents with cervical lymph-node enlargement and suppuration; a submandibular node abscess has been drained in **Fig. 10.14**.

Recurrent infections in early childhood may result in enamel hypoplasia (**Fig. 10.15**). The tooth loss here, however, was from a road traffic accident. CGD also predisposes to oral ulceration and periodontal destruction.

Other types of neutrophil defect also predispose to ulcers and accelerated periodontitis.

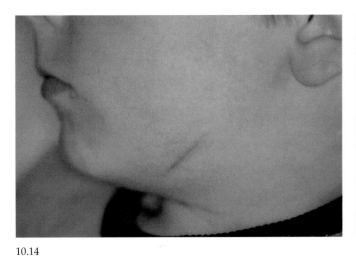

10.14

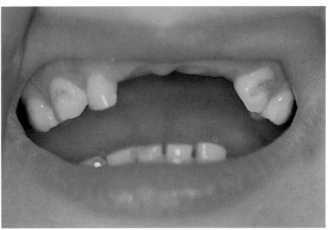

10.15

FANCONI'S ANAEMIA

Fanconi's anaemia is the most common of the inherited bone marrow failure disorders. It is clinically characterized by low birth weight and a variety of skeletal features (short stature, microcephaly, microphthalmia, microstomia or skeletal anomalies, particularly of the thumbs and radii), cutaneous features (patchy or generalized pigmentation) and/or genitourinary features (horseshoe or pelvic kidney, or maldescended testes) together with progressive marrow failure and a liability to leukaemia, squamous cell carcinoma and hepatocellular carcinoma. Oral features may include the oral mucosal features of anaemia, leukoplakia (**Fig. 10.16**), leukopenia, thrombocytopenia and a possible liability to ulcers, accelerated periodontitis and squamous cell carcinoma.

FOLATE DEFICIENCY

Folate deficiency secondary to coeliac disease, malnourishment (e.g. in anorexia nervosa) (**Fig. 10.17**) or methotrexate therapy commonly gives rise to superficial oral ulceration. Rarely there may be glossitis and angular cheilitis.

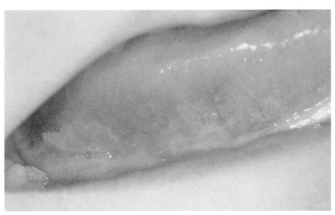

10.16

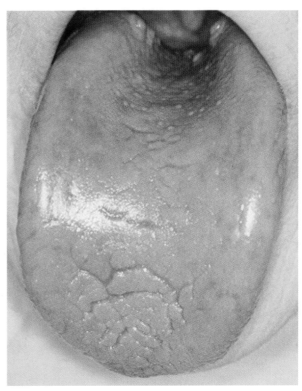

10.17

HAEMOGLOBINOPATHIES

Haemoglobinopathies such as sickle cell anaemia and thalassaemias may present with maxillary hyperplasia owing to marrow overgrowth (**Figs 10.18, 10.19**). Sickle cell disease may present with orofacial pain (due to infarcts) or occasionally with infections such as osteitis.

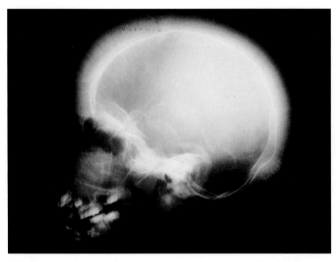

10.18

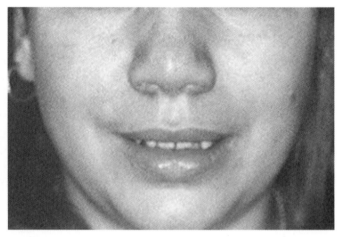

10.19

HAEMOPHILIAS

Haemophilia A (classic haemophilia) is ten times as common as haemophilia B (Christmas disease) where factor IX is deficient. Deep haemorrhage is a serious complication of both. Trauma predisposes to bleeding though it can be spontaneous.

Defects of blood coagulation factors, unlike thrombocytopenia, do not predispose to spontaneous gingival haemorrhage, oral petechiae or ecchymoses. Any breach of the mucosae, however, especially tooth extraction, can lead to persistent bleeding (**Figs 10.20, 10.21**), which is occasionally fatal. Haemorrhage after extraction here, a case of

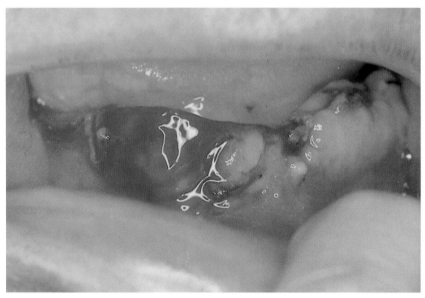

10.20

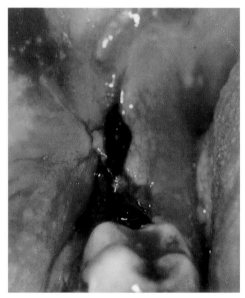

10.21

haemophilia A, was controlled with factor VIII replacement. Surgery must only be carried out with adequate factor VIII levels. Bleeding into tissues causes aesthetic problems but, more importantly joint damage (Figs 10.22–10.24); a main danger is that haemorrhage into the fascial spaces, especially from surgery in the lower molar region, can track into the neck and embarrass the airway.

Haemarthrosis (Figs 10.23 and 10.24) can be crippling. Tooth eruption and exfoliation are usually uneventful but, occasionally, there can be a small bleed into the follicle (Fig. 10.25).

HIV or hepatitis virus infection may arise in patients who were given blood transfusions or factor replacement before appropriate screening or heat-treated factors were available.

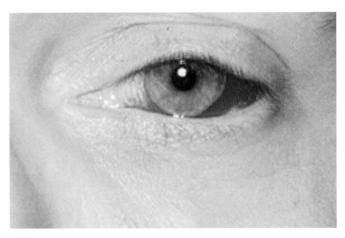

10.22

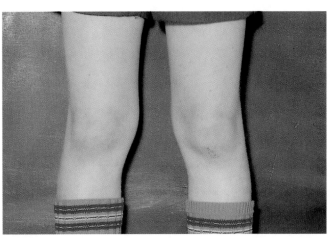

10.23

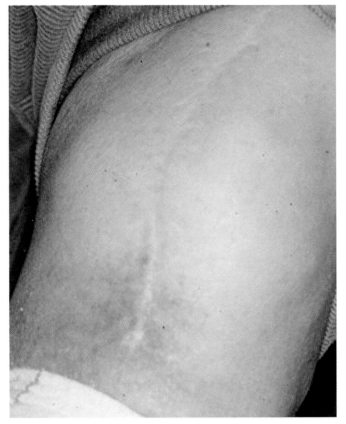

10.24

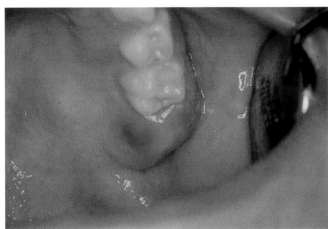

10.25

HYPOPLASMINOGENAEMIA

Deficiency in plasminogen may lead to abnormal fibrin depositions and gingival swelling and ulceration (**Figs 10.26–10.28**), sometimes with ligneous conjunctivitis, a rare form of chronic membranous conjunctivitis associated with fibrin deposits and often with associated lesions in the larynx, nose and cervix. Some patients develop corneal involvement and blindness while, others may also develop congenital occlusive hydrocephalus. Perhaps surprisingly, there is usually no tendency to thrombosis.

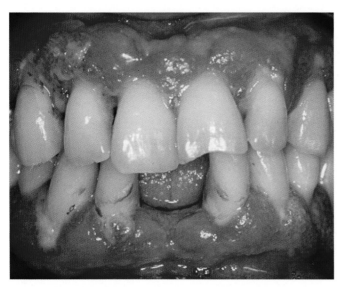

10.26

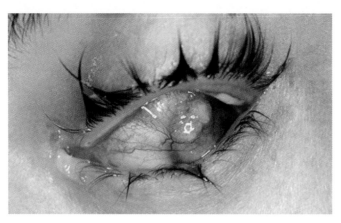

10.28

10.27

IRON DEFICIENCY ANAEMIA

The most common cause of iron deficiency in western countries is chronic haemorrhage. When bone marrow iron stores are depleted, there is a stage of iron deficiency without anaemia (sideropenia) before red cell changes are evident. Glossitis (**Fig. 10.29**) is one oral manifestation which may be seen in the pre-anaemic stage as well as in anaemia.

Angular stomatitis is soreness and sometimes fissuring at the commissures (**Figs 10.29–10.31**). Usually of local aetiology, and related to candidosis beneath an upper denture, it is occasionally precipitated by a deficiency of iron, folate or vitamin B.

Although deficiency of iron or other haematinics can cause a sore tongue with atrophic glossitis, many haematinic-deficient patients with a sore tongue have no obvious organic lesion. Oral ulceration is sometimes a manifestation of iron deficiency.

Spoon-shaped nails (koilonychia), which tend to split, are typical of iron deficiency anaemia (**Fig. 10.32** but rarely seen).

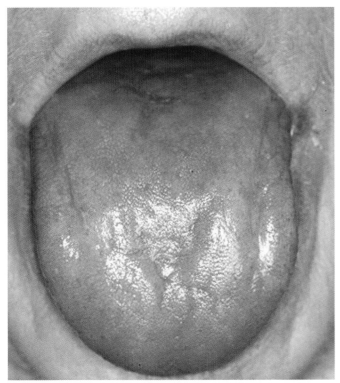

10.29

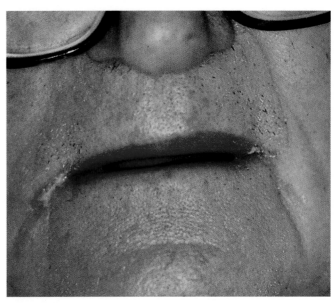

10.30

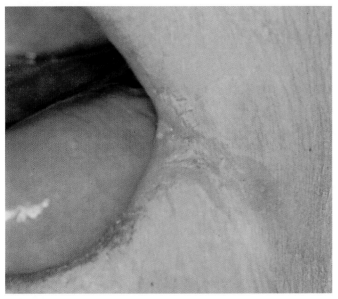

10.31

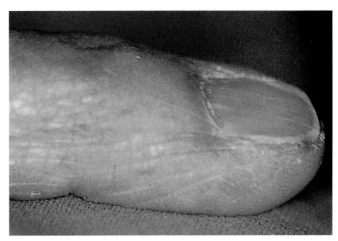

10.32

MYELODYSPLASTIC SYNDROME

In this group of disorders there is a functional neutropenia as a result of disordered granulopoiesis. The ulcers notably lack an inflammatory halo (**Figs 10.33, 10.34**). There may be a predisposition to acute myeloid leukaemia and, albeit rarely, associated gingival enlargement.

NEUTROPENIA

Neutropenia is characterized by severe neutropenia with an absolute neutrophil count below $0.5 \times 10^9/L$ and is associated with severe systemic bacterial infections. Neutropenias predispose to gingivitis, accelerated periodontal disease (**Figs 10.35 and 10.36**) and to oral ulceration (**Fig. 10.37**).

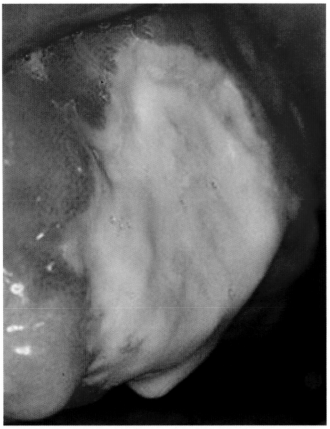

10.33

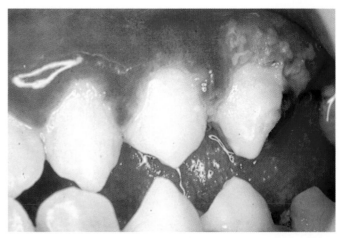

10.35

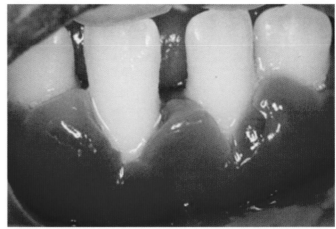

10.36

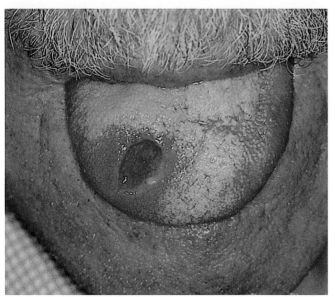

10.34

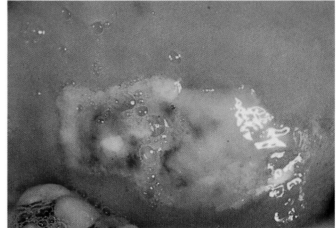

10.37

Cyclic neutropenia is a cyclical drop in polymorphonuclear neutrophil count, and sometimes other leukocytes, every 21 days. Destructive periodontal disease, recurrent ulcerative gingivitis and recurrent mouth ulcers are frequent manifestations (**Fig. 10.38**), together with recurrent pyogenic infections. Palatal ulceration (**Fig. 10.39**) is rare in aphthae and in this case suggested an immune defect, which proved to be neutropenia. Recurrent mouth ulcers in neutropenias are sometimes due to intraoral herpes simplex recurrences or other viral infections such as CMV (see **Fig. 9.33**).

Gangrene may be seen in patients with neutropenia or rare neutrophil defects such as acatalasia (seen mainly in Japan, Korea, Israel and Switzerland).

Leukopenia (particularly neutropenia) leads to decreased resistance to infection and manifests with ulceration, often associated with opportunistic organisms. Typically there is, as in agranulocytosis, only a minimal red inflammatory halo around the ulcers.

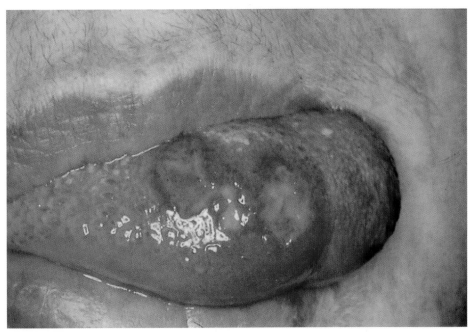

10.38

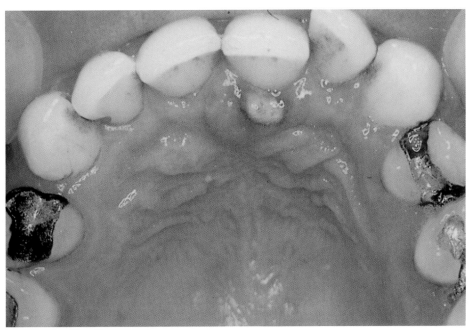

10.39

PERNICIOUS ANAEMIA

Pernicious anaemia is defined as severe lack of cobalamin due to gastric atrophy. It is more common in northern Europeans than other ethnic groups, being particularly common in middle-age to elderly females. Patients typically have antibodies to parietal cells, although a range of other relevant autoantibodies may also be detected. Pernicious anaemia is often associated with other autoimmune disorders and may rarely be a feature of candidosis endocrinopathy syndrome. The oral manifestations of pernicious anaemia include superficial oral ulceration, glossitis, Moeller's glossitis, angular cheilitis and, when profound, can give rise to severe oral epithelial dysplasia (**Figs 10.40–10.42**).

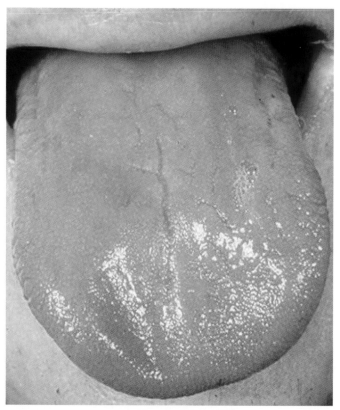

10.40

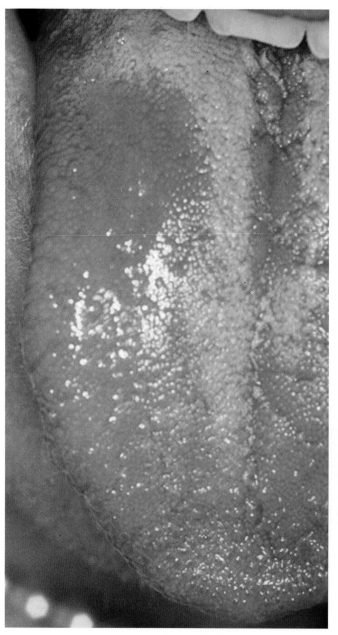

10.41

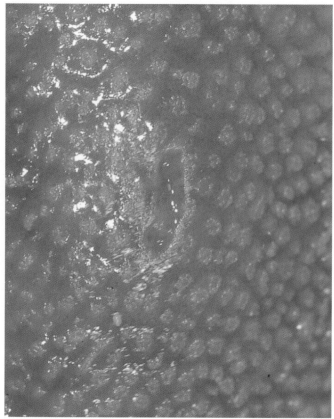

10.42

PLASMACYTOSIS

Idiopathic plasmacytosis is an uncommon disorder clinically characterized by the development of painful, diffuse, red granular lesions on the free and attached gingivae (**Fig. 10.43**). Plasmacytosis probably represents an atypical hypersensitivity reaction to a variety of agents including cinnamon in chewing gum, other confectionery and toothpastes. In the past, plasma-cell gingivitis was seen and probably again represented a hypersensitivity reaction. Gingival lesions can be localized or generalized and there can also be involvement of other oral mucosal surfaces, particularly the lips and tongue. Rarely, there is involvement of the palate, pharynx and supraglottic larynx (**Fig. 10.44**).

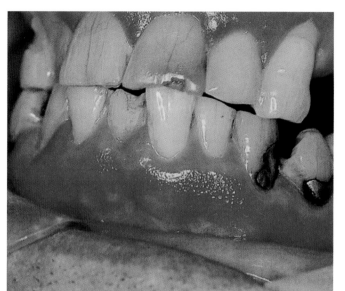

10.43

PLUMMER–VINSON SYNDROME
(Paterson–Brown–Kelly syndrome)

In this syndrome (sideropenic dysphagia) patients typically are middle-aged with dysphagia caused by an oesophageal web, often with candidosis, hypochromic microcytic anaemia, koilonychia and a depapillated tongue. There is a predisposition to postcricoid carcinoma and to oral carcinoma (**Fig. 10.45**).

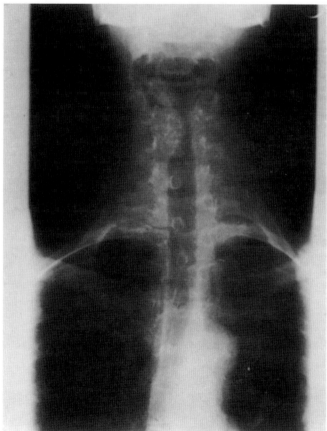

10.45

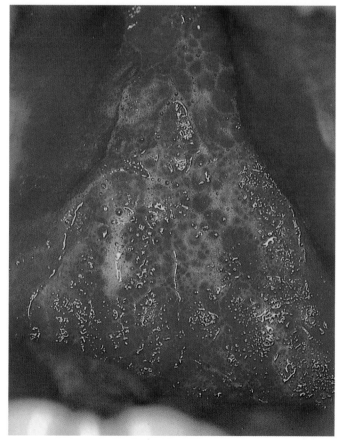

10.44

POLYCYTHAEMIA RUBRA VERA

Polycythaemia rubra vera is a primary myeloproliferative disorder characterized by increased numbers of red cells (giving a plethoric appearance; **Fig. 10.46**), increased granulocytes and increased but dysfunctional platelets. Oral purpura or haemorrhage may be seen and occasionally there may be pronounced gingival redness.

Cytotoxic therapy of the disease may lead to neutropenic oral ulceration and an increased bleeding tendency (**Fig. 10.47**). Secondary polycythaemia is associated with compensatory or inappropriate erythropoietin release in cardiorespiratory disease, heavy smoking or in association with a variety of tumours, such as renal carcinoma, cerebellar haemangioblastoma and malignant fibrous histiocytoma of the parotid gland.

PURPURA

Spontaneous gingival bleeding, oral petechiae and ecchymoses may appear (**Figs 10.48–10.50**), mainly at sites of trauma but they can be spontaneous. Petechiae appear mainly in the buccal mucosa, on the lateral margin of the tongue and at the junction of the hard and soft palates — sites readily traumatized. Spontaneous gingival bleeding is often an early feature in platelet deficiencies or defects. Postextraction bleeding may be a problem.

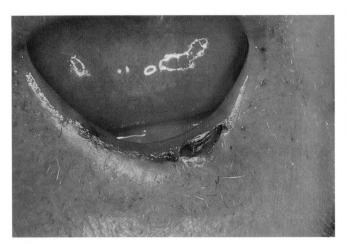

10.46

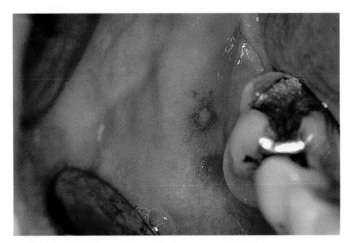

10.48

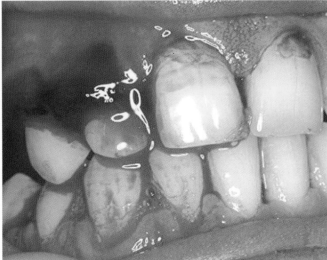

10.49

10.47

Petechiae and ecchymoses also appear readily on the skin (**Fig. 10.51**), especially if there is trauma. Even the pressure from a sphygmomanometer can cause petechiae during the measurement of blood pressure.

Localized oral purpura (angina bullosa haemorrhagica) is included here, but no thrombocytopenia is usually detectable. The cause of the blood blisters typically found on the palate of an older person is unclear, though a few cases appear after corticosteroid inhaler use (**Fig. 10.52**).

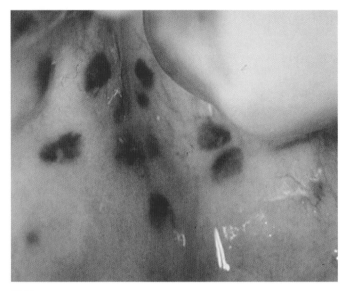

10.50

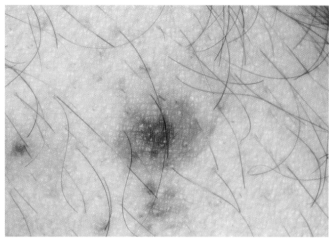

10.51

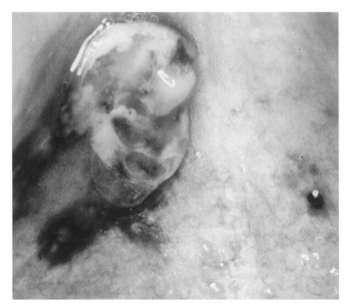

10.52

VON WILLEBRAND'S DISEASE

The combined factor VIII defect and platelet abnormality in von Willebrand's disease (**Figs 10.53–10.55**) is more common, and can sometimes be more serious, than classic haemophilia A (deficiency of factor VIII). This affects females as well as males and can lead to haemorrhage into the skin and mucosae.

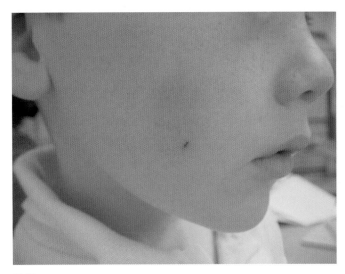

10.53

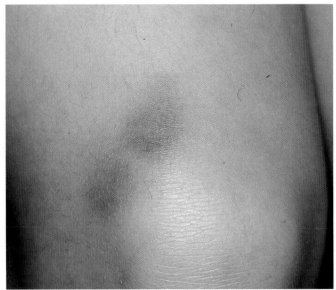

10.54

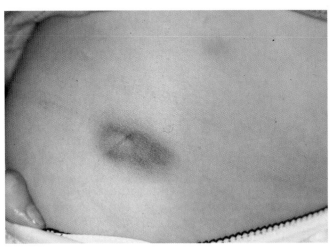

10.55

FURTHER READING

Barker GJ. Current practices in the oral management of the patient undergoing chemotherapy or bone marrow transplantation. Support Care Cancer 1999; 7(1): 17–20.

Bishop K, Briggs P, Kelleher M. Sickle cell disease; a diagnostic dilemma. Int Endodont J 1995; 28: 297–302.

Boyd D, Kinirons M. Dental caries experience of children with haemophilia in Northern Ireland. Int J Paediatr Dent 1997; 7: 149–53.

Brennan MT, Sankar V, Baccaglini L, et al. Oral manifestations in patients with aplastic anemia. Oral Surg Oral Med Oral Pathol Oral Radiol Endod 2001; 92(5): 503–8.

Chadwick B. Congenital coagulopathies. In Porter SR and Scully C (eds) Oral Health Care for Those with HIV Infection and Other Special Needs. Northwood, Science Reviews, 1995, pp. 85–92.

Duggal MS, Bedi R, Kinsey SE, Williams SA. The dental management of children with sickle cell disease and b thalassaemia: a review. Int J Paediat Dent 1996; 6: 227–34.

Field EA, Speechley JA, Rugman FR, et al. Oral signs and symptoms in patients with undiagnosed vitamin B12 deficiency. J Oral Pathol Med 1995; 24: 468–70.

Giuliani M, Favia GF, Lajolo C, Miani CM. Angina bullosa haemorrhagica: presentation of eight new cases and a review of the literature. Oral Dis 2002; 8(1): 54–8.

Kelleher M, Bishop K, Briggs P. Oral complications associated with sickle cell anemia: a review and case report. Oral Surg Oral Med Oral Pathol Oral Radiol Endod 1996; 82(2): 225–8.

Khan NA, McKerrow WS, Palmer TJ. Mucous membrane plasmacytosis of the upper aerodigestive tract. A case report with effective treatment. J Laryngol Otol 1997; 111: 293–5.

Lee MS, Lee ML, Fryer J, Saurajen A, Guay JL. Oral papillary plasmacytosis cleared by radiotherapy. Br J Dermatol 1996; 134: 945–8.

Lucas VS, Roberts GJ, Beighton D. Oral health of children undergoing allogeneic bone marrow transplantation. Bone Marrow Transplant 1998; 22: 801–8.

Marcovich CK, Davis MJ. Bone marrow transplants. Current applications and implications for oral health. NY State Dent J 1999; 65: 28–31.

Misch CM, Jolly RL, Williams DR, Chorazy CJ. Maxillary implant surgery on a patient with thalassemia: a case report. Oral Surg Oral Med Oral Pathol Oral Radiol Endod 1998; 86(4): 401–5.

O'Rourke CA, Hawley GM. Sickle cell disorder and orofacial pain in Jamaican patients. Br Dent J 1998; 185(2): 90–2.

Porter SR, Scully C. Gingival and oral mucosal ulceration associated with the myelodysplastic syndrome. Eur J Cancer B Oral Oncol 1994; 30B: 346–50.

Porter SR, Scully C, Standen GR. Autoimmune neutropenia manifesting as recurrent oral ulceration. Oral Surg Oral Med Oral Pathol 1994; 78: 178–80.

Schardt-Sacco D. Update on coagulopathies. Oral Surg Oral Med Oral Pathol Oral Radiol Endod 2000; 90: 559–63.

Scipio JE, Al-Bayaty HF, Murti PR, Matthews R. Facial swelling and gingival enlargement in a patient with sickle cell disease. Oral Dis 2001; 7(5): 306–9.

Scully C, Wolff A. Oral surgery in patients on anticoagulants. Oral surgery in patients on anticoagulant therapy. Oral Surg Oral Med Oral Pathol Oral Radiol Endod 2002; 94: 57–64.

Scully C, Gokbuget AY, Allen C, et al. Oral manifestations indicative of plasminogen deficiency (hypoplasminogenemia). Oral Surg Oral Med Oral Pathol 2001; 91: 344–7.

Scully C, Dis Dios P, Giangrande P, Lee C. Oral health care in hemophilia and other bleeding tendencies, World Federation on Hemophilia. Treatment of Hemophilia Monograph Series, No. 27, 2002.

Scully C, Watt-Smith P, Dios P, Giangrande PLF. Complications in HIV-infected and non-HIV-infected hemophiliacs and other patients after oral surgery. Intern J Oral Max Surg 2002; 31: 634–40.

Taylor LB, Nowak AJ, Giller RH, Casamassimo PS. Sickle cell anemia: a review of the dental concerns and a retrospective study of dental and bony changes. Spec Care Dentist 1995; 15(1): 38–42.

Wilde J, Cook RJ. Von Willebrand disease and its management in oral and maxillofacial surgery. Brit J Oral MaxFac Surg 1998; 36: 112–18.

Ziccardi VB, Feretti A, Schneider W. Management of sickle cell/beta thalassemia patient with severe odontogenic infection. NY State Dent J 1996; 62(8): 28–32.

11 MENTAL DISORDERS

- anorexia nervosa/bulimia
- atypical facial pain
- learning disability
- Munchausen's syndrome
- oral dysaesthesia
- psychogenic oral disease
- self-mutilation (oral artefactual disease).

ANOREXIA NERVOSA/BULIMIA

Anorexia nervosa is a syndrome characterized by severe weight loss due to self-starvation — a condition affecting mainly previously healthy adolescent girls.

The disorder, which is regarded as an hysterical neurosis, is associated with a preoccupation to be thin.

The body image appears to be so distorted that, even when emaciated, the patient still regards herself as too fat.

These patients usually refuse to eat or, if forced to do so, often induce vomiting. Menstrual upset is an early feature. Anorexia nervosa may be complicated by anaemia, endocrine disturbances, peripheral oedema and electrolyte depletion (especially hypokalaemia). Peripheral cyanosis and coldness with bradycardia and amenorrhoea are common, as are depression, which lacks the classic features of depression in adults, and obsessional features.

Tooth erosion (perimylolysis) (**Fig. 11.1** is an extreme example) may result from repeated vomiting. The erosion is usually most pronounced on lingual, palatal and occlusal surfaces. Self-mutilation (**Fig. 11.2**

shows gingival mutilation), ulcers in the palate caused by using the fingers to induce retching, and sialosis are the other main oral features seen in anorexia nervosa/bulimia. Oral ulcers or abrasions may be caused by fingers or other objects used to induce vomiting. Some patients cannot control their voluntary food restriction and have episodes in which they gorge food (bulimia) and then force vomiting.

Parotid enlargement (sialosis) and angular cheilitis may develop, as in other forms of starvation. The parotid swellings tend to subside if and when the patient returns to a normal diet.

Bulimics, in contrast to anoretics, may have normal or near-normal weight. Uncontrolled and unpredictable ingestion of huge amounts of foods (usually soft, sweet or starchy foods) is followed by vomiting. Bulimia may occur in isolation, or in anorexia nervosa, and appears to be a stress-related disorder.

Other features may include conjunctival suffusion, oesophageal tears (caused by retching) and Russell's sign (abrasions on the back of the hand or fingers caused by thrusting the hand to touch the throat to induce vomiting).

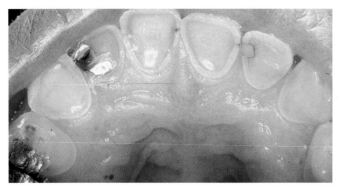

11.1

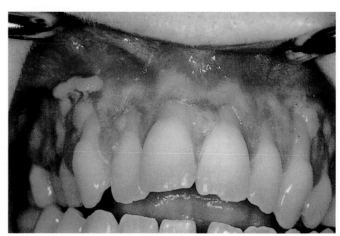

11.2

ATYPICAL FACIAL PAIN

Persistent, dull, boring pain, especially in the maxilla, in the absence of identifiable organic disease, is seen in some psychiatric disorders such as depression and, in others, may be a form of monosymptomatic hypochondriasis. Most patients affected with this atypical facial pain are females of middle age or older. **Figure 11.3** is an extreme example of a patient who is wearing a large bandage to help 'relieve' the pain, perhaps an attention-seeking device.

Patients with psychogenically related orofacial symptoms not infrequently bring in diaries, graphs or notes outlining their complaints ("la maladie du petit papiers"), which are often of pain, bad taste in the mouth, non-existent slime, lumps, dry or wet mouth, and are often multiple. A 'syndrome of oral complaints' has even been described.

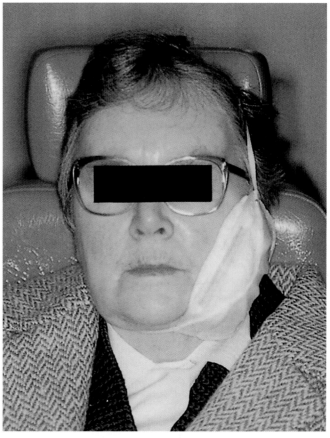

11.3

LEARNING DISABILITY

Persons with learning disability may find it difficult to maintain good oral hygiene, either because of the mental or sometimes physical disability. Tooth staining and marginal gingivitis are therefore common (**Fig. 11.4**).

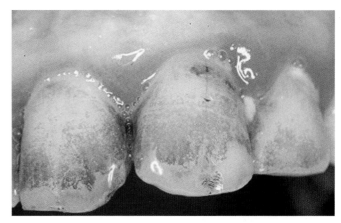

11.4

MUNCHAUSEN'S SYNDROME

Munchausen's syndrome is the term used for persons who fabricate symptoms so as to result in unwarranted operative intervention. Patients with this syndrome typically present with apparently acute illnesses supported by plausible histories, later often found to be full of falsifications. They have usually been seen by multiple clinicians and/or in several hospitals. Patients also frequently discharge themselves from care, sometimes after arguments with their clinical attendants.

The symptomatology of Munchausen's syndrome is highly varied but may be centred on particular areas, though few patients have been described with Munchausen's syndrome presenting with oral complaints. **Figure 11.5** shows one patient who complained of multiple odontalgia eventually persuading several clinicians to perform unnecessary interventions (**Fig. 11.6**).

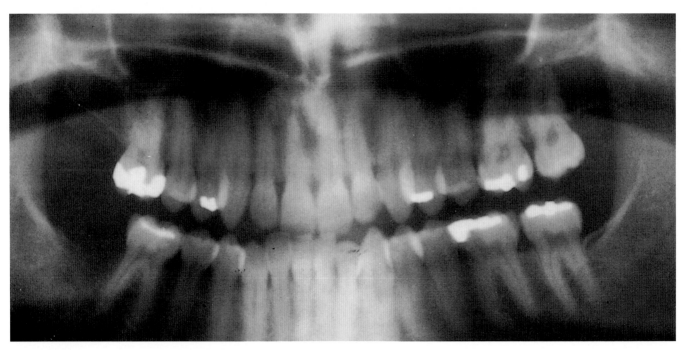

11.5

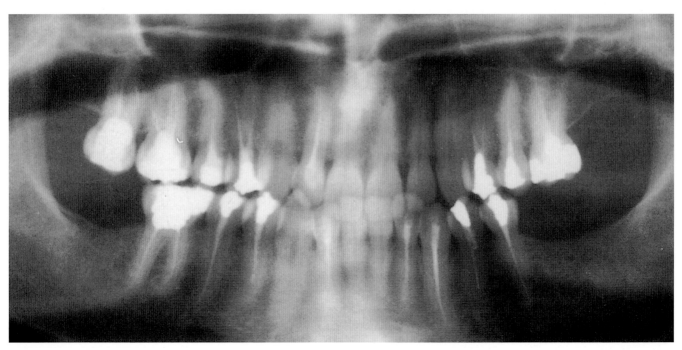

11.6

ORAL DYSAESTHESIA *(burning mouth syndrome; glossopyrosis; glossodynia)*

A burning sensation in the mouth, especially the tongue, may be caused by infection such as candidosis, vitamin or iron deficiency, diabetes, drugs such as captopril or lesions such as erythema migrans; dry mouth underlies some cases. In some patients, no organic cause can be established, the tongue appears normal (**Fig. 11.7**), and there may be a psychogenic basis, often a monosymptomatic hypochondriasis. Affected patients are often females of middle age or older and the burning sensation may be relieved by eating. Anxiety, for example about cancer, is found in many. Oral dysaesthesia may be one of the first clinical features of variant Creutzfeldt–Jakob disease.

PSYCHOGENIC ORAL DISEASE

A feature sometimes seen in tense or anxious patients is a remarkable degree of tongue protrusion to the extent that the epiglottis can be seen (**Fig. 11.8**). Others have pronounced occlusal lines (**Fig. 11.9**) and/or

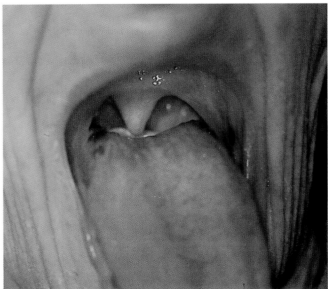

11.8

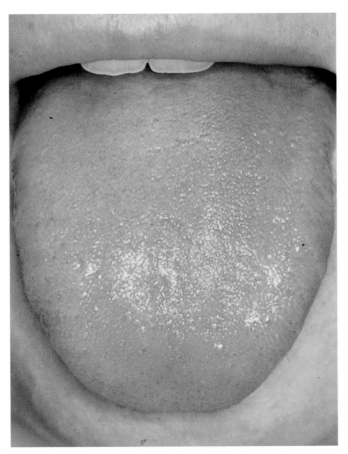

11.7

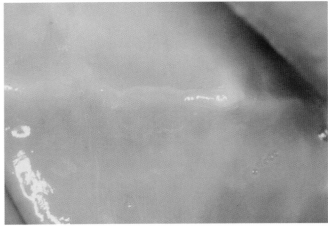

11.9

crenation or ulceration of the lateral border of the tongue (**Figs 11.10, 11.11**). Some suffer from para-function, bruxism, clenching (sometimes with masseteric hypertrophy), burning mouth syndrome or atypical facial pain, or have supposed xerostomia or abnormalities of taste — or a combination of these and other complaints. A few of these patients are depressed.

Patients with psychotic illness not infrequently neglect their oral health, occasionally to considerable degree (**Fig. 11.13**), and may have dyskinesias or pronounced xerostomia if on medication (see Chapter 17).

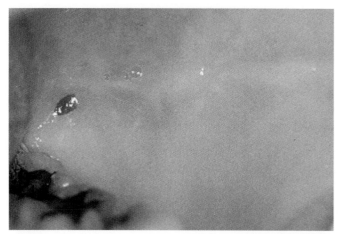

11.10

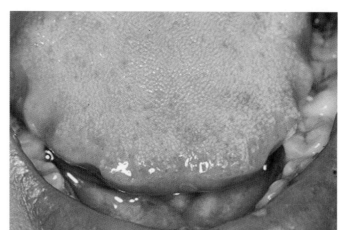

11.11

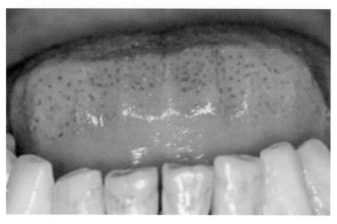

11.12

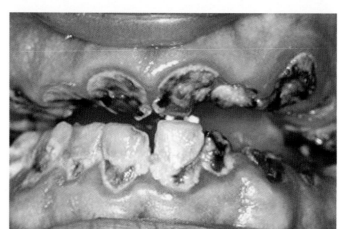

11.13

Bruxism may be seen in patients with learning disability, amfetamine or ecstasy abuse, or Rett's syndrome (see Chapter 28). Masseteric hypertrophy may result (**Fig. 11.14**) especially where there are parafunctional habits such as jaw-clenching.

A computed tomography scan shows the thickened masseters (**Fig. 11.15**). Attrition is common (**Fig. 11.16**; an extreme example in a patient with learning disability).

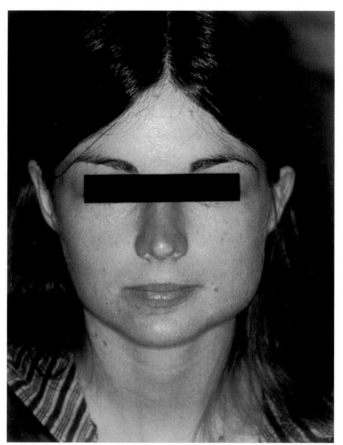

11.14

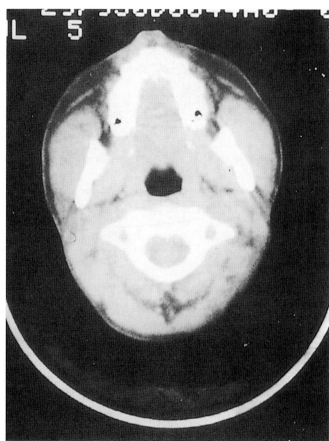

11.15

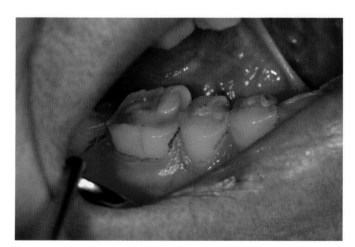

11.16

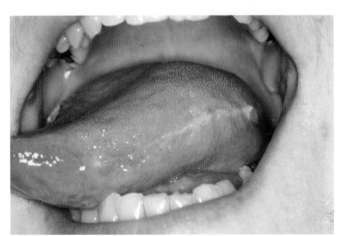

11.17

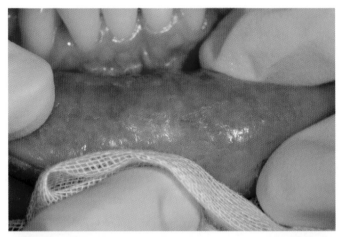

11.18

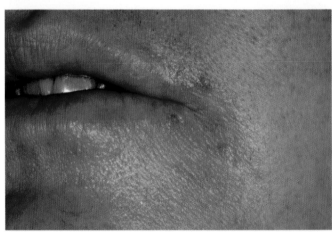

11.20

11.19

SELF-MUTILATION *(oral artefactual disease)*

Self-mutilation may be seen, to a minor degree, in anxious patients or those with psychogenic problems or learning disability. This may present with damage to the teeth, lips or tongue from chewing (**Figs 11.17–11.19**), or to the lips from licking (**Fig. 11.20**). Exfoliative cheilitis often has a psychogenic basis (**Figs 11.21, 11.22**). Self-mutilation may also be seen where there is sensory loss in the area and where there is congenital indifference to pain as in familial dysautonomia (Riley–Day syndrome, see Chapter 12). Factitious or artefactual lesions are seen in some mentally disturbed patients or those with learning disability, in Gilles de la Tourette's syndrome (tic, coprolalia and copropraxia) and in Lesch–Nyhan syndrome. Oral self-inflicted lesions are often bizarre, typically destructive and may involve hard or soft tissues. The lesions are typically in sites that can readily be reached by the dominant hand, for example, gingival lesions may be seen in the right labial aspect of the maxilla (see **Fig. 11.2**).

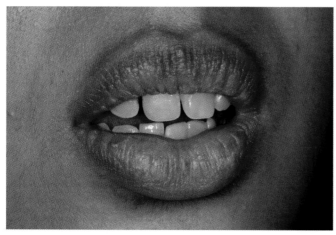

11.21

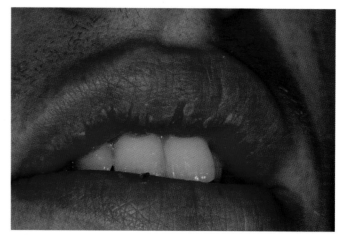

11.22

FURTHER READING

Bartoshuk LM, Grushka M, Duffy VB, Fast K, Lucchina L, Prutkin J, Snyder D. Burning mouth syndrome: damage to CN VII and pain phantoms in CN V. Chemical Senses 1999; 24: 609.

Becker AE, Grinspoon SK, Klibanski A, Herzog DB. Eating disorders. New Engl J Med 1999; 340(14): 1092–8.

Buchanan J, Zakrzewska J. Burning mouth syndrome. Clin Evid 2002; June: 1239–43.

Burchiel KJ. Facial pain syndromes: practical considerations. Clin Neurosurg 2000; 46: 435–45.

Dieterich M, Pfaffenrath V. Atypical facial pain. In Brandt T (ed) Neurological Disorders: Course and Treatment. New York, Academic Press, 1996, pp. 43–7.

Drage LA, Rogers RS, 3rd. Burning mouth syndrome. Dermatol Clin 2003; 21: 135–45.

Femiano F, Scully C, Gombos F. Idiopathic dysgeusia; an open trial of alpha lipoic acid (ALA) therapy. Int J Oral Maxillofac Surg 2002; 31: 625–8.

Genco RJ, Ho AW, Grossi SG, Dunford RG, Tedesco LA. Relationship of stress, distress and inadequate coping behaviours to periodontal disease. J Periodontol 1999; 70(7): 711–23.

Glaros AG. Emotional factors in temporomandibular joint disorders. J Indiana Dent Assoc 2000–01; 79(4): 20–3.

Hoek HW, Van Hoeken D. Review of the prevalence and incidence of eating disorders. Int J Eat Disord 2003; 34(4): 383–96.

Johansson AK, Johansson A, Birkhed D, Omar R, Baghdadi S, Carlsson GE. Dental erosion, soft-drink intake, and oral health in young Saudi men, and the development of a system for assessing erosive anterior tooth wear. Acta Odontol Scand 1996; 54(6): 369–78.

Milosevic A, Thomas J, Mitzman S. Satisfaction with dento-facial appearance in the eating disorders. Eur J Prosthodont Restor Dent 2003; 11(3): 125–8.

Ravaldi C, Vannacci A, Zucchi T, *et al.* Eating disorders and body image disturbances among ballet dancers, gymnasium users and body builders. Psychopathology 2003; 36(5): 247–54.

Scala A, Checchi L, Montevecchi M, Marini I, Giamberardino MA. Update on burning mouth syndrome: overview and patient management. Crit Rev Oral Biol Med 2003; 14: 275–91.

Scully C, Eveson JW, Porter SR. Munchausen's syndrome: oral presentations. Br Dent J 1995; 178: 65–7.

12 DISEASES OF THE NERVOUS SYSTEM

- abducent nerve lesion
- Bell's palsy
- cerebral palsy
- cerebrovascular accident
- congenital pain insensitivity
- epilepsy
- glossopharyngeal and vagus nerve palsy
- hypoglossal palsy
- lateral medullary syndrome
- Möbius' syndrome
- parkinsonism
- Riley–Day syndrome (and other dysautonomias)
- trigeminal neuralgia (paroxysmal trigeminal neuralgia)
- trigeminal sensory loss.

ABDUCENT NERVE LESION

The abducent nerve (cranial nerve VI) arises from the pons, has the longest intracranial course of any cranial nerve, and can be damaged by lesions in the posterior or middle cranial fossae, or the orbit. Abducent nerve palsy can be an early feature of an aneurysm on the circle of Willis.

The nerve supplies the lateral rectus muscle which abducts the eye. **Figure 12.1** shows a patient with a left abducent nerve palsy looking forwards. **Figure 12.2** demonstrates that when the patient tries to look to her left, the left eye cannot abduct.

BELL'S PALSY

Bell's palsy is an acute lower motor neurone (LMN) facial palsy initially regarded as of unknown aetiology, possibly infective, especially viral, and now known frequently to be caused by infection with herpes simplex virus (HSV). **Figures 12.3** and **12.4** show a patient during, and **Fig. 12.5** after, recovery from an attack of right-sided palsy.

Typically, Bell's palsy affects young or middle-aged patients and is acute and unilateral, often preceded by mild pain around the ear region

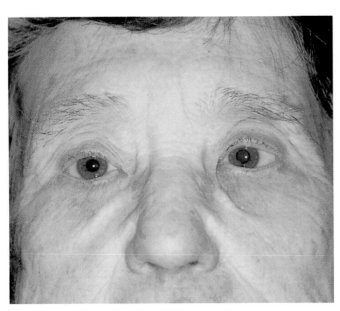

12.1

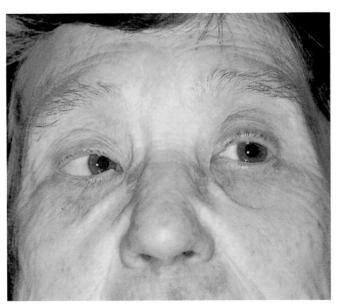

12.2

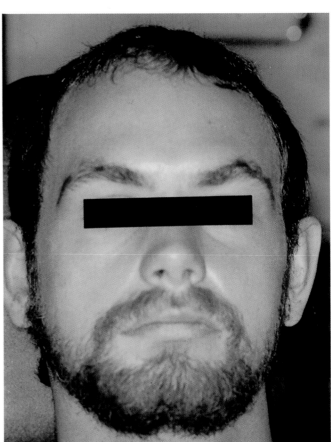

12.3

and sometimes a degree of hypo-aesthesia. The mouth droops on the side affected.

One complete side of the face is paralysed. Attempts to smile or whistle reveal the motionless affected side (**Fig. 12.4**); the eyelids cannot be closed tightly on that side. Absence of the efferent arc of the corneal reflex presents a hazard to the eye. LMN facial palsy is characterized by unilateral paralysis of all muscles of facial expression for voluntary and emotional responses. The forehead is unfurrowed and the patient unable to close the eye on that side. Upon attempted closure the eye rolls upwards (Bell's sign; **Fig. 12.6**).

Although usually a mononeuropathy, Bell's palsy may occasionally be part of a more widespread cranial or even peripheral polyneuropathy. There are a number of aetiological factors to exclude, including occasional associations with diabetes and with lymphoma. Facial palsy may also be caused by varicella-zoster virus (Ramsay Hunt's syndrome) or, by HIV, or seen in association with sarcoidosis (Heerfordt's syndrome). Melkersson–Rosenthal syndrome, neoplasms, Guillain–Barré syndrome, leprosy, Kawasaki's disease (mucocutaneous lymph node syndrome) or Lyme disease (tick-borne infection with *Borrelia burgdorferi*). Lower motor neurone facial palsy is rarely congenital (Möbius' syndrome, p. 255).

Most cases of Bell's palsy resolve spontaneously in a few weeks but it is often prudent to give a short course of systemic corticosteroids (and aciclovir if there is a possibility that HSV is involved), to try to avoid permanent nerve damage.

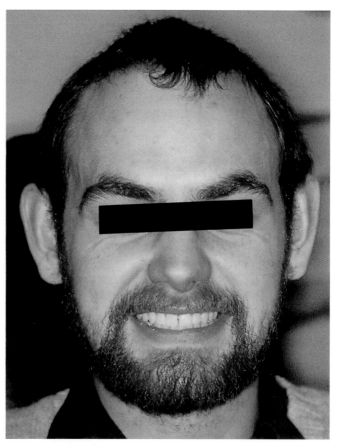

12.5

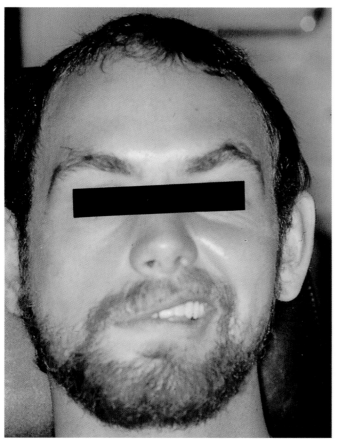

12.4

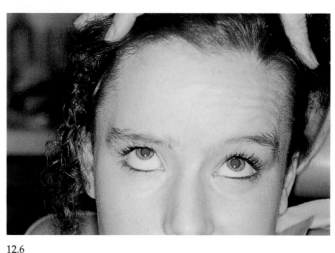

12.6

CEREBRAL PALSY

If muscle tone is increased, the term 'spastic' is used to describe the type of cerebral palsy (CP). Patients with spastic CP have stiff and jerky movements and difficulty moving from one position to another or letting go of something in their hand. This is the most common type of CP. About half of all people with CP have spastic CP.

Low muscle tone and poor coordination of movements in ataxic CP results in unsteadiness and shaking.

The term 'athetoid' is used to describe the type of CP when muscle tone is mixed: causing difficulty in holding themselves in an upright, steady position for sitting or walking, and frequent random, involuntary movements of their face, arms and upper body, making it difficult to hold things (like a toothbrush or fork). About a quarter of all people with CP have athetoid CP.

When muscle tone is reduced in some muscles and increased in others, the type of cerebral palsy is called 'mixed'. About a quarter of all people with CP have mixed CP.

Some persons with CP are unable to bite and chew foods, or they have trouble sucking through a straw or licking an ice-cream. Dysarthria is common, and epilepsy or learning disability may be seen, with attrition and sometimes dental damage or poor oral hygiene, and occasionally self-induced ulceration (**Fig. 12.7**).

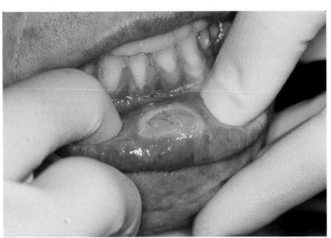

12.7

CEREBROVASCULAR ACCIDENT

Stroke is one of the main causes of facial palsy, when there is often unilateral facial palsy with ipsilateral hemiplegia. An upper motor neurone lesion, as in a stroke, causes paralysis mainly of the contralateral lower face although involuntary movement is preserved; for instance, laughing can still produce facial movement. Perhaps the greatest danger from facial palsy is to the eye on the affected side, since poor eyelid closure and defective corneal reflex exposes the cornea to damage (**Fig. 12.8**).

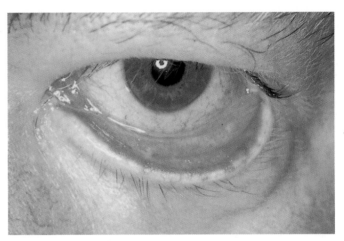

12.8

CONGENITAL PAIN INSENSITIVITY

Congenital insensitivity to pain is a rare disorder defined as the absence of normal subjective and objective responses to noxious stimuli in patients with intact central and peripheral nervous systems. Soft or hard tissue damage can result (**Fig. 12.9**).

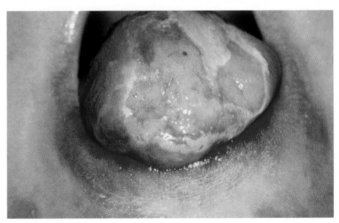

12.9

EPILEPSY

Epileptics often suffer repeated orofacial trauma causing soft tissue lacerations and scarring, and damage to the teeth and/or jaws (**Fig. 12.10**). Phenytoin can induce gingival swelling (**Fig. 12.10**). Anti-epileptic drugs such as phenytoin and sodium valproate given to pregnant mothers may cause fetal orofacial defects.

GLOSSOPHARYNGEAL AND VAGAL NERVE PALSY

In glossopharyngeal and vagus nerve palsy the palatal sensation and, therefore, the gag reflex are impaired. The uvula deviates away from the affected side (**Fig. 12.11**). This patient had deficits of cranial nerves IX to XII inclusive (bulbar palsy) from a posterior cranial fossa neoplasm.

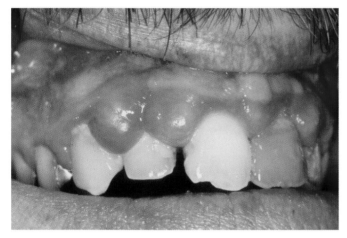

12.10

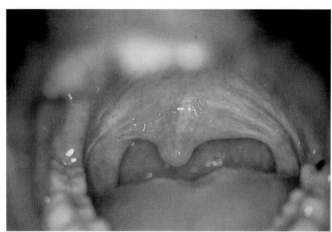

12.11

HYPOGLOSSAL PALSY

The hypoglossal nerve arises from the medulla and supplies motor fibres to most tongue muscles. Lower motor neurone lesions are rare but cause paralysis and wasting of the ipsilateral half of the tongue (**Fig. 12.12**); such lesions may become extreme (**Fig. 12.13**). On protrusion the tongue often deviates to the affected side. Lingual carcinoma may involve and damage the hypoglossal nerve.

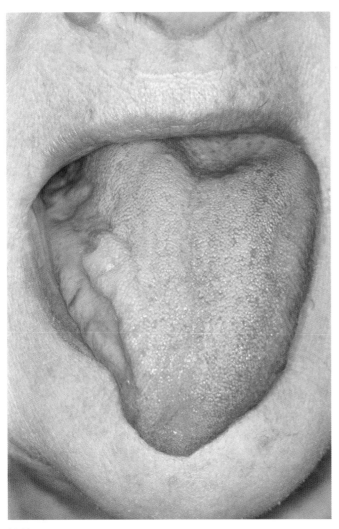

12.12

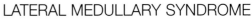

12.13

LATERAL MEDULLARY SYNDROME

Occlusion of the inferior artery of the lateral medulla oblongata (or occasionally of the posterior inferior cerebellar artery or vertebral artery) produces a syndrome of contralateral impairment of pain and thermal sense (damage to the spinothalamic tract), ipsilateral Horner's syndrome (damage to the sympathetic tract), hoarseness, dysphagia and ipsilateral palatal palsy, as shown in **Fig. 12.14** (IX and X cranial nerve palsies), sensory loss over the ipsilateral face (damage to V nerve nuclei), vestibular signs and loss of taste (damage to tractus solitarius).

Asymmetry of the soft palate is demonstrated in **Fig. 12.14** by the nasogastric tube which marks the midline.

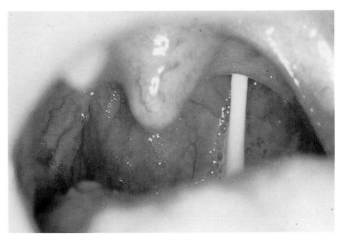

12.14

MÖBIUS' SYNDROME

Möbius' sequence/syndrome is a rare disorder characterized by congenital palsy of the abducens and facial nerves. The paralysis may be unilateral or bilateral, partial or complete, but is always nonprogressive. Affected patients have oculofacial palsy, profound lack of facial expression (**Fig. 12.15**), lower eyelid ectropion and conjunctivitis. Intraoral features may include hypodontia, microglossia and cleft palate. Systemic features include limb deformities (e.g. joint ankylosis, pectus excavatum, syndactyly and clubfoot), hearing impairment, external ear malformation and mild learning disability.

The addition of the congenital absence of pectoral muscles with ipsilateral hand deformities constitutes Poland–Möbius syndrome; while the precise cause remains unknown, defects on chromosomes 1, 3, 10 and 13 have been implicated.

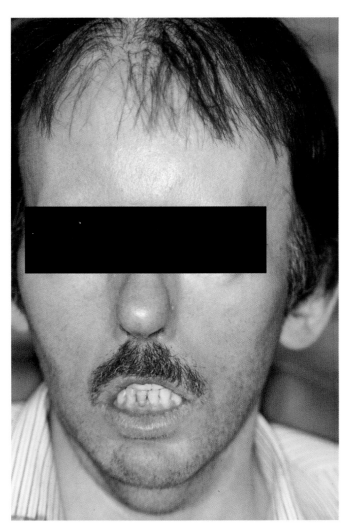

12.15

PARKINSONISM

There are no specific oral lesions in parkinsonism but there can be oral neglect and salivary dysfunction, or facial dyskinesias can result from drug therapy (see Section 1.5).

RILEY–DAY SYNDROME *(familial dysautonomia)*

Riley–Day syndrome is an autosomal recessive disorder which arises almost exclusively in Ashkenazi Jews. It is characterized clinically by widespread autonomic dysfunction in combination with loss of pain and temperature sensation.

A wide range of orofacial features have been described and include traumatic injury to oral tissues (**Fig. 12.16**), attrition, intentional or accidental extraction of teeth, absent pulpal vitality, retrognathism, dental crowding, masseteric hypertophy, lack of fungiform papillae and taste buds on the tongue, and hypersalivation.

Clinical problems manifest from birth, initially presenting with feeding difficulties, uncoordinated swallowing, gastro-oesophageal reflux and vomiting, which can lead to aspiration pneumonia. Cardiovascular manifestations include postural hypotension, intermittent tachycardias and hypertension. Repeated syncopal episodes in combination with poor pain sensibility can result in frequent traumatic injury. Ocular disease is common, lacrimation is diminished, with a lack of overflow tears during emotional crying, and corneal damage is likely due to reduced corneal sensation. Although causing profound disability in early life, most affected individuals survive to early adulthood. The precise molecular anomaly is not known but the candidate gene may lie on chromosome 9q31.

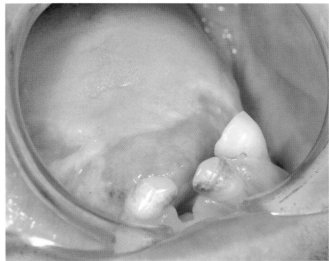

12.16

There is a wide spectrum of primary autonomic neuropathies, those with cholinergic involvement are the most likely to give rise to salivary gland dysfunction. Selective cholinergic dysautonomia, is characterized by involvement of peripheral parasympathetic and sudomotor sympathetic fibres, but preserved function of sympathetic adrenergic and somatic peripheral nerve fibres. Selective cholinergic dysautonomia may follow a viral illness and often presents with gastrointestinal motility dysfunction, although other likely manifestations are visual disturbance, difficult micturition and lack of saliva and tears. The oral manifestations are those of long-standing xerostomia and these include oral mucosal dryness (**Fig. 12.17**) and liability to caries (**Fig. 12.18**).

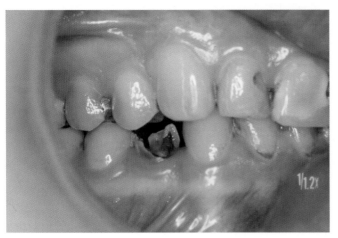

12.17

12.18

TRIGEMINAL NEURALGIA *(paroxysmal trigeminal neuralgia)*

Neuralgia in the trigeminal region can have many causes but most are of uncertain aetiology — benign paroxysmal trigeminal neuralgia. However, this diagnosis is only reached after exclusion of organic lesions such as multiple sclerosis, intracranial neoplasms and vascular anomalies, and connective tissue disorders.

Benign paroxysmal trigeminal neuralgia affects mainly the middle aged or elderly and causes intermittent lancinating pain, usually in one division or branch in the sensory distribution of the trigeminal nerve. There may be a trigger zone on the face or in the mouth, and patients are then understandably reluctant to touch the area, as in **Fig. 12.19**, which shows a patient who was reluctant to shave his left upper lip.

Treatment is usually medical (typically carbamazepine and more recently gabapentin) but intervention such as cryoanalgesia may be required. Neurosurgery is rarely required and then may leave a sensory deficit. The patient in **Fig. 12.20** was left with a numb left cheek and nose after neurosurgery and constantly traumatizes the area.

Vascular decompression of the trigeminal nerve produces good results with a relatively low complication rate.

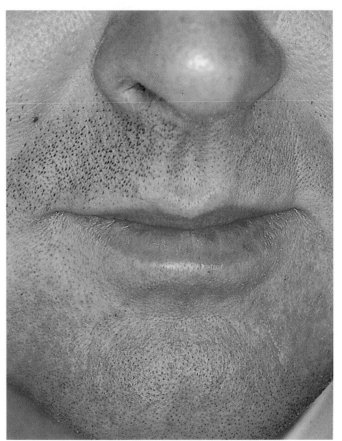

12.19

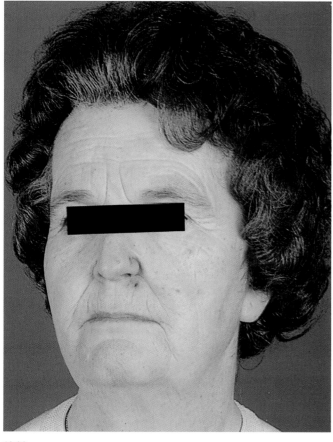

12.20

TRIGEMINAL SENSORY LOSS

The most common cause of trigeminal sensory loss is trauma, often iatrogenic, for example local anaesthesia, after which the patient accidentally traumatizes the lip (**Fig. 12.21**). Removal of lower third molars, mandibular osteotomies and cancer resections are the other main iatrogenic causes.

Sensory loss may be central in origin (cerebrovascular disease and anomalies, multiple sclerosis, syringobulbia, cerebral neoplasm or trauma) or peripheral (trauma, neoplasm or infection). **Figures 12.22** and **12.23** show a patient who had a cerebral neoplasm resulting in lesions of cranial nerves V and VI. Subsequently she repeatedly traumatized her nose and mouth on the right side. Trophic ulceration has also been reported.

The trigeminal nerve emerges from the pons and runs through the posterior and middle cranial fossa and can be damaged by disease affecting these areas. Causes include tumours, multiple sclerosis, infections, sarcoidosis, bone disease, drugs, neuropathy, a premonitory feature in the occasional patient with trigeminal neuralgia, an acute spontaneously resolving idiopathic neuropathy (benign trigeminal sensory neuropathy), and neuropathy associated with HIV or other viral infections, connective tissue diseases or other autoimmune states.

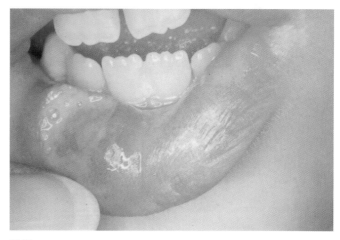

12.21

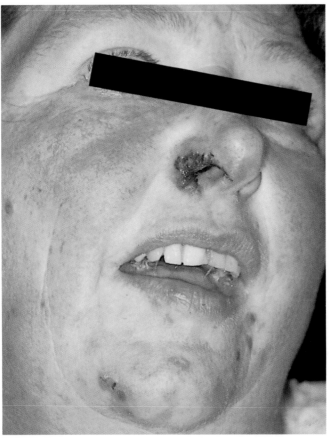

12.22

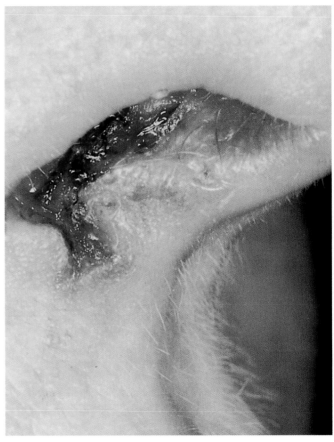

12.23

FURTHER READING

Baringer JR. Herpes simplex virus and Bell's palsy. Ann Intern Med 1996; 124: 63–5.

Biswas A, Prasad A, Anand KS. Trigeminal neuropathy in NIDDM. J Assoc Physicians India 1999; 47(11): 1125–6.

Brandt T, Illingworth RD, Peatfield RC. Trigeminal and glossopharyngeal neuralgia. In Brandt T. Neurological Disorders: Course and Treatment. New York, Academic Press, 1996, pp. 49–58.

Brandt T, Peatfield RC. Cluster headache and chronic paroxysmal hemicrania. In Brandt T (ed) Neurological Disorders: Course and Treatment. New York, Academic Press, 1996, pp. 17–27.

Fiske J, Boyle C. Epilepsy and oral care. Dent Update 2002; 29: 180–7.

Hodgson TA, Haricharan AK, Barrett AW, Porter SR. Microcystic adnexal carcinoma: an unusual cause of swelling and paraesthesia of the lower lip. Oral Oncol 2003; 39: 195–8.

Hupp WS. Seizure disorders. Oral Surg Oral Med Oral Pathol Oral Radiol Endod. 2001; 92: 593–6.

Israel HA, Scrivani SJ. The interdisciplinary approach to oral, facial and head pain. J Am Dent Assoc 2000; 131(7): 919–26.

James DJ. All that palsies is not Bell's. J R Soc Med 1996; 89: 184–7.

Kang YK, Lee EH, Hwang M. Pure trigeminal motor neuropathy: a case report. Arch Phys Med Rehabil 2000; 81(7): 995–8.

Kapur N, Kamel IR, Herlich A. Oral and craniofacial pain: diagnosis, pathophysiology, and treatment. Int Anesthesiol Clin 2003; 41: 115–50.

Kost RG, Straus SE. Postherpetic neuralgia – pathogenesis, treatment, and prevention. N Engl J Med 1996; 335: 32–42.

Meeks SL, Buatti JM, Foote KD, Friedman WA, Bova FJ. Calculation of cranial nerve complication probability for acoustic neuroma radiosurgery. Int J Radiat Oncol Biol Phys 2000; 47(3): 597–602.

Olesen J, Diener HC. Tension-type and cervicogenic headache. In Brandt T (ed) Neurological Disorders: Course and Treatment. New York, Academic Press, 1996, pp. 29–35.

Penarrocha M, Bagan JV, Penarrocha MA, Silvestre FJ. Cluster headache and cocaine use. Oral Surg 2000; 90: 271–4.

Penarrocha M, Bagan JV, Alfaro A, Penarrocha M. Acyclovir treatment in 2 patients with benign trigeminal sensory neuropathy. J Oral Maxillofac Surg 2001; 59(4): 453–6.

Qasho R, Vangelista T, Rocchi G, Ferrante L, Delfini R. Abducens nerve paresis as first symptom of trigeminal neurinoma. Report of two cases and review of the literature. J Neurosurg Sci 1999; 43(3): 223–8.

Ribeiro RA, Romano AR, Birman EG, Mayer MP. Oral manifestations in Rett syndrome: a study of 17 cases. Pediatr Dent 1997; 19(5): 349–52.

Ruboyianes JM, Trent CS, Adour KK, et al. Bell's palsy treatment with acyclovir and prednisone compared with prednisone alone: a double-blind, randomized, controlled trial. Ann Otol Rhinol Laryngol 1996; 105: 371–8.

Sawaya RA. Trigeminal neuralgia associated with sinusitis. ORL J Otorhinol Relat Spec 2000; 62(3): 160–3.

Schiffman SS. Taste and smell losses in normal aging and disease. JAMA 1997; 278: 1357–62.

Schrader V, Sumner A. Idiopathic (Bell's) facial palsy. In Brandt T (ed) Neurological Disorders: Course and Treatment. New York, Academic Press, 1996, pp. 113–16.

Scully C, Diz Dios P. Oral dyskinesias and palsies. In Alio Sanz JJ (ed) Rapport XV Congress of International Association of Disability and Oral Health. Aula Medica, Madrid 2000, pp. 306–29.

Scully C, Shotts R. The mouth in neurological disorders. Practitioner 2001; 245: 539–49.

Shankland WE 2nd. The trigeminal nerve. Part I: An over-view. Cranio 2000; 18(4): 238–48.

Shotts RH, Porter SR, Kumar N, Scully C. Longstanding trigeminal sensory neuropathy of nontraumatic cause. Oral Surg Oral Med Oral Pathol Oral Radiol Endod 1999; 87: 572–6.

Tacconi L, Miles JB. Bilateral trigeminal neuralgia: a therapeutic dilemma. Br J Neurosurg 2000; 14(1): 33–9.

Vickers ER, Cousins MJ. Neuropathic orofacial pain. Part 2 — Diagnostic procedures, treatment guidelines and case reports. Aust Endod J 2000; 26(2): 53–63.

Voss NF, Vrionis FD, Heilman CB, Robertson JH. Meningiomas of the cerebellopontine angle. Surg Neurol 2000; 53(5): 439–46.

Watt-Smith S, Mehta K, Scully C. Mefloquine-induced trigeminal sensory neuropathy. Oral Surg Oral Med Oral Pathol Oral Radiol Endod 2001; 92: 163–5.

Wingerchuk, Nyquist PA, Rodriguez M, Dodick DW. Extratrigeminal short-lasting unilateral neuralgiform headache with conjunctival injection and tearing (SUNCT): new pathophysiologic entity or variation on a theme? Cephalalgia 2000; 20(2): 127–9.

Zakrzewska JM. Facial pain: neurological and non-neurological. J Neurol Neurosurg Psychiatry 2002; 72: ii27–ii32.

Zakrzewska JM. Trigeminal neuralgia. Clin Evid 2002; (7): 1221–31.

Zakrzewska JM. Cluster headache; review of the literature. Brit J Oral MaxFac Surg 2002; 39: 103–13.

Zakrzewska JM, Harrison SD (eds). Assessment and Management of Orofacial Pain (Pain Research and Clinical Management vol 14). Elsevier, 2002.

13 DISEASES OF THE CIRCULATORY SYSTEM

- calibre-persistent artery
- cardiac transplantation
- giant cell arteritis (cranial or temporal arteritis; Horton's disease)
- hereditary haemorrhagic telangiectasia (Rendu–Osler–Weber syndrome)
- ischaemic and other heart diseases
- midline granuloma (idiopathic midfacial granuloma syndrome)
- periarteritis nodosa (polyarteritis nodosa)
- varices
- Wegener's granulomatosis.

CALIBRE-PERSISTENT ARTERY

A 'calibre-persistent artery' is defined as an artery with a diameter larger than normal and which lies near a mucosal or external surface. Most are seen in the lower lip and are asymptomatic. However, they may occasionally cause chronic ulceration, which can be mistaken for cancer (**Fig. 13.1**).

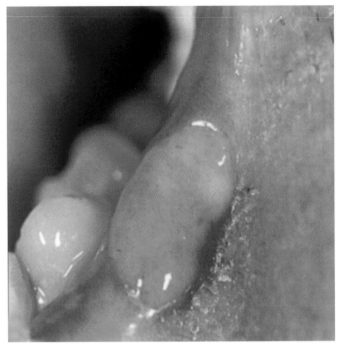

13.1

CARDIAC TRANSPLANTATION

Oral complications are mainly those related to the immunosuppression used to prevent rejection, and may include infections such as candidosis

(**Fig. 13.2**), herpes simplex virus-related ulceration (**Fig. 13.3**) and hairy leukoplakia, as in persons with other organ transplants.

Drugs used after cardiac transplantation may also produce other oral adverse side-effects. The most common is gingival swelling

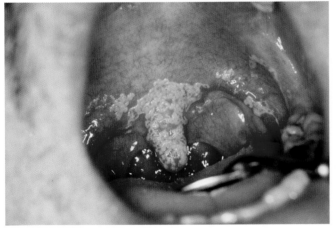

13.2

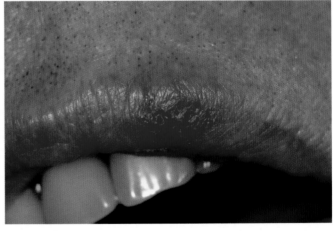

13.3

(ciclosporin and/or nifedipine; **Fig. 13.4**) but other cardioactive drugs can produce dry mouth, ulcers, lichenoid and other lesions (see Chapter 29).

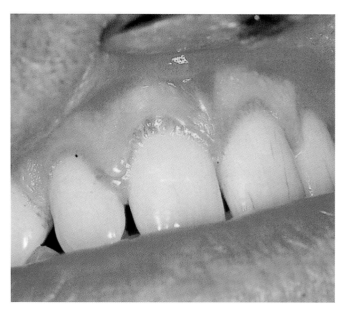

13.4

GIANT CELL ARTERITIS *(cranial or temporal arteritis; Horton's disease)*

Giant cell arteritis is a granulomatous condition which involves medium and larger arteries, mainly in the head and neck and particularly branches of the aortic arch. It is found mainly in older women and is closely related to polymyalgia rheumatica.

The main manifestations (in the head and neck) include temporal pain, tenderness and headache, with neuro-ophthalmic features, particularly sudden blindness. Patients may also have jaw or masseteric pain, or may have pain in the tongue, particularly during chewing (claudication). Lingual arteritis is common, presenting as pain or ulceration (**Fig. 13.5**).

Although the tongue has an excellent blood supply and usually survives, lingual necrosis has now been described in several patients with giant cell arteritis. The lingual necrosis is almost invariably unilateral, and only very rare cases of bilateral necrosis (**Fig. 13.6**) have been reported. Labial gangrene (**Fig. 13.7**) is another rare complication of giant cell arteritis. Low-grade fever, anorexia, weight loss, generalized aches and pains and a raised erythrocyte sedimentation rate may be seen. Systemic corticosteroids are indicated to prevent retinal damage.

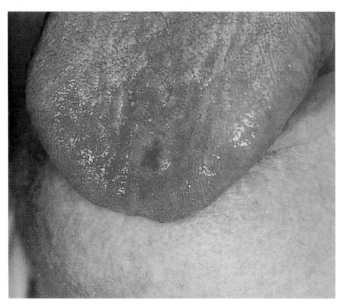

13.5

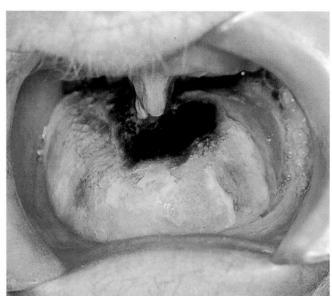

13.6

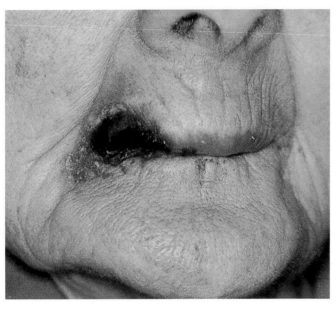

13.7

HEREDITARY HAEMORRHAGIC TELANGIECTASIA *(Rendu–Osler–Weber syndrome)*

Hereditary haemorrhagic telangiectasia (HHT) is an autosomal dominant condition characterized by mucosal and cutaneous telangiectases which may not be present at birth but appear on the lips and periorally (**Fig. 13.8**). Occasional telangiectases appear on the extremities, particularly on the palmar surfaces of the digits (**Fig. 13.9**), and on the conjunctiva (**Fig. 13.10**), nasal and gastro-intestinal mucosae.

The mucosal telangiectases found in the mouth (**Fig. 13.11**), nasal and alimentary mucosa may lead to repeated haemorrhage, and eventually to severe anaemia and, therefore, even cardiac failure.

Retinal telangiectases predispose to intraocular bleeding. Pulmonary arteriovenous fistulae, central nervous system and hepatic vascular anomalies predispose to complications, and HHT has occasional associations with von Willebrand's disease and IgA deficiency.

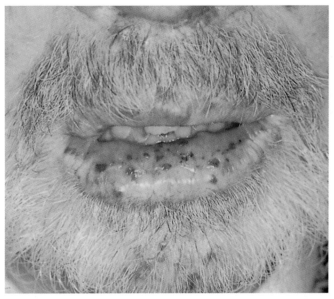

13.8

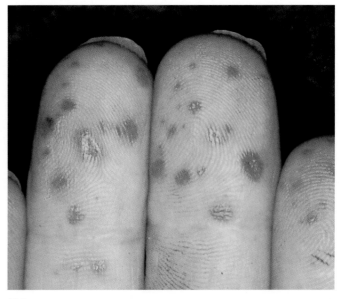

13.9

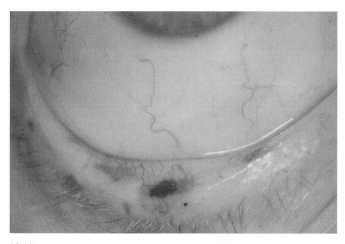

13.10

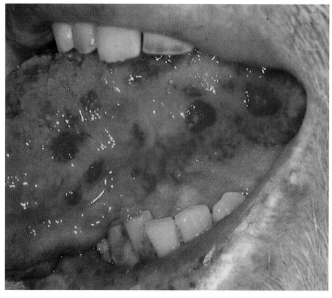

13.11

ISCHAEMIC AND OTHER HEART DISEASES

Central cyanosis is readily demonstrable in the oral soft tissues (**Fig. 13.12;** see also **Fig. 28.69**). Angina occasionally produces pain that radiates to the jaw or palate. Cardioactive drugs can produce gingival swelling, dry mouth, ulcers, lichenoid and other lesions (see Chapter 29).

Use of calcium-channel blockers such as nifedipine may lead to gingival swelling (**Fig. 13.4**). Nicorandil may cause oral ulceration (see Chapter 29), beta-blockers may cause lichenoid lesions or dry mouth (see Chapter 29), and ACE inhibitors may cause angioedema, burning sensation, dry mouth, taste disturbances, lichenoid lesions and pemphigus-like disease (see Chapter 29).

MIDLINE GRANULOMA *(idiopathic midfacial granuloma syndrome)*

This is a group of rare disorders, now recognized as lymphomas, mainly T-cell, which start in the nasal or paranasal tissues but cause destruction of the facial bones (**Fig. 13.13**). This clinical syndrome can result from Stewart's granuloma, lymphomatoid granulomatosis or polymorphic reticulosis. A similar clinical picture may rarely arise with cocaine abuse.

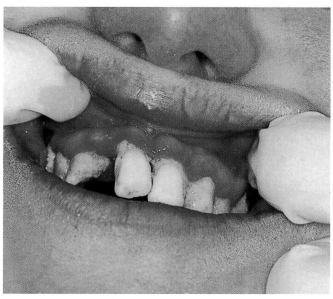

13.12

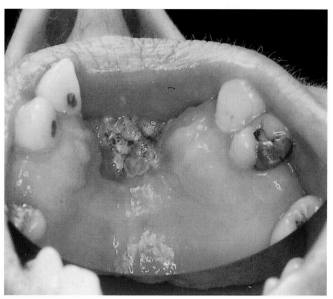

13.13

PERIARTERITIS NODOSA *(polyarteritis nodosa)*

Periarteritis nodosa is a necrotizing vasculitis affecting small- and medium-sized arteries, mainly seen in males and often related to previous infection with hepatitis B virus. Arthralgia, angina, hypertension and renal disease are the main features. Oral nodules, bleeding or ulcers (**Figs 13.14, 13.15**) may be seen.

VARICES

Dilated lingual veins give rise to varices, common in the elderly (**Fig. 13.16**), and are of no special significance. There are occasional associations with varices elsewhere in the body, including the jejunum and scrotum.

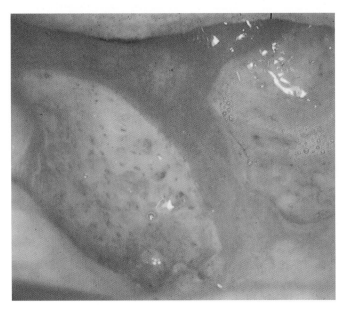

13.14

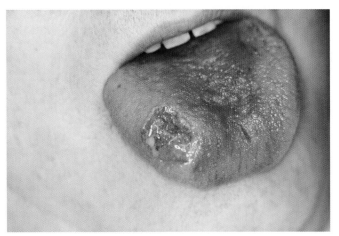

13.15

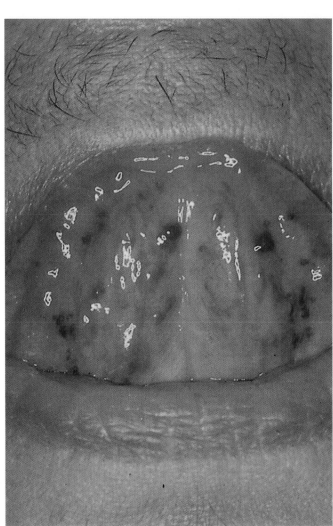

13.16

WEGENER'S GRANULOMATOSIS

Wegener's granulomatosis is a rare disorder of uncertain aetiology though sometimes associated with *Staphylococcus aureus*, which presents with generalized necrotizing vasculitis, granulomatous lesions in the respiratory tract, and, later, focal necrotizing glomerulonephritis. Antineutrophil cytoplasmic antibodies (ANCA) against proteinase 3 are characteristic.

Up to 5% of patients with Wegener's granulomatosis have oral lesions, the most pathognomonic of which is gingival swelling with a particular resemblance to a ripe strawberry (gingival hyperplasia with petechiae; **Fig. 13.17**). Mucosal ulcers (**Fig. 13.18**) or delayed wound healing are the other main oral features.

Occasionally, a limited form of the disease, involving only one or two organ systems, is seen.

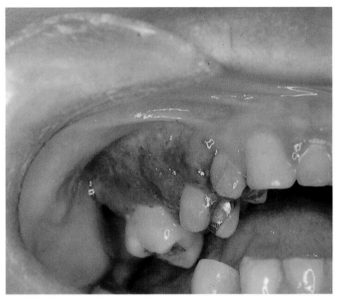

13.17

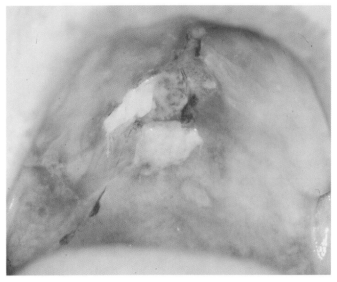

13.18

FURTHER READING

al-Sarheed M, Angeletou A, Ashley PF, Lucas VS, Whitehead B, Roberts GJ. An investigation of the oral status and reported oral care of children with heart and heart-lung transplants. Int J Paediatr Dent 2000; 10(4): 298–305.

Blanchaert RH Jr. Ischemic heart disease. Oral Surg Oral Med Oral Pathol Oral Radiol Endod 1999; 87(3): 281–3.

Carmona IT, Dios PD, Scully C. An update on the controversies in bacterial endocarditis of oral origin. Oral Surg Oral Med Oral Pathol Oral Radiol Endod 2002; 93: 660–70.

Crean SJ, Adams R, Bennett J. Sublingual gland involvement in systemic Wegener's granulomatosis: a case report. Int J Oral Maxillofac Surg 2002; 31: 104–6.

Glueck CJ, McMahon RE, Bouquot J, Stroop D, Tracy T, Wang P, Rabinovich B. Thrombophilia, hypofibrinolysis, and alveolar osteonecrosis of the jaws. Oral Surg Oral Med Oral Pathol 1996; 81: 557–66.

Herman WW, Konzelman JL. Angina: an update for dentistry. J Am Dent Assoc 1996; 127: 98–104.

Hsi ED, Singleton TP, Swinnen L, Dunphy CH, Alkan S. Mucosa-associated lymphoid tissue-type lymphomas occurring in post-transplantation patients. Am J Surg Pathol 2000; 24(1): 100–6.

Joshipura KJ, Rimm EB, Douglass CW, et al. Poor oral health and coronary heart disease. J Dent Res 1996; 75: 1631–6.

Joshipura KJ, Douglass CW, Willett WC. Possible explanations for the tooth loss and cardiovascular disease relationship. Ann Periodontol 1998; 3(1): 175–83.

Jowett NI, Cabot LB. Patients with cardiac disease; considerations for the dental practitioner. Brit Dent J 2000; 189: 297–302.

Larsson B, Johansson I, Hallmans G, Ericson T. Relationship between dental caries and risk factors for atherosclerosis in Swedish adolescents? Commun Dent Oral Epidemiol 1995; 23: 205–10.

Lilly J, Juhlin T, Lew D, Vincent S, Lilly G. Wegener's granulomatosis presenting as oral lesions: a case report. Oral Surg Oral Med Oral Pathol Oral Radiol Endod 1998; 85: 153–7.

Loesche WJ, Schork A, Terpenning MS, Chen YM, Dominguez BL, Grossman N. Assessing the relationship between dental disease and coronary heart disease in elderly US veterans. J Am Dent Assoc 1998; 129(3): 301–11.

Lowry LY, Welbury RR, Seymour RA, Waterhouse PJ, Hamilton JR. Gingival overgrowth in paediatric cardiac transplant patients: a study of 19 patients aged between 2 and 16 years. Int J Paediatr Dent 1995; 5(4): 217–22.

Meyer U, Kleinheinz J, Handschel J, Kruse-Losler B, Weingart D, Joos U. Oral findings in three different groups of immunocompromised patients. J Oral Pathol Med 2000; 29: 153–8.

Niederman R, Joshipura K. Cause celebre; oral health and heart disease. Evidence-based Dentistry 2000; 2: 59–60.

Prusinski L, Eisold JF. Hyperlipoproteinemic states and ischemic heart disease. Dent Clin North Am 1996; 40(3): 563–84.

Rahilly G, Rahilly M. A case of palatal Wegener's granulomatosis. Oral Dis 2000; 6: 259–61.

Scully C, Roberts G, Shotts R. The mouth in heart disease. Practitioner 2001; 245: 432–7.

Thomason JM, Seymour RA, Murphy P, Brigham KM, Jones P. Aspirin-induced post-gingivectomy haemorrhage: a timely reminder. J Clin Periodontol 1997; 24(2): 136–8.

14 DISEASES OF THE RESPIRATORY SYSTEM

- antral carcinoma
- asthma
- cystic fibrosis
- fascial space infections
- influenza
- lung cancer
- lymphonodular pharyngitis
- maxillary sinusitis
- quinsy (peritonsillar abscess)
- tonsillitis
- tuberculosis.

Note that any form of respiratory, tonsillar or pharyngeal infection can cause halitosis.

ANTRAL CARCINOMA

Carcinoma of the maxillary antrum is a rare neoplasm, found especially in those who work with wood, for example in the furniture industry, and in those who work in the shoe and boot industry. Snuff use also appears to predispose to antral carcinoma.

Initially asymptomatic, antral carcinoma eventually invades the palate, nose or orbit. It often presents clinically as a swelling in the palate or alveolus, usually in the premolar molar region (**Figs 14.1–14.3**). The swelling may ulcerate. The globe on the affected side is displaced superiorly, and these is a blood-stained nasal discharge (**Fig. 14.1**). Occipitomental radiography, CT or MRI show opacity and invasion with loss of the bony walls of the antrum (see **Fig. 14.3**).

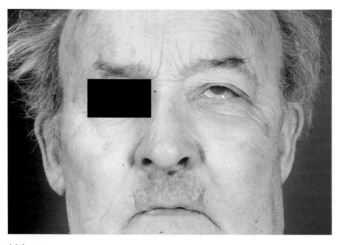

14.1

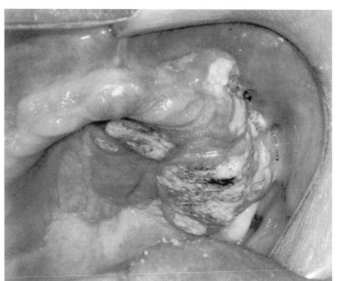

14.2

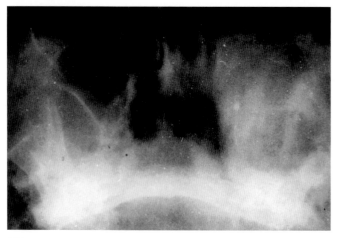

14.3

ASTHMA

There are no oral complications of asthma, but corticosteroid inhaler use may precipitate candidosis and some medications are cariogenic.

CYSTIC FIBROSIS

Cystic fibrosis, which produces serious pulmonary and pancreatic disease, may result in sinusitis and xerostomia the use of tetracyclines may cause tooth discoloration (**Fig. 14.4**). Finger clubbing is common (**Fig. 14.5**).

FASCIAL SPACE INFECTIONS

Ludwig's angina is a bacterial infection of the sublingual and submandibular fascial spaces, usually of odontogenic origin. It manifests with pain, submandibular swelling, dysphagia and fever and may be a hazard to the airway (**Fig. 14.6**).

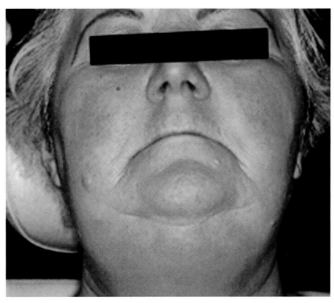

14.6

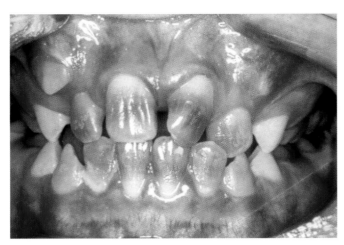

14.4

INFLUENZA

Oral lesions have not often been formally reported in influenza but ulcers (**Fig. 14.7**), pericoronitis, gingivitis and soft palate hyperaemia have been described.

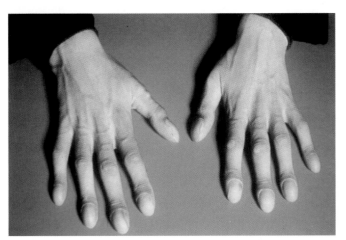

14.5

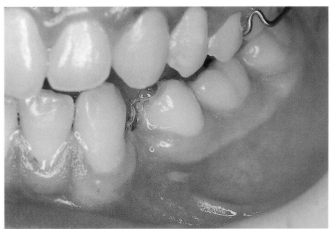

14.7

LUNG CANCER

The prevalence of lung cancer and other aerodigestive tract cancer is increased in patients with oral carcinoma.

Oral changes are rare in lung cancer but may include metastases usually to the jaws (**Fig. 14.8**), pain (sometimes mimicking temporomandibular pain-dysfunction), trigeminal neuropathy or, because of ectopic ACTH production, hyperpigmentation (particularly of the soft palate).

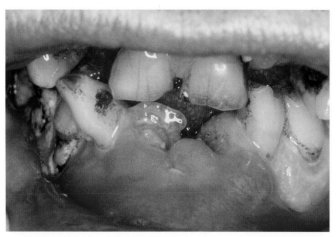

14.8

LYMPHONODULAR PHARYNGITIS

Lymphonodular pharyngitis is an acute infection with Coxsackievirus associated with strain A10. Similar to herpangina, lymphonodular pharyngitis presents with fever and multiple small (2–5 mm) yellowish papules on the soft palate and oropharynx (**Fig. 14.9**).

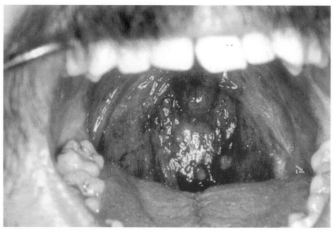

14.9

MAXILLARY SINUSITIS

Acute maxillary sinusitis is usually preceded by an upper respiratory tract viral infection but occasionally follows an oroantral fistula or displacement of a tooth or root into the sinus (antrum). Pain is felt over the sinus, especially on moving the head, the cheek may be tender to palpate and the ipsilateral premolars and molars may be tender to percussion. There may be halitosis. Transillumination or occipitomental radiography show opacities in the affected sinuses (bilateral in **Fig. 14.10**).

Tilting the head (**Fig. 14.11**) shows that the bilateral sinus opacities in this case are fluid.

Sinusitis is also a complication of cystic fibrosis, Kartagener's syndrome (immobile cilia and dextrocardia), HIV disease and various other immunodeficiencies. Kartagener's syndrome and immunodeficiencies may also cause enhanced gingivitis and periodontitis.

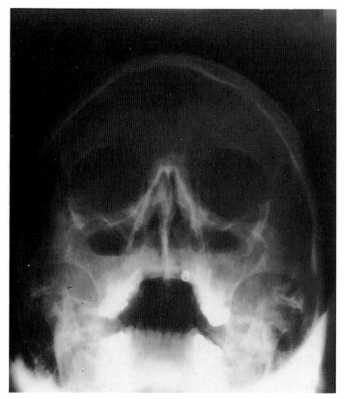

14.10

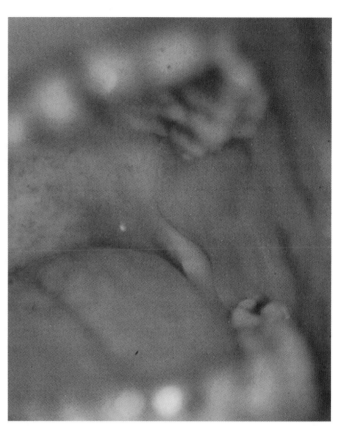

14.11

QUINSY *(peritonsillar abscess)*

Peritonsillar abscess, although usually following *Streptococcus pyogenes* infection, typically contains a variety of oropharyngeal micro-organisms. The abscess causes severe pain, dysphagia and trismus before pointing (**Fig. 14.12**) and discharging.

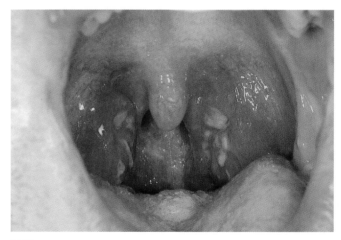

14.12

TONSILLITIS

Caused by *Streptococcus pyogenes* (Lancefield Group A β-haemolytic streptococcus), the incubation period of 2–4 days is followed by sore throat, dysphagia and fever. Usually children are affected. The uvula, tonsils and pharynx are diffusely red, with punctate white or yellow tonsillar exudates (**Fig. 14.13**). Complications are rare but can include otitis media, quinsy, sinusitis, rheumatic fever or glomerulonephritis. Tonsillar exudates are also seen in infectious mononucleosis.

TUBERCULOSIS

For tuberculosis, see Chapter 3.

14.13

FURTHER READING

Bagg J. Common infectious diseases. Dent Clin North Am 1996; 40: 385–93.

Barasch A, Gordon S, Geist RY, Geist JR. Necrotizing stomatitis: report of 3 *Pseudomonas aeruginosa*-positive patients. Oral Surg Oral Med Oral Pathol Oral Radiol Endod 2003; 96(2): 136–40.

Cohen R. Obstructive sleep apnea. Oral Surg Oral Med Oral Pathol Oral Radiol Endod 1998; 85: 388–92.

Copp PE. The asthmatic dental and oral surgery patient. A review of management considerations. Ont Dent 1995; 72: 33–42.

Harlow RF, Rutkauskas JS. Tuberculosis risk in the hospital dental practice. Spec Care Dentist 1995; 15(2): 50–5.

Kargul B, Tanboga I, Ergeneli S, Karakoc F, Dagli E. Inhaler medicament effects on saliva and plaque pH in asthmatic children. J Clin Pediatr Dent 1998; 22: 137–40.

Laurikainen K, Kuusisto P. Comparison of the oral health status and salivary flow rate of asthmatic patients with those of nonasthmatic adults – results of a pilot study. Allergy 1998; 53: 316–19.

Lee KC, Schecter G. Tuberculous infections of the head and neck. ENT J 1995; 74: 395–9.

Levin JA, Glick M. Dental management of patients with asthma. Compend Contin Educ Dent 1996; 17: 284–92.

Limeback H. Implications of oral infections on systemic diseases in the institutionalized elderly with a special focus on pneumonia. Ann Periodontol 1998; 3: 262–75.

Mathieu D, Neviere R, Teillon C, et al. Cervical necrotizing fasciitis; clinical manifestations and management. Clin Infect Dis 1995; 21: 51–6.

Menzies D, Fanning A, Yuan L, Fitzgerald M. Tuberculosis among health care workers. N Engl J Med 1995; 332: 92–8.

Mojon P, Budtz-Jorgensen E, Michel JP, Limeback H. Oral health and history of respiratory tract infection in frail institutionalised elders. Gerodontology 1997; 14: 9–16.

Murphy DC, Younai FS. Obstacles encountered in application of the Centers for Disease Control and Prevention guidelines for control of tuberculosis in a large dental center. Am J Infect Control 1997; 25(3): 275–82.

Nakamura S, Inui M, Nakase M, Kamei T, Higuchi Y, Goto A, Tagawa T. Clostridial deep neck infection developed after extraction of a tooth: a case report and review of the literature in Japan. Oral Dis 2002; 8: 224–6.

Parry JA, Harrison VE, Barnard KM. Recognizing and caring for the medically compromised child: 1. Disorders of the cardiovascular and respiratory systems. Dent Update 1998; 25: 325–31.

Phelan JA, Jimenez V, Tompkins DC. Tuberculosis. Dent Clin North Am 1996; 40(2): 327–41.

Scannapieco FA, Mylotte JM. Relationships between periodontal disease and bacterial pneumonia. J Periodontol 1996; 67: 1114–22.

Scannapieco FA, Papandonatos GD, Dunford RG. Associations between oral conditions and respiratory disease in a national sample survey population. Ann Periodontol 1998; 3: 251–6.

Schiodt M. Deep cervical infections – an uncommon but significant problem. Oral Dis 2002; 8(4): 180–2.

Scully C. The mycobacterioses. In Millard HD and Mason DK (eds), 1993 World Workshop on Oral Medicine. Ann Arbor, University of Michigan Press, 1995, pp. 57–61.

Sollecito TP, Tino G. Asthma. Oral Surg Oral Med Oral Pathol Oral Radiol Endod 2001; 92: 485–90.

Spitalnic SJ, Sucov A. Ludwig's angina: case report and review. J Emerg Med 1995; 13(4): 499–503.

Strull GE, Dym H. Tuberculosis: diagnosis and treatment of resurgent disease. J Oral Maxillofac Surg 1995; 53: 1334–40.

Umeda M, Minamikawa T, Komatsubara H, Shibuya Y, Yokoo S, Komori T. Necrotizing fasciitis caused by dental infection: a retrospective analysis of 9 cases and a review of the literature. Oral Surg Oral Med Oral Pathol Oral Radiol Endod 2003; 95(3): 283–90.

Younai FS, Murphy DC. TB and dentistry. NY State Dent J 1997; 63(1): 49–53.

Zhu JF, Hidalgo HA, Holmgreen WC, Redding SW, Hu J, Henry RJ. Dental management of children with asthma. Pediatr Dent 1996; 18: 363–70.

15 DISORDERS OF TEETH

- abrasion
- amelogenesis imperfecta
- ankylosis
- anomalies of tooth shape
- attrition
- dental caries
- dentinogenesis imperfecta
- dilaceration
- enamel cleft
- enamel hypoplasia
- enamel nodule (enameloma; enamel pearl)
- erosion
- fluorosis
- hypercementosis
- hyperdontia
- hyperplastic pulpitis (pulp polyp)
- hypodontia
- impacted teeth
- localized damage
- malocclusion
- natal teeth
- nonvital teeth
- odontomes
- periapical abscess (dental abscess; odontogenic abscess)
- periapical cyst (radicular or dental cyst)
- prominent tubercules or cusps
- residual cyst
- resorption
- retained primary tooth
- retained root
- taurodontism
- teratoma
- tooth extrinsic staining
- tooth intrinsic staining.

ABRASION

Abrasion is the wearing away of tooth substance by a habit such as toothbrushing. Brushing with a hard brush and coarse dentifrice may abrade the neck of the tooth. The gingiva recedes but is otherwise healthy; the cementum and dentine wear but the harder enamel survives, resulting in a notch. There may be cervical hypersensitivity and, eventually, the tooth may fracture (**Fig. 15.1**). The term 'abfraction' is used to describe the pathologic loss of both enamel and dentine caused by biomechanical loading forces, such as those produced by swallowing and clenching or chewing. The abfractive lesions appear to be caused by flexure and ultimate material fatigue of susceptible teeth at locations away from the point of loading. The breakdown is dependent on the magnitude, duration, direction, frequency and location of the forces.

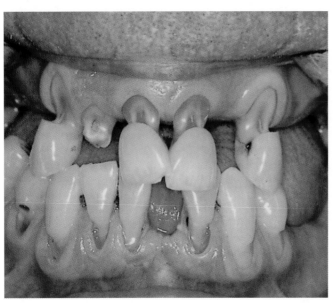

15.1

AMELOGENESIS IMPERFECTA

Amelogenesis imperfecta is the term applied to a group of rare genetically determined disorders of enamel formation. There are three main types

- *hypoplastic type* — hereditary enamel hypoplasia; the enamel is thin.
- *hypocalcified type* — the enamel is of normal thickness but weak and soft.
- *hypomaturation type* — the enamel can be pierced with a probe.

Figure 15.2 shows a primary dentition affected by amelogenesis imperfecta. **Figure 15.3** is a sibling of the patient in **Fig. 15.2**, showing

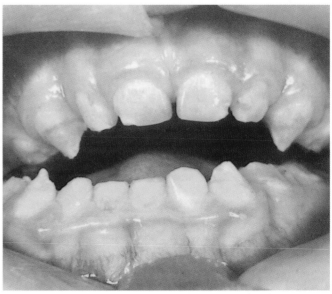

15.2

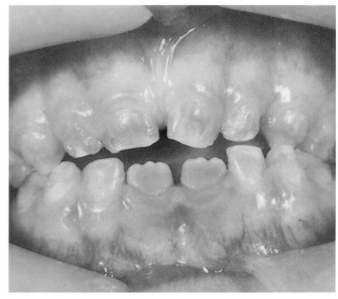

15.3

the genetic basis and demonstrating that the primary and secondary dentitions (the permanent central incisors are erupting) are both affected. **Figure 15.4** shows an example of hereditary enamel hypoplasia of an autosomal dominant type. The enamel matrix is defective although calcification is normal (note the vertical ridging). **Figure 15.5** shows a more extreme example: a sex-linked dominant type. Pitting and grooving is seen in some types of hereditary enamel hypoplasia (**Fig. 15.6**). **Figure 15.7** shows a more extreme example of the type of hereditary enamel hypoplasia shown in **Fig. 15.6**.

Radiographs show enamel deficiencies in hereditary enamel hypoplasia (**Figs 15.8, 15.9**).

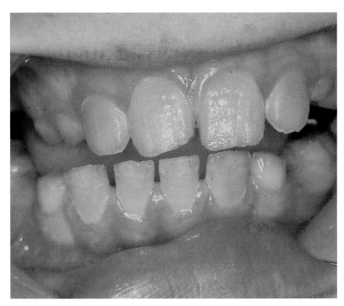

15.4

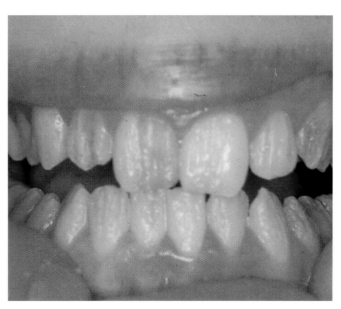

15.5

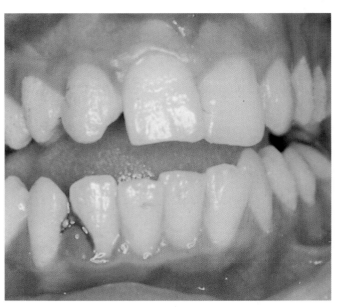

15.6

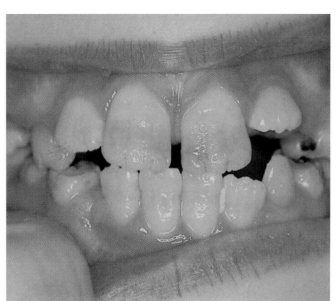

15.7

In hereditary enamel hypocalcification the matrix is normal but calcification defective and thus the soft enamel may wear away rapidly to leave only the dentine core (**Fig. 15.10**). In **Fig. 15.11**, there is almost complete breakdown of the dentition and incidental calculus deposition.

Figures 15.12–15.14 show opaque white flecks or patches in an autosomal dominant variety of amelogenesis imperfecta ('snow-capped' teeth) whilst **Fig. 15.15** shows a variant affecting permanent first molars only.

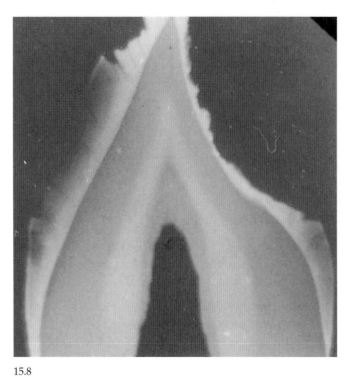

15.8

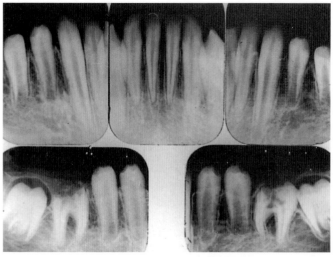

15.9

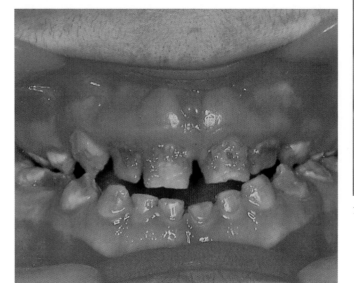

15.10

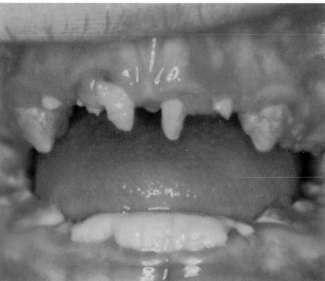

15.11

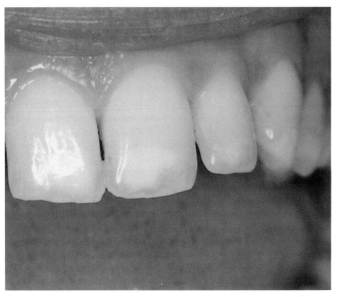

15.12

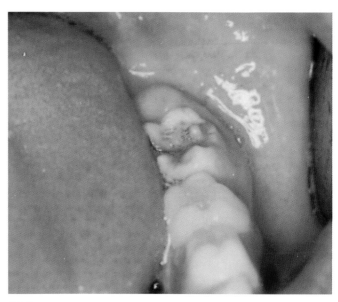

15.15

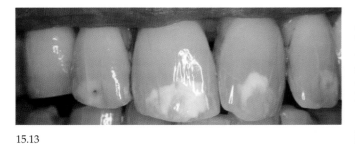

15.13

ANKYLOSIS

Teeth that are single standing molars are often ankylosed as are those that are hypercementosed. Deciduous molars may be retained and in infraocclusion ("submerged") because the permanent successor is absent. (**Figure 15.16** shows bony ankylosis and no evidence of a periodontal ligament.)

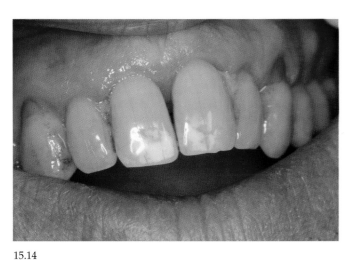

15.14

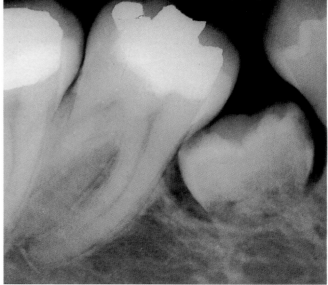

15.16

ANOMALIES OF TOOTH SHAPE

Peg-shaped teeth is the most common anomaly of tooth shape and may produce a cosmetic problem (**Figs 15.17, 15.18**).

Fusion (the union of two normally separate, adjacent tooth germs) gives rise to a large tooth; therefore there is a tooth missing from the series (**Fig. 15.19**) unless the fusion is with a supernumerary tooth.

Fusion may be complete along the length of the teeth (**Fig. 15.20**) or may involve roots alone, and it may give rise to poor aesthetics (**Fig. 15.21**) and sometimes malocclusions.

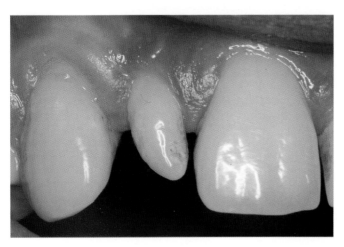

15.17

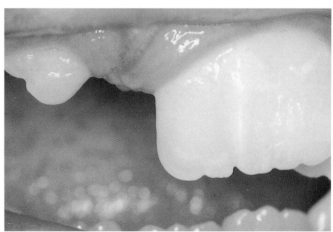

15.19

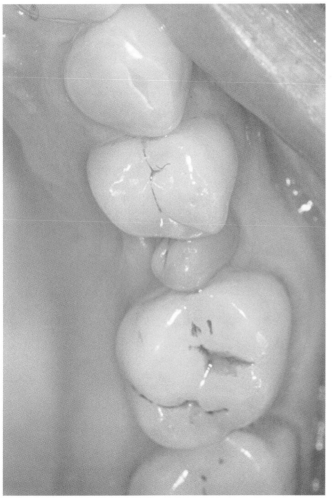

15.18

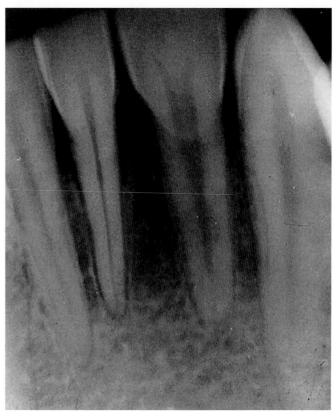

15.20

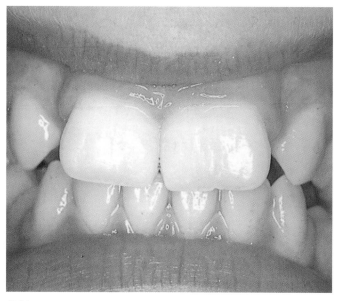

15.21

ATTRITION

Attrition is the wearing away of tooth substance by mastication. It is most obvious where the diet is coarse, where the teeth are of abnormal composition (such as amelogenesis imperfecta) or where there is a parafunctional habit such as bruxism (**Figs 15.22–15.25**). It is rarely found in post-traumatic stress disorder (PTSD), amphetamine or ecstasy use, profound vegetative states, Rett syndrome (see Chapter 28), Riley–Day syndrome (see Chapter 13) or fragile X syndrome (Chapter 28). The incisal edges and cusps wear and there is more loss of dentine than enamel, leading to a flat or hollowed surface. Unless attrition is rapid, the pulp is protected by obliteration with secondary dentine.

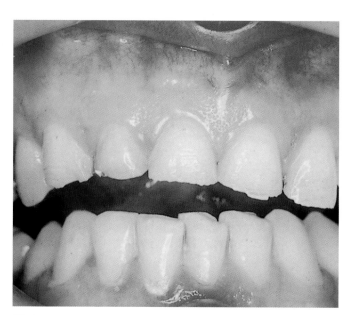

15.22

15.23

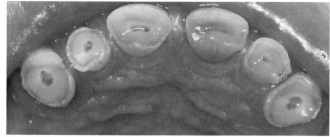

15.24

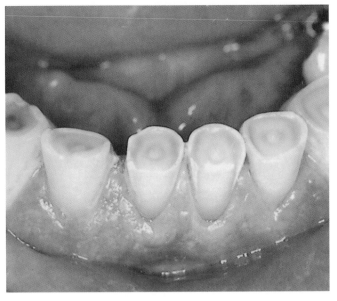

15.25

DENTAL CARIES

Decalcification beneath the bacterial plaque that accumulates in stagnation areas, such as close to the gingival margin, produces an opaque whitish band (**Fig. 15.26**). At this early stage, where there is no cavitation, the lesion is reversible if diet is changed and fermentable carbohydrates reduced or excluded; fluoride aids remineralization.

The carious enamel breaks down to form a cavity, as shown in **Fig. 15.27**, an upper deciduous canine tooth with early caries.

This may progress, such as in **Fig. 15.28**, where the enamel has been undermined and fractured away. The carious dentine is discoloured and this shows through the enamel. Pulpal involvement is inevitable in such carious teeth.

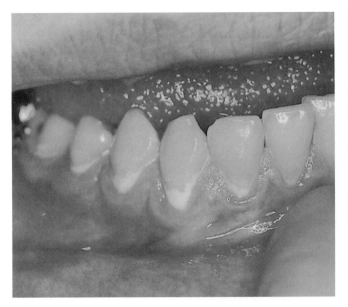

15.26

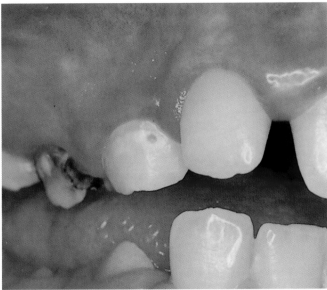

15.27

Rampant caries, affecting mainly the upper incisors is typically seen in children using a sugar/fruit juice mix in a bottle to aid sleep at night (**Fig. 15.29**).

Change in dietary habits (particularly a reduction in frequency of fermentable carbohydrate intake), fluoride treatment and improved oral hygiene can arrest the progress of caries. Lesions then darken and become static, as seen in this example at the cervical margins (**Fig. 15.30**).

Any change in local environment that makes the various lesions self-cleansing, for example loss of a tooth adjacent to an interproximal lesion or fracture of cusps overlying a lesion, may cause arrest of the caries (**Fig. 15.31**). Even completely fractured carious teeth may become

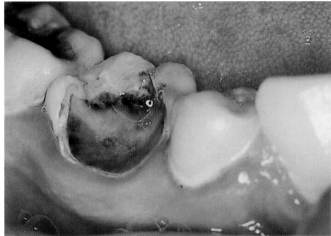
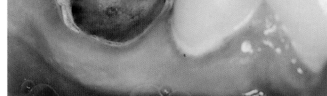

15.28

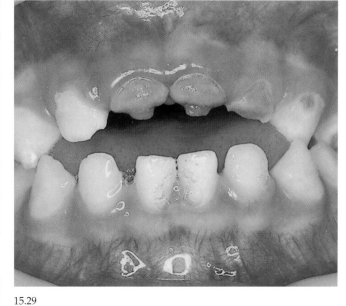

15.29

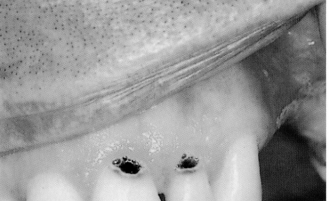

15.30

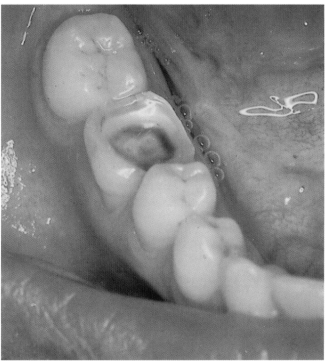

15.31

self-cleansing (**Fig. 15.32**). In contrast, xerostomia for any reason significantly predisposes to caries.

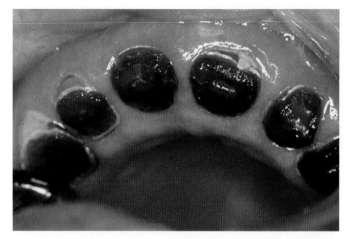

15.32

DENTINOGENESIS IMPERFECTA

Dentinogenesis imperfecta is an autosomal dominant condition in which the dentine is abnormal in structure and is translucent. The deciduous dentition is often more severely affected than the permanent. There are four recognized types of dentinogenesis imperfecta:

- Type I (this may be seen in osteogenesis imperfecta). This manifests with translucent teeth, which may vary from grey to blue or brown in colour (**Fig. 15.33**). **Figure 15.34** shows Type I dentinogenesis imperfecta. The tooth crowns are bulbous and the roots short. The enamel, though normal, is poorly adherent to the abnormal dentine; it chips and wears (**Fig. 15.35**) and thus ultimately the teeth are worn flat by attrition (**Fig. 15.36**). Fortunately, the pulp chambers are obliterated by secondary dentine and, therefore, the pulps do not become exposed and infected. Radiographs show flame-shaped pulp chambers and narrow pulp canals. There may be several pulp stones

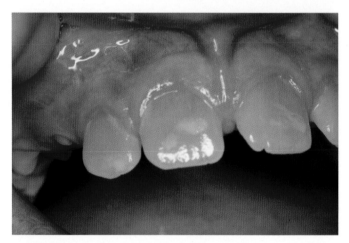

15.33

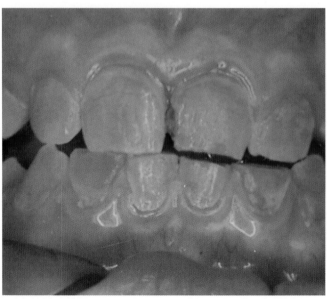

15.34

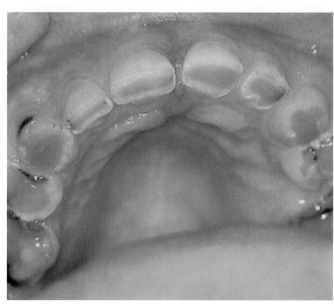

15.35

in most teeth. Pulp obliteration can be seen (**Fig. 15.37**). The roots, however, fracture easily.

- Type II (hereditary opalescent dentine). In this type the deciduous dentition is often more severely affected than the permanent (**Fig. 15.38**).
- Type III (associated with osteogenesis imperfecta).

Dentinogenesis imperfecta appears more frequently in those patients with osteogenesis imperfecta who have normal rather than blue sclerae (**Fig. 15.39**).

In Type IV dentinogenesis imperfecta ('shell teeth'), dentine formation ceases after the initial mantle layer, leaving teeth that are shell like (**Fig. 15.40**).

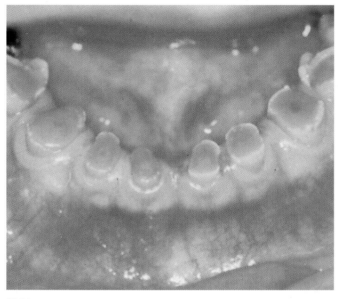

15.36

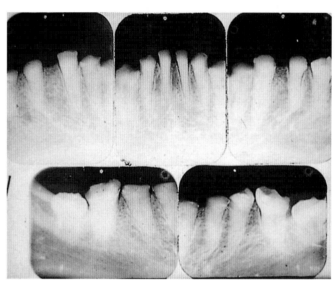

15.37

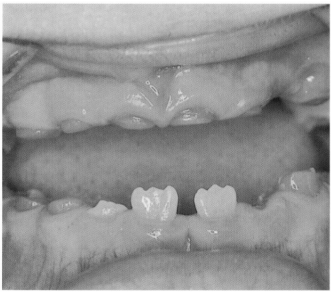

15.38

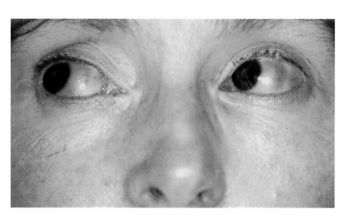

15.39

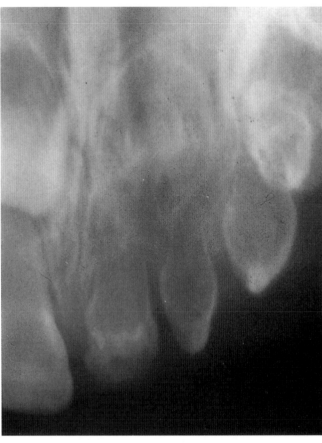

15.40

DILACERATION

Trauma to a developing tooth may produce distortion and dilaceration — a bend — in the root (**Figs 15.41, 15.42**).

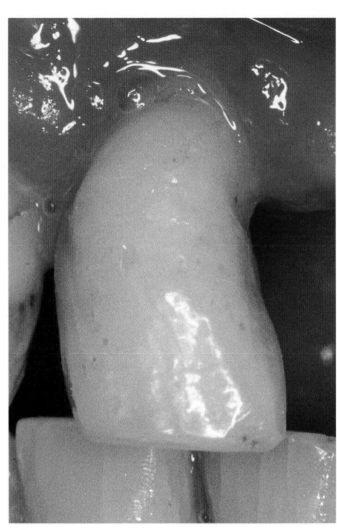

15.41

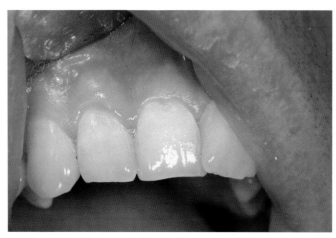

ENAMEL CLEFT

An enamel cleft is a morphological anomaly usually seen at the cervical margin of the tooth (**Fig. 15.43**).

15.43

15.42

ENAMEL HYPOPLASIA

Enamel hypoplasia may be caused by disturbed tooth morphogenesis from a number of identifiable disorders *in utero* or early childhood but it may also appear in the absence of any identifiable cause.

Intrauterine infections such as rubella, or metabolic disturbances such as jaundice, may cause hypoplasia of the deciduous dentition, producing a linear pattern of defects corresponding to the site of amelogenesis at the time ('chronological' hypoplasia). In **Fig. 15.44**, mottling and hypoplasia of the deciduous dentition has been caused by intrauterine pseudohypoparathyroidism.

Tooth development can also be disturbed by constitutional disturbances in childhood, such as fevers, coeliac disease, cystic fibrosis, gastroenteritis and radiotherapy or chemotherapy. Horizontal pits or grooves are usually seen in the incisal third of the crowns of permanent teeth (**Fig. 15.45**).

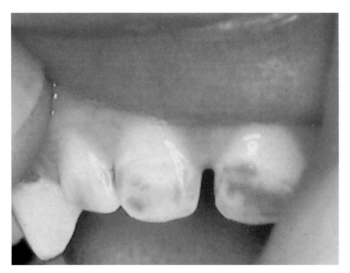

15.44

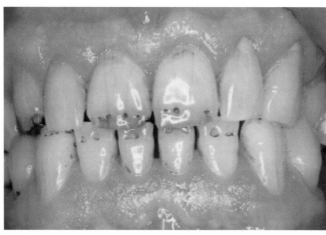

15.45

Isolated hypoplasia *(Turner's tooth)*
Infection of, or trauma to, a deciduous tooth, may cause hypoplasia of the developing and vulnerable underlying permanent successor (**Fig. 15.46**).

In **Fig. 15.47**, the lower second premolar was deformed after an abscess on the predecessor deciduous molar. The malformed Turner's tooth has subsequently become carious.

In **Fig. 15.48**, comparison of a normal premolar (on the reader's left) with a Turner's tooth shows the degree of deformity that can result.

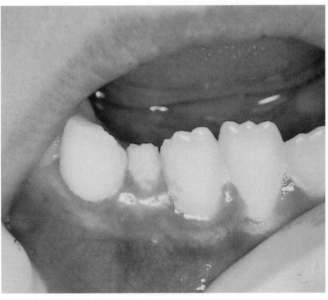

15.46

15.47

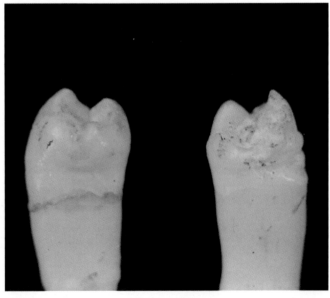

15.48

ENAMEL NODULE *(enameloma; enamel pearl)*
A small circular mass of enamel is seen on the tooth surface near the cemento-enamel junction (**Fig. 15.49**).

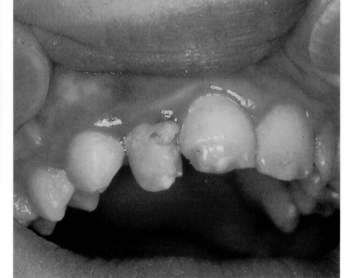

15.49

Sometimes the enamel nodule contains dentine and pulp. Nodules are most common on maxillary teeth (**Fig. 15.50**).

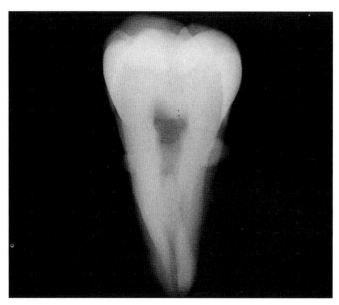

15.50

EROSION

Erosion is the loss of tooth substance caused by acids. For example, the habitual sucking of oranges may cause erosion (**Fig. 15.51**). Citrus drinks, apple juice, carbonated beverages (colas and other fizzy drinks, and sports drinks), alcoholic drinks or gastric acid may produce such lesions. Rarely, the acidic nature of some drugs (such as inhaled anti-asthmatic drugs) or occupational exposure to acids may produce erosion, and even the low pH of indoor swimming pools may be a cause.

Erosion is also seen where there is gastric regurgitation, such as in alcoholism or anorexia nervosa/bulimia. Repeated gastric regurgitation over a prolonged period may cause erosion, mainly of the palatal surfaces of the upper teeth. **Figure 15.52** shows a patient with recurrent gastric regurgitation and extreme erosion along with attrition.

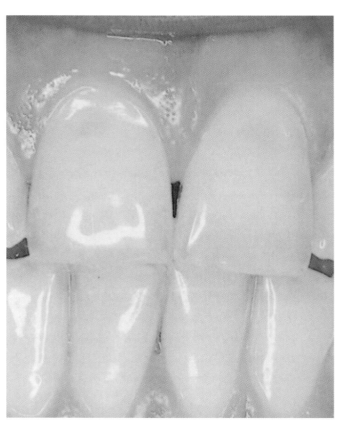

15.51

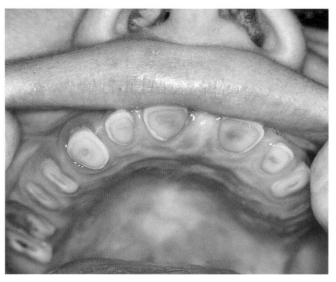

15.52

FLUOROSIS

Fluoride reduces caries. Mottling of the enamel may be seen where the fluoride in drinking water exceeds about 2 ppm or excess fluoride is taken via other sources, although in its mildest form it may not produce a cosmetic defect. Mottling in mild fluorosis is usually seen as white flecks or patches (**Fig. 15.53**). The mottling here is enough to require the cosmetic crowning of the upper anterior teeth. An example of more severe mottling is shown in **Fig. 15.54**.

Severe fluorosis causes opacity, brown and white staining and pitting of the entire enamel (**Fig. 15.55**). This can be difficult to differentiate clinically from amelogenesis imperfecta.

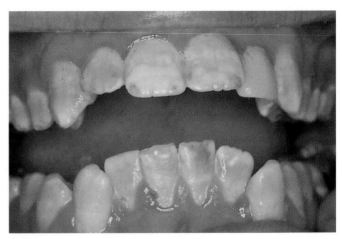

15.54

HYPERCEMENTOSIS

Hypercementosis is usually a consequence of periapical periodontitis, although it may affect isolated functionless teeth. A rare cause is Paget's disease of bone (**Fig. 15.56**).

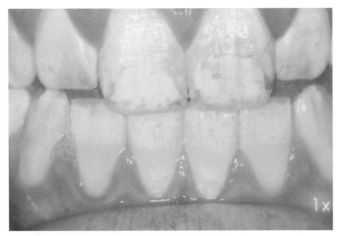

15.53

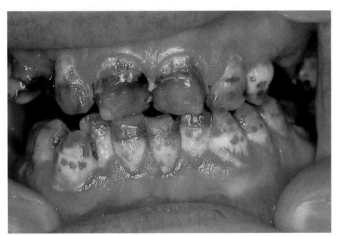

15.55

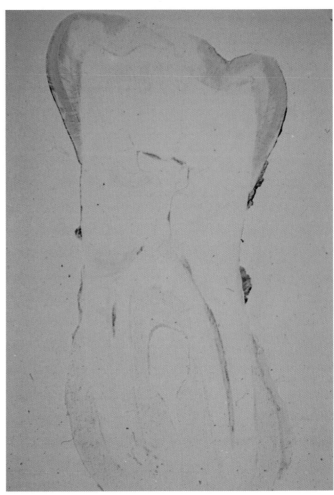

15.56

HYPERDONTIA

Additional teeth are most common in the upper incisor region, where they are usually of a simple conical shape (supernumerary) (**Fig. 15.57**). If midline (**Fig. 15.58**) the tooth is termed a mesiodens. Although a mesiodens may erupt, sometimes it is inverted.

Supernumerary teeth may cause malocclusion, occasionally impede tooth eruption or, rarely, are the site of cyst formation. Additional teeth often erupt in an abnormal position (**Figs 15.59 and 15.60**). This malocclusion may predispose to caries or periodontal disease. Extramaxillary molars often resemble normal teeth and are thus termed supplemental teeth (or sometimes distodens; **Fig. 15.61**).

Supernumerary teeth are usually seen in otherwise healthy patients. Occasionally, however, hyperdontia is a manifestation of a systemic disorder such as cleidocranial dysplasia or Gardner's syndrome.

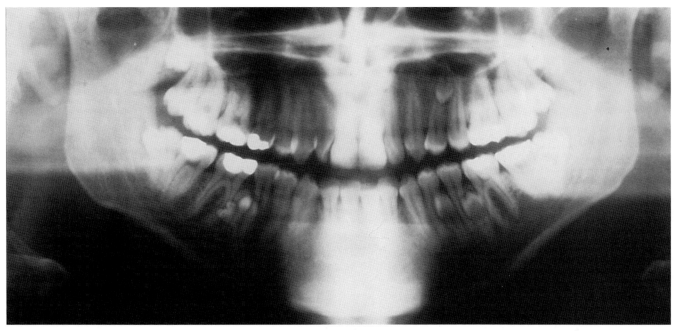

15.57

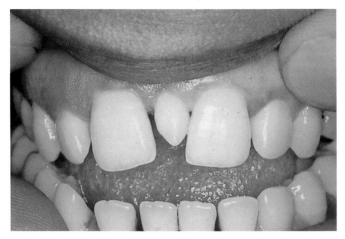

15.58

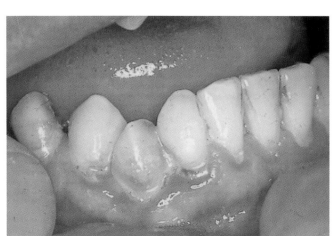

15.59

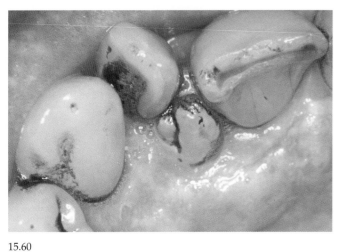

15.60

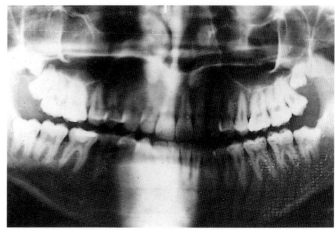

15.61

HYPERPLASTIC PULPITIS *(pulp polyp)*

Only when the coronal pulp is widely exposed and there is a very good blood supply, such as in children with incompletely formed roots and open apices, does the pulp survive trauma or infection. The pulp becomes hyperplastic and epithelialized (**Fig. 15.62**).

HYPODONTIA

Hypodontia may be *apparent* because teeth are impacted and thus fail to erupt. Rarely, eruption is delayed because of systemic disease, such as Down's syndrome or cleidocranial dysplasia, or because of damage to the tooth germs from radio- or chemotherapy (see Chapter 31).

Isolated true hypodontia is fairly common, may have a genetic basis and affects mainly the permanent dentition, particularly the third molars, second premolars or upper lateral incisors (**Fig. 15.63**). In

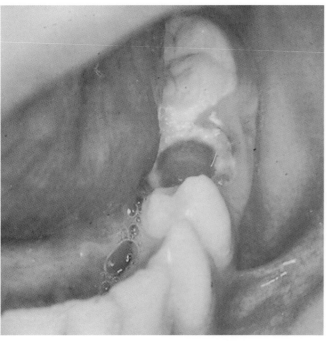

15.62

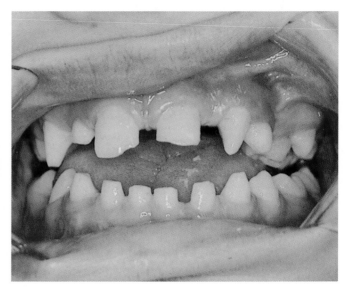

15.63

hypodontia, when the permanent successor is missing, a common occurrence is the retention of the deciduous tooth (**Fig. 15.64**). The upper deciduous lateral incisors are retained in **Fig. 18.63**.

Figures 15.65–15.67 show the congenital absence of several teeth. In **Fig. 15.65** the retained lower deciduous central incisors are discoloured because they are nonvital, having been worn down by attrition which has caused pulpal exposure, as shown, and pulp necrosis. The permanent central incisors in **Fig. 15.66** are congenitally absent as is the incisor in **Fig. 15.67**.

Figure 15.68 is a radiograph showing several missing teeth in an otherwise healthy person.

Hypodontia is a feature of local growth disorders, such as cleft palate, and of several systemic disorders. In some systemic disorders, such as cleidocranial dysplasia, the teeth are present but fail to erupt; in others, such as ectodermal dysplasia (**Fig. 15.69**) or incontinentia pigmenti, they are truly missing. Rarely, all teeth are absent (anodontia).

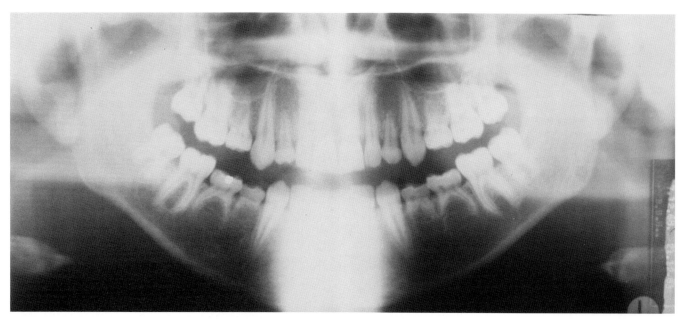

15.64

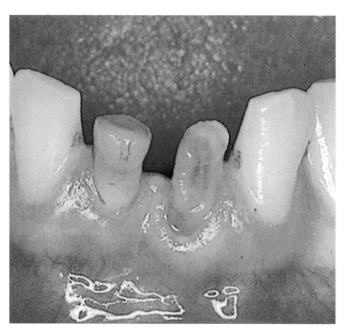

15.65

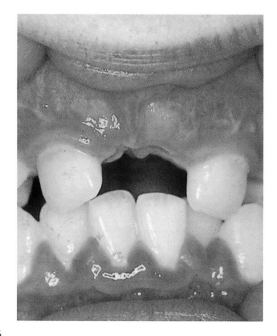

15.66

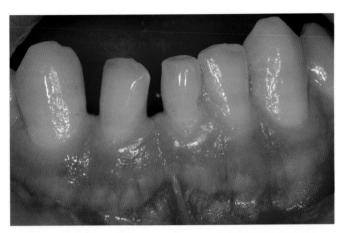

15.67

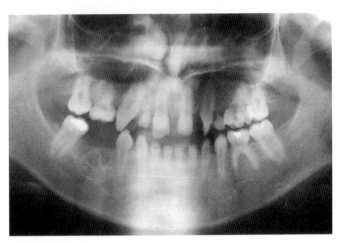

15.68

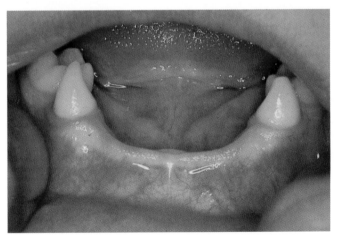

15.69

IMPACTED TEETH

Teeth impact, that is fail to erupt fully, because of insufficient space in the dental arch. Lower third molars (as here) are the most common teeth to impact (**Fig. 15.70**). Canines, second premolars and second molars, as well as other teeth may also impact.

Impacted teeth may well be asymptomatic but occasionally cause pain, usually from caries or pericoronitis, or are the site of dentigerous cyst formation. There is no evidence they contribute to malocclusion.

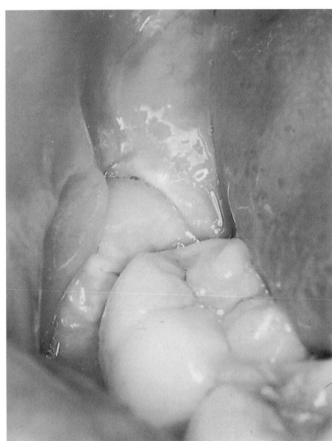

15.70

LOCALIZED DAMAGE

Seamstress' notch — holding pins, nails, etc., between the teeth can produce a variety of lesions. The patient seen in **Fig. 15.71** held pins in her teeth during her work as a seamstress.

Localized damage may be produced for aesthetic reasons, according to custom (**Fig. 15.72**; there is also a degree of fluorosis in this case). Cracked teeth are more common than often believed and may cause severe pain (**Figs 15.73–15.76**).

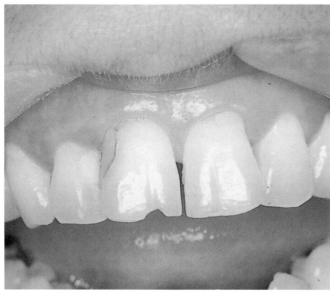

15.71

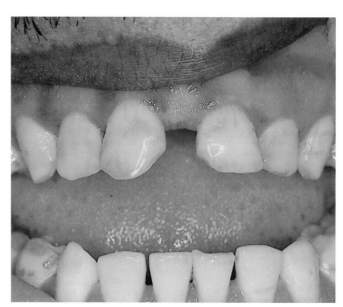

15.72

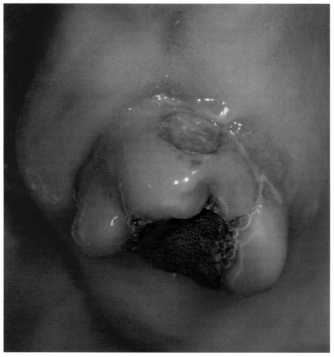

15.73

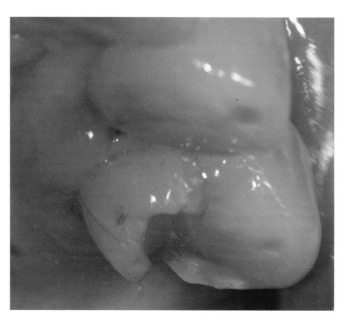

15.74

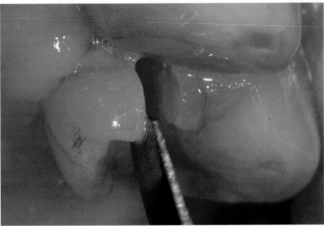

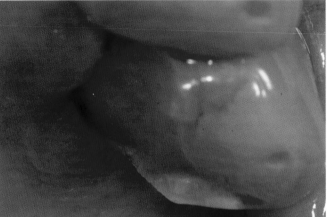

15.75

15.76

MALOCCLUSION

Figure 15.77 shows the typical bird face of mandibular retrusion.

Maxillary protrusion is seen in **Fig. 15.78**. This type of malocclusion is termed class II division I. **Figure 15.79** is a case of mandibular protrusion (class III malocclusion) — the Hapsburg chin of a prognathic mandible. In mandibular protrusion, the teeth often show reverse overjet with the upper incisors occluding lingual to the lower teeth (**Fig. 15.80**).

Another form of malocclusion is open bite (**Fig. 15.81**). Many of the teeth are in occlusion but some fail to meet.

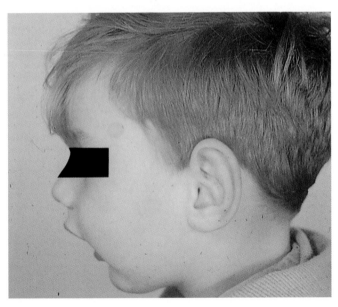

15.77

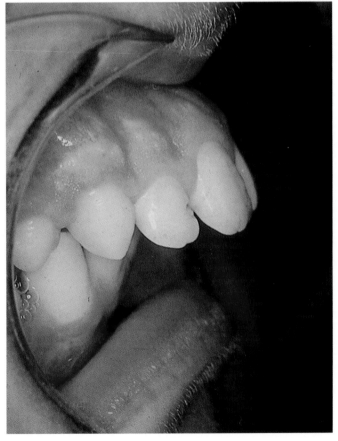

15.78

Anterior open bites are characterized by posterior teeth in occlusion but anteriors not. It may be caused by increased height of the lower face, tongue posture, dentoalveolar factors, trauma or thumb sucking. The upper lateral incisors are also congenitally absent in this patient.

Obvious malocclusion and anterior open bite can be caused by thumb sucking (Figs 15.82, 15.83).

Finally, the permanent canine normally erupts slightly later than the premolar and lateral incisor and, if there is a lack of space in the dental arch (dentoalveolar disproportion), it may be crowded out (Fig. 15.84). Second premolars and third molars are the other teeth that may suffer this fate. Any of these teeth, especially lower third molars, may then impact.

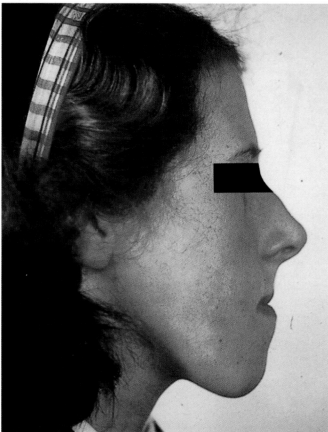

15.79

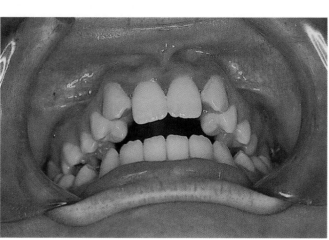

15.81

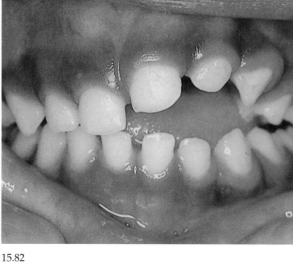

15.80

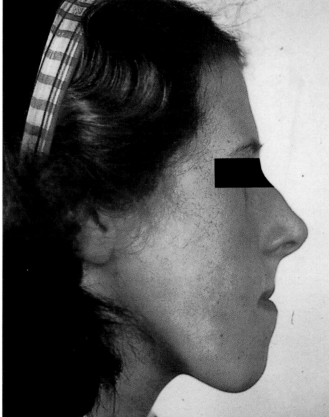

15.82

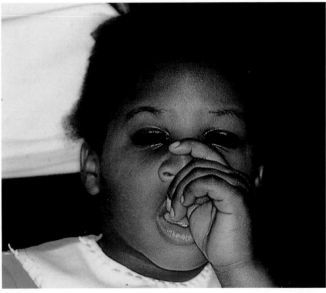

15.83

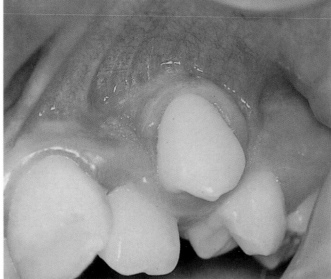

15.84

NATAL TEETH

Rarely, teeth are present at or soon after birth (natal teeth); they have even been described at 26 weeks' gestation. Natal teeth may cause no trouble or they may ulcerate the tongue (**Fig. 15.85**) or the breast if suckling. Usually the teeth involved are lower incisors of the normal primary dentition but occasionally they are supernumeraries. Rarely, there are associations with Ellis–van Creveld syndrome, pachyonychia congenita, Hallermann–Streiff syndrome or steatocystoma multiplex.

If there are problems from natal teeth, radiographs should be taken before extractions are contemplated (**Fig. 15.86**); extractions are best restricted to those teeth that are supernumeraries or are very loose and in danger of being inhaled.

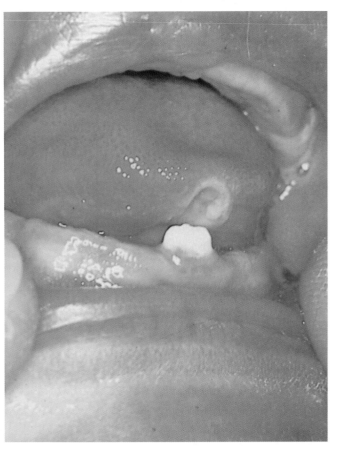

15.85

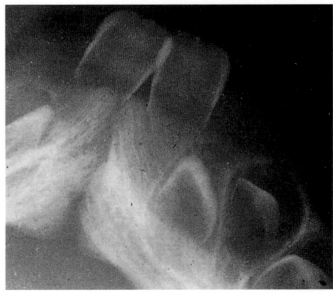

15.86

NONVITAL TEETH

Trauma or caries may result in nonvital teeth, which with time tend to discolour and become brownish (**Figs. 15.87 and 15.65**).

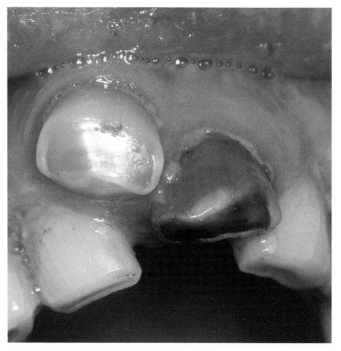

15.87

ODONTOMES

Odontomes are developmental malformations of dental tissue. They are hamartomatous and thus develop in childhood and early adulthood.

Gemination *(geminated odontome)*
Gemination is a result of the incomplete attempted division of a tooth germ. Usually seen in the incisor region, the crowns may be separate or divided by a shallow groove (**Fig. 15.88**) but the root is shared.

It is often difficult to differentiate gemination from fusion (**Fig. 15.89**) and therefore the terms 'double tooth' or 'twinning' are sometimes used. Double teeth are seen most commonly in the incisor and canine regions (**Fig. 15.90**) and may be seen in the deciduous or permanent dentitions.

Invaginated odontome *(dilated odontome; dens in dente)*
The invagination of enamel and dentine in the dens in dente may also dilate the affected tooth (**Fig. 15.91**). Ameloblasts invaginate during

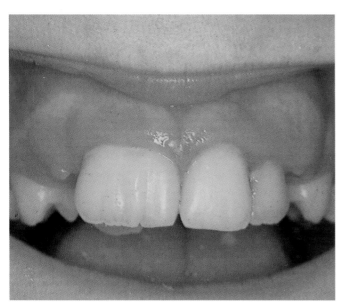

15.88

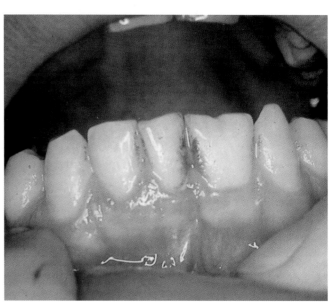

15.89

development to form a pouch of enamel such that a radiograph shows what resembles a tooth within a tooth (**Fig. 15.92**). This odontome is prone to caries development in the abnormal pouch.

Evaginated odontome (*dens evaginatus*)
A small occlusal nodule is seen, especially in mongoloid races (**Fig. 15.93**). Since the nodule contains a pulp horn, pulpitis is not uncommon when there is attrition.

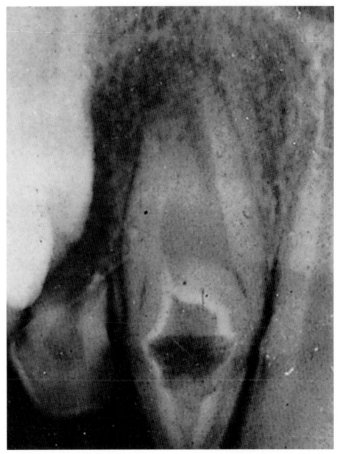

15.92

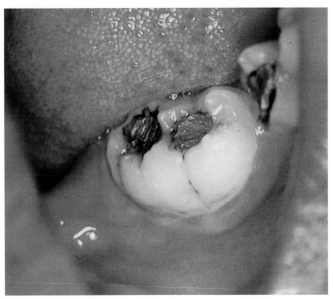

15.90

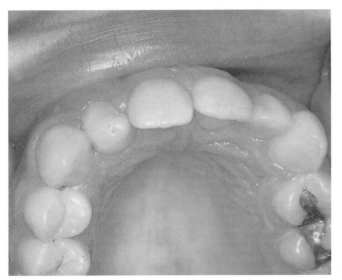

15.91

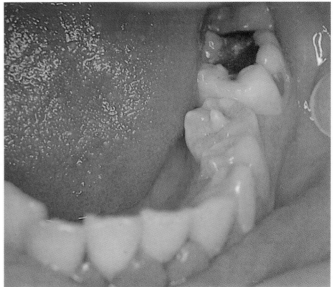

15.93

Compound odontomes

Compound odontomes manifest as regularly shaped solitary or multiple small tooth-like denticles. They are usually unerupted and asymptomatic, being found incidentally on radiograph, although they may give rise to the delayed or abnormal eruption of adjacent teeth, and rarely dentigerous cyst formation (**Fig. 15.94**).

Complex odontomes

Complex odontomes do not resemble teeth, having a much more irregular, sometimes cauliflower-like appearance. Both compound and complex odontomes contain all the normal dental tissues, are more commonly found in the anterior jaws and are liable to dental decay if erupted (**Fig. 15.95**).

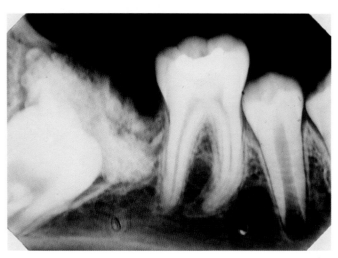

15.95

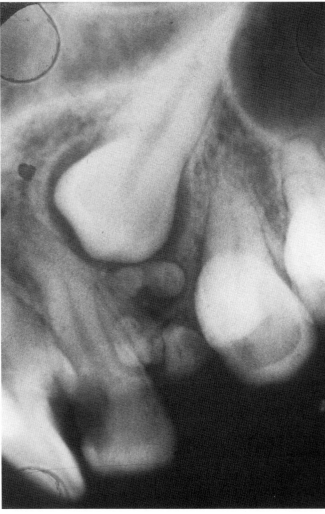

15.94

PERIAPICAL ABSCESS *(dental abscess; odontogenic abscess)*

An abscess is often a sequel of pulpitis caused by dental caries but may arise in relation to any nonvital tooth. A mixed bacterial flora is implicated although the role of anaerobes such as *Fusobacterium* and *Bacteroides* species is increasingly recognized. Pain and facial swelling, in **Figs 15.96–15.98**, from abscesses on a lower molar, are characteristic.

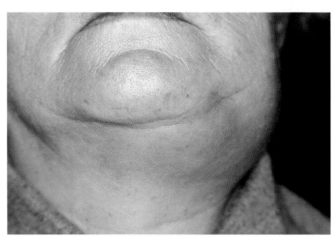

15.96

Figure 15.99 shows inflammatory swelling resulting from a dental abscess on a lower incisor. However, not all dental abscesses cause facial swelling.

Figure 15.100 shows a periapical abscess on an upper premolar causing infraorbital swelling.

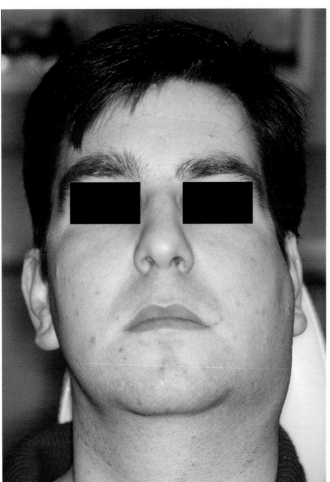

15.97

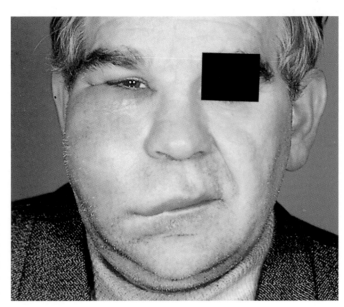

15.98

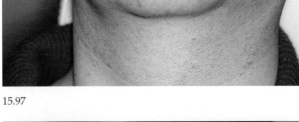

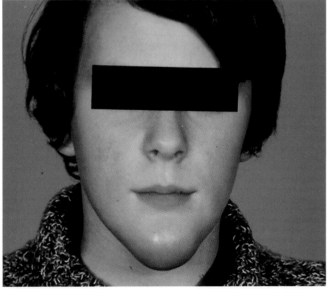

15.99

15.100

Figure 15.101 shows swelling of the infraorbital region and upper lip from a periapical abscess on an upper canine.

Most dental abscesses also produce an intraoral swelling, typically on the labial or buccal gingiva. In **Fig. 15.102**, the large, tender, inflammatory swelling, which is about to discharge, is related to pulp exposure from attrition.

Although most periapical abscesses cause swelling buccally, abscesses on maxillary lateral incisors (**Fig. 15.103**) and those arising from the palatal roots of the first molar tend to present palatally. The lateral incisor involved here has a deep, carious palatal pit, which caused pulp necrosis.

Bone destruction caused by a periapical abscess (**Fig. 15.104**) on the carious lower permanent molar shows well on this radiograph.

In **Fig. 15.105**, the periapical abscess resulted from trauma, rendering the upper deciduous incisor nonvital.

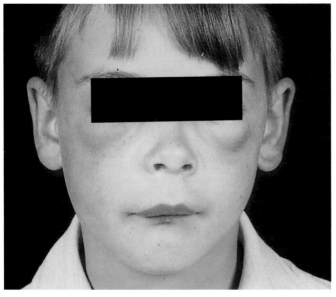

15.101

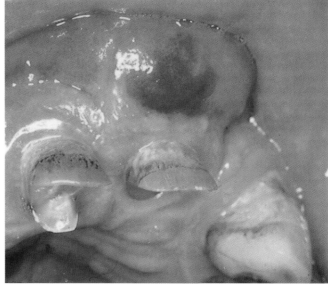

15.102

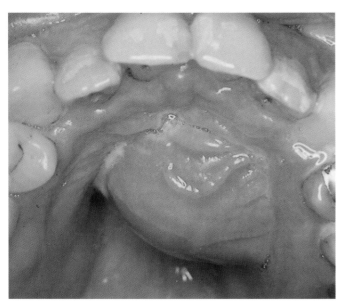

15.103

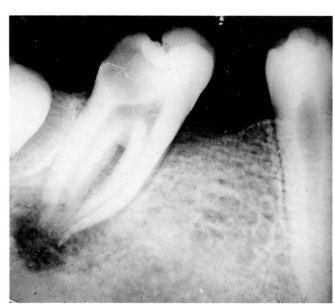

15.104

Once the abscess discharges, the acute inflammation, pain and swelling resolve and a chronic abscess develops discharging from a sinus, usually buccally (**Fig. 15.106**).

Extraction or endodontic therapy of a tooth affected with a periapical abscess removes the source of infection. **Figure 15.107** shows the pus discharging through the extraction socket.

Facial swelling is common (**Figs 15.108–15.110**).

The patient in **Figs. 15.108–15.110** is shown pre-operatively (**Fig. 15.108**), peri-operatively (**Fig. 15.109**) and after drainage of the abscess (**Fig. 15.110**). Most abscesses discharge into the mouth (**Figs. 15.111 and 15.112**). Occasionally, abscesses — especially those of lower incisors or molars — discharge extraorally (**Figs 15.113–15.116**).

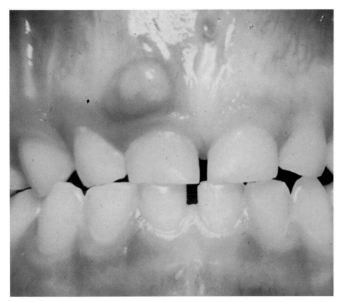

15.105

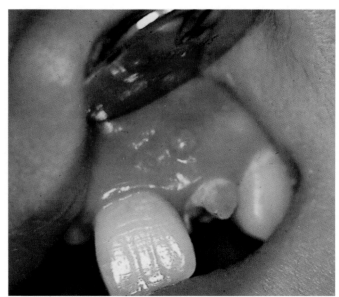

15.106

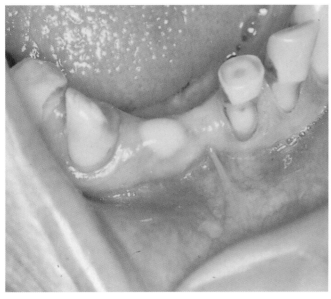

15.107

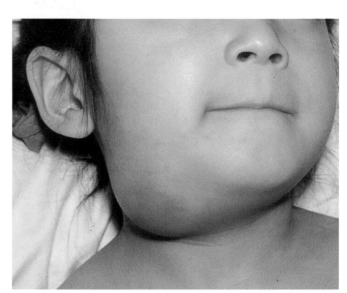

15.108

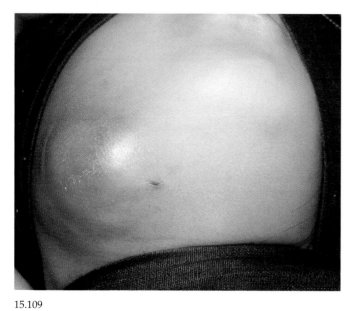

15.109

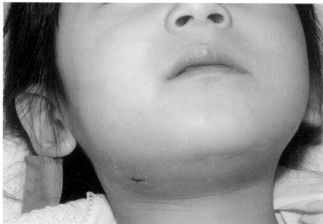

15.110

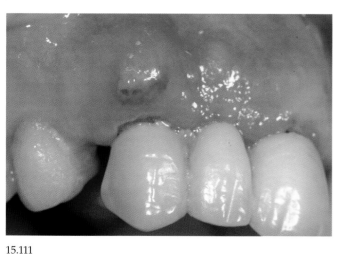

15.111

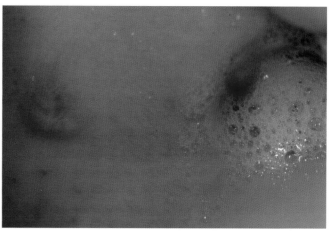

15.112

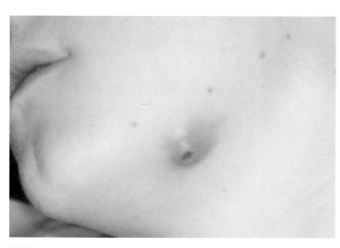

15.113

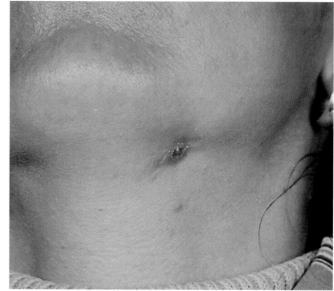

15.114

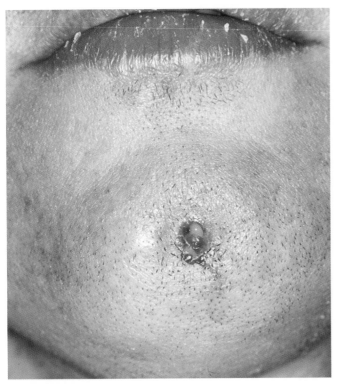

15.115

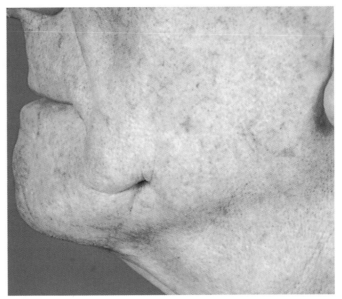

15.116

PERIAPICAL CYST *(radicular or dental cyst)*

A granuloma may arise at the apex of a nonvital tooth and may occasionally develop into a cyst from proliferation of epithelial rests in the area (cell rests of Malassez). In **Fig. 15.117** there is a retained root in the maxilla with swelling from a cyst. Many periapical cysts involve upper lateral incisors since these not infrequently become carious and the pulp can be involved relatively rapidly.

Most odontogenic cysts are periapical cysts. A periapical cyst may well be asymptomatic and often is a chance radiographic finding. It may present as a swelling (usually in the labial sulcus) or may become infected and present as an abscess. In **Fig. 15.118** there is a cyst on the incisor root.

A small periapical cyst may remain attached to, and be extracted with, the causal root or tooth, or resolve with endodontic therapy.

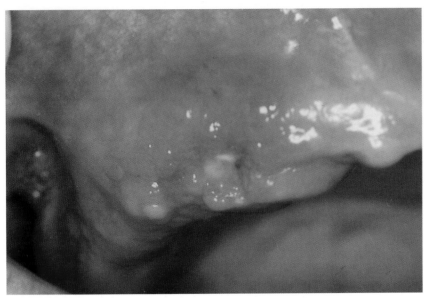

15.117

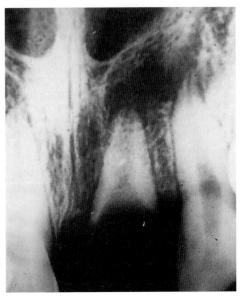

15.118

PROMINENT TUBERCULES OR CUSPS

Cusp of Carabelli

This is an anatomical variant — a palatal cusp on the upper first molar (**Fig. 15.119**).

Paramolar

This is shown in **Fig. 15.120**.

RESIDUAL CYST

A periapical cyst left *in situ* after the causal root or tooth is removed may continue to expand and is termed a residual cyst. This may produce a bluish swelling (**Fig. 15.121**). A residual cyst is almost invariably unilocular but may expand to an appreciable size. It may be asymptomatic, detected as a swelling, a chance radiographic finding (**Fig. 15.122**), a pathological fracture or it may rarely become infected and present as an abscess.

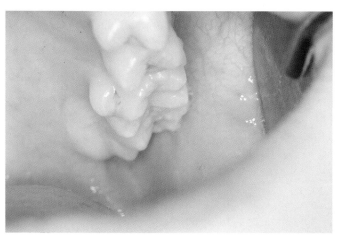

15.119

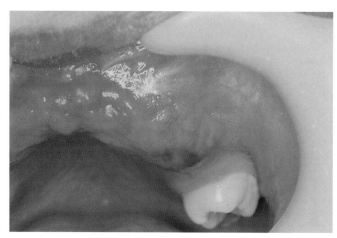

15.121

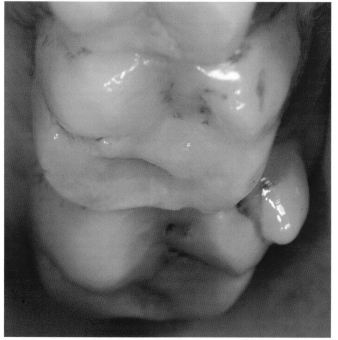

15.120

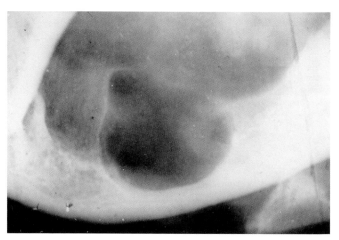

15.122

RESORPTION

Internal resorption *(pink spot)*

In pink spot, dentine is spontaneously resorbed from within and the pulp is eventually exposed (**Fig. 15.123**). Here, the dark brown lesion on the premolar is a result of interproximal caries that has arrested. The lesion on the second molar is a cavity from which the restoration has been lost.

External resorption

Resorption may progress from the external surface, eventually to involve the pulp. In **Fig. 15.124** the maxillary incisor is involved. The canine has a composite restoration. The white semilunar line is decalcification that occurred some years earlier, when the oral hygiene was not so good and the gingiva not so far receded. In rare cases, multiple teeth are involved (**Fig. 15.125**).

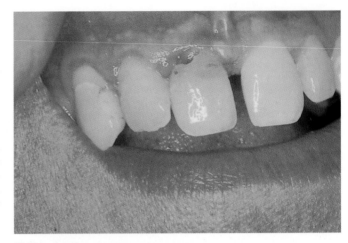

15.124

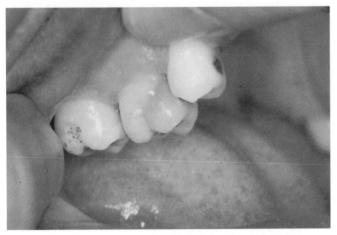

15.123

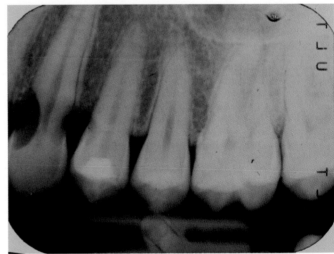

15.125

RETAINED PRIMARY TOOTH

The common cause for primary teeth to be retained is the absence of a successor. Usually this is of little consequence but occasionally, particularly in the case of lower deciduous molars, the tooth fails to maintain its occlusal relationship (infraocclusion or submergence; **Fig. 15.126**).

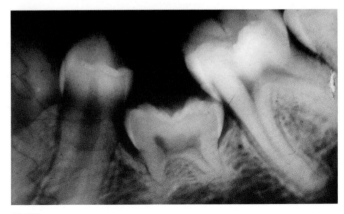

15.126

RETAINED ROOT

Retained roots are often asymptomatic (**Fig. 15.127**) but may give rise to a periapical abscess (**Fig. 15.128** shows the cyst sac on an extracted root). Occasionally roots 'erupt' under a denture (**Fig. 15.129**) or form a cyst.

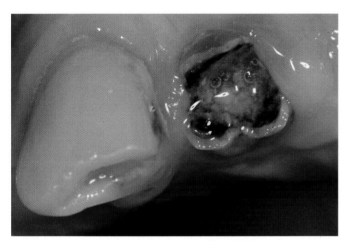

15.127

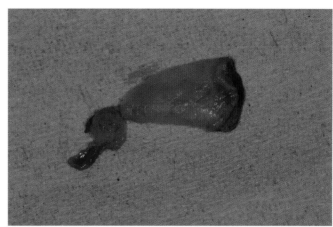

15.128

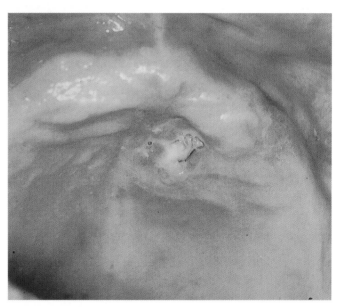

15.129

TAURODONTISM

Taurodontism is the term applied to teeth that clinically look normal but on radiograph resemble those of ungulates (hence the Latin origin, *taurus*, a bull) — the crown is long and the roots short (**Fig. 15.130**). Taurodont teeth lack a pronounced constriction at the neck of the tooth and are parallel sided. The floor of the pulp chamber is lower than normal and the pulp appears extremely large (**Fig. 15.131**). Taurodontism usually affects permanent molars, especially the lower second molar, and sometimes only one in the arch but it may affect teeth in the deciduous dentition.

Taurodontism is usually a simple racial trait. However, it may rarely be associated with chromosome anomalies such as Klinefelter's syndrome, tricho-dento-osseous syndrome, orofacio-digital syndrome, ectodermal dysplasia or amelogenesis imperfecta. In tricho-dento-osseous syndrome there is also enamel hypoplasia, curly hair and thickening of cortical bone.

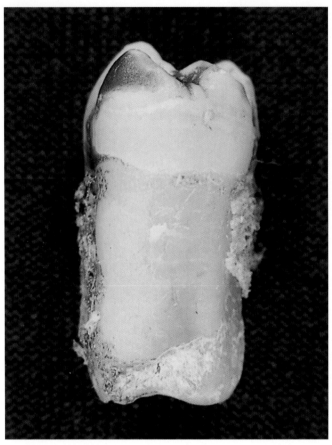

15.130

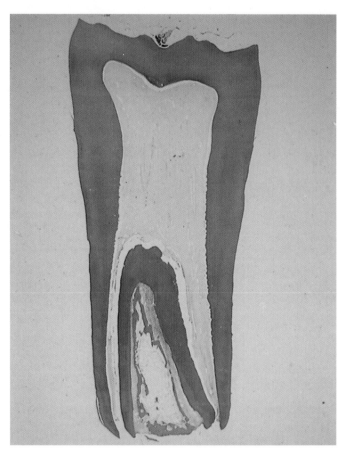

15.131

TERATOMA

Cystic ovarian teratomas (dermoid) may contain well-formed teeth (**Fig. 15.132**).

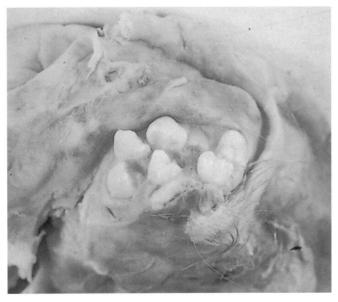

15.132

TOOTH EXTRINSIC STAINING

Extrinsic staining of the teeth can be of various colours and is more likely to appear where oral hygiene is poor or where coloured foods or drinks are taken.

Orange stain (**Fig. 15.133**) is believed to be caused by chromogenic bacteria. Similar effects can result from prolonged antimicrobial exposure.

Brown stain is shown in **Fig. 15.134**. Extrinsic staining is concentrated mainly where plaque accumulates, such as between the teeth and close to the gingival margins, and in pits and fissures. Brown stain can be caused by stannous fluoride toothpastes, chlorhexidine and other substances. Chlorhexidine is an effective oral antiseptic and binds to dental pellicle where it can produce discoloration, especially in drinkers of tea, coffee or red wine.

Black stain is often of unknown aetiology and is unusual in that it seems to be associated, by an unknown mechanism, with caries resistance. It is seen in clean mouths. Black-staining of the teeth is carried out deliberately for cosmetic reasons in some communities. In **Fig. 15.135**, the black staining is caused by smoking.

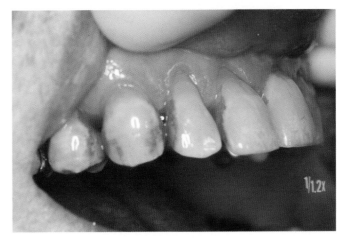

15.134

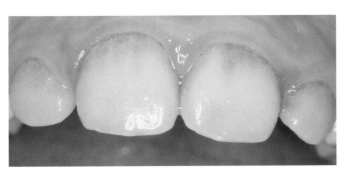

15.133

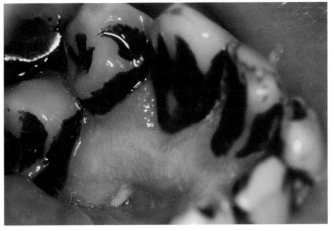

15.135

'Nicotine' stain (**Fig. 15.135**) is caused by cigarette smoking or tobacco chewing, especially in a person with poor oral hygiene. Dentine also stains dark brown. Tobacco use predisposes to oral keratoses and cancer. Staining can also be produced by chewing habits such as use of betel or khat (**Fig. 15.136**).

Iron stain (**Fig. 15.137**) may result from iron preparations taken orally. Green stain is more common, especially in children with poor oral hygiene, and may result from the breakdown of blood pigment after gingival haemorrhage or from chromogenic bacteria.

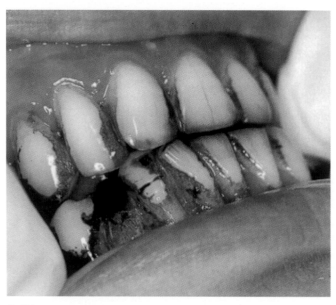

15.136

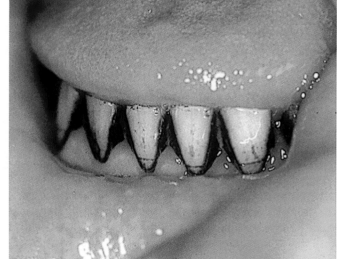

15.137

TOOTH INTRINSIC STAINING

Bile pigment staining

Infants with hyperbilirubinaemia now often survive and may receive liver transplants. The more classic haemolytic disease of the newborn (icterus gravis neonatorum) caused by rhesus incompatibility is now rare. Jaundice in either case may cause enamel hypoplasia in the deciduous dentition, which may have a greenish color (**Fig. 15.138**).

Porphyria

Disorders of haem synthesis, such as congenital erythropoietic porphyria is a rare cause of yellow to brown-red tooth discoloration.

Tetracycline staining

Tetracyclines given systemically cross the placenta, enter breast milk and, if entering the circulation by these routes or by being given to a child, are taken up by developing teeth (**Fig. 15.139**) and by bone. If tetracyclines are given to pregnant or nursing mothers or to

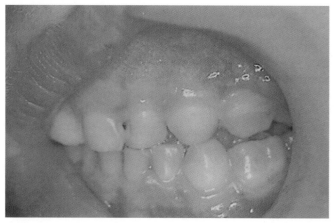

15.138

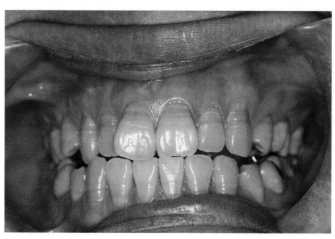

15.139

children under the age of 8 years, the tooth crowns may become discoloured, initially being yellow but darkening with time (**Fig. 15.140**).

Staining of the permanent dentition — yellow and brown bands of staining — is most obvious at the necks of the teeth where the thinner enamel allows the colour of the stained dentine to show through. Staining is greater in light-exposed anterior teeth and with larger doses of tetracyclines, and is worse with, for example, tetracycline than oxytetracycline.

More severe staining of the permanent dentition is seen in **Fig. 15.141**; the tooth of normal colour is supernumerary and clearly developed at a time after tetracyclines had been given.

Even in older children, tetracyclines cause staining but by then most tooth crowns have been formed. The staining then usually affects the third molar only (**Fig. 15.142**) or the roots, as in the lower third molar (**Fig. 15.143**).

Affected teeth may fluoresce bright yellow under UV light and this helps to distinguish tetracycline staining from dentinogenesis

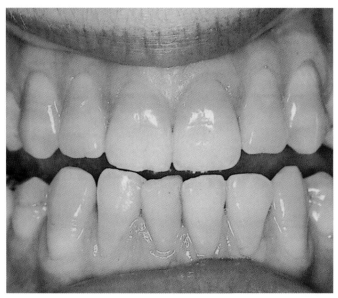

15.140

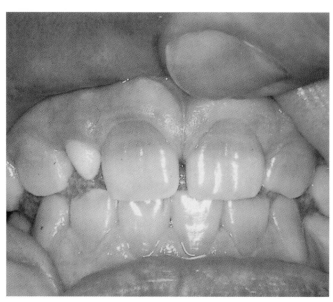

15.141

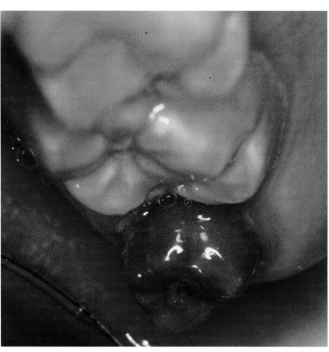

15.142

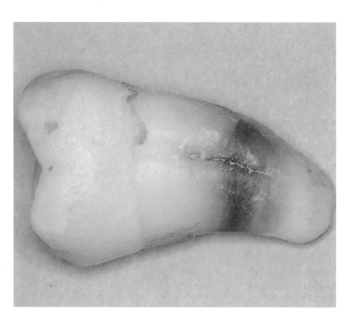

15.143

imperfecta. Fluorescence is also seen in undecalcified sections viewed under UV light (**Fig. 15.144**). Nitrofurantoin has also been reported to cause tooth discoloration.

Caries is the common cause of tooth discolouration. Isolated teeth that discolour are usually carious or nonvital. Pulp necrosis from caries or trauma is the usual cause of a tooth that progressively darkens, sometimes to a brownish colour (see **Fig. 15.65**), and the tooth also becomes more brittle.

Metal staining

This is a rare cause of colour change affecting many teeth; it is occupational, affecting workers with chromium or lead.

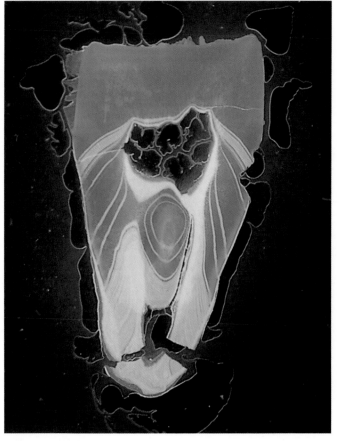

15.144

FURTHER READING

Addy M, Hunter ML. Can tooth brushing damage your health? Effects on oral and dental tissues. Int Dent J 2003; 53 Suppl 3: 177–86.

Aldred MJ, Savarirayan R, Crawford PJ. Amelogenesis imperfecta: a classification and catalogue for the 21st century. Oral Dis 2003; 9(1): 19–23.

Becktor KB, Reibel J, Vedel B, Kjaer I. Segmental odontomaxillary dysplasia: clinical, radiological and histological aspects of four cases. Oral Dis 2002; 8(2): 106–10.

Brkic H, Filipovic-Zore I, Kokic N. The treatment options of dens invaginatus complications in children: report of 3 cases. J Dent Child (Chic) 2003; 70(1): 77–81.

Chu FC, Li TK, Lui VK, Newsome PR, Chow RL, Cheung LK. Prevalence of impacted teeth and associated pathologies — a radiographic study of the Hong Kong Chinese population. Hong Kong Med J 2003; 9(3): 158–63.

Chugal NM, Clive JM, Spangberg LS. Endodontic infection: some biologic and treatment factors associated with outcome. Oral Surg Oral Med Oral Pathol Oral Radiol Endod 2003; 96(1): 81–90.

Cousin GC. Potentially fatal oro-facial infections: five cautionary tales. J R Coll Surg Edinb 2002; 47: 585–6.

Drogemuller C, Distl O, Leeb T. X-linked anhidrotic ectodermal dysplasia (ED1) in men, mice, and cattle. Genet Sel Evol 2003; 35 Suppl 1: S137–45.

Faine MP. Recognition and management of eating disorders in the dental office. Dent Clin North Am 2003; 47(2): 395–410.

Gaynor WN. Dens evaginatus — how does it present and how should it be managed? NZ Dent J 2002; 98(434): 104–7.

Hart PS, Hart TC, Simmer JP, Wright JT. A nomenclature for X-linked amelogenesis imperfecta. Arch Oral Biol 2002; 47: 255–60.

Hung HC, Willett W, Ascherio A, Rosner BA, Rimm E, Joshipura KJ. Tooth loss and dietary intake. J Am Dent Assoc 2003; 134(9): 1185–92.

Johansson AK. On dental erosion and associated factors. Swed Dent J Suppl 2002; 156: 1–77.

Kantaputra PN. Dentinogenesis imperfecta-associated syndromes. Am J Med Genet 2001; 104: 75–8.

Knouse MC, Madeira RG, Celani VJ. *Pseudomonas aeruginosa* causing a right carotid artery mycotic aneurysm after a dental extraction procedure. Mayo Clin Proc 2002; 77: 1125–30.

Kurisu K, Tabata MJ. Human genes for dental anomalies. Oral Dis 1997; 3: 223–8.

Lamartine J. Towards a new classification of ectodermal dysplasias. Clin Exp Dermatol 2003; 28(4): 351–5.

Navazesh M, Mulligan R. Systemic dissemination as a result of oral infection in individuals 50 years of age and older. Spec Care Dentist 1995; 15(1): 11–19.

Nordgarden H, Jensen JL, Storhaug K. Oligodontia is associated with extra-oral ectodermal symptoms and low whole salivary flow rates. Oral Dis 2001; 7(4): 226–32.

Nunn JH, Carter NE, Gillgrass TJ, Hobson RS, Jepson NJ, Meechan JG, Nohl FS. The interdisciplinary management of hypodontia: background and role of paediatric dentistry. Br Dent J 2003; 194(5): 245–51.

Paine ML, Wang HJ, Luo W, Krebsbach PH, Snead ML. A transgenic animal model resembling amelogenesis imperfecta related to ameloblastin overexpression. J Biol Chem 2003; 278(21): 19447–52.

Sandor GK, Low DE, Judd PL, Davidson RJ. Antimicrobial treatment options in the management of odontogenic infections. J Can Dent Assoc 1998; 64(7): 508–14.

Silvestri AR Jr, Singh I. The unresolved problem of the third molar: would people be better off without it? J Am Dent Assoc 2003; 134(4): 450–5.

Touger-Decker R, van Loveren C. Sugars and dental caries. Am J Clin Nutr 2003; 78(4): 881S–892S.

Vieira AR. Oral clefts and syndromic forms of tooth agenesis as models for genetics of isolated tooth agenesis. J Dent Res 2003; 82(3): 162–5.

16 GINGIVAL AND PERIODONTAL DISEASE

- abscesses
- chronic hyperplastic gingivitis
- chronic marginal gingivitis
- dental bacterial plaque
- dental calculus
- desquamative gingivitis
- drug-induced swelling
- fibrous epulis
- giant cell granuloma (giant cell epulis)
- gingival cyst
- gingival fibromatosis
- gingival recession
- keratosis (leukoplakia)
- materia alba
- pericoronitis
- periodontitis
- pigmentation
- plasma cell gingivitis
- pyogenic granuloma
- tumours
- traumatic occlusion.

ABSCESSES

Gingival infection, or a foreign body, may initiate a gingival abscess. **Figure 16.1** is the result of cement pushed into the tissues during cementing the crown on the central incisor.

Lateral periodontal abscess (parodontal abscess) is seen almost exclusively in patients with severe periodontitis but it may follow impaction of a foreign body or be related to a lateral root canal on a nonvital tooth. Debris and pus cannot escape easily from the pocket and therefore an abscess (**Fig. 16.2**), with pain and swelling, results.

Lateral periodontal abscesses usually discharge either through the pocket or buccally, but more coronally than a periapical abscess (**Fig. 16.3**).

In **Fig. 16.4** the probe has been gently inserted into a pocket to show continuity with the labial sinus.

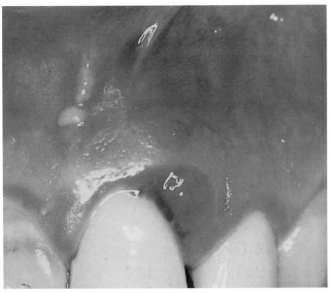

16.1

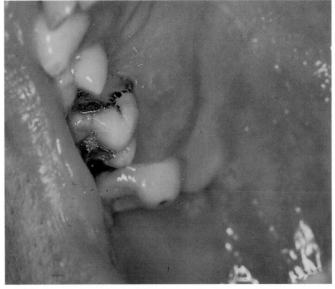

16.2

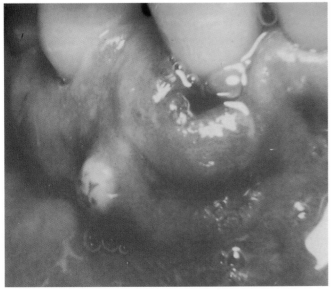

16.3

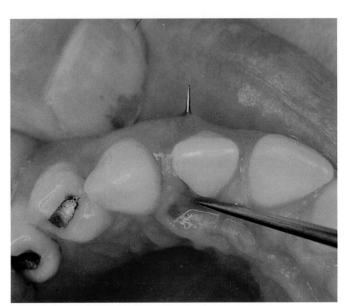

16.4

CHRONIC HYPERPLASTIC GINGIVITIS

Gingivitis may be hyperplastic, especially where there is mechanical irritation or mouth breathing, sometimes with the use of the oral contraceptive or other drugs or, rarely, vitamin C deficiency. Mouth breathing and poor oral and appliance hygiene are responsible in **Fig. 16.5.**

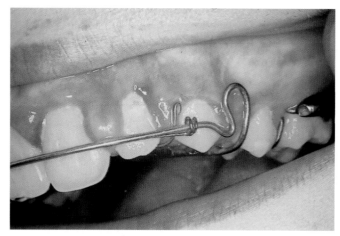

16.5

CHRONIC MARGINAL GINGIVITIS

Most of the population have a degree of gingivitis. Chronic marginal gingivitis (**Fig. 16.6**) is caused by the accumulation of dental bacterial plaque on the tooth close to the gingiva. If plaque is not removed it calcifies, to become calculus, which aggravates the condition by facilitating plaque accumulation. Inflammation of the margins of the gingiva is painless and often the only features are gingival bleeding on eating or brushing, some halitosis, erythema, swelling (**Figs 16.7–16.9**), and bleeding on probing. If left uncorrected this may slowly and painlessly progress to periodontitis and tooth loss.

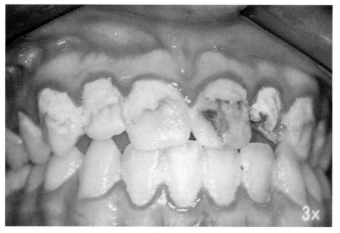

16.6

16.7

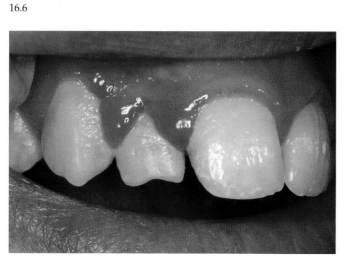

16.8

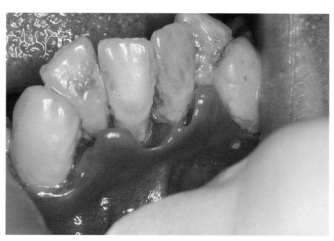

16.9

DENTAL BACTERIAL PLAQUE

Plaque is not especially obvious clinically (**Fig. 16.10**) although teeth covered with plaque lack the lustre of clean teeth. Various solutions can be used to disclose the plaque (**Figs 16.10, 16.11**).

Even after thorough toothbrushing, plaque often remains between the teeth unless they are flossed.

DENTAL CALCULUS

If plaque is not removed it readily calcifies to produce calculus (tartar; **Fig. 16.12**), especially in sites close to salivary duct orifices, lingual to the lower incisors (**Fig. 16.13**) and buccal to the upper molars.

The calculus is covered with plaque, cannot be removed by toothbrushing and is associated with periodontal disease (**Fig. 16.14**).

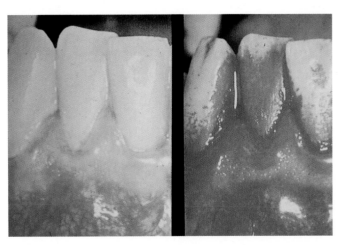

16.10

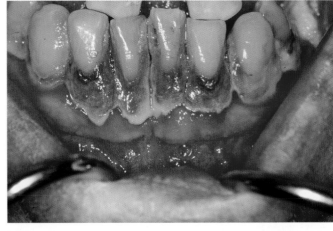

16.12

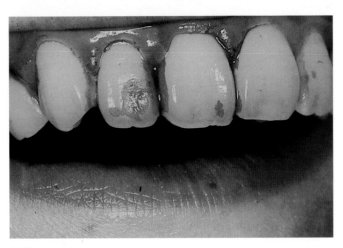

16.11

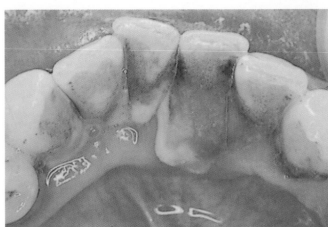

16.13

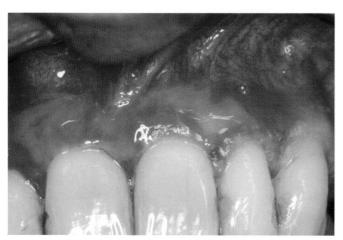

16.14

DESQUAMATIVE GINGIVITIS

Desquamative gingivitis differs from marginal gingivitis in that there is erythema over the attached gingiva, extending into the vestibule; indeed, the gingival margins may be spared (**Fig. 16.15**). Mainly seen in middle-aged or elderly females, desquamative gingivitis is typically caused by lichen planus, pemphigoid or, occasionally, by pemphigus or other vesiculobullous disorders (see Chapter 18).

16.15

DRUG-INDUCED SWELLING

A number of drugs may induce gingival swelling but those most commonly implicated are phenytoin, ciclosporin and calcium channel blockers (**Figs 16.16, 16.17**).

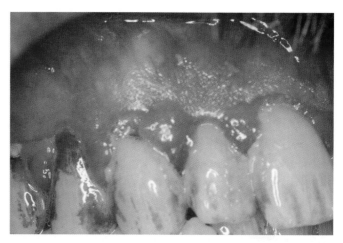

16.16

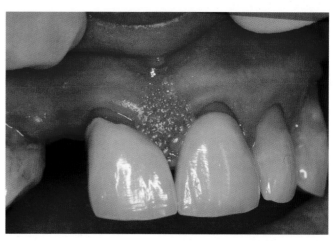

16.17

FIBROUS EPULIS

An epulis is a discrete gingival swelling. Low-grade gingival irritation can produce a fibrous epulis, a benign process (**Fig. 16.18**).

Most epulides are seen in the anterior part of the mouth and most are fibrous epulides.

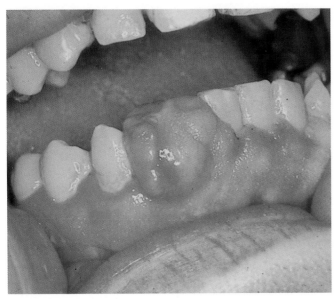

16.18

GIANT CELL GRANULOMA *(giant cell epulis)*

This is a non-neoplastic swelling of proliferating fibroblasts in a highly vascular stroma containing many multinucleate giant cells. It is most common in children (**Fig. 16.19**) after tooth extraction.

Giant cell epulides are usually deep red or purple; Kaposi's sarcoma and epithelioid angiomatosis may have a similar appearance.

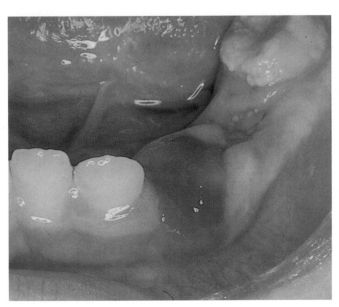

16.19

GINGIVAL CYST

Small white nodules are extremely common on the alveolar ridge (**Fig. 16.20**) and midline palate of the newborn. Sometimes termed Epstein's pearls or Bohn's nodules, they usually disappear spontaneously by rupturing or involution within a month or so. There may be an association of gingival cysts with milia (superficial epidermal inclusion cysts).

Oral cysts are otherwise rare in neonates, although they may be present at the base of the tongue where they can cause stridor.

Gingival cysts are rare in adults (**Fig. 16.21**). They are often solitary and found typically in the mandibular canine or premolar region as small, painless swellings of the attached or free gingiva, especially near the interdental papilla.

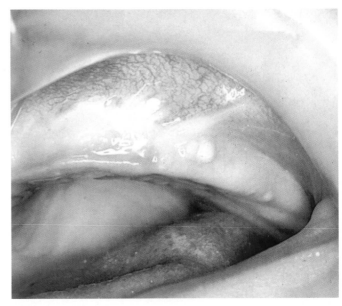

16.20

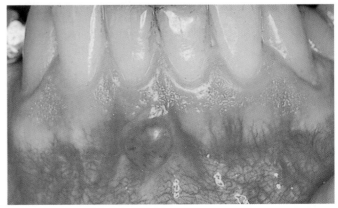

16.21

GINGIVAL FIBROMATOSIS

Enlarged maxillary tuberosities are a localized form of gingival fibromatosis (**Fig. 16.22**). Occasionally fibromatosis is found in the posterior mandibular region (**Fig. 16.23**).

Hereditary gingival fibromatosis is a familial condition in which generalized gingival fibromatosis (**Fig. 16.24**) is often associated with hirsutism. Hereditary gingival fibromatosis usually becomes most apparent at the time teeth are erupting. Rarely, the fibromatosis is one feature of a multisystem syndrome (see Table 28.1).

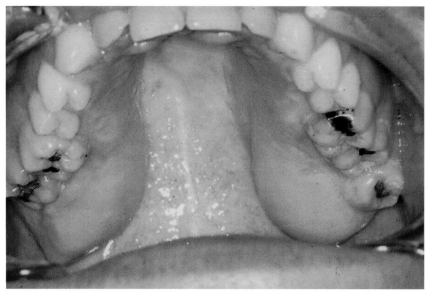

16.22

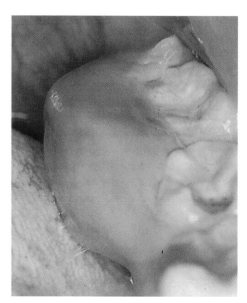

16.23

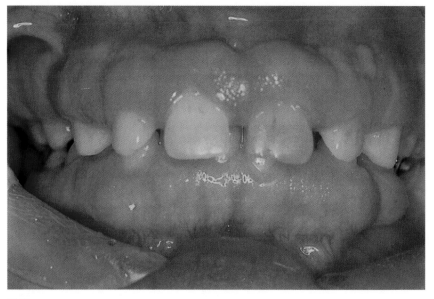

16.24

GINGIVAL RECESSION

Recession may be because of periodontitis, trauma from an occlusion or toothbrushing, artefactual or caused, for example, by the use of snuff or smokeless tobacco.

Isolated recession has exposed the root of the lower lateral incisor in **Fig. 16.25.** Incidentally the central incisor has an artificial crown.

Self-induced ulcers of the gingival margin are not rare (**Figs 16.26, 11.2**). The upper canine region seems a common site, and this artefactual gingival recession may be a form of Munchausen's syndrome.

KERATOSIS *(leukoplakia)*

Keratosis (hyperkeratinization) is fairly common on edentulous ridges and often produced by friction from chewing on the ridge (**Fig. 16.27**), by smoking or tobacco chewing or by papillomavirus (**Fig. 16.28**) but some cases are idiopathic.

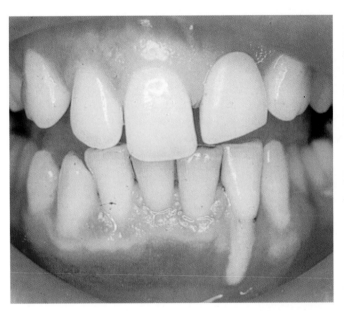

16.25

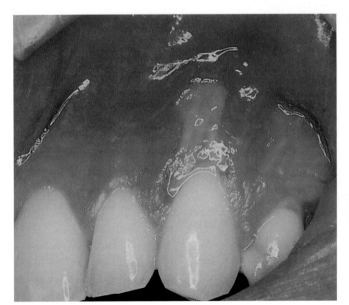

16.26

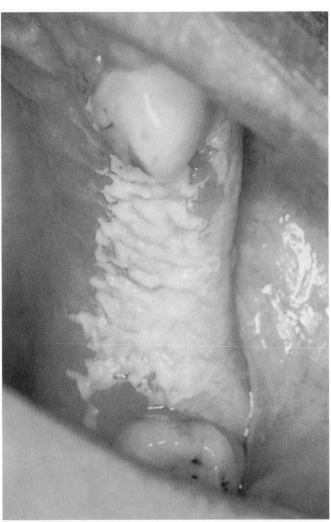

16.27

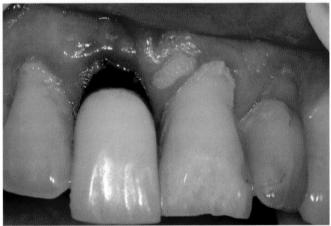

16.28

MATERIA ALBA

This is white debris due to squames and food debris (**Figs. 16.14, 16.29**). A more extreme example is shown in **Fig. 11.13** — a patient with learning disability whose teeth were virtually never cleaned. The teeth are covered with calculus, plaque and debris from food.

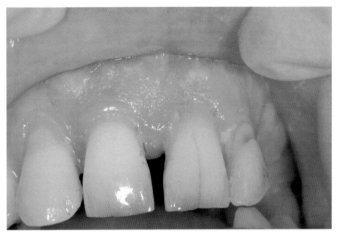

16.29

PERICORONITIS

Inflammation of the operculum over an erupting or impacted tooth is common (**Fig. 16.30**). The lower third molar is the site most commonly affected and patients complain of pain, trismus, swelling and halitosis. There may be fever and regional lymphadenitis, and the operculum is swollen, red and often ulcerated.

Acute pericoronitis appears in relation to the accumulation of plaque and trauma from the opposing tooth. Immune defects may predispose. A mixed flora is implicated and *Fusobacterium* and *Bacteroides* (*Porphyromonas*) are recognized to be important. Pus usually drains from beneath the operculum but may, in a migratory abscess of the buccal sulcus, track anteriorly (**Fig. 16.31**).

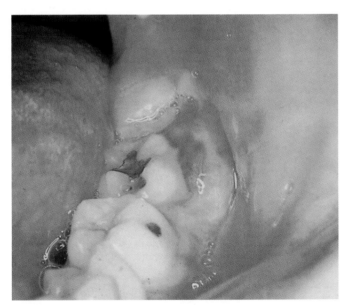

16.30

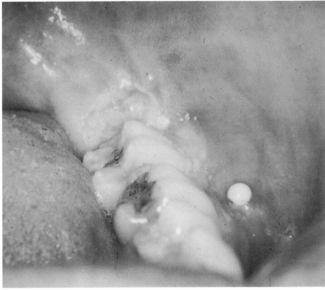

16.31

PERIODONTITIS

Chronic periodontitis is common, related to plaque accumulation and often smoking, and progresses from marginal gingivitis. The features are often those of marginal gingivitis but, with destruction of alveolar bone support, there is increasing tooth mobility, teeth may drift, and there is deep pocket formation (**Fig. 16.32**).

In accelerated (aggressive) periodontitis, patients still develop periodontitis despite good control of plaque (**Fig. 16.33**). A range of systemic causes may underlie this accelerated periodontitis, notably diabetes mellitus, white cell dyscrasias (including neutrophil defects and neutropenias), HIV and other immune defects including cathepsin C deficiency.

Rapidly progressive periodontitis (**Fig. 16.34**) is the term previously applied to adults — typically females in their early 30s — who, despite good oral hygiene and general health, develop periodontitis. Minor neutrophil defects may be responsible.

In the previously termed localized juvenile periodontitis, localized destruction, classically in the permanent incisor (**Fig. 16.35**) and first molar regions is seen in some adolescents or young adults in the absence of poor oral hygiene or gross systemic disease. Juvenile

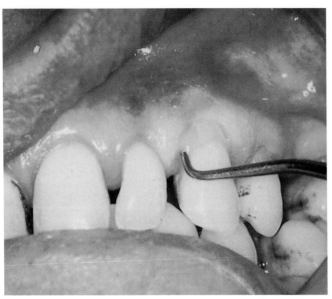

16.32

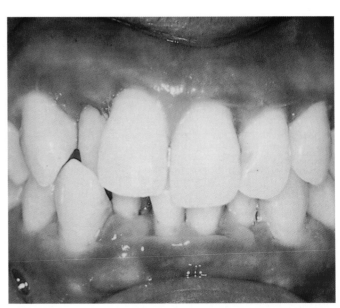

16.33

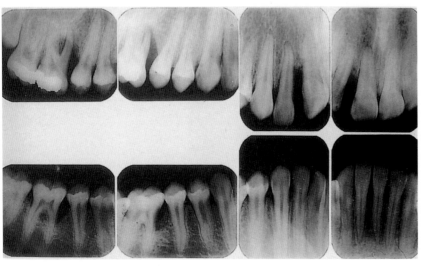

16.34

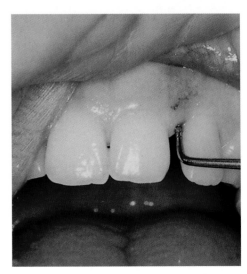

16.35

periodontitis (periodontosis) is seen especially in females and Afro-Asians, and may be associated with minor defects of neutrophil function and micro-organisms such as *Actinobacillus actinomycetemcomitans* and *Capnocytophaga*. Similar periodontal destruction can be seen in Down's syndrome, type VIII Ehlers–Danlos syndrome, HIV infection and hypophosphatasia (**Fig. 16.36**).

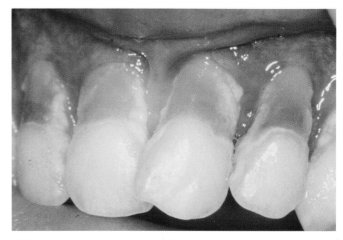

16.36

PIGMENTATION

Racial pigmentation is common on the gingivae in persons of Asian, African or Mediterranean heritage (**Figs 16.37–16.39**).

Hyperpigmentation may be seen in amalgam tattoos (**Fig 29.8**). Minocycline may cause black pigmentation of the bone, which may show through the gingivae (**Fig. 16.41**). Rarely, pigmentation of the gingivae can be a feature of congenital biliary atresia.

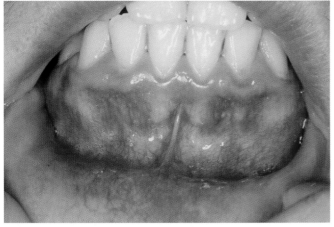

16.37

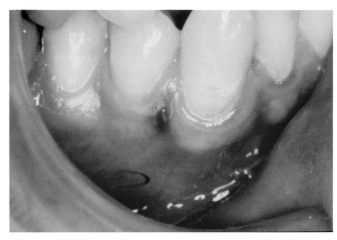

16.38

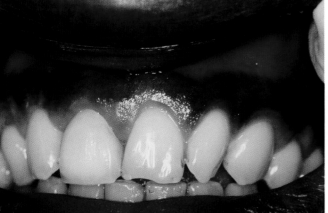

16.39

16.40

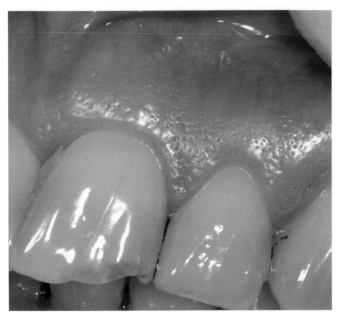

16.41

PYOGENIC GRANULOMA

Pyogenic granulomas are an exaggerated response to minor trauma. They tend to be soft, fleshy, rough-surfaced vascular lesions which bleed readily (**Fig. 16.43**). The gingiva is the most common site, the granuloma often arising on the buccal aspect from the interdental papilla and especially where there is a slight malocclusion leading to plaque accumulation. Most pyogenic granulomas are seen in the maxilla, anteriorly (**Fig. 16.44**, see also Chapter 18).

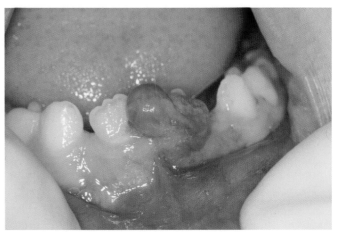

16.43

PLASMA CELL GINGIVITIS

This is a chronic erythematous swelling characterized histologically by a dense plasma cell infiltrate, often related to exposure to cinnamon, as in some chewing gums and oral health care products (**Fig. 16.42**).

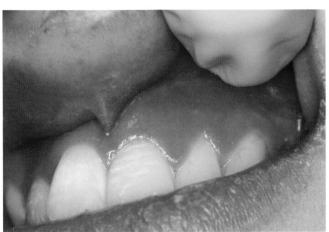

16.42

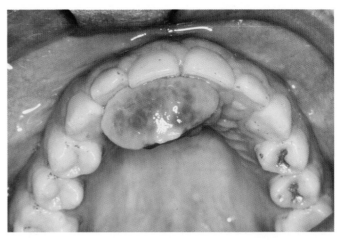

16.44

TUMOURS

Gingival carcinomas (**Fig. 16.45**), lymphomas, Kaposi's sarcoma and Wegener's granulomatosis are among the main neoplasms affecting the gingivae (see also Chapter 6).

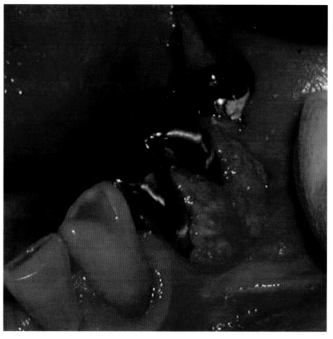

16.45

TRAUMATIC OCCLUSION

Trauma can damage the periodontium, often through excessive occlusal stresses and sometimes through direct damage. In **Fig. 16.46** both upper and lower incisors are retroclined and the upper incisors are traumatizing the lower labial gingiva (class II division II malocclusion; **Fig. 16.47**).

There is stripping of the periodontium labial to the lower incisors. The upper incisor periodontium may also be traumatized palatally by the lower incisors.

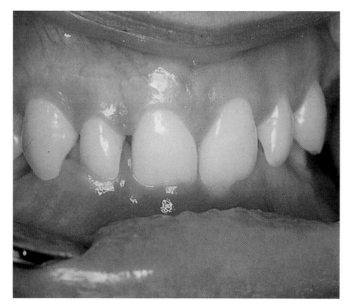

16.46

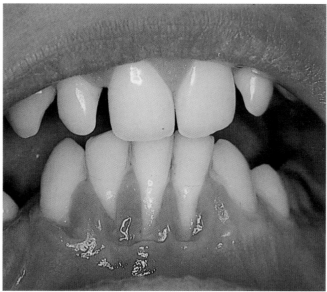

16.47

FURTHER READING

Arowojolu MO, Dosumu EB, Onyeaso CO, Lawoyin JO. Effects of some risk factors and immunodeficiencies on the periodontium — a review. Afr J Med Med Sci 2002; 31(3): 195–9.

Baehni PC, Takeuchi Y. Anti-plaque agents in the prevention of biofilm-associated oral diseases. Oral Dis 2003; 9 (Suppl 1): 23–9.

Bjelland S, Bray P, Gupta N, Hirscht R. Dentists, diabetes and periodontitis. Aust Dent J 2002; 47(3): 202–7.

Deas DE, Mackey SA, McDonnell HT. Systemic disease and periodontitis: manifestations of neutrophil dysfunction. Periodontol 2000 2003; 32: 82–104.

Dorfer CE. Antimicrobials for the treatment of aggressive periodontitis. Oral Dis 2003; 9 (Suppl 1): 51–3.

Etienne D. Locally delivered antimicrobials for the treatment of chronic periodontitis. Oral Dis 2003; 9 (Suppl 1): 45–50.

Lorenzana ER, Rees TD, Glass M, Detweiler JG. Chronic ulcerative stomatitis: a case report. J Periodontol 2000; 71: 104–11.

Madianos PN, Bobetsis GA, Kinane DF. Is periodontitis associated with an increased risk of coronary heart disease and preterm and/or low birth weight births? J Clin Periodontol 2002; 29 (Suppl 3): 22–36.

Mignogna MD, Lo Muzio L, Bucci E. Clinical features of gingival pemphigus vulgaris. J Clin Periodontol 2001; 28: 489–93.

Mombelli A. Periodontitis as an infectious disease: specific features and their implications. Oral Dis 2003; 9 (Suppl 1): 6–10.

Mombelli A, Casagni F, Madianos PN. Can presence or absence of periodontal pathogens distinguish between subjects with chronic and aggressive periodontitis? A systematic review. J Clin Periodontol 2002; 29 (Suppl 3): 10–21.

Nares S. The genetic relationship to periodontal disease. Periodontol 2000 2003; 32: 36–49.

Nunn ME. Understanding the etiology of periodontitis: an overview of periodontal risk factors. Periodontol 2000 2003; 32: 11–23.

Page RC. The etiology and pathogenesis of periodontitis. Compend Contin Educ Dent 2002; 23 (Suppl 5): 11–14.

Reibel J. Tobacco and oral diseases. Update on the evidence, with recommendations. Med Princ Pract 2003; 12 (Suppl 1): 22–32.

Ritchie CS, Kinane DF. Nutrition, inflammation, and periodontal disease. Nutrition 2003; 19(5): 475–6.

Ryder MI. An update on HIV and periodontal disease. J Periodontol 2002; 73(9): 1071–8.

Scully C, Porter SR. The clinical spectrum of desquamative gingivitis. Semin Cutan Med Surg 1997; 16: 308–13.

Simonian K. The role of herpesviruses in periodontal disease. J West Soc Periodontol Periodontal Abstr 2003; 51(1): 5–9.

Skaleric U, Kovac-Kavcic M. Some risk factors for the progression of periodontal disease. J Int Acad Periodontol 2000; 2(1): 19–23.

Wiebe CB, Silver JG, Larjava HS. Early onset periodontitis associated with Weary–Kindler syndrome: a case report. J Periodontol 1996; 67: 1004–10.

17 SALIVARY DISORDERS

- acute bacterial sialadenitis (acute suppurative sialadenitis)
- adenomatoid hyperplasia
- mucoceles
- necrotizing sialometaplasia
- obstructive sialadenitis
- salivary fistula
- sialosis (sialadenosis)
- tumours
- xerostomia.

ACUTE BACTERIAL SIALADENITIS *(acute suppurative sialadenitis)*

Acute bacterial sialadenitis is almost invariably a mixed infection, often including penicillin-resistant *Staphylococcus aureus* which ascends the duct because of xerostomia or a ductal anomaly. There is severe pain over the gland and often trismus if the parotid is affected. The gland is swollen (**Fig. 17.1**) and there is erythema over the gland (**Fig. 17.2**) which is tender to palpation.

Enteric Gram-negative rods have a high oropharyngeal colonization in hospitalized persons; these rods and pseudomonads have been implicated in a few cases of sialadenitis: indeed a wide range of bacteria have occasionally been implicated in the aetiology of acute bacterial sialadentis.

Purulent saliva (**Fig. 17.3**) or frank pus may be expressed from the duct of the affected gland — in this case the parotid. Normal parotid salivation (**Fig. 17.4**, shown here for comparison with **Fig. 17.3**, shows clear, watery, normal parotid saliva flowing from Stensen's duct).

Recurrent sialadenitis

In children, there is a rare form of recurrent parotitis that is of uncertain aetiology, possibly viral, and mainly seen in boys. It is characterized by

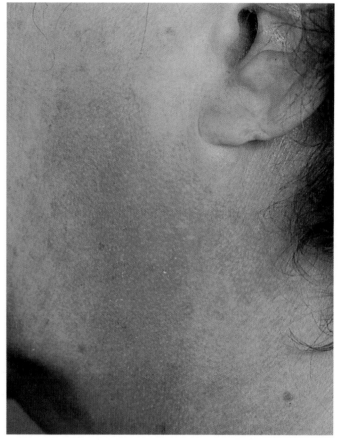

17.2

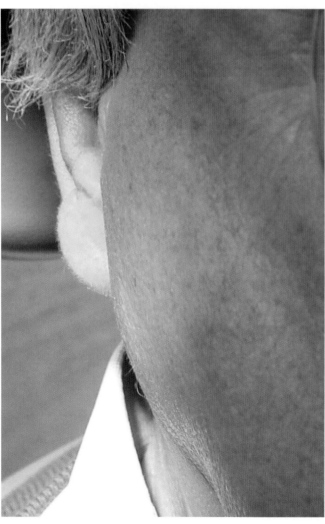

17.1

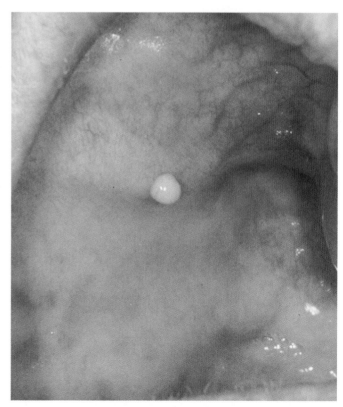

17.3

recurrent painful swelling, usually unilaterally. Peak incidence is between ages 3–6 years. The condition resolves spontaneously at puberty in most cases.

MUCOCELES

Mucoceles are common, especially inside the lower lip. The mucocele is a dome-shaped, fluctuant, bluish, nontender, submucosal swelling with a normal overlying mucosa (**Figs 17.6–17.10**). As an aid to diagnosis, the mucocele can be punctured to reveal the inspissated saliva (**Fig. 17.10**).

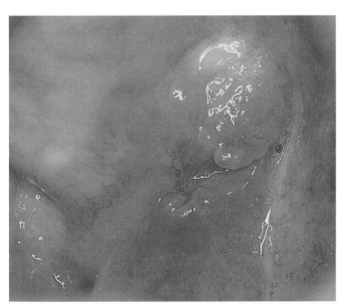

17.4

ADENOMATOID HYPERPLASIA

Adenomatoid hyperplasia is a rare, idiopathic, noninflammatory, non-neoplastic and benign lesion of the minor salivary glands, which typically presents with a tumour-like mass in the palate (**Fig. 17.5**). The lesion is usually a painless, sessile, firm or soft swelling of normal colour, indeterminate duration and located in the hard palate, although other intra-oral sites have occasionally been reported. Most patients have been males, usually middle aged or older. The aetiology is quite unclear though most patients are smokers.

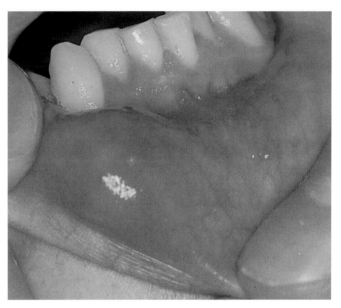

17.6

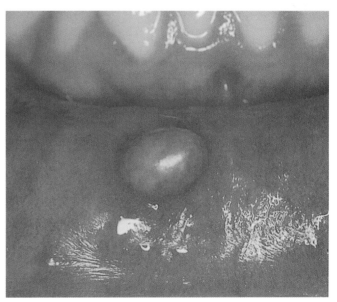

17.7

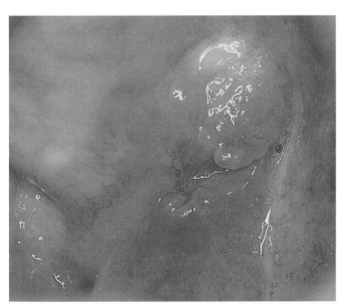

17.5

Extravasation mucoceles

These are caused by saliva extravasating into the tissues from a damaged salivary duct; they are most common and seen in the lower labial and ventral lingual mucosa.

Superficial mucoceles

These may be caused by small extravasations intraepithelially or occasionally subepithelially. Seen typically in females of middle or later age, often in the palate (**Fig. 17.11**) or buccal mucosae, they are most frequent in patients with oral lichen planus.

Retention mucoceles

These are uncommon and seen particularly in the sublingual gland (**Fig. 17.12**). Cysts may occasionally develop within salivary neoplasms.

Mucoceles arising from the sublingual gland are termed ranulas because of their resemblance to a frog's belly. Rarely, a ranula extends through the mylohyoid muscle (a plunging ranula).

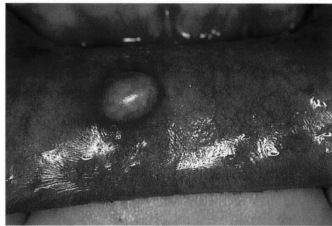

17.9

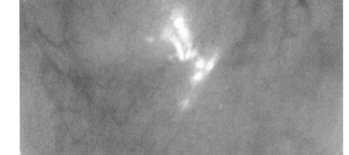

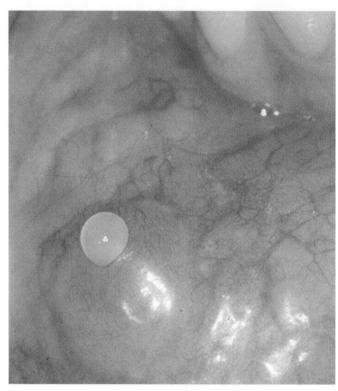

17.8

17.10

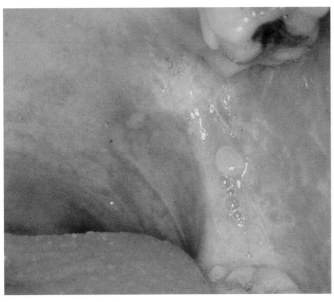

17.11

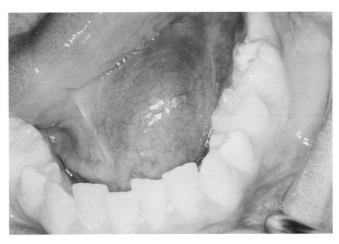

17.12

NECROTIZING SIALOMETAPLASIA

Necrotizing sialometaplasia is a rare ulcerative lesion of unknown aetiology, possibly the result of infarction, seen especially in the hard palate in adult males, most of whom are smokers. It may resemble a carcinoma clinically and histologically. **Figure 17.13** shows chronic swelling of the palate which ulcerated and then healed slowly over 1–2 months.

OBSTRUCTIVE SIALADENITIS

Salivary calculi are not uncommon and sometimes asymptomatic but the typical presentation is pain in, and swelling of, the gland around meal times.

Submandibular duct

Submandibular duct calculi are the most common. Calculi are usually yellow or white and can sometimes be seen in the duct (**Figs 17.14, 17.15**) or may be palpable. Not all are radiopaque. Quite large calculi

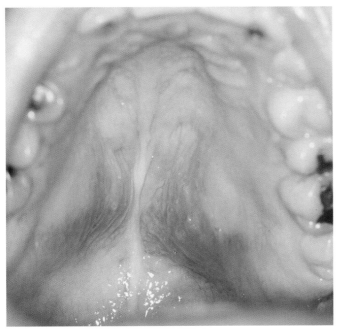

17.13

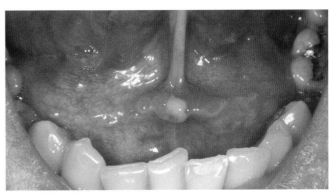

17.14

(**Fig. 17.16**) can form and calculi may be multiple. Chronic sialadenitis may develop if a salivary obstruction is not removed.

Parotid duct

This is less common in the parotid and less often radiopaque but obstruction (**Fig. 17.17**) can also be caused by mucus plugs, strictures or the oedema associated with ulceration of the parotid papilla. Rarely, salivary obstruction has other aetiologies.

Minor salivary gland

Minor salivary gland stones are rare (**Fig. 17.18**).

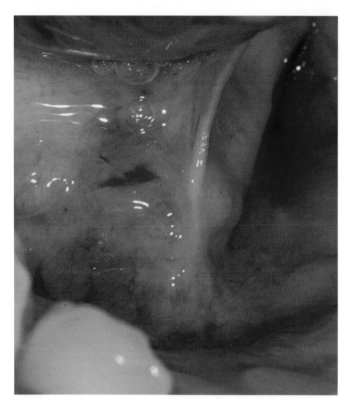

17.15

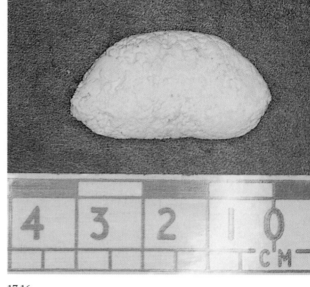

17.16

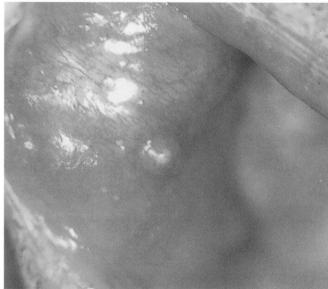

17.18

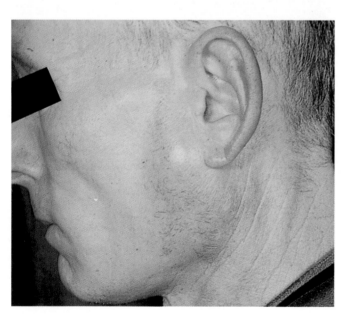

17.17

SALIVARY FISTULA

Internal fistulae (**Fig. 17.19**) may be congenital or acquired and are inconsequential.

External fistulae usually follow trauma in an accident, assault or after surgery, and are disconcerting and unpleasant for the patient.

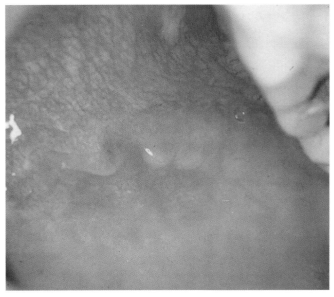

17.19

SIALOSIS *(sialadenosis)*

Sialosis is painless, bilateral chronic swelling of the salivary glands, typically the parotids (**Figs 17.20, 17.21**) without xerostomia. The cause appears to be an autonomic neuropathy with serous cell hypertrophy and striated duct atrophy related to drugs (e.g. methyldopa), endocrinopathies (e.g. diabetes mellitus and acromegaly), alcoholic liver cirrhosis, or malnutrition such as in bulimia. Although sialosis is benign and usually idiopathic, it is important to exclude underlying causes.

Salivary glands, especially the submandibular, may also swell in cystic fibrosis and most affected children also have antral polyps.

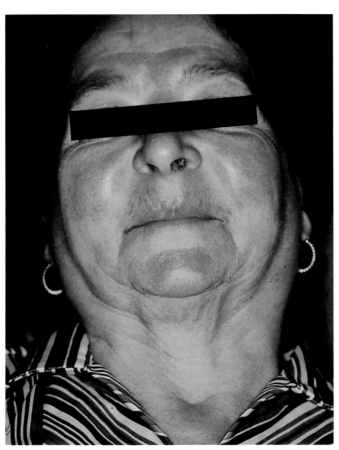

17.20

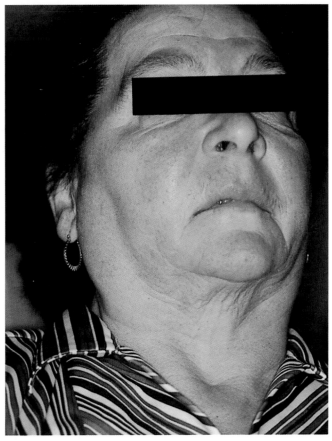

17.21

TUMOURS

Salivary gland neoplasms are usually pleomorphic adenomas mainly affecting the parotid glands (**Fig. 17.22**), but minor glands may also be the location for benign or malignant neoplasms (**Fig. 17.23**).

XEROSTOMIA

In xerostomia there is reduced salivation (hyposalivation); the dry mucosa may become tacky and the lips can adhere to each other (**Fig. 17.24**). An examining dental mirror may often stick to the mucosa. There may be a lack of salivary pooling in the floor of the mouth — any saliva present tends to be viscous, show spinbarkeit and appear frothy (**Figs 17.25, 17.26**) and saliva flows poorly, if at all, from the ducts of the

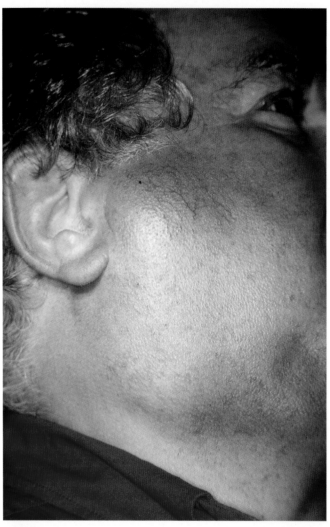

17.22

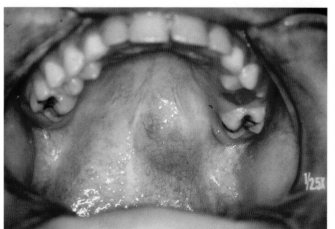

17.23

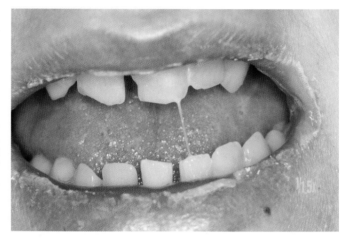

17.24

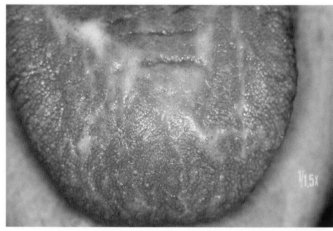

17.25

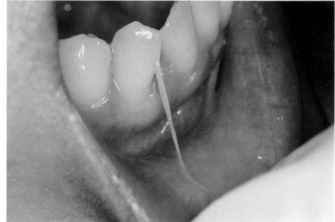

17.26

major glands on stimulation or palpation. Food may accumulate on the hard and soft tissues. Complications such as caries (particularly cervical), candidosis or acute bacterial sialadenitis may arise.

The main causes of dry mouth are drugs (those with anticholinergic or sympathomimetic activity: see 1.5), irradiation of the salivary glands, Sjögren's syndrome), HIV disease, HCV infection, sarcoidosis and dehydration, such as in diabetes.

Many patients complain of a dry mouth and yet lack objective evidence of xerostomia (**Fig. 17.27**).

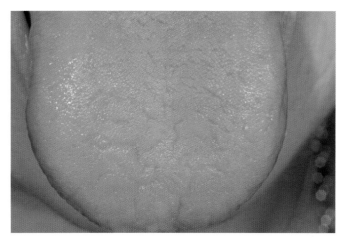

17.27

FURTHER READING

Bsoul SA, Flint DJ, Terezhalmy GT, Moore WS. Sialolithiasis. Quintessence Int 2003; 34(4): 316–17.

Delbem AC, Cunha RF, Vieira AE, Ribeiro LL. Treatment of mucus retention phenomena in children by the micro-marsupialization technique: case reports. Pediatr Dent 2000; 22(2): 155–8.

Ellis SG, Lee NJ, Peckitt NS. Mucous retention cyst of the soft palate: a case presentation. Dent Update 1995; 22(10): 421–2.

Escudier MP, Brown JE, Drage NA, McGurk M. Extracorporeal shockwave lithotripsy in the management of salivary calculi. Br J Surg 2003; 90(4): 482–5.

Greer JE, Eltorky M, Robbins KT. A feasibility study of salivary gland autograft transplantation for xerostomia. Head Neck 2000; 22(3): 241–6.

Guggenheimer J, Moore PA. Xerostomia: etiology, recognition and treatment. J Am Dent Assoc 2003; 134(1): 61–9.

Harrison HD. Sublingual gland is origin of cervical extravasation mucocele. Oral Surg Oral Med Oral Pathol Oral Radiol Endod 2000; 90(4): 404–5.

Hassan R, Asfar SK, Scully C. Salivary mega-calculus. Medicina Oral 2000; 5: 54–6.

Kastin B, Mandel L. Alcoholic sialosis. NY State Dent J 2000; 66(6): 22–4.

Kim D, Uy C, Mandel L. Sialosis of unknown origin. NY State Dent J 1998; 64(7): 38–40.

Lindman JP, Woolley AL. Multiple intraparenchymal parotid calculi: a case report and review of the literature. Ear Nose Throat J 2003; 82(8): 615–17.

Longman LP, Higham SM, Rai K, Edgar WM, Field EA. Salivary gland hypofunction in elderly patients attending a xerostomia clinic. Gerodontology 1995; 12(12): 67–72.

Longman LP, Higham SM, Bucknall R, Kaye SB, Edgar WM, Field EA. Signs and symptoms in patients with salivary gland hypofunction. Postgrad Med J 1997; 73(856): 93–7.

Marchal F, Dulguerov P. Sialolithiasis management: the state of the art. Arch Otolaryngol Head Neck Surg 2003; 129(9): 951–6.

Pape SA, MacLeod RI, McLean NR, Soames JV. Sialadenosis of the salivary glands. Br J Plast Surg 1995; 48(6): 419–22.

Porter SR, Scully C, Kainth B, Ward-Booth P. Multiple salivary mucoceles in a young boy. Int J Paediatr Dent 1998; 8: 149–51.

Porter, SR, Scully, C, Hegarty, A. An update of the aetiology and management of xerostomia. Oral Surg Oral Med Oral Pathol Oral Radiol Endod 2004; 97: 28–46.

Scully C. Drug effects on salivary glands: dry mouth. Oral Dis 2003; 9(4): 165–76.

Ship JA. Diagnosing, managing, and preventing salivary gland disorders. Oral Dis 2002; 8(2): 77–89.

Soundy TJ, Lucas AR, Suman VJ, Melton LJ 3rd. Bulimia nervosa in Rochester, Minnesota from 1980 to 1990. Psychol Med 1995; 25(5): 1065–71.

Sutay S, Erdag TK, Ikiz AO, Guneri EA. Large submandibular gland calculus with perforation of the floor of the mouth. Otolaryngol Head Neck Surg 2003; 128(4): 587–8.

18 MUCOSAL DISORDERS

- aphthae (recurrent aphthae; recurrent aphthous stomatitis; RAS)
- Behçet's syndrome (Behçet's disease)
- black hairy tongue
- cheek chewing
- cheilitis
- denture-induced hyperplasia (epulis fissuratum)
- dermoid cyst
- eosinophilic ulcer (eosinophilic granuloma of oral mucosa)
- ephelis (freckle)
- erythema migrans (geographic tongue; benign migratory glossitis; migratory stomatitis)
- erythroplasia (erythroplakia)
- fibrous lump (fibroepithelial polyp)
- foliate papillitis
- furred tongue
- glossitis
- glossodynia (glossopyrosis)
- keratosis (leukoplakia)
- leukoedema
- linea alba (occlusal line)
- lingual abscess
- lingual haematoma
- lingual laceration
- lingual hemihypertrophy
- lip chapping
- lip fissure
- lip horn
- melanotic macules
- naevi
- oral submucous fibrosis
- papillary hyperplasia
- papillomatosis
- pigmentation
- pyogenic granuloma
- stomatitis nicotina (smoker's palate)
- tattoos
- traumatic ulcers
- verrucous hyperplasia
- verrucous xanthoma.

APHTHAE *(recurrent aphthae; recurrent aphthous stomatitis; RAS)*

Recurrent aphthae are typically ovoid or round ulcers with a yellow floor and pronounced inflammatory halo (**Fig. 18.1**). Episodes usually begin in childhood and the natural history is of spontaneous remission after some years; the aetiology is unknown. Minor aphthae (Mikulicz's aphthae) are small, 2–4 mm in diameter (**Figs 18.2–18.8**), last 7–10 days, tend not to be seen on the gingivae, palate or dorsum of the tongue, and heal with no obvious scarring. Most patients develop no more than six ulcers at any single episode.

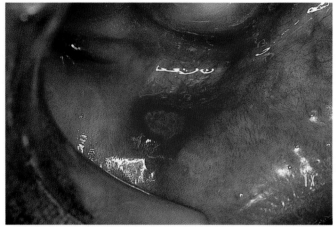

18.2

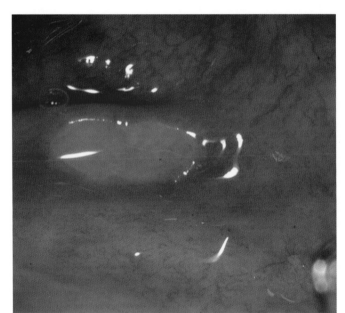

18.1

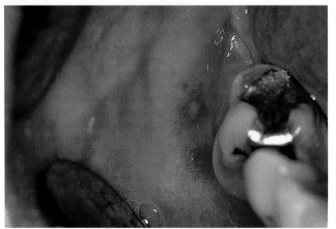

18.3

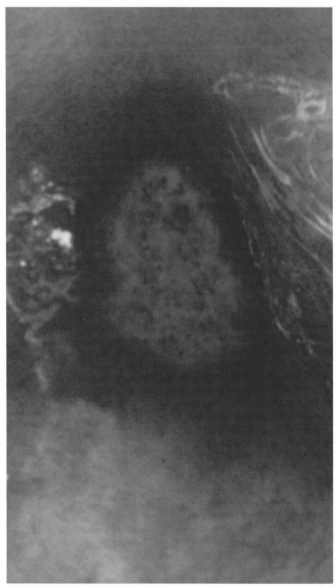

18.4

Most patients with RAS are otherwise apparently well but a significant proportion of those referred to a hospital clinic prove to be deficient in a haematinic such as iron, folate or vitamin B_{12}, a few have coeliac disease and there are also occasional associations with menstruation, stress, food allergy, sodium lauryl sulphate, malabsorption states and immunodeficiencies. Most patients with aphthae are nonsmokers and others may develop aphthae for the first time on ceasing smoking.

Aphthae may occasionally be a manifestation of Behçet's syndrome (see below) or Sweet's syndrome, and aphthous-like ulcers may occasionally be a manifestation of HIV disease, cyclic or chronic neutropenia, or a similar syndrome with periodic fever, adenitis and pharyngitis (PFAPA) but with no neutropenia.

Major aphthae are recurrent, often ovoid ulcers with an inflammatory halo but they are less common, much larger (**Fig. 18.9**), more persistent than minor aphthae, and can affect the dorsum of the tongue and soft palate (**Figs 18.10–18.12**) as well as other sites.

Sometimes termed Sutton's ulcers or periadenitis mucosa necrotica recurrens (PMNR), major aphthae can be well over 1 cm in diameter

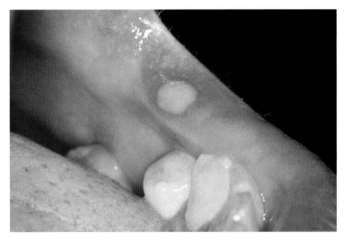

18.5

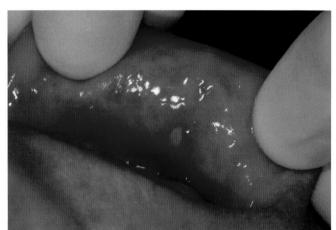

18.6

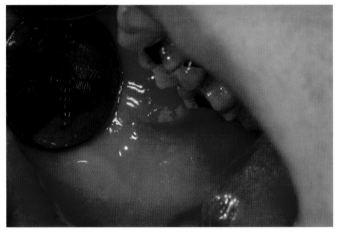

18.7

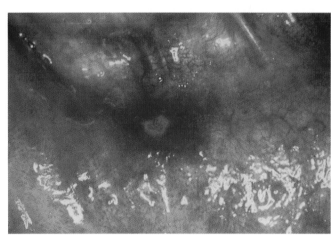

18.8

and can take several months to heal. In any one episode there are usually fewer than six ulcers. Major aphthae may leave obvious scars on healing (**Figs 18.13, 18.14**).

Herpetiform aphthae are so termed because the patients have a myriad of small ulcers that clinically resemble those of herpetic stomatitis (**Figs 18.15, 18.16**). It is, however, a distinct entity, lacking the associated fever, gingivitis and lymph node involvement of primary herpetic stomatitis.

Pinpoint herpetiform aphthae (Cooke's aphthae) enlarge and fuse to produce irregular ulcers. These aphthae affect females more than males, present at a slightly later age (often from 30 years of age) than other forms of RAS, and affect any site in the mouth.

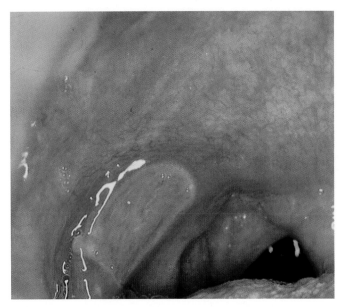

18.9

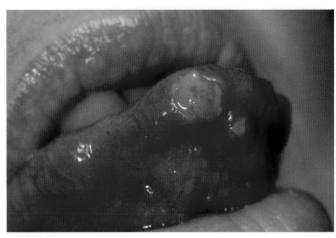

18.10

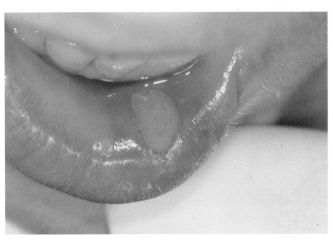

18.11

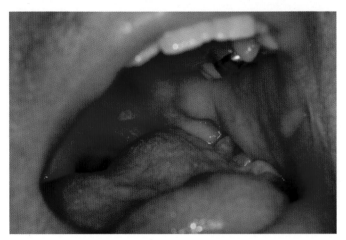

18.12

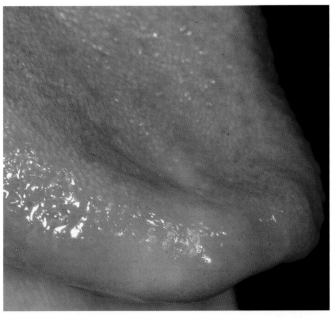

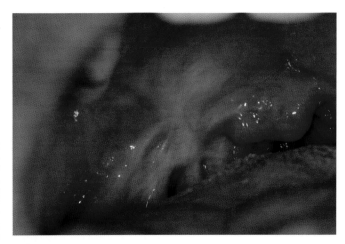

18.14

18.13

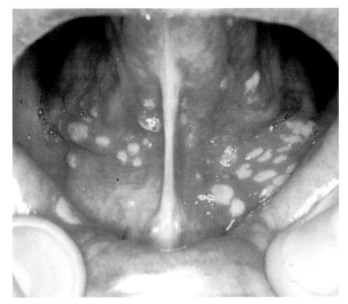

18.15

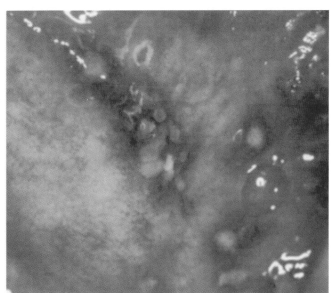

18.16

BEHÇET'S SYNDROME *(Behçet's disease)*

Aphthae of any of the types previously described usually occur in isolation in apparently healthy persons. A minority are a manifestation of Behçet's syndrome (**Figs 18.17, 18.18**), where aphthae are associated with genital ulcers and uveitis.

Behçet's syndrome is a multisystem disease affecting the mouth in most cases. Genital ulcers in this syndrome often closely resemble oral aphthae (**Fig. 18.19**). Other sites commonly affected are the eyes, skin and joints although Behçet's syndrome is not the only cause of this constellation of lesions. Other causes, such as ulcerative colitis, Crohn's disease, mixed connective tissue disease, lupus erythematosus Sweet's syndrome and Reiter's syndrome, should be excluded.

Behçet's syndrome is most common in people from Japan, China, North and South Korea and the Middle East.

Uveitis — posterior uveitis (**Fig. 18.20**; retinal vasculitis) — is one of the more important ocular lesions of Behçet's syndrome but anterior uveitis and other changes occur. The left pupil in **Fig. 18.20** has been dilated for fundoscopy. Ocular and arthritic symptoms are more common in males. Neurological involvement may cause headache and psychiatric, motor or sensory manifestations.

Erythema nodosum can be a feature of Behçet's syndrome (**Fig. 18.21**), particularly in females.

Of the various rashes seen in Behçet's syndrome, an acneiform pustular rash (**Fig. 18.22**) is the most common. Patients with Behçet's syndrome may develop pustules at the site of venepuncture (pathergy) but this feature is uncommon in British patients.

Although large-joint arthropathy is not uncommon in Behçet's syndrome, an overlap syndrome with relapsing polychondritis has also been described (mouth and genital ulcers with inflamed cartilage — MAGIC — syndrome).

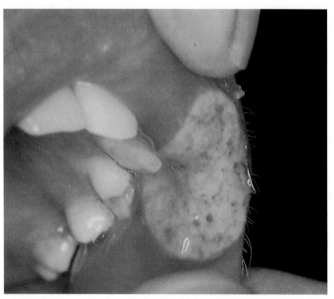

18.17

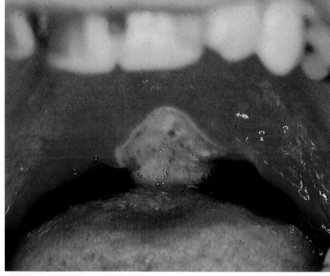

18.18

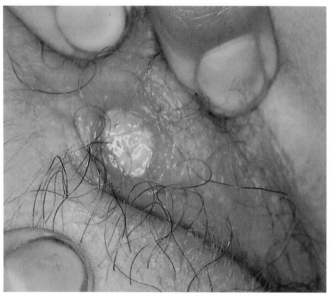

18.19

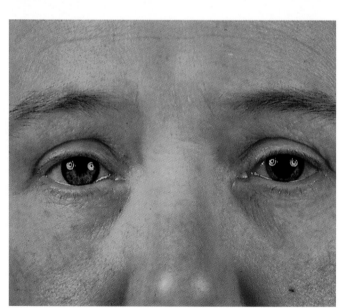

18.20

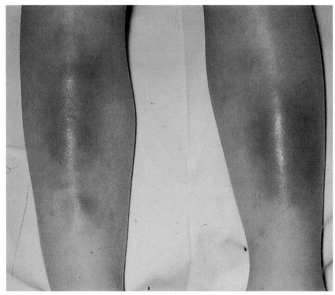

18.21

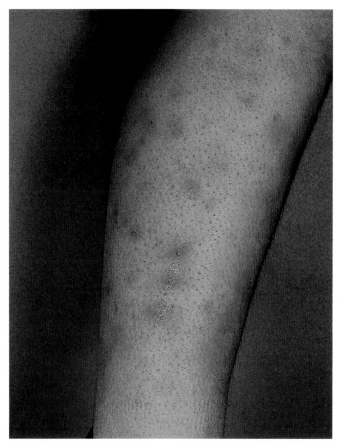

18.22

BLACK HAIRY TONGUE

Overgrowth of the filiform papillae, with proliferation of chromogenic bacteria may cause a black hairy tongue (**Figs 18.23–18.25**). The patient in **Fig. 18.24** also has a cleft lip and palate.

Although often idiopathic, a brown hairy tongue may be seen for any of the reasons discussed above. Mouthwashes, antibiotics, tobacco, dry mouth or gastrointestinal disease may predispose.

White or coloured lesions of the tongue are also sometimes seen in immunocompromised patients. It is now evident that any of a range of micro-organisms may become opportunistic pathogens in such patients. For example, a soil saprophytic fungus *Ramichloridium schulzeri* has been described as causing a 'golden' tongue.

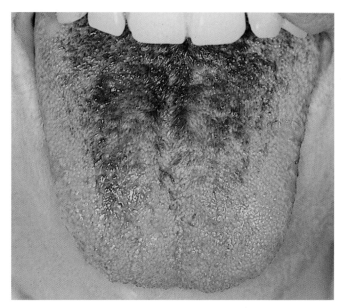

18.23

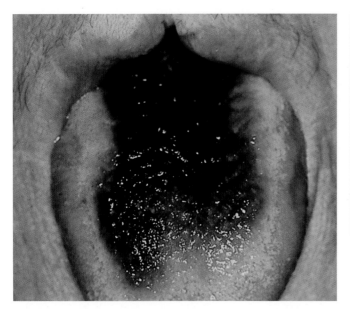

18.24

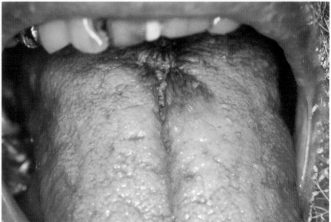

18.25

CHEEK CHEWING

The mucosa in cheek chewing is shredded with a shaggy white appearance similar to that of white sponge naevus but restricted to areas close to the occlusal line (**Figs 18.26, 18.27**) or the lower labial mucosa.

Lip biting *(morsicatio buccarum)*
Lip biting is a common habit (**Fig. 18.28**), particularly in anxiety states, and may be associated with a few traumatic petechiae.

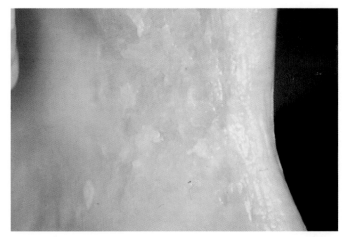

18.26

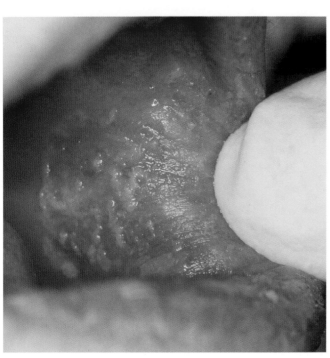

18.27

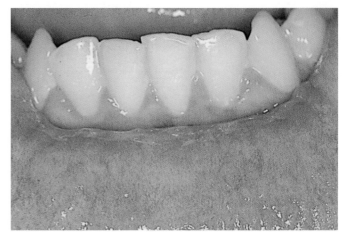

18.28

CHEILITIS

Cheilitis is inflammation of the lips, often caused by allergens (see Chapter 29). Cheilitis can also be caused by a number of other factors such as sun exposure (**Fig. 18.29**) and lip licking; children in particular may develop a habit of licking the lips and adjacent skin, leading to erythematous lesions (**Fig. 18.30**). Candidosis may infect some of these lesions (**Fig. 18.31**).

Exfoliative cheilitis is persistent scaling of the vermilion of the lips and is seen mainly in adolescent or young adult females (**Fig. 18.32**). It may have a somewhat cyclical nature but is of unknown, possibly factitious, aetiology. The lips scale and peel and can be covered with a shaggy yellowish coating.

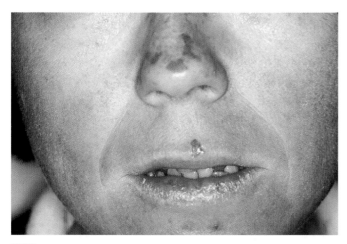

18.29

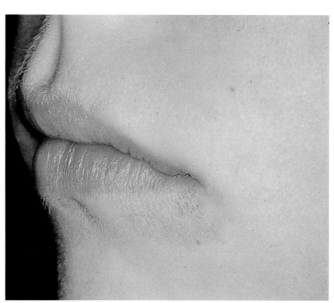

18.30

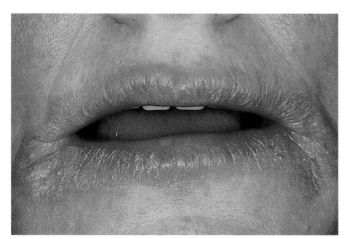

18.31

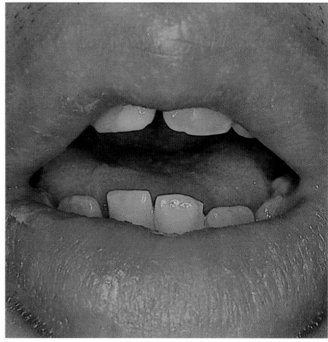

18.32

Cheilitis glandularis is shown in **Fig. 18.33**. The black puncta in this case, inside the upper lip, were associated with swelling and a thick mucinous exudate from the minor salivary glands. This lesion, of unknown aetiology, may be premalignant and usually affects the lower lip.

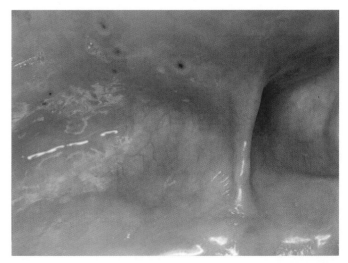

18.33

DENTURE-INDUCED HYPERPLASIA
(epulis fissuratum)

A denture margin (flange) may cause ulceration, and chronic irritation may produce hyperplasia (**Fig. 18.34**).

In **Fig. 18.35** the denture fits neatly into the groove between the hyperplastic leaves of tissue (this is the same patient as **Fig. 18.34**). The lesion is common over the genial tubercles (**Fig. 18.36**).

This condition is quite benign but, very occasionally, hyperplasia results from a lesion proliferating beneath and impinging on a denture flange.

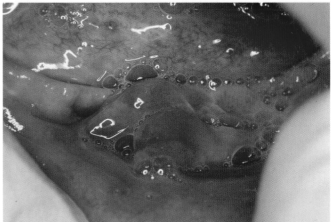

18.35

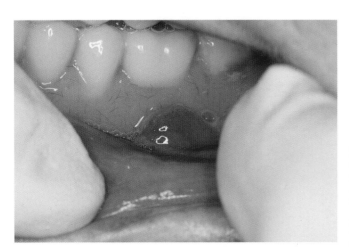

18.34

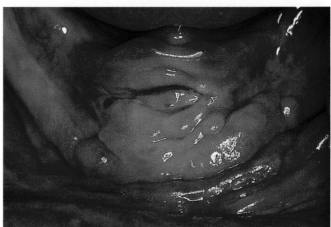

18.36

DERMOID CYST

Dermoid cyst is an uncommon midline entity, often presenting with a slowly growing swelling beneath the chin (**Fig. 18.37**). Found in the floor of the mouth (**Fig. 18.38**), the dermoid cyst sometimes resembles a ranula.

EOSINOPHILIC ULCER *(eosinophilic granuloma of oral mucosa)*

Eosinophilic granuloma of the oral mucosa is a rare chronic lesion typically found on the tongues of males (**Fig. 18.39**), and supposed to have a traumatic aetiology. Numerous eosinophils are seen on biopsy examination, though a T-lymphocyte aetiology is now suspected.

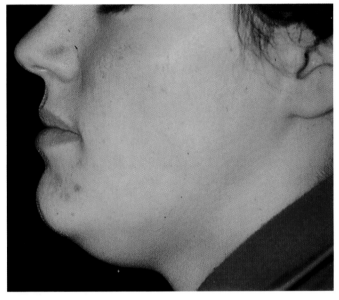

18.37

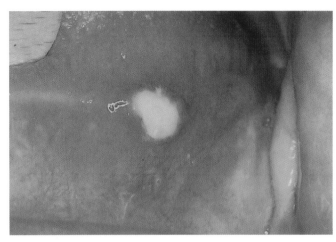

18.39

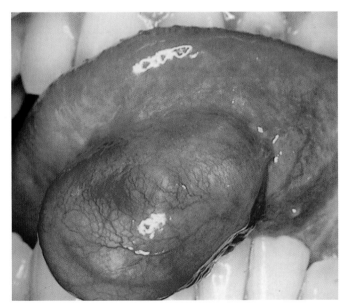

18.38

EPHELIS *(freckle)*

These circumscribed melanotic macules, typically smaller than 0.5 cm, appear on sun-exposed areas in childhood, owing to a local increase in melanin production, in a normal number of melanocytes. Although usually affecting the skin, ephelides may occasionally involve the lip or mucous membranes (**Figs 18.40, 18.41**).

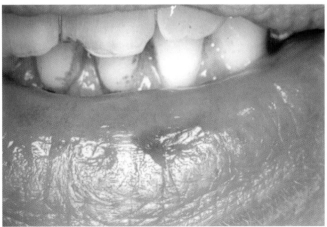

18.40

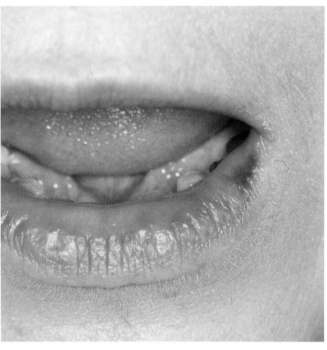

18.41

ERYTHEMA MIGRANS *(geographic tongue; benign migratory glossitis; migratory stomatitis)*

Erythema migrans is common, especially on the tongue but uncommon elsewhere. Often asymptomatic, the lesions are characterized by a somewhat serpiginous yellow-white lesion with surrounding erythema, which can simulate snailtrack ulcers (**Figs 18.40–18.43**).

The lesions change in shape and site over hours (**Figs 18.46–18.48**) and are totally benign. They may represent a variant of psoriasis.

Erythema migrans is a benign condition, of unknown aetiology, in which the filiform papillae desquamate in irregular demarcated areas. Patients with a fissured (scrotal) tongue often have erythema migrans. Most patients with erythema migrans are otherwise healthy but it may

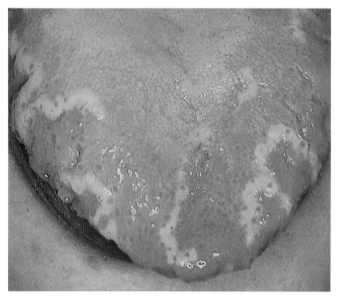

18.42

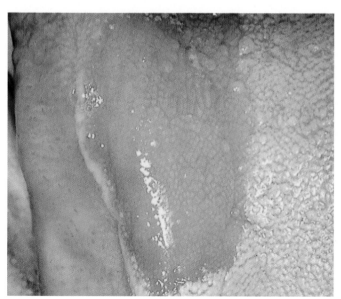

18.43

be a *forme fruste* of psoriasis and may be confused with Reiter's syndrome.

If the tongue is furred, the lesions of erythema migrans can appear quite pronounced. Though the configuration of the lesions can change over a few hours, there are rare examples where the lesion is persistent and unchanging (erythema migrans perstans is the rather inappropriate term used; **Fig. 18.49**).

The patient seen in **Fig. 18.50** (the same patient as in **Fig. 18.49**) had a virtually identical lesion over 4 years; biopsy confirmed that this was erythema migrans.

Occasionally, erythema migrans affects sites other than the tongue (geographic stomatitis; **Figs 18.51–18.53**).

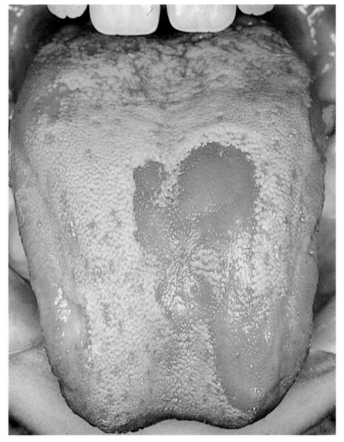

18.44

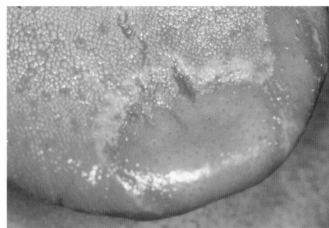

18.45

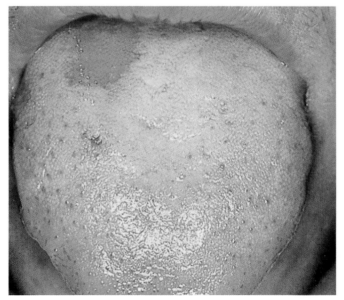

18.46

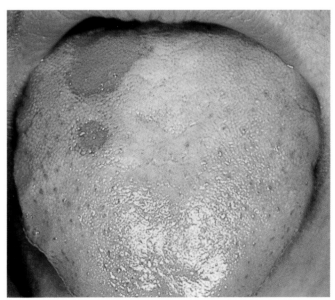

18.47

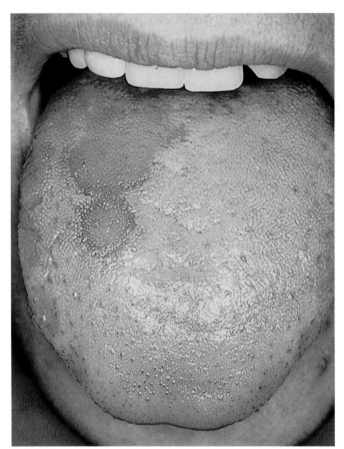

18.48

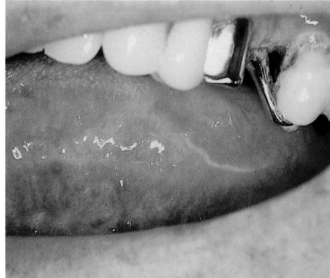

18.49

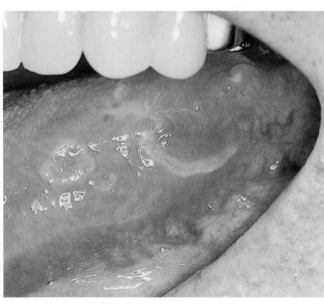

18.50

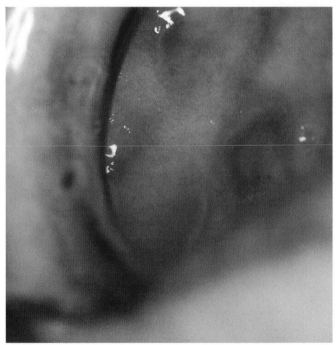

18.51

ERYTHROPLASIA *(erythroplakia)*

Less common than leukoplakia, erythroplasia (**Figs 18.54, 18.55**) is characterized by epithelial atrophy and pronounced dysplasia. Erythroplasia is seen mainly in elderly males, in the buccal mucosa or palate and is often carcinoma-in-situ.

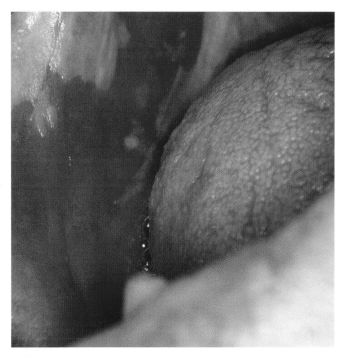

18.54

18.52

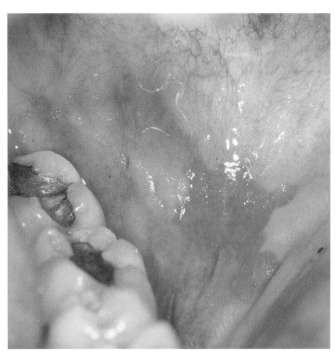

18.55

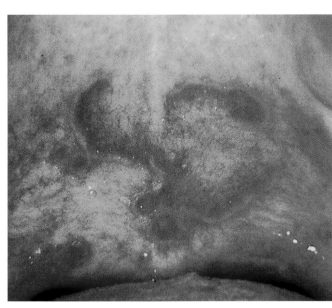

18.53

FIBROUS LUMP *(fibroepithelial polyp)*

Fibrous lumps may be related to irritation but this is not always evident (**Figs 18.56–18.59**). This is the so-called 'leaf fibroma', although it is not actually a true fibroma is totally benign. Fibrous lumps on the margin of the tongue may also be benign although biopsy is prudent to establish the diagnosis.

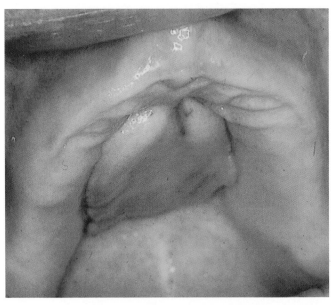

18.56

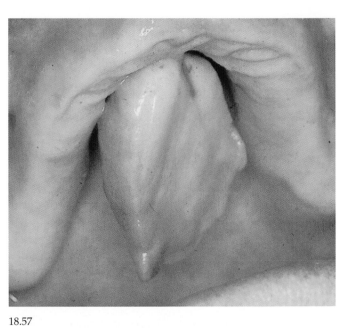

18.57

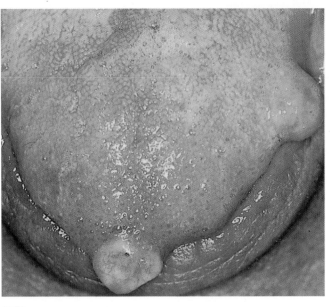

18.58

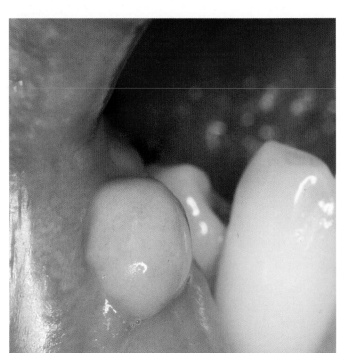

18.59

FOLIATE PAPILLITIS

The size and shape of the foliate papillae are variable and occasionally they swell if irritated mechanically or if there is an upper respiratory infection (**Fig. 18.60**). Located at a site of high predilection for lingual carcinoma, they may give rise to anxiety about cancer.

Inflammation of the lingual tonsils may also give rise to concern as it may present with pain and dysphagia.

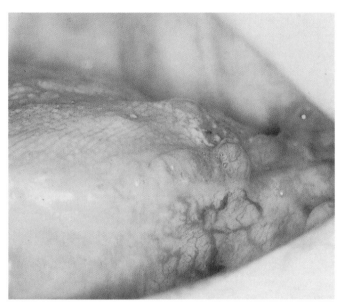

18.60

FURRED TONGUE

The tongue is rarely furred in a healthy child but may be lightly furred in a healthy adult, especially if the oral hygiene is poor, the patient smokes, wears full dentures or if the diet is soft. Any febrile illness (**Fig. 18.61**) may also cause a furred tongue.

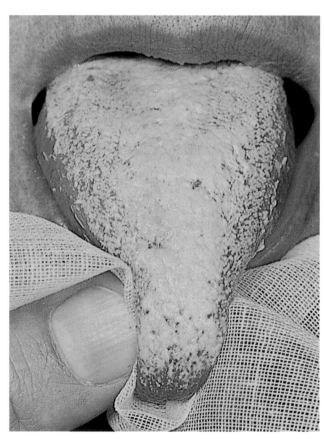

18.61

GLOSSITIS

Lingual papillary atrophy is usually due to haematinic deficiency (**Fig. 18.62**), but atrophy may be seen after repeated ulceration, burns or irradiation.

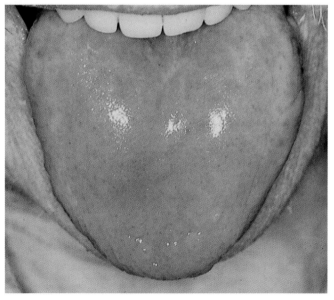

18.62

GLOSSODYNIA *(glossopyrosis)*

Most patients with glossodynia have no identifiable organic lesion of the tongue (**Fig. 18.63**) and the discomfort usually has a psychogenic basis.

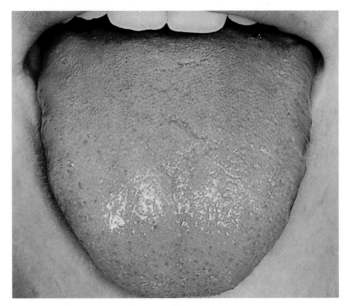

18.63

KERATOSIS *(leukoplakia)*

Hyperkeratosis in the mouth can present as a white lesion (**Fig. 18.64**). Most keratoses are flat, smooth-surfaced (homogeneous) and benign.

In **Fig. 18.65** the homogeneous leukoplakia of the lower lip was seen in a heavy smoker. Smoking and tobacco-related habits are, with friction, the most common identifiable causes of keratoses. Sanguinaria may cause a white lesion.

Figure 18.66 shows homogeneous keratosis in the buccal mucosa, which is a common site.

Keratoses may be extremely pronounced (**Fig. 18.67**). In **Figs 18.68** and **18.69**, the keratosis has two components: a diffuse overall keratosis and a more verrucous area centrally.

Verrucous or nodular keratoses (**Fig. 18.70**) have a malignant potential higher than that of homogeneous keratoses. In **Figs 18.71** and **18.72**, the lesions developed into carcinoma, as shown.

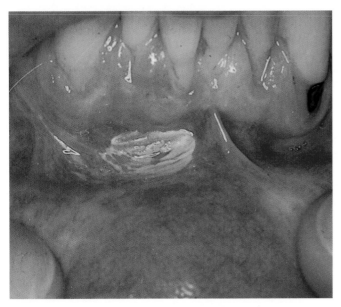

18.64

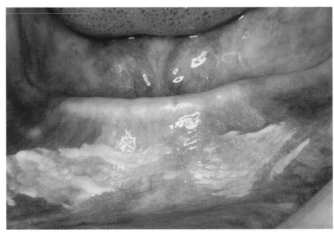

18.65

Speckled leukoplakias have the highest premalignant potential of the keratoses. Keratoses such as these (**Figs 18.73, 18.74**) may have a candidal association, although these are typically located at the commissures. The patient in **Fig. 18.75** developed a carcinoma.

A recently described variant termed proliferative verrucous leukoplakia is seen especially in the buccal mucosa in older women and about one half develop carcinoma. Keratosis on the ventrum of the tongue and floor of the mouth has a higher premalignant potential than similar lesions elsewhere (**Figs 18.76–18.79**).

The sublingual keratosis, which is seen especially in middle-aged or older women, is usually bilateral, but not invariably. The surface may have a so-called 'ebbing tide' appearance, resembling the appearance of sand on the beach as the tide ebbs, and the lesion may be a mixture of white and red lesions: a speckled leukoplakia. The red areas are most sinister.

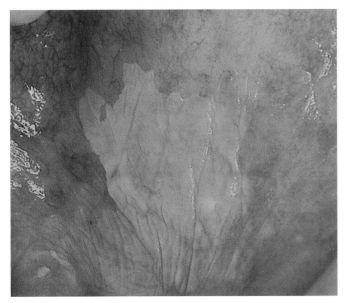

18.66

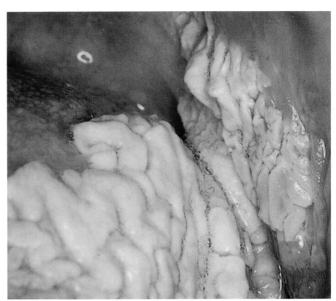

18.67

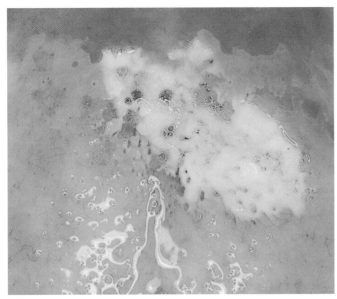

18.68

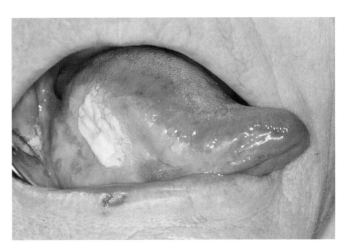

18.69

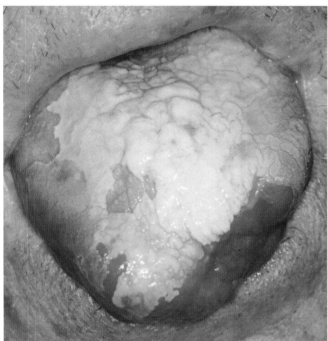

18.70

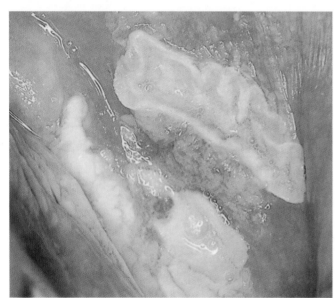

18.72

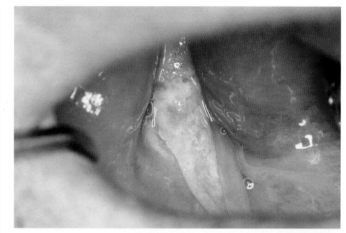

18.71

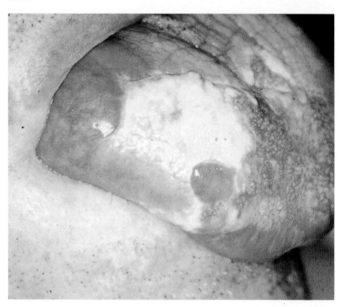

18.73

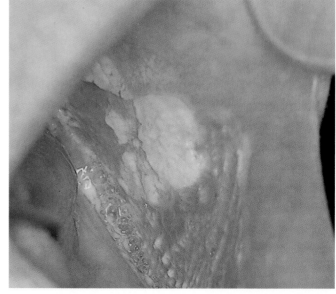

18.74

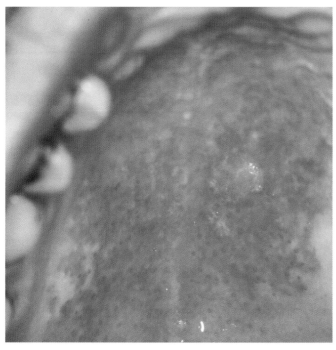

18.75

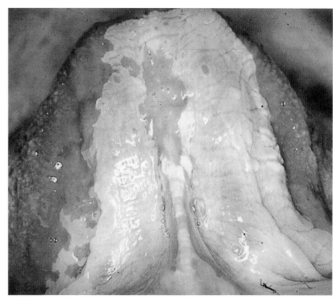

18.76

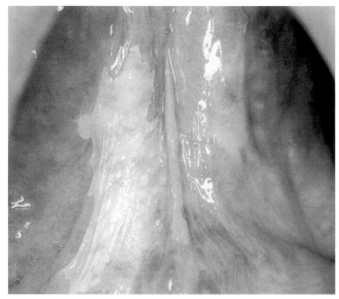

18.77

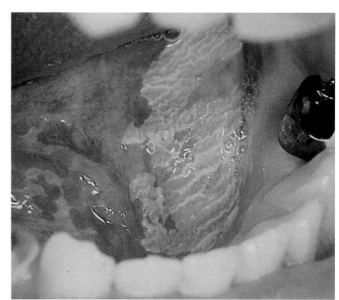

18.78

Leukoplakia and glossitis on the dorsum of the tongue may sometimes have a syphilitic origin (**Fig. 3.31**).

Some keratoses are induced by friction (**Fig. 18.79**; an extreme example resulting from over-zealous brushing) or tobacco (**Fig. 18.80**) and appear to be benign.

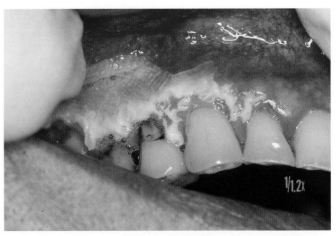

18.80

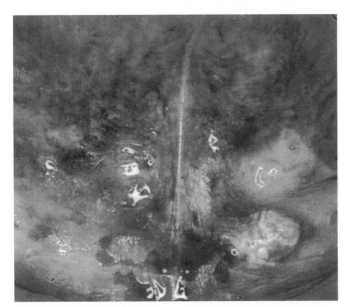

18.79

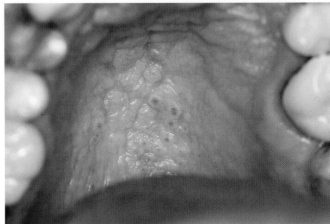

18.81

LEUKOEDEMA

Leukoedema is the term given to the clinical appearance of a milky whitish wrinkled film in the buccal mucosa (**Fig. 18.82**). It is a normal variant common in people of colour (see Chapter 28) and disappears if the mucosa is stretched when the cheek is pushed in from outside (as demonstrated posteriorly to the left here).

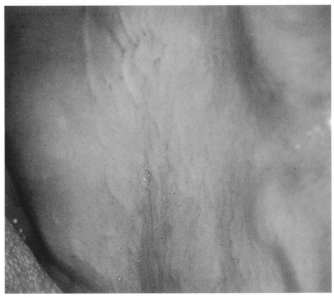

18.82

LINEA ALBA *(occlusal line)*

A horizontal whitish line at the level where the teeth occlude (**Fig. 18.83**) is a common benign lesion, more obvious in patients with parafunctional habits such as jaw clenching or tooth grinding, and in those with temporomandibular joint pain-dysfunction syndrome. There may also be similar lesions on, or crenation of, the lateral margins of the tongue in the same patient (Chapter 11).

LINGUAL ABSCESS

Lingual abscesses are uncommon but may follow a penetrating injury (**Fig. 18.84**), a tracking dental abscess, or infection of a lesion such as a neoplasm, cyst or haematoma.

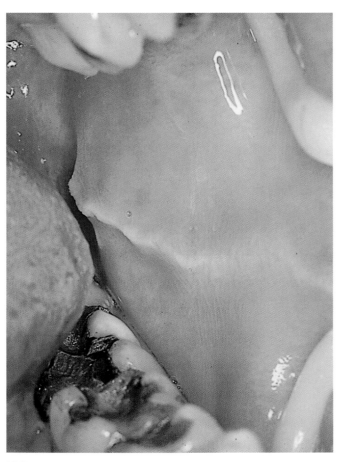

18.83

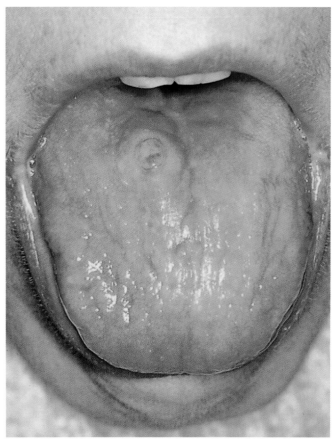

18.84

LINGUAL HAEMATOMA

Trauma to the tongue, especially in a patient with a bleeding tendency (**Fig. 18.85**), may produce a haematoma.

LINGUAL LACERATION

Figure 18.86 shows a laceration of the tongue by the teeth of a child who fell on his chin. **Figure 18.87** shows a laceration that was not sutured and has resulted in the appearance of a false bifid tongue.

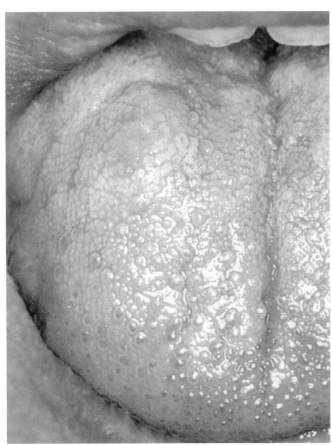

18.85

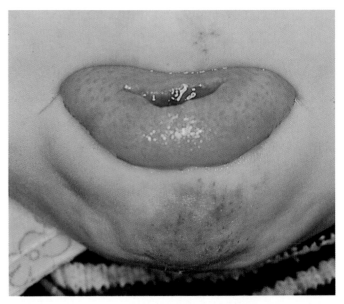

18.86

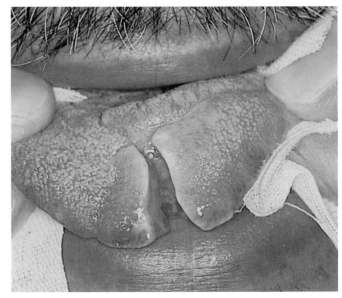

18.87

LINGUAL HEMIHYPERTROPHY

Hypertrophy of the right side of the tongue (**Fig. 18.88**). The whitish lines on the tongue are caused by strands of saliva, as this patient also has xerostomia.

LIP FISSURE

A fissure may develop in the lip where a patient, typically a child, is mouth breathing (**Figs 18.90, 18.91**); lip fissures are common in Down

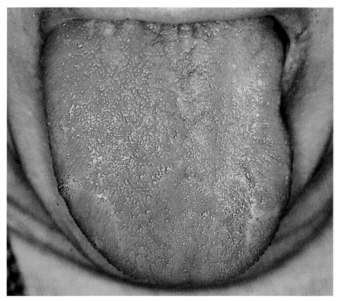

18.88

LIP CHAPPING

Chapping of the lips is mild exfoliation (**Fig. 18.89**) related to extremes of temperature, mouth breathing, lip licking and chewing, or xerostomia. Similar effects may be drug-induced, especially by etretinate and other retinoids.

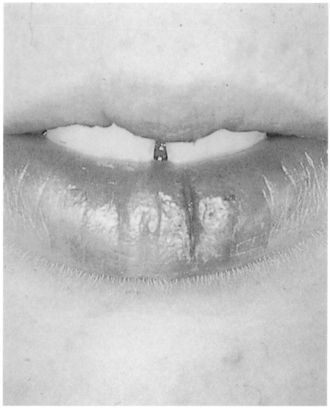

18.90

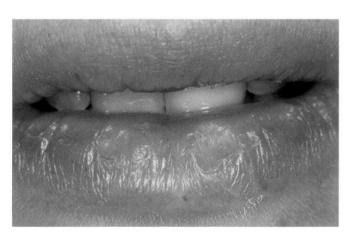

18.89

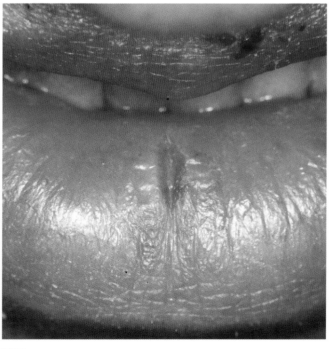

18.91

syndrome (**Fig. 18.92**). In others there may be a hereditary predisposition for weakness in the first branchial arch fusion. The lips may also crack in this way if swollen, for example in oral Crohn's disease.

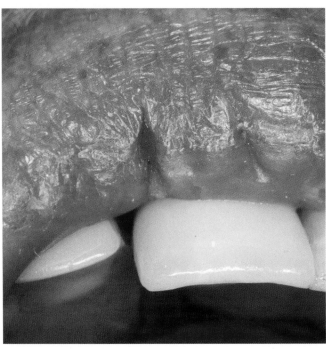

18.92

LIP HORN

Cutaneous horn is a relatively uncommon lesion consisting of keratotic material resembling that of an animal horn. It is more common in Caucasians and in older age groups. The primary underlying lesion may be benign, premalignant or malignant. There have been rare reports associated with oral leukoplakia. Treatment is excisional biopsy with a narrow margin for histopathological evaluation (**Fig. 18.93**).

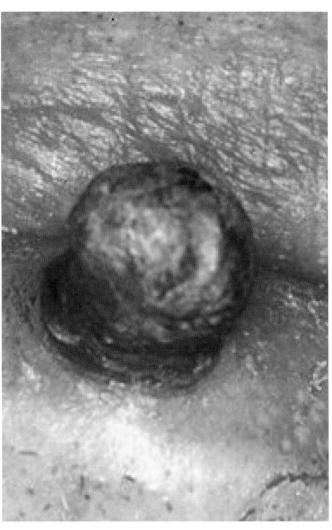

18.93

MELANOTIC MACULES

Oral melanotic macules are brown or black macules (**Figs 18.94, 18.95**). They are seen typically on the lips, especially in females. They are benign and are unrelated to racial pigmentation.

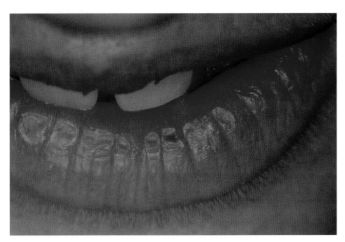

18.94

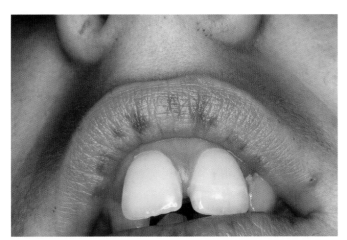

18.95

NAEVI

Oral pigmented naevi include the intramucosal naevus and blue naevus (**Fig. 18.96**). Naevi of Ota, seen mainly in young female Japanese, affect the first or second divisions of the trigeminal nerve with pigmentation of the choroid and iris (oculodermal melanocytosis; see also Chapter 28).

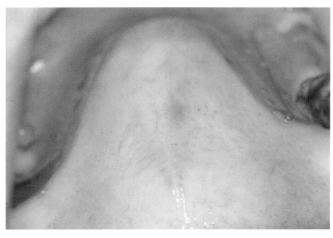

18.96

ORAL SUBMUCOUS FIBROSIS

Oral submucous fibrosis (OSMF) is a chronic disorder affecting the oral and sometimes pharyngeal mucosa, characterized by pain, the development of epithelial atrophy and fibrosis leading to stiffening of the mucosa and restricted mouth opening (**Figs 18.97, 18.98**).

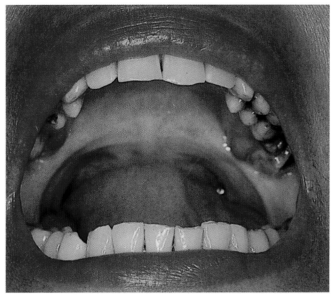

18.97

The mucosa is pale and tight with vertical submucosal fibrous bands; it may develop carcinoma. Seen in persons who use betel (*Areca catechu*) nuts, the lesions of OSMF appear to be due to constituents such as copper, alkaloids, tannin and catechin. OSMF is seen mainly in Asians and there may be a genetic predisposition.

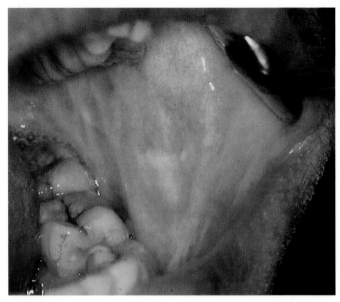

18.98

PAPILLARY HYPERPLASIA

Papillary hyperplasia of the palate is a benign condition of unknown aetiology (**Figs 18.99, 18.100**), but is often more obvious where a denture is worn and where there is denture-induced stomatitis. Papillary hyperplasia can also appear in the absence of dentures and a similar lesion is rarely induced by phenytoin or ciclosporin.

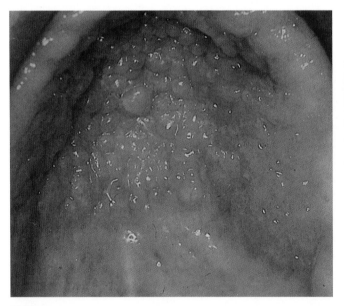

18.99

18.100

PAPILLOMATOSIS

Papillomatous lesions in the vault of the palate may occasionally result from obstructed ducts of minor salivary glands (**Fig. 18.101**).

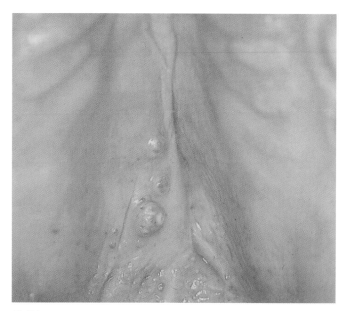

18.101

PIGMENTATION

There is no direct correlation between skin colour and gingival pigmentation. Pigmentation is often clearly visible on the attached gingiva (**Fig. 18.102**).

Pigmentary incontinence may rarely be seen in lichen planus and can persist after the lichen planus has resolved (**Fig. 18.103**; see also **Fig. 23.39**).

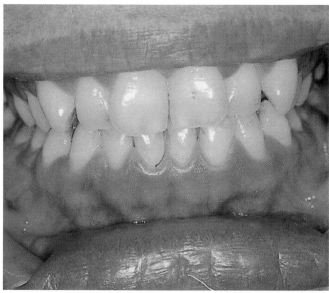

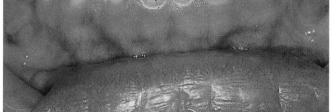

18.102

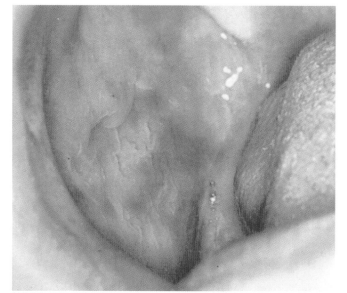

18.103

PYOGENIC GRANULOMA

Pyogenic granuloma is a vascular lesion reaction, induced by trauma or infection, which is a painless, red, proliferative and friable lesion that bleeds readily.

The head and neck region, especially the lip, is a common location. Pyogenic granuloma usually affects the lip, gingiva or tongue, and may grow to 1 cm or more in diameter. Clinically, a pyogenic granuloma may occasionally resemble a capillary haemangioma (**Figs 18.104–18.106**).

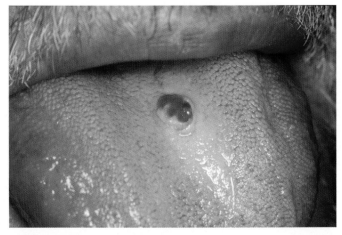

18.105

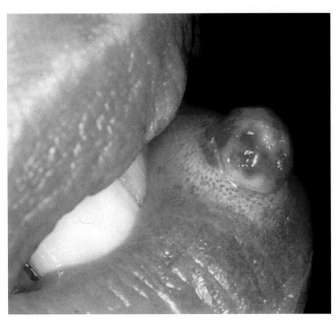

18.104

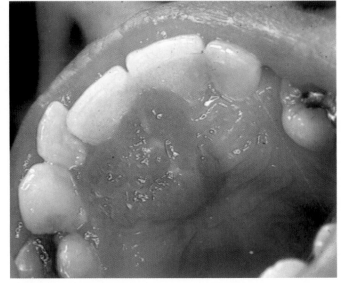

18.106

STOMATITIS NICOTINA (smoker's palate)

Stomatitis nicotina is a fairly common lesion, seen typically in middle-aged or elderly pipe smokers. The palate is diffusely white and the orifices of the minor salivary glands are obvious as red spots (**Figs 18.107–18.109**).

In **Fig. 18.108**, a close-up view shows the typical features and the heavily tobacco-stained teeth. Smoker's keratosis is usually a benign lesion that regresses if smoking is stopped. The obvious red area in **Fig. 18.109** proved, however, to be dysplastic.

If a denture is worn, the mucosa is protected by the denture and appears normal in contrast to the nondenture-bearing area (**Fig. 18.109**).

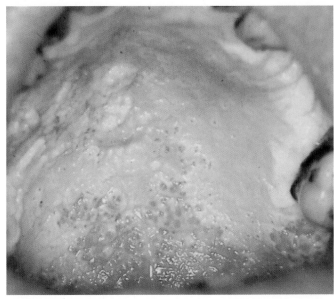

18.107

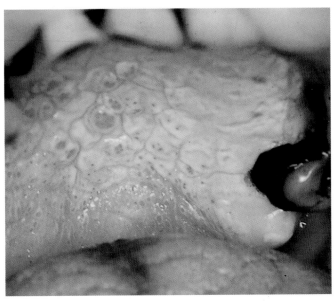

18.108

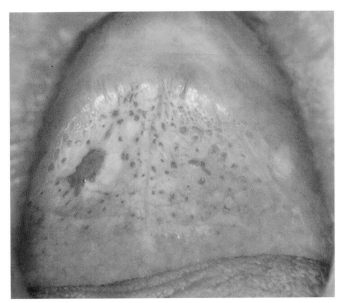

18.109

TATTOOS

A foreign-body tattoo is shown in **Fig. 18.110**: there is pigmentation after foreign material (metal) was left in the lip after an accident. Pigmentation due to amalgam (**Fig. 18.111**) is more common.

Melanosis is seen in smokers (**Fig. 18.112**) and is caused by pigmentary incontinence following chronic irritation, which may mimic amalgam tattoo.

Pigmentation of the soft palate may be seen in conditions with ectopic production of adrenocorticotrophic hormone, for example, bronchogenic carcinoma.

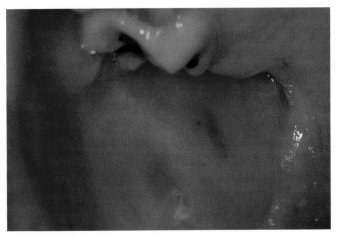

18.111

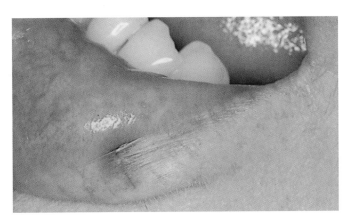

18.110

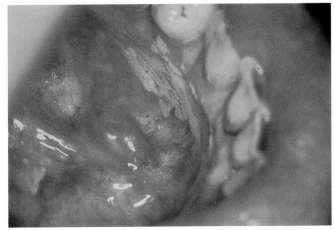

18.112

TRAUMATIC ULCERS

Traumatic ulcers are common, usually caused by accidental biting, hard foods, appliances such as dentures or orthodontic appliances, or following dental treatment (**Figs 18.113–18.118**). **Figure 18.113** shows an unusual self-induced ulcer on the tongue of a child.

Less common causes are shown in the following figures. **Figure 18.114** shows small bruises and ulcers which have followed a blow on the lip in child abuse syndrome (nonaccidental injury). Bruised and swollen lips, lacerated fraenum (see **Fig. 18.115**) and even subluxed teeth or a fractured mandible can be features.

The lingual fraenum can be traumatized by repeated rubbing over the lower incisor teeth (cunnilingus tongue is shown in **Fig. 18.116**). A similar lesion can be seen in children with recurrent bouts of coughing as in whooping cough, termed Riga–Fedes disease.

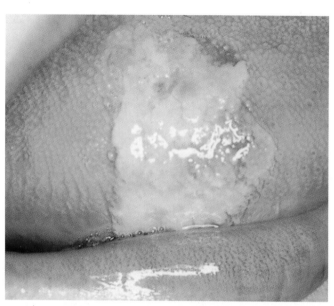

18.113

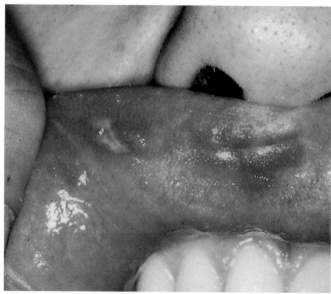

18.114

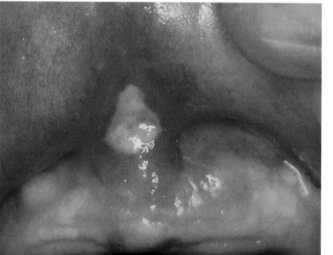

18.115

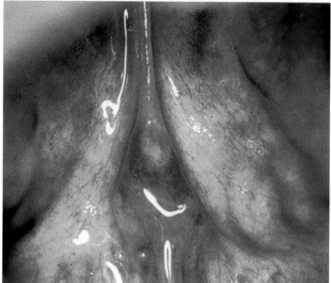

18.116

Traumatic ulceration of the soft palate is fairly uncommon. Trauma from an erect penis together with oral suction can produce ulceration, bruising and petechiae (fellatio palate is shown in **Fig. 18.117**).

Neonates occasionally develop an ulcer at a similar site (Bednar's ulcer), which it is thought may be caused by trauma from the examining finger of the paediatrician. Chronic self-induced traumatic ulcers (see **Fig. 18.118**) may be seen in self-mutilation in a disturbed patient or in learning disability and may present with surrounding keratosis.

VERRUCOUS HYPERPLASIA

Within the histologic spectrum seen in proliferative verrucous hyperplasia, usually as a function of time, are: (1) verrucous hyperplasia (VH), a histologically defined lesion (**Fig. 18.119**); (2) varying degrees of dysplasia; and (3) three forms of squamous cell carcinoma: verrucous, conventional and, according to some, papillary squamous cell carcinoma.

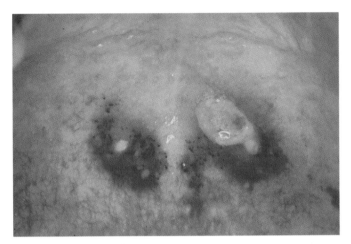

18.117

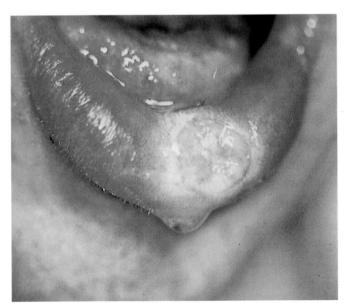

18.118

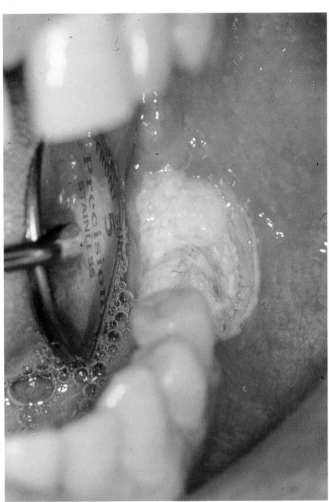

18.119

VERRUCOUS XANTHOMA

Verrucous xanthoma (**Figs 18.120, 18.121**) is a rare, benign lesion with a sessile or pedunculated base presenting as a red or pink, papillary/ granular/verrucous mucosal growth, occurring most commonly at the gingival margin or on other areas of the masticatory oral mucosa. Vacuolated, foam or xanthoma cells of the monocyte/macrophage lineage replace the connective tissue between epithelial ridges.

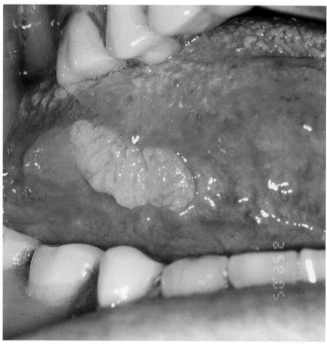

18.120

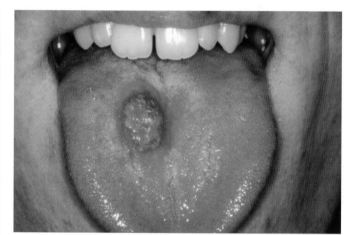

18.121

FURTHER READING

Aoki T, Tanaka T, Akifuji Y, *et al*. Beneficial effects of interferon-alpha in a case with Behcet's disease. Intern Med 2000; 39(8): 667–9.

Barnes CG. Behcet's syndrome — classification criteria. Ann Med Interne (Paris) 1999; 150: 477–82.

Berlucchi M, Meini A, Plebani A, Bonvini MG, Lombardi D, Nicolai P. Update on treatment of Marshall's syndrome (PFAPA syndrome): report of five cases with review of the literature. Ann Otol Rhinol Laryngol 2003; 112: 365–9.

Brown RS, Krakow AM. Median rhomboid glossitis and a 'kissing' lesion of the palate. Oral Surg Oral Med Oral Pathol Oral Radiol Endod 1996; 82: 472–3.

Burton J, Scully C. The lips. In Champion RH, Burton J and Ebling FJG (eds) Textbook of Dermatology, 6th edn, Oxford, Blackwell, 1998.

Chams-Davatchi C, Shizarpour M, Davatchi F, *et al*. Comparison of oral aphthae in Behcet's disease and idiopathic recurrent aphthous stomatitis. Adv Exp Med Biol 2003; 528: 317–20.

Chorzelski TP, Olszewska M, Jarzabek-Chorzelska M, Jablonska S. Is chronic ulcerative stomatitis an entity? Clinical and immunological findings in 18 cases. Euro J Dermat 1998; 8: 261–5.

Dahn KA, Glode MP, Chan KH. Periodic fever and pharyngitis in young children: a new disease for the otolaryngologist? Arch Otolaryngol Head Neck Surg 2000; 126(9): 1146–9.

DiAlberti L, Porter SR, Speight PM, *et al*. Presence of human herpesvirus-8 variants in the oral ulcer tissues of HIV-infected individuals. J Infect Dis 1997; 175: 703–7.

Feder HM Jr. Periodic fever, aphthous stomatitis, pharyngitis, adenitis: a clinical review of a new syndrome. Curr Opin Pediatr 2000; 12(3): 253–6.

Femiano F, Gombos F, Scully C. Recurrent aphthous stomatitis unresponsive to topical corticosteroids: a study of the comparative therapeutic effects of systemic prednisone and systemic sulodexide. Int J Dermatol 2003; 42: 394–7.

Herranz P, Arribas JR, Navarro A, *et al*. Successful treatment of aphthous ulcerations in AIDS patients using topical granulocyte-macrophage colony-stimulating factor. Br J Dermatol 2000; 142(1): 171–6.

Jaber MA, Porter SR, Gilthorpe MS, Bedi R, Scully C. Risk factors for oral epithelial dysplasia — the role of smoking and alcohol. Oral Oncol 1999; 35: 151–6.

Jaber MA, Porter SR, Speight P, Eveson JW, Scully C. Oral epithelial dysplasia: clinical characteristics of western European residents. Oral Oncol 2003; 39: 589–96.

Laskin DM, Giglio JA, Rippert ET. Differential diagnosis of tongue lesions. Quintessence Int 2003; 34(5): 331–42.

Lodi G, Sardella A, Bez C, Demarosi F, Carrassi A. Systematic review of randomized trials for the treatment of oral leukoplakia. J Dent Educ 2002; 66: 896–902.

McBride DR. Management of aphthous ulcers. Am Fam Physician 2000; 62(1): 149–54, 160.

McCarty MA, Garton RA, Jorizzo JL. Complex aphthosis and Behcet's disease. Dermatol Clin 2003; 21: 41–8, vi.

McCullough M, Jaber M, Barrett AW, Bain L, Speight PM, Porter SR. Oral epithelial dysplasia: clinical characteristics of western European residents. Oral Oncol 2003; 39: 589–96.

Petti S. Pooled estimate of world leukoplakia prevalence: a systematic review. Oral Oncol 2003; 39(8): 770–80.

Porter S, Scully C. Aphthous ulcers: recurrent. Clin Evid 2002; 7: 1232–8.

Porter SR, Cawson RA, Scully C, Eveson JW. Multiple hamartoma syndromes presenting with oral lesions. Oral Surg Oral Med Oral Pathol Oral Radiol Endod 1996; 82: 295–301.

Porter SR, Scully C, Pedersen A. Recurrent aphthous stomatitis. Crit Rev Oral Biol Med 1998; 9: 306–21.

Porter SR, Hegarty A, Kaliakatsou F, Hodgson TA, Scully C. Recurrent aphthous stomatitis. Clin Dermatol 2000; 18: 569–78.

Porter SR, Scully C. Aphthous ulcers: recurrent. Clinical Evidence 2000; 5: 606–12, 2001; 6: 1037–41, 2001; 7: 1232–38; Clinical Evidence Concise 2002; 7: 234.

Reibel J. Prognosis of oral pre-malignant lesions: significance of clinical, histopathological, and molecular biological characteristics. Crit Rev Oral Biol Med 2003; 14: 47–62.

Scully C. Prevention of oral mucosal disease. In Murray JJ (ed.), Prevention of Oral and Dental Disease, 3rd edn, Oxford, Oxford University Press, 1995; pp. 160–72.

Scully C. The oral cavity. In Champion RH, Burton J and Ebling FJG (eds) Textbook of Dermatology, 6th edn, Oxford, Blackwell 2004.

Scully C, Gorsky M, Lozada-Nur F. Aphthous ulcerations, In Camisa C (ed.) Diagnosis and Treatment of Oral Lesions. Dermatologic Therapy 2002; 15: 185–205.

Scully C, Gorsky M, Lozada-Nur F. The diagnosis and management of recurrent aphthous stomatitis: a consensus approach. J Am Dent Assoc 2003; 134: 200–7.

Scully C, Sudbo J, Speight PM. Progress in determining the malignant potential of oral lesions. J Oral Pathol Med 2003; 32: 251–6.

Shotts RH, Scully C, Avery CM, Porter SR. Nicorandil-induced severe oral ulceration: a newly recognized drug reaction. Oral Surg Oral Med Oral Pathol Oral Radiol Endod 1999; 87: 706–7.

Shotts R, Scully C. How to identify and deal with tongue problems. Pulse 2002; 62: 73–6.

19 GASTROINTESTINAL DISORDERS

- Crohn's disease
- gastric regurgitation
- gastrointestinal neoplasms
- gluten-sensitive enteropathy (coeliac disease)
- Melkersson–Rosenthal syndrome
- orofacial granulomatosis
- peptic ulceration
- tylosis
- ulcerative colitis.

CROHN'S DISEASE

Crohn's disease is a chronic inflammatory bowel disease of unknown aetiology, affecting mainly the ileum although any part of the gastrointestinal tract can be involved, including, in up to 10% of cases, the mouth. Noncaseating granulomas are also seen in sarcoid and it is possible that oral Crohn's disease is actually a similar but distinct condition since biopsy shows lymphoedema and granulomas. The majority of patients with 'oral Crohn's disease' do not have identifiable gastrointestinal lesions and some seem to have lesions as a consequence of food or food additive 'allergy'. Agents implicated include benzoates and cinnamon aldehyde. Some use the term 'orofacial granulomatosis' when similar manifestations are seen in the absence of intestinal disease. Swelling of the lips, and angular stomatitis, are common (**Fig. 19.1**).

Facial swelling (**Fig. 19.2**) may be seen and gingival swelling may also be a feature (**Fig. 19.3**). Skip lesions may be seen (**Fig. 19.4**). Mucosal

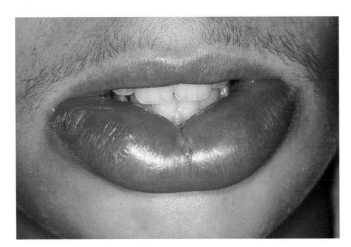

19.1

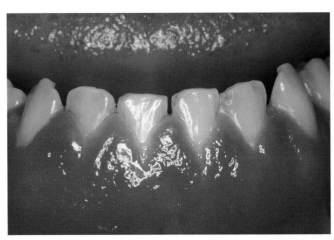

19.3

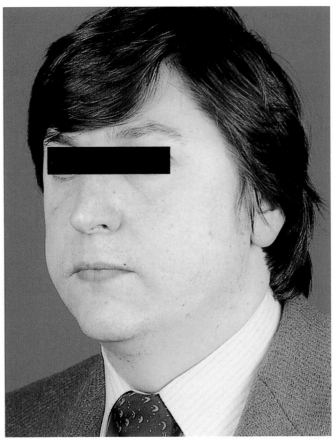

19.2

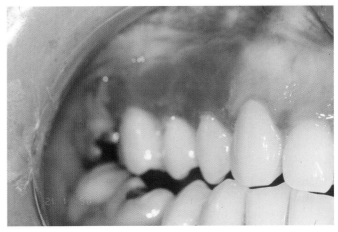

19.4

tags are a feature in some patients (**Fig. 19.5**) and folding of the oral mucosa may lead to a 'cobblestone' appearance (**Figs 19.6, 19.7**).

Persistent irregular ulcers with bordering hyperplastic areas (**Fig. 19.8**) or ulcers that can mimic classic aphthae (**Fig. 19.9**), are common features. Angular stomatitis (**Fig. 19.10**) may be seen. Pyostomatitis vegetans may also be seen but this is usually associated with ulcerative colitis.

Perianal tags are also seen in Crohn's disease (**Fig. 19.11**).

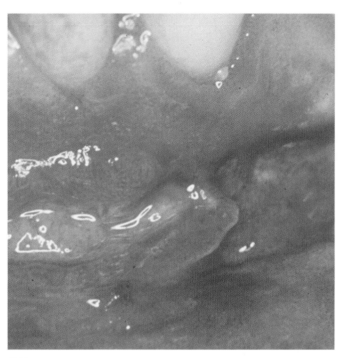

19.5

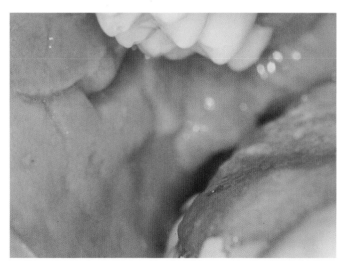

19.6

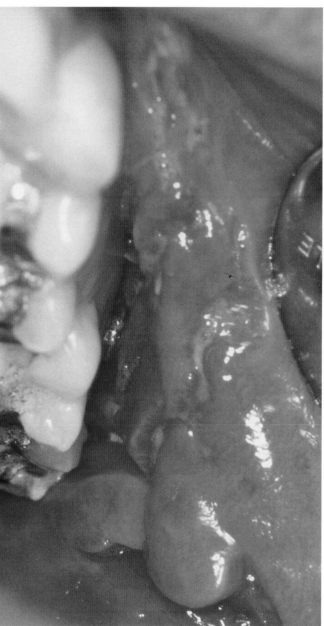

19.7

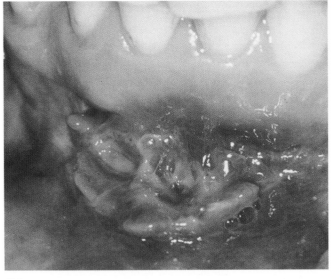

19.8

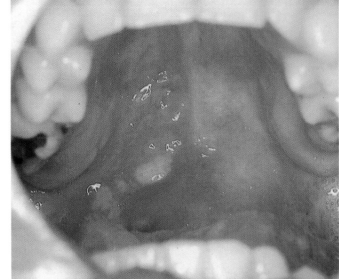

19.9

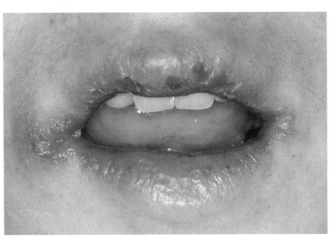

19.10

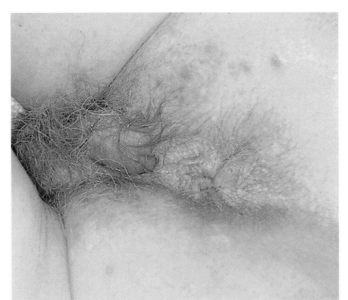

19.11

GASTRIC REGURGITATION

Gastroesophageal reflux is the apparently effortless passage of gastric contents into the oesophagus due to impairment of the antireflux mechanism at the gastroesophageal junction. Reflux is facilitated by the presence of a gradient in pressure between the positive pressure within the abdominal cavity and the negative pressure within the intrathoracic cavity. Effortless reflux of stomach contents is noted in approximately 50% of healthy newborn infants. In the majority of affected children it resolves over the first year of life, especially in the second 6 months when the dietary intake of solids increases and sitting and standing are achieved. In all children, occasional reflux after a meal is a normal event. Regurgitation of gastric contents in adults may be seen in obese patients, hiatus hernia, pregnancy and some asthmatic drugs. Pathological reflux is defined as being secondary to an underlying disorder or when the reflux is complicated by failure to thrive, oesophagitis or respiratory conditions such as asthma or aspiration pneumonia. Dental erosion may result (**Figs 19.12, 19.13 and 15.52**).

GASTROINTESTINAL NEOPLASMS

Metastases from gastrointestinal neoplasms occasionally affect the cervical lymph nodes or oral tissues (see Chapter 6). Acanthosis nigricans is usually a benign lesion affecting localized areas of the skin in persons with obesity and/or high insulin levels but it may be an indicator of underlying malignancy — a paraneoplastic syndrome — and may affect the mouth, mainly as papillomatous lesions seen at any site but, unlike some other similar mucosal disorders, may also involve the gingivae, lips and palate (**Fig. 19.14**). Acanthosis nigricans with florid cutaneous and mucosal papillomatosis is frequently associated with internal malignancy, most often (90%) with an abdominal adenocarcinoma and most commonly with gastric or gallbladder adenocarcinoma (**Fig. 19.15**; this is the same patient as in **Fig. 19.14**, showing cholangiocarcinoma).

Acanthosis nigricans may also affect the conjunctiva, anus, vagina, oesophagus, pharynx or intestines.

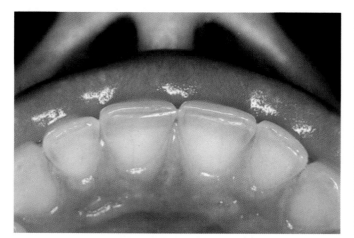

19.12

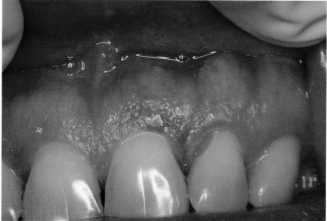

19.14

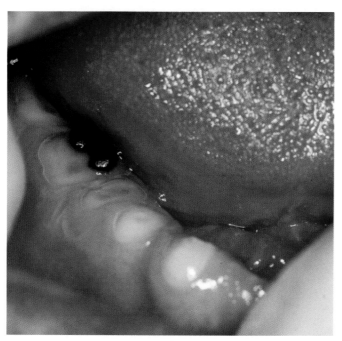

19.13

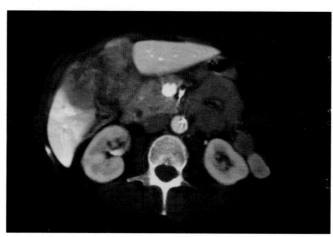

19.15

GLUTEN-SENSITIVE ENTEROPATHY
(coeliac disease)

Coeliac disease is commonly associated with enamel defects, which can also be seen in healthy first-degree relatives; patients may also develop glossitis or angular stomatitis. Up to 3% of patients seen as outpatients with aphthae prove to have coeliac disease (**Fig. 19.16**).

Patients with dermatitis herpetiformis often also suffer from coeliac disease.

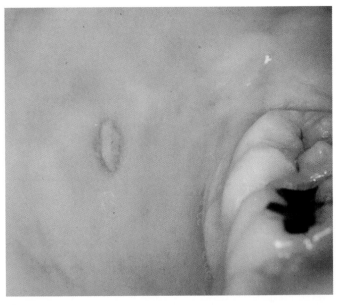

19.16

MELKERSSON–ROSENTHAL SYNDROME

Melkersson–Rosenthal syndrome is the association of orofacial swelling, fissured tongue (30%) and unilateral lower motor neurone facial palsy (**Figs 19.17, 19.18**). It appears to be related to cheilitis granulomatosa, oral Crohn's disease, sarcoidosis and orofacial granulomatosis.

The swelling is nontender and will not pit on pressure. Intraorally, swellings may involve the buccal mucosa and gingiva and there may be ulceration.

Partial forms of the syndrome are not infrequent.

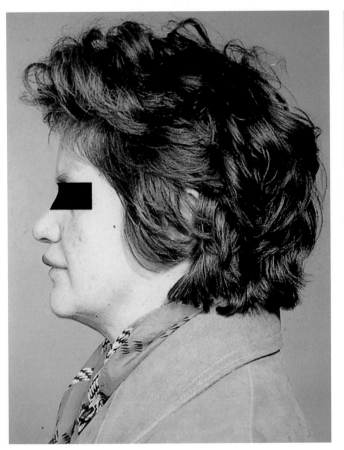

19.17

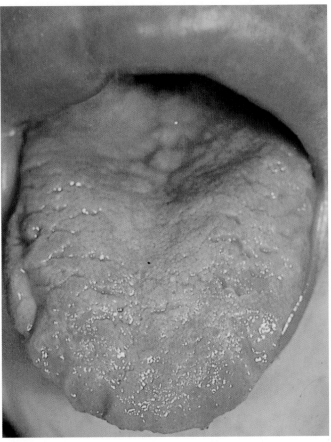

19.18

OROFACIAL GRANULOMATOSIS

The clinical features seen in Crohn's disease may be present in the absence of identifiable intestinal disease (**Figs 19.19–19.21**). Termed orofacial granulomatosis (OFG), this is uncommon but increasing and seen mainly in adolescents and young adults. The aetiology is unknown. A minority eventually prove indeed to have gastrointestinal Crohn's or sarcoidosis but in others there is a postulated reaction to food or food additives or possibly to other antigens such as paratuberculosis. OFG can manifest with facial and/or labial swelling, angular stomatitis and/or cracked lips, ulcers, mucosal tags, cobblestoning or gingival swelling. Miescher's cheilitis is where lip swelling is seen in isolation.

The patient in **Fig. 19.19**, for example, had a somewhat swollen lower lip with a cobblestoned mucosa, and proved to be reacting to cinnamon.

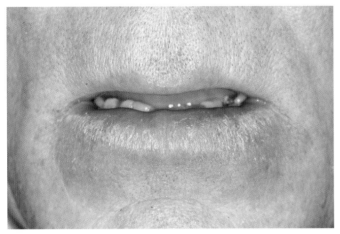

19.19

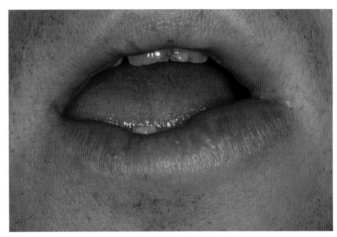

19.20

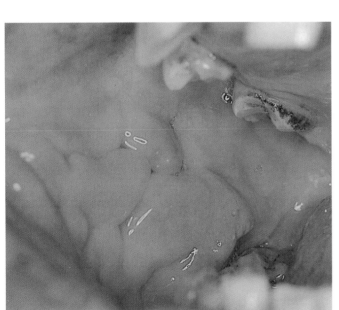

19.21

PEPTIC ULCERATION

Peptic ulceration *per se* has no known oral manifestations but drugs such as omeprazole may produce dry mouth, and lansoprazole may produce dry mouth and/or tongue discoloration.

TYLOSIS

Tylosis, a diffuse keratosis occurring especially on the palms and soles and inherited as an autosomal dominant trait, may occasionally be associated with oral leukoplakias but is more classically associated with oesophageal carcinoma (**Fig. 19.22**).

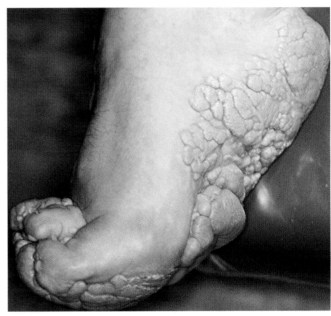

19.22

ULCERATIVE COLITIS

Oral lesions in ulcerative colitis include ulcers and pustules (pyostomatitis vegetans) which may also be found in Crohn's disease or overlap syndromes.

Ulceration may be widespread with multiple small pustules (**Figs 19.23, 19.24**) and produce an unusual type of desquamative gingivitis (**Fig. 19.25**), or occasionally it presents with discrete areas (**Fig. 19.26**). Such an aphthous type of ulcer may be a manifestation of pyostomatitis gangrenosum. Irregular ulceration may clinically resemble a 'snailtrack' ulcer, resulting from fusion of the ulcerated pustules (**Fig. 19.28**). There may be associated pyoderma gangrenosum (**Fig. 19.29**).

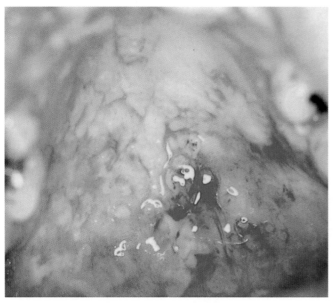

19.23

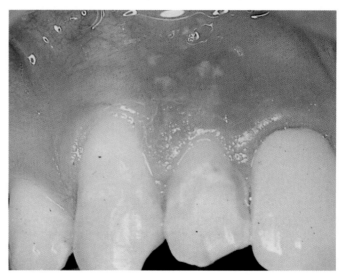

19.24

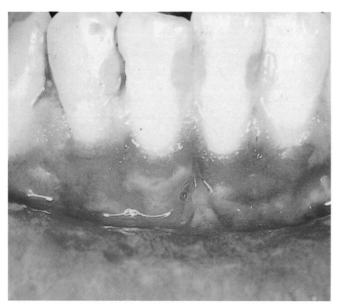

19.25

19.26

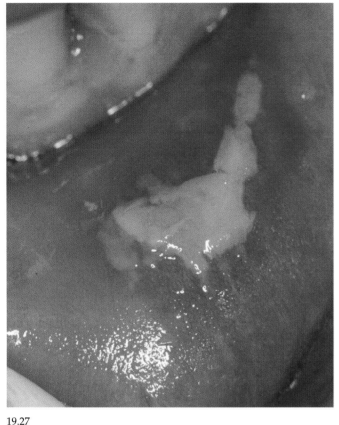

19.27

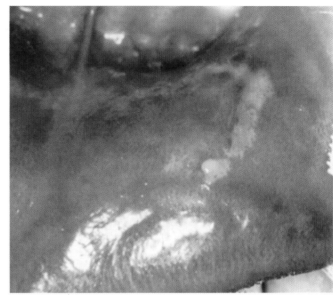

19.28

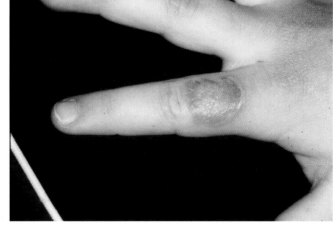

19.29

FURTHER READING

Eveson JW. Granulomatous disorders of the oral mucosa. Semin Diagn Pathol 1996; 13(2): 118–27.

Greenfield S, Apolone G, McNeil BJ, Cleary PD. The importance of co-existent disease in the occurrence of postoperative complications and one-year recovery in patients undergoing total hip replacement. Comorbidity and outcomes after hip replacement. Med Care 1993; 31: 141–54.

Hardo PG, Tugnait A, Hassan F, et al. Helicobacter pylori infection and dental care. Gut 1995; 37(1): 44–6.

Hegarty A, Hodgson T, Porter S. Thalidomide for the treatment of recalcitrant oral Crohn's disease and orofacial granulomatosis. Oral Surg Oral Med Oral Pathol Oral Radiol Endod 2003; 95: 576–85.

Hegarty AM, Barrett AW, Scully C. *Pyostomatitis vegetans*. Clinical and Experimental Dermatology 2004; 28: 1–7.

Hugot J-P, Laurent P, Gower Rousseau C, et al. Mapping of a susceptibility locus for Crohn's disease on chromosome 16. Nature 1996; 379: 821–3.

Kalmar JR. Crohn's disease: orofacial considerations and disease pathogenesis. Periodontol 2000 1994; 6: 101–15.

Katz J, Shenkman A, Stavropoulos F, Melzer E. Oral signs and symptoms in relation to disease activity and site of involvement in patients with inflammatory bowel disease. Oral Dis 2003; 9(1): 34–40.

Marsh MN. The natural history of gluten sensitivity: defining, refining and redefining. Q J Med 1995; 85: 9–11.

Mignogna MD, Fedele S, Lo Russo L, Lo Muzio L. The multiform and variable patterns of onset of orofacial granulomatosis. J Oral Pathol Med 2003; 32: 200–5.

Mizuno Y, Nishida J, Ebihara Y. Dental diseases and gastroenterology. Bull Tokyo Dent Coll 1997; 38(4): 261–7.

Pavli P, Cavanaugh J, Grimm M. Inflammatory bowel disease: germs or genes? Lancet 1996; 347: 1198.

Rees TD. Orofacial granulomatosis and related conditions. Periodontol 2000 1999; 21: 145–57.

Romero-Gomez M, Larraona JL. Pancreatic abscess due to *Streptococcus*.

Scheper HJ, Brand HS. Oral aspects of Crohn's disease. Int Dent J 2002; 52(3): 163–72.

Scully C. Gastroenterological diseases and the mouth. Practitioner 2001; 245; 215–22.

Silva MAGS, Damante JH, Stipp ACM, Tolentino MM, Carlotto PR, Fleury RN. Gastroesophageal reflux disease; new oral findings. Oral Surg Oral Med Oral Pathol Oral Radiol Endod 2001; 91: 301–10.

Soll AH. Medical treatment of peptic ulcer disease. J Am Med Assoc 1996; 275: 622–9.

Stratakis CA, Carney JA, Lin J-P, *et al.* Carney complex, a familial multiple neoplasia and lentiginosis syndrome. J Clin Invest 1996; 97: 699–705.

Targan SR, Murphy LK. Clarifying the causes of Crohn's. Nature Med 1995; 1: 1241–3.

van der Waal RI, Schulten EA, van der Meij EH, van de Scheur MR, Starink TM, van der Waal I. Cheilitis granulomatosa: overview of 13 patients with long-term follow-up — results of management. Int J Dermatol 2002; 41: 225–9.

von Wowern SN, Klausen B, Moller EH [Bone loss and oral health status in patients on home parenteral nutrition]. Ugeskr Laeger 1997; 159(33): 4982–5.

Walmsley RS, Ibbotson JP, Chahal H, *et al.* Antibodies against *Mycobacterium paratuberculosis* in Crohn's disease. Q J Med 1996; 89: 217–21.

20 DISEASES OF THE LIVER

- alcoholic cirrhosis
- biliary atresia
- chronic active hepatitis
- liver transplantation
- primary biliary cirrhosis
- viral hepatitis.

ALCOHOLISM AND CIRRHOSIS

Sialosis (**Fig. 20.1**), and tooth erosion from gastric acid regurgitation are fairly common oral features of alcoholism, and alcohol use predisposes to oral carcinoma and potentially malignant lesions such as leukoplakia. Jaundice (**Fig. 20.2**) and hyperpigmentation may be seen. Liver failure may cause hepatic fetor with pronounced halitosis.

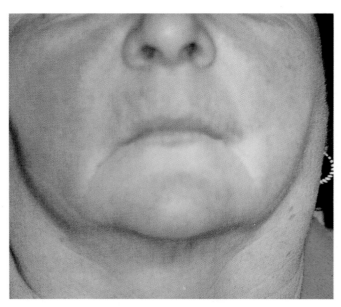

20.1

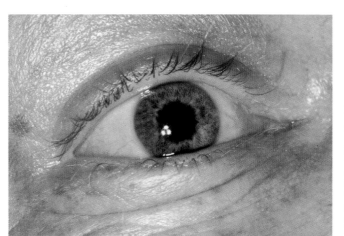

20.2

BILIARY ATRESIA

Oral manifestations in patients with biliary atresia may include enamel hypoplasia, delayed tooth eruption and green teeth (**Fig. 20.3**; see also **Fig. 15.138**) or gingival discoloration.

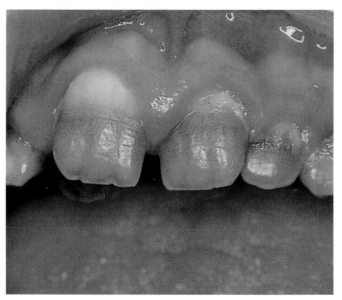

20.3

CHRONIC ACTIVE HEPATITIS

Chronic active hepatitis can manifest with lichen planus (**Fig. 20.4**). In some patients, particularly those of southern European or Japanese extraction, there often appears to be an association between oral lichen planus and infection with hepatitis C virus (HCV) or hepatitis B virus.

A sicca-like syndrome may also be associated with HCV infection.

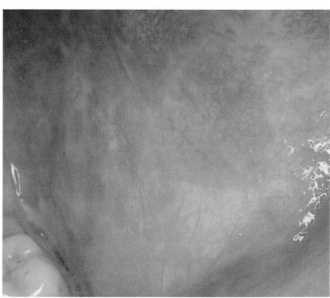

20.4

LIVER TRANSPLANTATION

Immunosuppressant agents used in liver transplant patients may be associated with oral adverse effects such as viral infections with herpes simplex (**Fig. 20.5**) or hairy leukoplakia, or with mycoses such as candidosis or aspergillosis or mucormycosis or occasionally with neoplasms (**Fig. 20.6**). Drug use may induce gingival swelling.

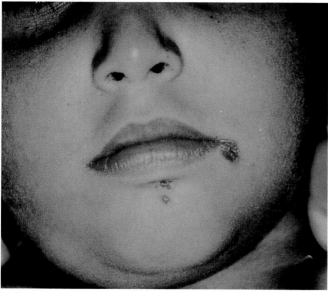

20.5

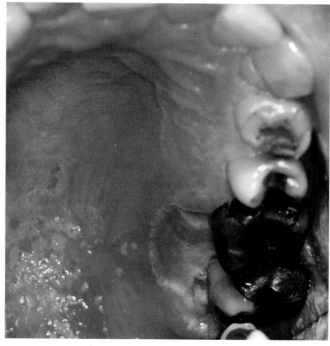

20.6

PRIMARY BILIARY CIRRHOSIS

Primary biliary cirrhosis (PBC) — an autoimmune, chronic, destructive, nonsuppurative cholangitis characterized by progressive inflammatory destruction of intrahepatic bile ducts — may present with icterus and telangiectasia (**Fig. 20.7**). Telangiectasia may be seen on the skin (**Fig. 20.8**), lips (**Fig. 20.9**) and intraorally (**Fig. 20.10**); over 90% of patients are female. PBC may be associated with a sicca syndrome of

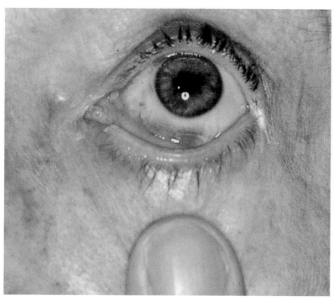

20.7

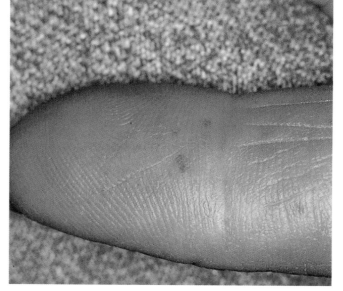

20.8

dry mouth (**Fig. 20.11**) and dry eyes, and a variety of other autoimmune disorders such as scleroderma, CRST syndrome (calcinosis cutis, Raynaud's phenomenon, sclerodactyly and telangiectasia), CREST syndrome (CRST syndrome plus oesophageal dysmotility) or rheumatoid arthritis. Over 90% of PBC patients have serum antimitochondrial antibodies, and some also express antibodies directed against ribosomal, smooth-muscle, nuclear, double-stranded deoxyribonucleic acid and thyroid components.

Other oral conditions that may be associated with PBC include lichenoid lesions, gingival xanthomatosis, green staining of teeth and mucosa and enamel hypoplasia.

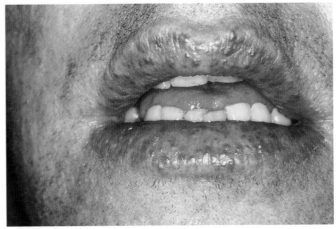

20.9

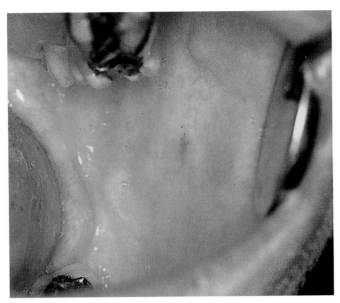

20.10

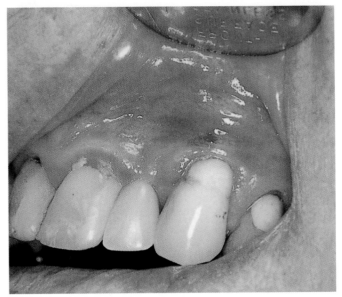

20.11

VIRAL HEPATITIS

Salivary enlargement and xerostomia may arise in HCV disease. Associations between HCV infection and lichen planus have been described although this is localized to southern Europe and Japan. Interferon-α therapy may give rise to oral lichen planus; lichen planus in response to hepatitis B vaccination has also been reported.

FURTHER READING

Bagan JV, Alapont L, del Olmo JA, Rodrigo JM, Lloria E, Jimenez Y. Dental findings in patients with liver cirrhosis. A study of 100 cases. Bull Group Int Rech Sci Stomatol Odontol 1996; 39: 77–9.

Bagg J. Viral hepatitis. In Porter SR and Scully C (eds) Oral Health Care for Those with HIV Infection and Other Special Needs. Northwood, Science Reviews, 1995, pp. 75–80.

Carrozzo M, Gandolfo S. Oral diseases possibly associated with hepatitis C virus. Crit Rev Oral Biol Med 2003; 14: 115–27.

Demas PN, McClain JR. Hepatitis: implications for dental care. Oral Surg Oral Med Oral Pathol Oral Radiol Endod 1999; 88: 2–4.

Di Bisceglie AM. Hepatitis G virus infection: a work in progress. Ann Intern Med 1996; 125: 772–3.

Douglas LR, Douglass JB, Sieck JO, Smith PJ. Oral management of the patient with end-stage liver disease and the liver transplant patient. Oral Surg Oral Med Oral Pathol Oral Radiol Endod 1998; 86: 55–64.

Glick M. Medical considerations for dental care of patients with alcohol-related liver disease. J Am Dent Assoc 1997; 128: 61–70.

Henderson L, Muir M, Mills PR, et al. Oral health of patients with hepatitis C virus infection: a pilot study. Oral Dis 2001; 7(5): 271–5.

Hosey MT, Gordon G, Kelly DA, et al. Oral findings in children with liver transplants. Int J Paediatr Dent 1996; 5: 29–34.

Lodi G, Porter SR, Scully C. Hepatitis C virus infection: review and implications for the dentist. Oral Surg Oral Med Oral Pathol Oral Radiol Endod 1998; 86: 8–22.

Lodi G, Carrassi A, Scully C, Porter SR. Hepatitis G virus: relevance to oral health care. Oral Surg Oral Med Oral Pathol Oral Radiol Endod 1999; 88: 568–72.

Lodi G, Bez C, Porter SR, Scully C, Epstein JB. Infectious hepatitis C, hepatitis G, and TT virus: review and implications for dentists. Special Care Dentistry 2002; 22: 53–8.

Novacek G, Plachetzky U, Potzi R, Lentner S, Slavicek R, Gangl A, Ferenci P. Dental and periodontal disease in patients with cirrhosis — role of etiology of liver disease. J Hepatol 1995; 22: 576–82.

Nunn J. Hepatic disease. In Porter SR and Scully C (eds) Oral Health Care for Those with HIV Infection and Other Special Needs. Northwood, Science Reviews, 1995, pp. 153–5.

Porter SR, Scully C. Innovations and Developments in Non-Invasive Oral Health Care. Northwood, Science Reviews, 1996.

Roy KM, Bagg J, McCarron B, Good T, Cameron S, Pithie A. Predominance of HCV type 2a in saliva from intravenous drug users. J Med Virol 1998; 54: 271–5.

Scully C. The dental profession. In Collins CH and Kennedy DA (eds) Occupational Blood Borne Infections. CAB International, 1997, pp. 133–58.

Zaia AA, Graner E, Almeida OPD, Scully C. Oral changes associated with biliary atresia and liver transplantation. J Clin Paed Dent 1993; 18: 39–42.

21 DISEASES OF THE GENITO-URINARY SYSTEM

- chronic renal failure
- hypophosphataemia (vitamin D-resistant rickets; renal rickets)
- renal transplantation.

394

CHRONIC RENAL FAILURE

In chronic renal failure, complaints of an unpleasant taste, halitosis and dry mouth are common. There may be obvious signs of pallor from the associated chronic anaemia (**Fig. 21.1**), or petechiae and spontaneous bleeding from the associated platelet dysfunction.

Oral lesions may include ulcers and mixed bacterial plaques (**Fig. 21.2**), candidosis and other white lesions. Patients with uraemia may present with uraemic stomatitis, with white lesions of the tongue (**Fig. 21.3**) and sometimes hairy leukoplakia or mucosal hyperpigmentation. After renal dialysis or transplantation, the lesions may resolve (**Fig. 21.4**).

Skeletal changes, which seem especially to affect the jaws, include localized radiolucencies and changes in trabecular pattern in patients on chronic haemodialysis. The dental pulp chambers tend to narrow.

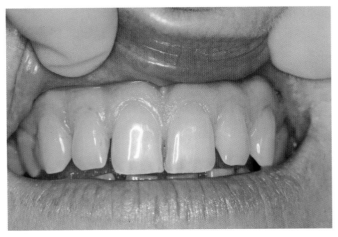

21.1

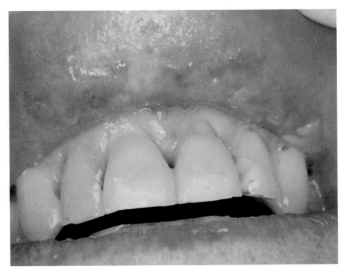

21.2

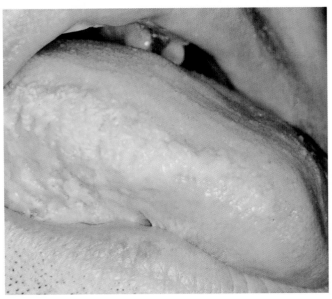

21.3

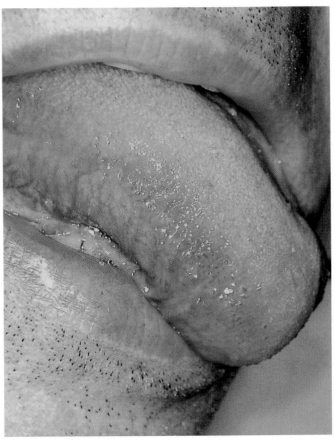

21.4

HYPOPHOSPHATAEMIA
(vitamin D-resistant rickets; renal rickets)

Hypophosphataemia is a sex-linked disorder characterized by a renal tubular defect of phosphate resorption due to end-organ resistance to vitamin D. Teeth may be hypoplastic (**Fig. 21.5**; incidentally, the upper lateral incisor is absent). The condition may be genetically linked: **Fig. 21.6** is the brother of the patient in **Fig. 21.5**.

Tooth eruption may be retarded, and the teeth have large pulp chambers (**Fig. 21.7**) and abnormal calcification of the dentine. Therefore, even minimal caries or attrition can produce pulpitis, hence periapical abscesses are common (**Fig. 21.8**). Radiography shows the generalized nature of the problem (**Fig. 21.9**).

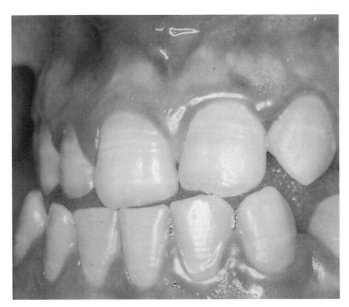

21.5

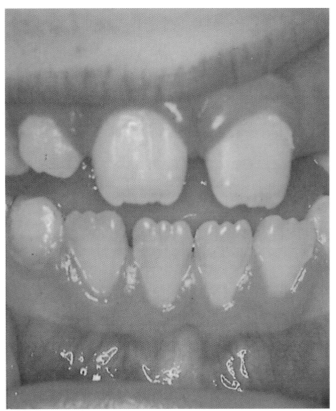

21.6

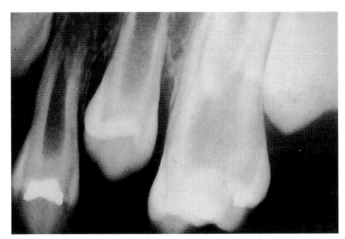

21.7

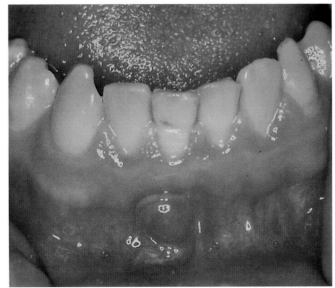

21.8

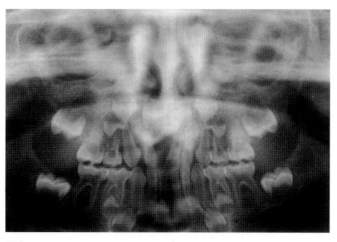

21.9

RENAL TRANSPLANTATION

Renal transplant patients, being chronically immunosuppressed can develop oral candidosis (**Fig. 21.10**), hairy leukoplakia, Kaposi's sarcoma and carcinoma of the lip, while gingival swelling may be related to use of ciclosporin or a calcium channel blocker such as nifedipine (**Fig 21.11**). Many patients are controlled with both ciclosporin and nifedipine.

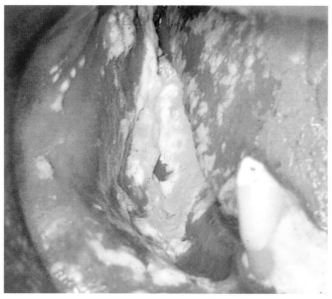

21.10

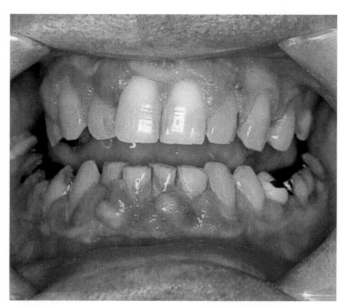

21.11

FURTHER READING

De Rossi SS, Glick M. Dental considerations for the patient with renal disease receiving hemodialysis. J Am Dent Assoc 1996; 127: 211–19.

Ferguson CA, Whyman RA. Dental management of people with renal disease and renal transplants. NZ Dent J 1998; 94: 125–30.

Gavalda C, Bagan JV, Scully C, Silvestre FJ, Milian MA, Jimenez Y. Renal hemodialysis patients: oral, salivary, dental and periodontal findings in 105 adult cases. Oral Diseases 1999; 5: 299–302.

Kantarci A, Cebeci I, Tuncer O, Carin M, Firatli E. Clinical effects of periodontal therapy on the severity of cyclosporin A-induced gingival hyperplasia. J Periodontol 1999; 70: 587–93.

Kerr AR. Update on renal disease for the dental practitioner. Oral Surg Oral Med Oral Pathol Oral Radiol Endod 2001; 92: 9–16.

Kho HS, Lee SW, Chung SC, Kim YK. Oral manifestations and salivary flow rate, pH, and buffer capacity in patients with end-stage renal disease undergoing hemodialysis. Oral Surg Oral Med Oral Pathol Oral Radiol Endod 1999; 88: 316–19.

King GN, Healy CM, Glover MT, *et al.* Increased prevalence of dysplastic and malignant lip lesions in renal transplant recipients. N Engl J Med 1995; 332: 1052–7.

London NJ, Farmery SM, Will EJ, *et al.* Risk of neoplasia in renal transplant patients. Lancet 1995; 346: 403–6.

Naugle K, Darby ML, Bauman DB, Lineberger LT, Powers R. The oral health status of individuals on renal dialysis. Ann Periodontol 1998; 3: 197–205.

Naylor GD, Fredericks MR. Pharmacologic considerations in the dental management of the patient with disorders of the renal system. Dent Clin North Am 1996; 40: 665–83.

Nunn J. Renal disease. In Porter SR and Scully C (eds) Oral Health Care for Those with HIV Infection and Other Special Needs. Northwood, Science Reviews, 1995, pp. 143–52.

Somacarrera ML, Lucas M, Cuervas-Mons V, Hernandez G. Oral care planning and handling of immunosuppressed heart, liver, and kidney transplant patients. Spec Care Dentist 1996; 16(6): 242–6.

Somacarrera ML, Lucas M, Scully, C, Barrios C. Effectiveness of periodontal treatments on cyclosporine-induced gingival overgrowth in transplant patients. Br Dent J 1997; 183: 89–94.

Spratt H, Boomer S, Irwin CR, Marley JJ, James JA, Maxwell P, Middleton D, Linden GJ. Cyclosporin associated gingival overgrowth in renal transplant recipients. Oral Dis 1999; 5(1): 27–31.

Zambrano M, Nikitakis NG, Sanchez-Quevedo MC, Sauk JJ, Sedano H, Rivera H. Oral and dental manifestations of vitamin D-dependent rickets type I: report of a pediatric case. Oral Surg Oral Med Oral Pathol Oral Radiol Endod 2003; 95(6): 705–9.

22 COMPLICATIONS OF PREGNANCY, CHILDBIRTH, PUERPERIUM AND THE MENOPAUSE

- chloasma
- gingivitis during menstruation
- menopause

- pregnancy epulis (pregnancy granuloma)
- pregnancy gingivitis.

CHLOASMA

Chloasma is facial pigmentation seen in pregnancy (**Fig. 22.1**) and related to the endocrine changes experienced. The hyperpigmented patches seen over the cheeks, temples or forehead tend to resolve after parturition.

Similar changes may be seen after use of petroleum jelly or some photosensitizing facial creams (chloasma cosmeticum).

Facial telangiectasia may appear in pregnancy or in those on synthetic oestrogens.

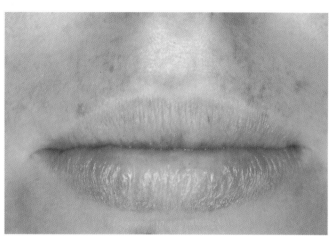

22.1

GINGIVITIS DURING MENSTRUATION

Where there is gingivitis, for example where plaque accumulates on crowded teeth (**Fig. 22.2**), there may be an exacerbation premenstrually or on use of the contraceptive pill.

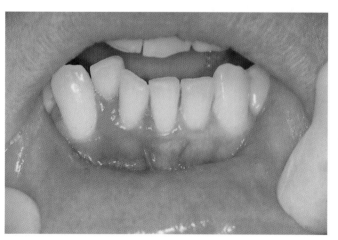

22.2

MENOPAUSE

Dryness of the mouth, desquamative gingivitis, atypical facial pain and oral dysaesthesias are particularly common at this time but there is little evidence of a relation to steroid sex hormones.

Oestrogen replacement therapy may be beneficial in preventing tooth loss but it affects oral bone in a manner similar to the way it affects other sites. HRT appears to lessen gingival bleeding and tooth loss in older women as well as alveolar bone resorption.

PREGNANCY EPULIS
(pregnancy granuloma)

Pyogenic granulomas are common in pregnancy, are typically on the gingivae and are then termed pregnancy epulides (**Figs 22.3–22.5**); they are benign but may bleed. Pregnancy epulides, if excised during pregnancy, tend to recur whereas they tend to resolve spontaneously after parturition.

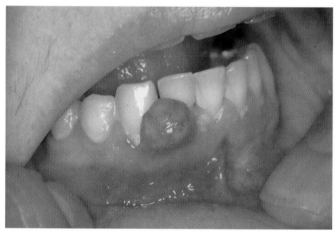

22.3

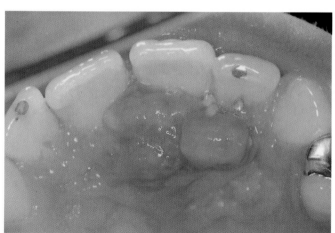

22.4

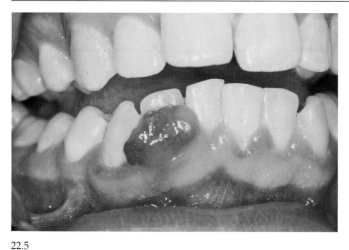

22.5

PREGNANCY GINGIVITIS

Gingivitis is most prevalent in pregnancy if oral hygiene is poor. A highly vascular marginal gingivitis (**Fig. 22.6**) appears at the second month of pregnancy, reaches a maximum intensity by the eighth month, and then regresses.

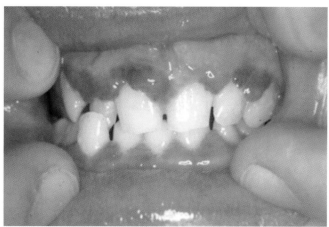

22.6

FURTHER READING

Birkenfeld L, Yemini M, Kase NG, Birkenfeld A. Menopause-related oral alveolar bone resorption: a review of relatively unexplored consequences of estrogen deficiency. Menopause 1999; 6(2): 129–33.

Dasanayake AP. Poor periodontal health of the pregnant woman as a risk factor for low birth weight. Ann Periodontol 1998; 3(1): 206–12.

Frutos R, Rodriguez S, Miralles-Jorda L, Machuca G. Oral manifestations and dental treatment in menopause. Med Oral 2002; 7(1): 26–30, 31–5.

Guthmiller JM, Hassebroek-Johnson JR, Weenig DR, Johnson GK, Kirchner HL, Kohout FJ, Hunter SK. Periodontal disease in pregnancy complicated by type 1 diabetes mellitus. J Periodontol 2001; 72(11): 1485–90.

Harris MN, Desai R, Chuang TY, Hood AF, Mirowski GW. Lobular capillary hemangiomas: An epidemiologic report, with emphasis on cutaneous lesions. J Am Acad Dermatol 2000; 42(6): 1012–16.

Kinane DF. Aetiology and pathogenesis of periodontal disease. Ann R Australas Coll Dent Surg 2000; 15: 42–50.

Laine M, Leimola-Virtanen R. Effect of hormone replacement therapy on salivary flow rate, buffer effect and pH in perimenopausal and post-menopausal women. Arch Oral Biol 1996; 41: 91–6.

Laine MA. Effect of pregnancy on periodontal and dental health. Acta Odontol Scand 2002; 60(5): 257–64.

Paganini-Hill A. The benefits of estrogen replacement therapy on oral health. The Leisure World cohort. Arch Intern Med 1995; 155(21): 2325–9.

Pilgram TK, Hildebolt CF, Yokoyama-Crothers N, et al. Relationships between longitudinal changes in radiographic alveolar bone height and probing depth measurements: data from postmenopausal women. J Periodontol 1999; 70(8): 829–33.

Shaw GM, Lammer EJ, Wasserman CR, O'Malley CD, Tolarova MM. Risks of orofacial clefts in children born to women using multivitamins containing folic acid periconceptually. Lancet 1995; 346: 393–6.

Weyant RJ, Pearlstein ME, Churak AP, Forrest K, Famili P, Cauley JA. The association between osteopenia and periodontal attachment loss in older women. J Periodontol 1999; 70(9): 982–91.

Yalcin F, Eskinazi E, Soydinc M, et al. The effect of sociocultural status on periodontal conditions in pregnancy. J Periodontol 2002; 73(2): 178–82.

23 DISEASES OF THE SKIN AND SUBCUTANEOUS TISSUES

- acanthosis nigricans
- acute lymphadenitis
- carbuncle
- dermatitis herpetiformis (Duhring's disease)
- discoid lupus erythematosus
- epidermolysis bullosa acquisita
- erythema multiforme
- impetigo
- lichen planus
- lichen sclerosus
- linear IgA disease
- localized oral purpura (angina bullosa haemorrhagica)
- necrotizing fasciitis
- pemphigoid
- pemphigus
- pigmented purpuric stomatitis
- psoriasis
- Stevens–Johnson syndrome (erythema multiforme exudativum)
- toxic epidermal necrolysis
- vitiligo.

ACANTHOSIS NIGRICANS

Acanthosis nigricans is a rare disorder characterized by hyperkeratosis and pigmentation. One type is congenital (autosomal dominant) and benign. A 'malignant' type of acanthosis nigricans precedes, accompanies or follows the detection of an internal malignancy, especially gastric adenocarcinoma (Chapter 19). Acanthosis nigricans can also be drug induced (diethylstilboestrol; nicotinic acid), associated with insulin resistance and other endocrinopathies, or with various other rare syndromes such as Prader–Willi, Crouzon's or Bloom's syndromes.

Acanthosis nigricans is characterized by grey-brown pigmentation, hyperkeratosis and subsequent exaggeration of skinfold markings of the axillae, neck (**Fig. 23.1**), anogenital areas, groin, flexures and submammary sites. In addition, there may be symmetrical velvety papulomatous plaques of the same sites.

Mucosal involvement is variable but in up to 40% of acanthosis nigricans patients there can be oral manifestations such as velvet-like oedematous mucosae, papillomatous proliferation of the lips (**Fig. 23.2**) and tongue and occasionally diffuse hyperpigmentation. The lips and tongue are most frequently involved. Thickening of the mucosa with a papilliferous surface (**Figs 23.3, 23.4**) characterizes acanthosis nigricans.

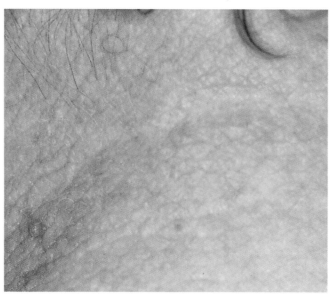

23.1

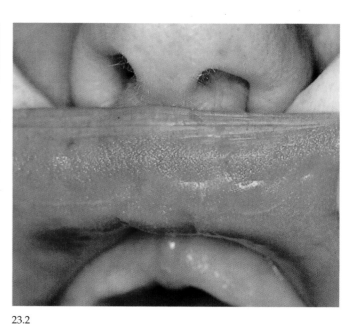

23.2

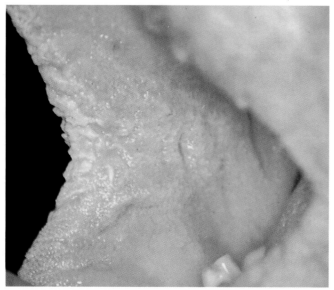

23.3

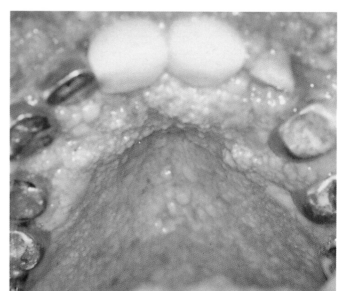

23.4

ACUTE LYMPHADENITIS

Lymphadenitis is infection of a lymph node, usually a consequence of the spread of infection from a focus in the drainage area. Cervical lymphadenitis is therefore common in persons with dental abscess, pericoronitis or other oral bacterial infection. It is also seen in viral stomatitides and may be seen in many systemic infections such as HIV, infectious mononucleosis, etc.

Occasionally a facial lymph node (**Fig. 23.5**), submandibular or other node is infected but the source remains unidentified. Such idiopathic submandibular abscesses are usually seen in preschool children who are apparently healthy. *Staphylococcus aureus* is usually implicated and it is presumed that a small lesion in the nose, mouth or scalp is the focus. Parotid (**Fig. 23.6**) or facial (**Fig. 23.7**) lymph nodes may occasionally become infected, typically from a cutaneous lesion, which may be hidden in the scalp.

Cervical lymph nodes may also be enlarged in the absence of an identifiable local infective lesion in malignant disease, connective tissue diseases, sarcoidosis, mycobacterioses, in other infections, and for other reasons (Chapter 1).

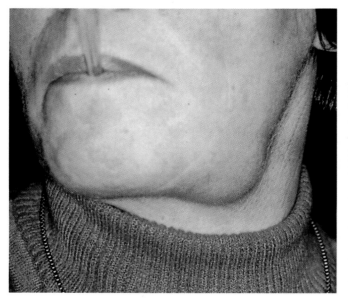

23.5

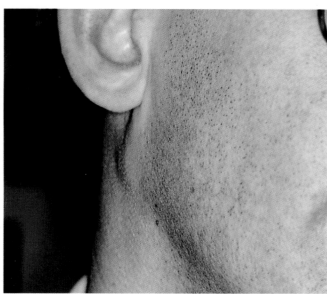

23.6

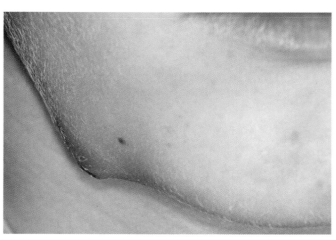

23.7

CARBUNCLE

Carbuncles are deep infections, usually with *Staphylococcus aureus*. Carbuncles are not seen in the mouth but may rarely affect the lip with tender red swelling and eventual suppuration (**Figs 23.8–23.11**).

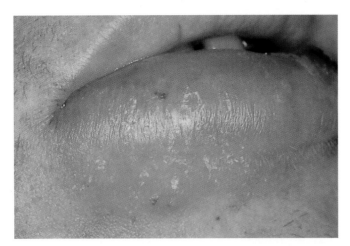

23.8

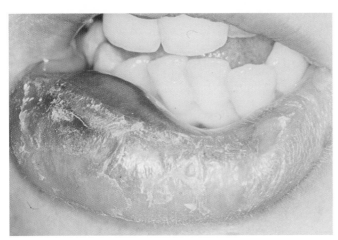

23.9

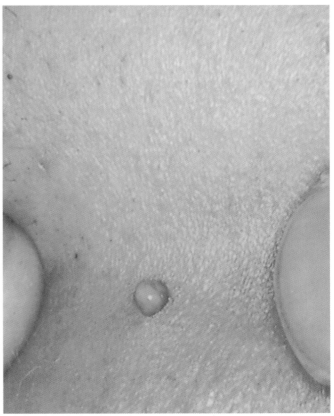

23.10

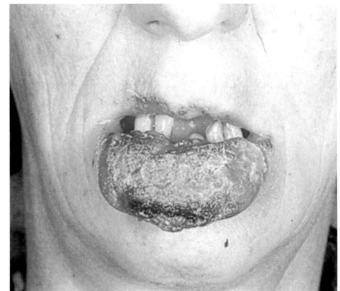

23.11

DERMATITIS HERPETIFORMIS
(Duhring's disease)

Dermatitis herpetiformis (DH) is an uncommon skin disease, often associated with gluten-sensitive enteropathy, and most common in adult males. Oral lesions, seen in up to 10% of patients, start as vesicles that rupture to leave nonspecific ulcers (**Fig. 23.12**) and some patients develop a desquamative gingivitis or hyperkeratotic areas (**Fig. 23.13**). Coeliac-disease type enamel hypoplasia may be seen.

The typical rash is very itchy and consists of multiple, tense vesicles on the elbows, shoulders and other extensor surfaces (**Fig. 23.14**). Granular deposits of IgA are seen in the epithelial basement membrane zone.

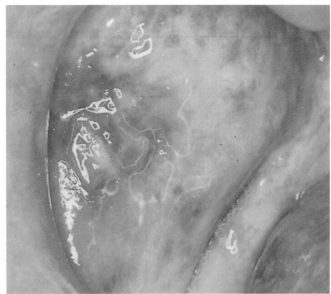

23.13

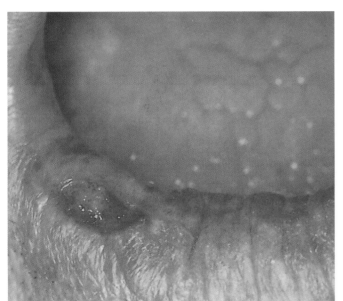

23.12

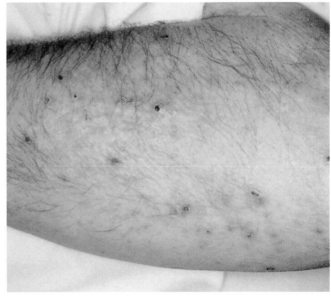

23.14

DISCOID LUPUS ERYTHEMATOSUS

Discoid lupus erythematosus (DLE) is an immunologically mediated disorder characterized by a rash on the face, scalp, ears and hands, consisting of red patches with scaling and follicular plugging. There may be scaly lesions on the vermilion and perioral skin (**Figs 23.15, 23.16**). The oral lesions can be difficult to differentiate clinically from lichen planus but they may ulcerate (**Fig. 23.17**), and there is a malignant predisposition, especially in males with lesions on the lip.

The typical oral lesions, seen in up to 25% of patients, are found mainly in the buccal mucosa and have an irregular white border, with telangiectasia, surrounding a central atrophic area in which there are small white papules (**Fig. 23.18**). Palatal lesions are far more common in DLE than in lichen planus. Discoid lupus may be drug induced, particularly with procainamide and hydralazine, although about 70 other agents can give rise to drug-induced lupus.

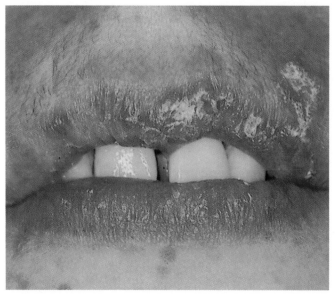

23.15

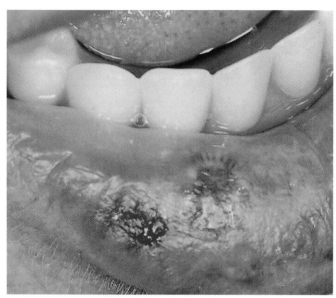

23.16

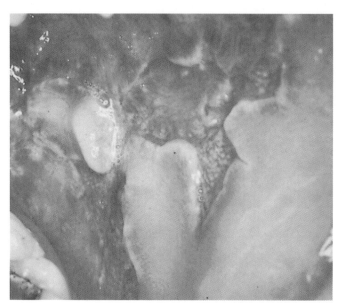

23.17

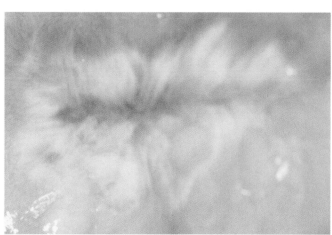

23.18

EPIDERMOLYSIS BULLOSA ACQUISITA

Epidermolysis bullosa is rarely acquired but may then present with features resembling pemphigoid or localized oral purpura (**Figs 23.19, 23.20**) but with cutaneous lesions in areas subject to trauma.

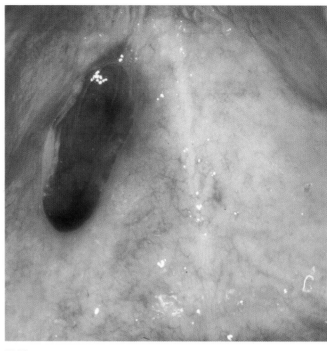

23.20

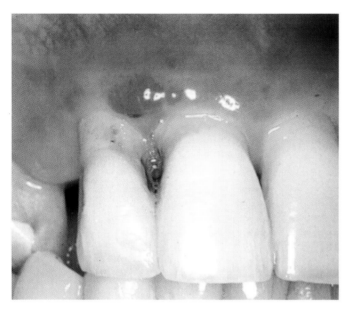

23.19

ERYTHEMA MULTIFORME

Erythema multiforme is an allergic type of reaction which presents in minor or major forms. Although the aetiology is unclear in some patients, in many the disorder is precipitated by infections (such as herpes simplex or mycoplasma), by drugs (sulfonamides, barbiturates, hydantoins and others) or by a range of other triggers, even HIV infection and menstruation. Most patients are males, typically adolescents or young adults, and there are periods of remission.

Erythema multiforme minor typically affects the skin of the back and palms and sometimes the anterior oral mucosa.

Erythema multiforme major (Stevens–Johnson syndrome) affects any mucosae, skin and other sites.

The virtually pathognomonic feature of either form of erythema multiforme is swollen, blood-stained or crusted lips (**Fig. 23.21**). Oral lesions progress through macules to blisters and ulceration, typically most pronounced in the anterior parts of the mouth (**Fig. 23.22**). Early

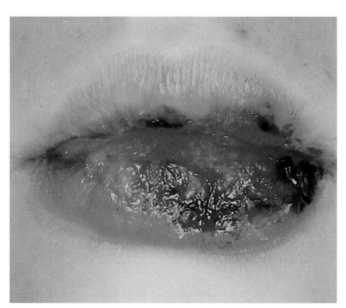

23.21

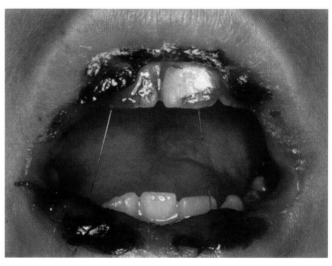

23.22

lesions may be macular and develop the appearance of an archery target (hence target lesions; **Figs 23.23, 23.24**). Extensive oral ulceration may eventually be seen (**Figs 23.25–23.27**).

Most patients only have oral lesions but in some other squamous epithelia are involved. Rashes of various types (hence 'erythema multiforme') are seen (**Fig. 23.28**). **Figure 23.29** shows a close-up of the same patient as in **Fig. 23.28** showing a vesiculobullous rash — the blisters are collapsed and scabbed centrally.

More pronounced blisters in erythema multiforme may resemble pemphigoid (**Fig. 23.30**).

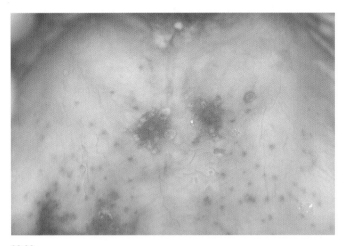

23.23

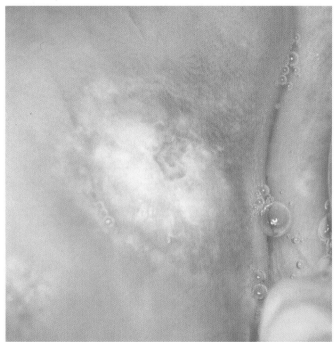

23.24

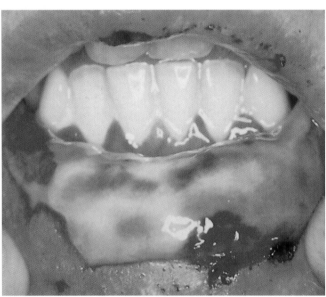

23.25

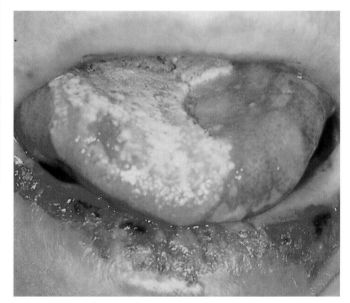

23.26

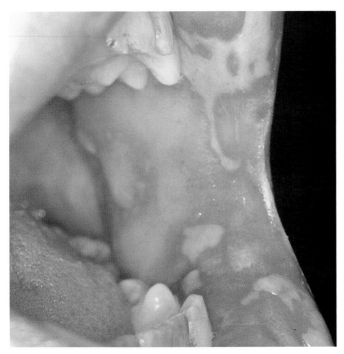

23.27

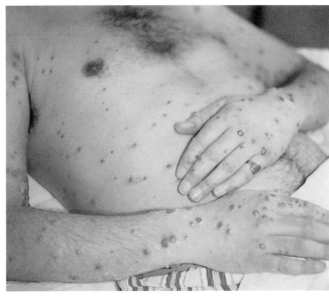

23.28

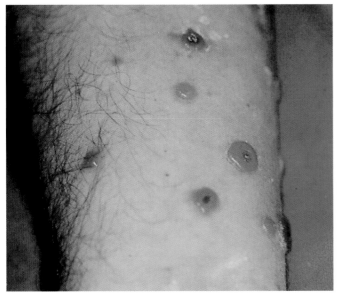

23.29

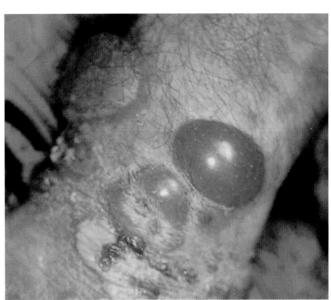

23.30

The characteristic rash consists of 'target' or 'iris' lesions in which the central lesion has a surrounding ring of erythema (**Fig. 23.31**). **Figure 23.32** shows a later stage of target lesions showing darkening and loss of distinction.

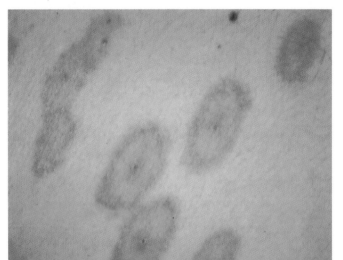

23.31

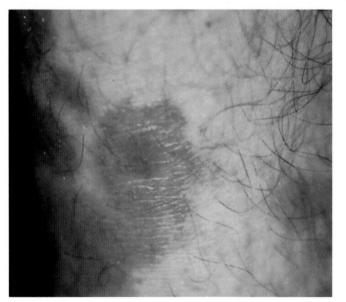

23.32

IMPETIGO

Perioral lesions such as herpes labialis or chickenpox may be secondarily infected with staphylococci or streptococci, resulting in impetigo (**Fig. 23.33**). Alternatively, there may be a primary infection or spread of impetigo from elsewhere.

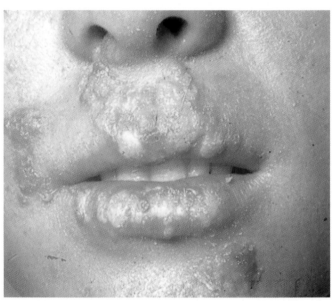

23.33

LICHEN PLANUS

Lichen planus (LP) is common, mostly idiopathic and often asymptomatic. Lesions are typically bilateral and white lesions in the mouth are the typical features (**Figs 23.34–23.61**).

Of the many types of lichen planus described in the literature, papular and striated (reticular) LP are the most common (see **Fig. 23.34**).

White papules are typically seen in the buccal mucosa bilaterally. Other types as follows:

- *Reticular types* (see **Figs 23.34–23.39**) *and mixed papular and reticular types* may be seen.
- *Plaque type LP* (see **Figs 23.40–23.42**), especially in smokers, can give rise to confluent white patches difficult to distinguish clinically from keratoses (leukoplakia).

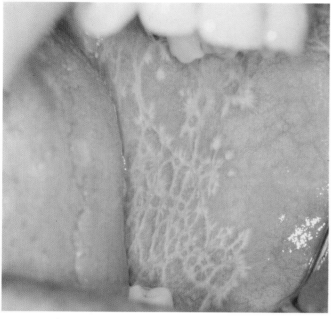

23.34

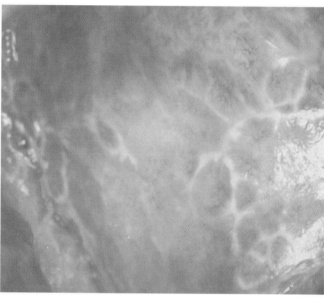

23.35

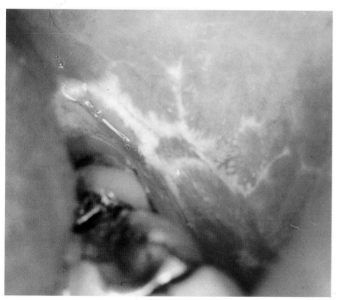

23.36

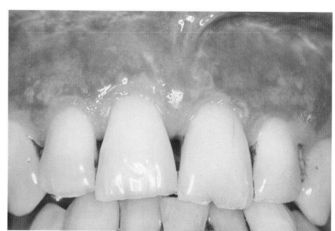

23.37

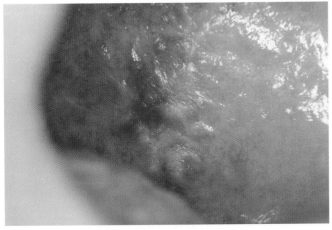

23.38

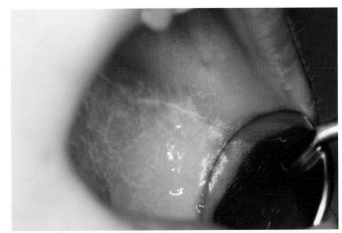

23.39

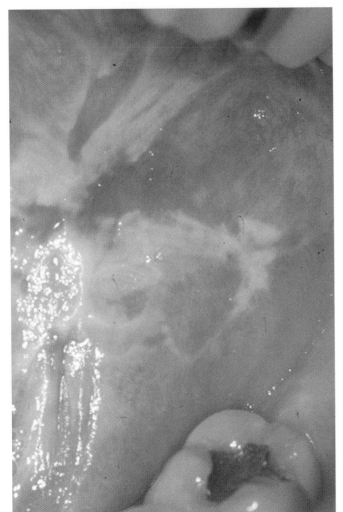

23.40

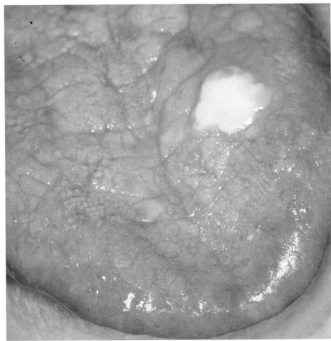

23.41

- *Erosive LP* (see **Figs 23.43, 23.44**) presents with irregular, often wide-spread persistent erosions, usually in the buccal and/or lingual mucosa, and can cause pronounced discomfort. The erosions may be irregular, often shaped like a holly leaf and there may be associated white lesions.
- *Atrophic forms of LP* (see **Figs 23.45, 23.46**) present with red lesions, often with a whitish border, and can resemble lupus erythematosus. Erosions may arise in these lesions.

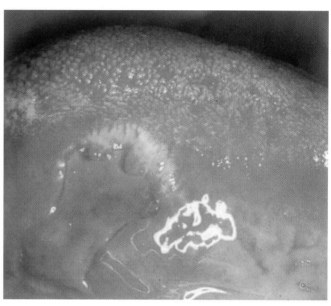

23.43

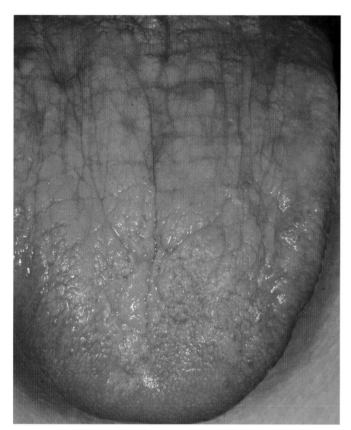

23.42

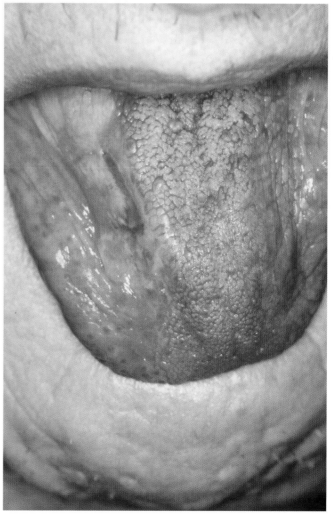

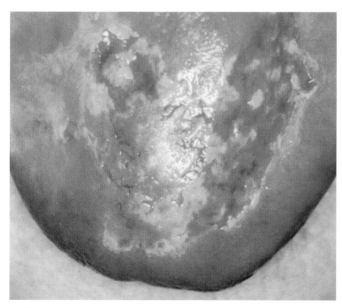

23.45

23.44

The buccal mucosa is the most common site for LP (see **Fig. 23.47**) but lesions may involve the tongue (see **Figs 23.48** and **23.49**), gingivae (**Figs 23.50–23.53**) or other areas. **Figures 23.54–23.59** show further examples of this common condition, to illustrate the variety of presentations. Oral lesions of LP are often persistent and patients typically have lesions for many years.

Erosive, atrophic and other nonreticular forms of LP may be potentially malignant in less than 3% of cases (**Figs 23.60, 23.61** are early

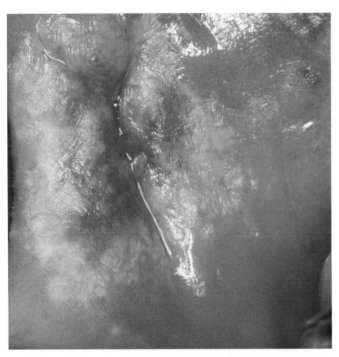

23.46

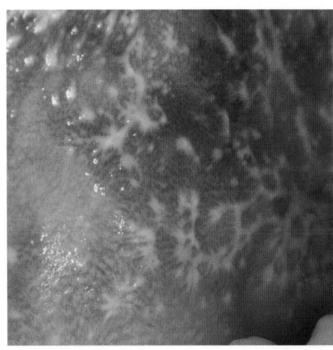

23.47

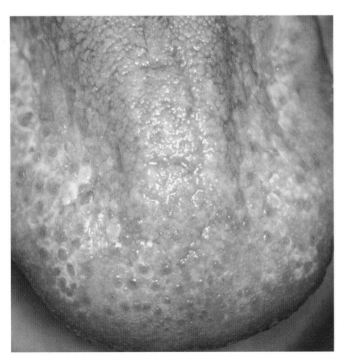

23.48

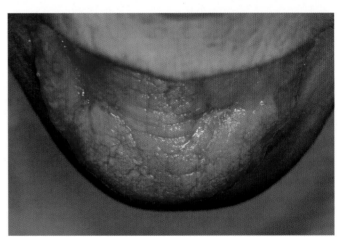

23.49

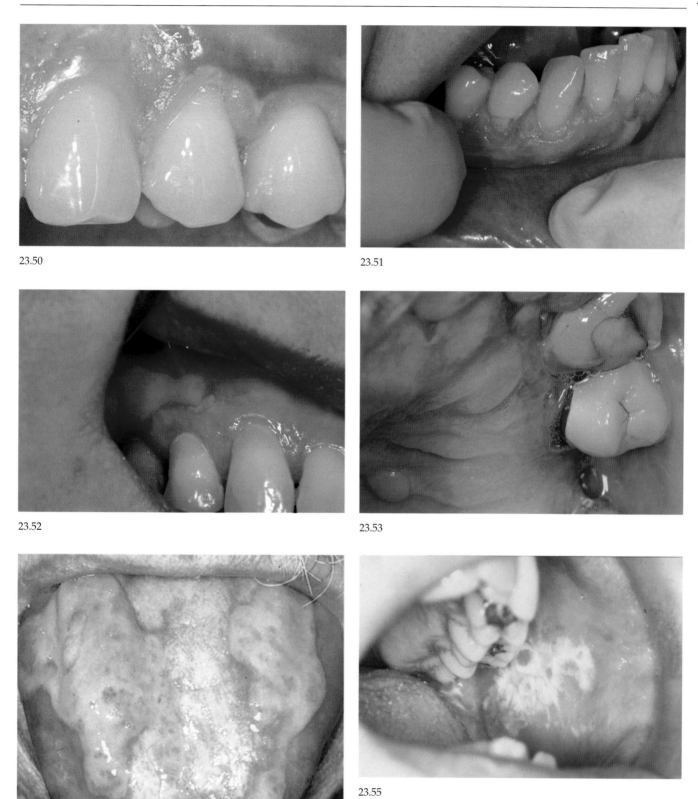

23.50

23.51

23.52

23.53

23.54

23.55

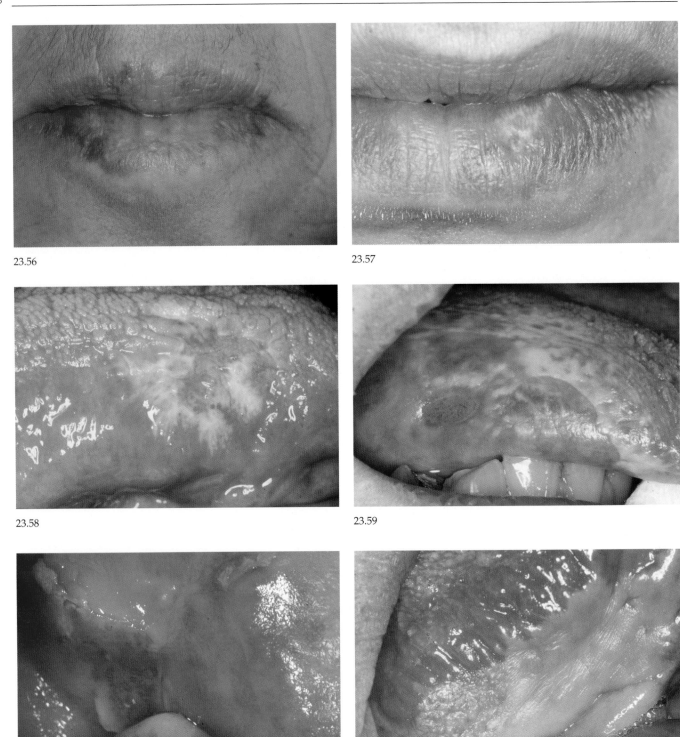

23.56

23.57

23.58

23.59

23.60

23.61

carcinoma) though some of these may represent associated lichenoid dysplasia or erythroplasia.

Cutaneous lesions of LP, if present, are typically purple, polygonal, pruritic papules on the flexor surfaces of the wrists (**Figs 23.62–23.71**). White striae may be seen on the surfaces of the papules (see **Figs. 23.66–23.68**): Wickham's striae.

Cutaneous lesions may be widespread (see **Fig. 23.69**) and cause extreme itching. Rubbing or scratching the skin may produce a row of lesions, termed the Koebner phenomenon (**Fig. 23.70**).

Lesions are also common over the shins (see **Fig. 23.65**) and may also be seen elsewhere but are rare on the face. Alopecia may be seen in LP.

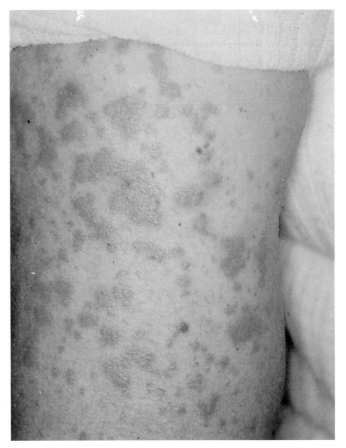

23.63

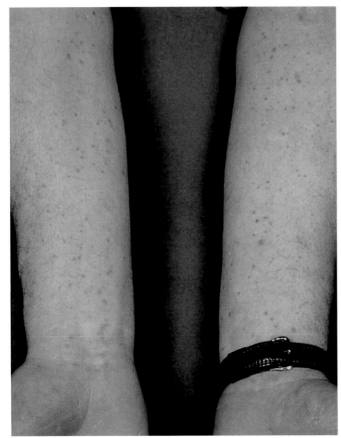

23.62

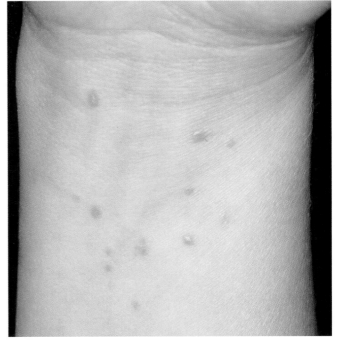

23.64

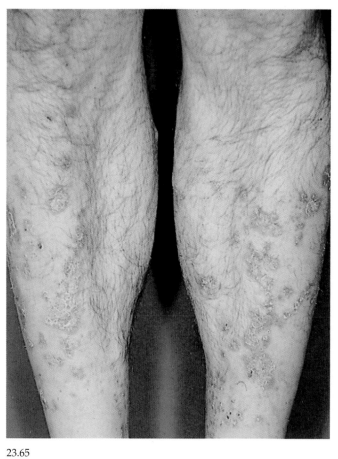

23.65

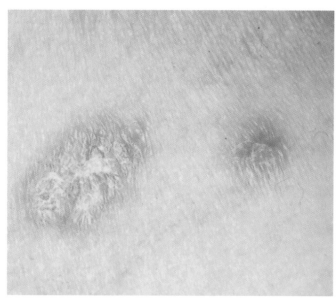

23.66

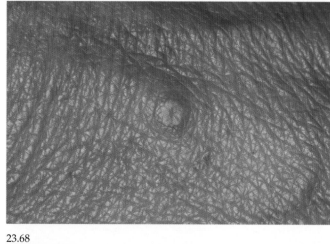

23.68

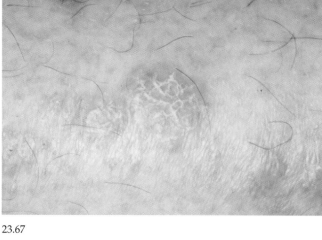

23.67

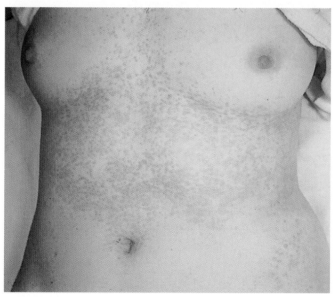

23.69

Lichen Planus Nail involvement may produce longitudinal ridging (**Figs 23.72, 23.73**) and other changes.

Lesions that resemble LP clinically and histologically may be induced by various identifiable factors. These lesions are termed 'lichenoid lesions' (**Fig. 23.74**) and may be caused by antihypertensives, oral hypoglycaemics, nonsteroidal anti-inflammatory agents (and a range of other drugs), metal restorative materials used in dentistry or HIV disease or perhaps hepatitis C virus. These lesions are a frequent complication of chronic graft-versus-host disease. The only true test of their nature is to observe the sequelae of removal of potential precipitating factors.

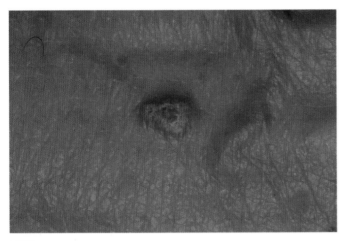

23.70

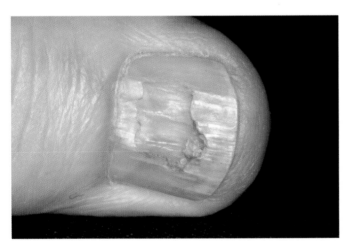

23.72

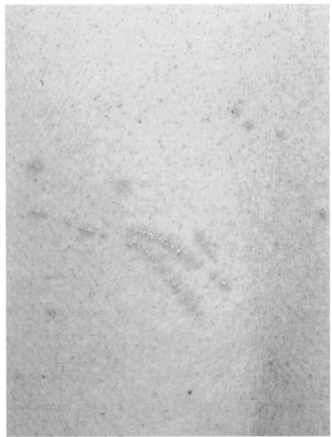

23.71

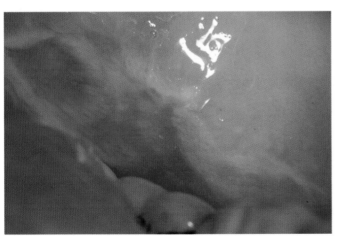

23.74

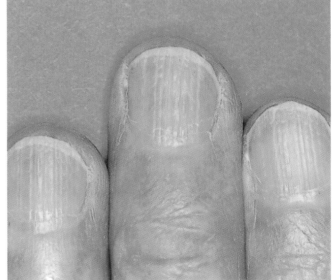

23.73

Lichen planus has occasional overlaps with other disorders such as pemphigoid, lichen sclerosis or lupus erythematosis, and occasional associations with other diseases, especially with diabetes mellitus and autoimmune disorders, and possibly other hepatitis viruses.

Chronic ulcerative stomatitis

Chronic ulcerative stomatitis is a rare disorder in which lesions appear clinically similar to erosive lichen planus but prove, on immunostaining, to be associated with stratified squamous epithelium-specific antinuclear antibodies.

LICHEN SCLEROSIS

Lichen sclerosis et atrophicus (LSA) is a relatively rare idiopathic dermatosis characterized by white, macular lesions on the skin, and is usually associated with an atrophic mucosa (**Fig. 23.75**) with or without concurrent genital or skin lesions. There are some patients who have an overlap syndrome with lichen planus.

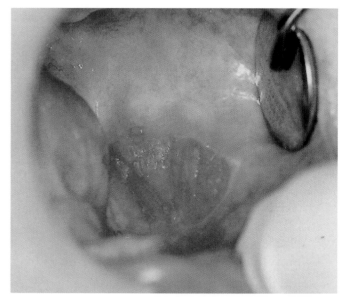

23.75

LINEAR IgA DISEASE

Linear IgA disease is a subepithelial immune-mediated blistering disease, a variant of dermatitis herpetiformis, in which the IgA deposits are linear rather than granular at the epithelial basement membrane zone. Oral vesicles or ulcers may be seen as well as desquamative gingivitis (**Figs 23.76–23.78**). Drugs such as vanucomycin may produce similar lesions.

Chronic bullous dermatosis of childhood (CBDC) is a rare related disorder, seen in young children, which may produce similar oral lesions.

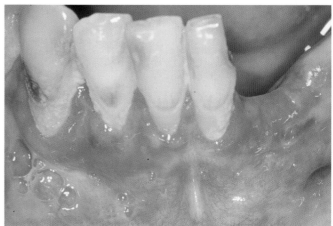

23.77

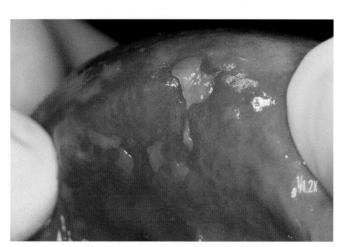

23.76

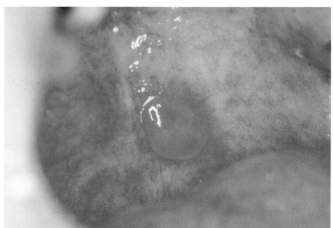

23.78

LOCALIZED ORAL PURPURA *(angina bullosa haemorrhagica)*

Localized oral purpura is a fairly common condition that mimics pemphigoid, although it is not associated with any defined immunopathogenesis. Patients present with blood blisters, typically on the soft palate, often after eating (**Fig. 23.79**) or sometimes after use of corticosteroid inhalers. There is subepithelial vesiculation (**Fig. 10.52**) and an ulcer eventually forms — this type of ulcer has been described as a 'sunburst ulcer' (**Fig. 23.80**).

This condition must be differentiated from pemphigoid, and acquired epidermolysis bullosa in particular (see **Table 1.1**).

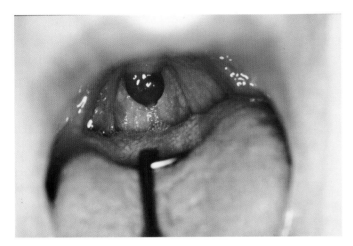

23.79

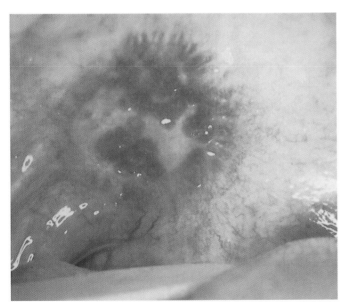

23.80

NECROTIZING FASCIITIS

Necrotizing fasciitis is due to group A streptococci or a mixture of other bacteria which gain access to tissues usually via a skin cut or surgical wound but sometimes via an oral infection or wound. It is seen most commonly on the head and neck (**Figs 23.81, 23.82**) or the limbs.

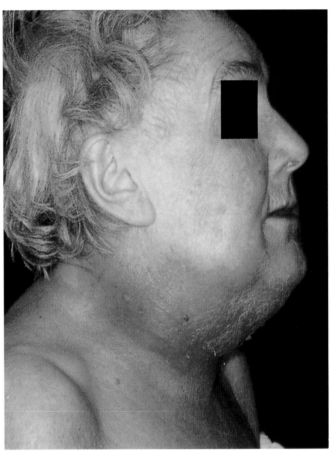

23.81

Necrotizing fasciitis usually presents with a hot, tender area of swelling which is erythematous or dusky. Bullae and necrosis of the underlying tissue may intervene, and the overlying skin may become anaesthetic.

The lesion spreads rapidly, the patient is usually severely ill and toxic, and there is a mortality of over 45% reported in some series. Similar conditions include progressive bacterial synergistic gangrene and gangrenous cellulitis due to other pathogens such as *Pseudomonas* species or zygomycete fungi (causing mucormycosis), mainly seen in the immunocompromised patient.

PEMPHIGOID

Various forms of pemphigoid can cause oral lesions but these are most common in mucous membrane and ocular forms.

Mucous membrane pemphigoid is a sub-epithelial immune-mediated blistering disease, a disorder of stratified squamous epithelia in which there are usually IgG autoantibodies against epithelial basement membrane zone.

Mucous membrane pemphigoid often causes oral lesions and although intact vesicles or bullae may be seen (**Figs 23.83–23.85**), they eventually break down to leave irregular ulcers (**Figs 23.86–23.87**).

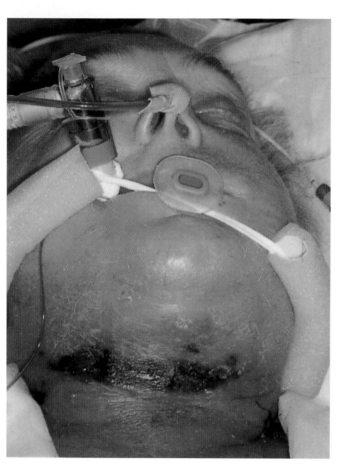

23.82

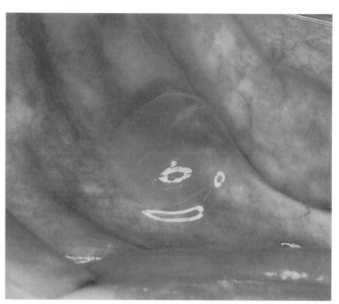

23.83

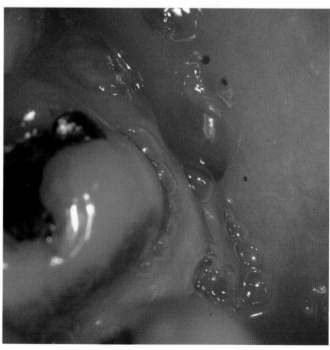

23.84

Although typically arising idiopathically mucous membrane pemphigoid may be drug induced, particularly by penicillamine.

Lesions typically affect the buccal mucosa, palate and gingiva. Mucous membrane pemphigoid is a frequent cause of desquamative gingivitis, which presents with patches of sore erythema (**Figs**

23.87–23.90). In contrast to marginal gingivitis, in desquamative gingivitis the interdental papillae and gingival margins may appear normal. Occasionally there is frank gingival ulceration.

Conjunctival involvement may lead to scarring and to symblepharon (**Fig. 23.90**), or ankyloblepharon (**Fig. 23.91**). Ocular involvement is

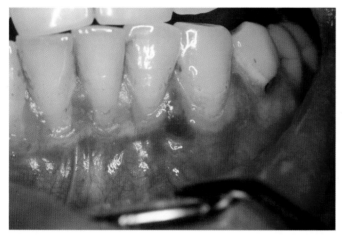

23.85

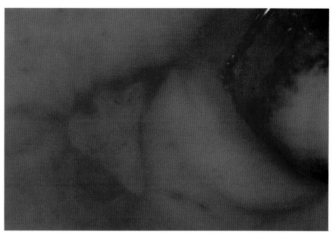

23.86

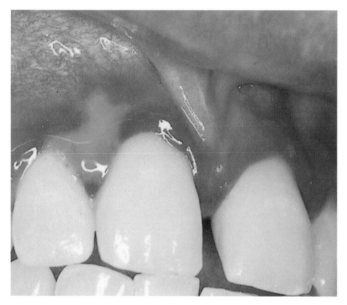

23.87

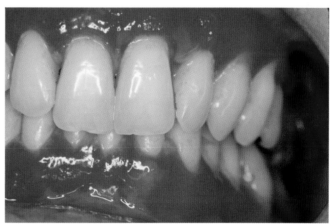

23.88

426

potentially serious since it may culminate in blindness. The eyes are dry and the cornea becomes opaque (**Fig. 23.92**). Other squamous epithelia may be involved and genital or laryngeal involvement may lead to stenosis; skin lesions are uncommon.

In bullous pemphigoid, skin lesions are far more common than oral. However, vesicles, bullae and erosions may be seen (**Fig. 23.93**).

The skin vesicles and bullae of pemphigoid tend to be more tense than those of pemphigus and are most often seen on the abdomen, groin axillae and flexures (**Fig. 23.94**).

Bullous pemphigoid is occasionally drug induced or secondary to UV light exposure. Brunsting–Perry disease is a mild variant of bullous pemphigoid.

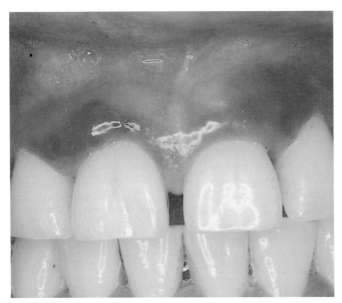

23.89

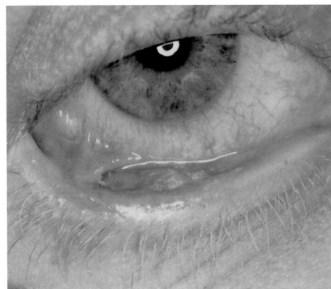

23.90

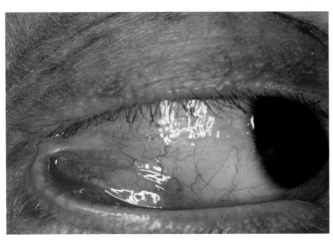

23.91

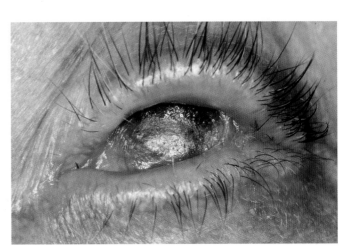

23.92

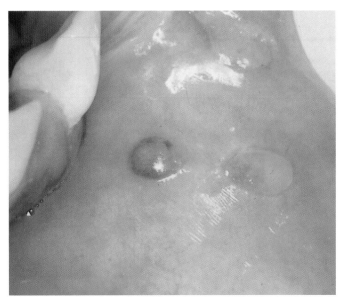

23.93

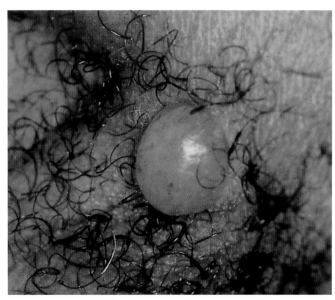

23.94

PEMPHIGUS

Pemphigus is the term given to a group of potentially lethal disorders, all characterized by autoantibodies directed against intercellular substance of stratified squamous epithelium, and seen especially in the middle aged or elderly. The autoantibodies are usually IgG. Pemphigus vulgaris is the most common type, involving the mouth, although still an uncommon disease, and is associated with antibodies against desmoglein. Pemphigus vegetans may involve the mouth but oral lesions of the foliaceus and erythematosus types of pemphigus are very rare. Occasional cases of pemphigus are paraneoplastic, or drug-related (e.g. to penicillamine or rifampicin).

In pemphigus, oral lesions commonly precede skin manifestations. Oral vesicles or blisters are rarely seen intact, as they break down rapidly to superficial irregular erosions which are initially red and later become ulcers covered with a fibrin slough as in **Figs 23.95–23.98**. Widespread erosions may be seen, especially where the mucosa is traumatized in the buccal mucosa, palate or gingiva, and gingival involvement can lead to a form of desquamative gingivitis (**Fig. 23.99**).

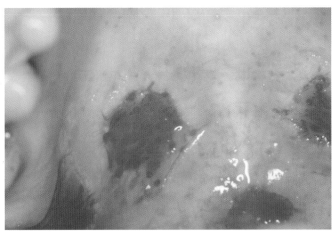

23.95

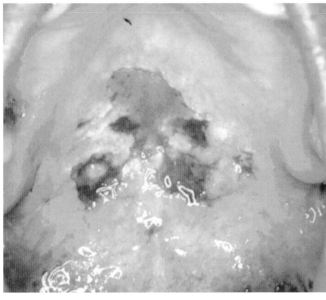

23.96

Pemphigus can affect other stratified squamous epithelium such as the anterior nasal mucosa, conjunctivae and skin (**Figs 23.100–23.105**).

Skin blisters tend to be flaccid, and appear at sites of trauma (Nikolsky's sign) (see **Fig. 23.102**; these lesions, on the anterior chest wall, were produced by the edge of a brassiere). The skin blisters break down to leave extensive scabbed lesions (see **Figs 23.103, 23.104**).

The axilla and groin are other lesion sites (see **Fig. 23.104**). Rarely, the nail beds are involved (see **Fig. 23.105**). Other types of pemphigus are as follows:

- *Pemphigus vegetans* (Neumann's type) follows a similar course to pemphigus vulgaris, whereas the Hallopeau type is more benign.

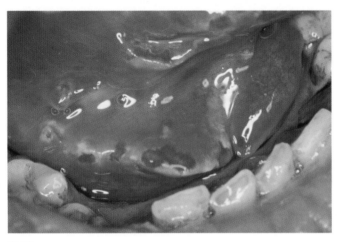

23.97

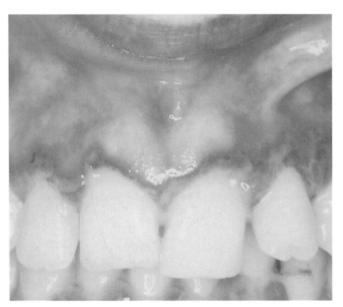

23.99

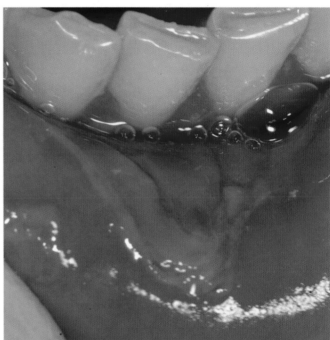

23.98

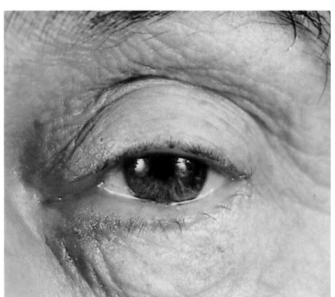

23.100

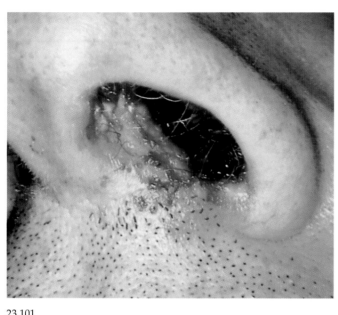

23.101

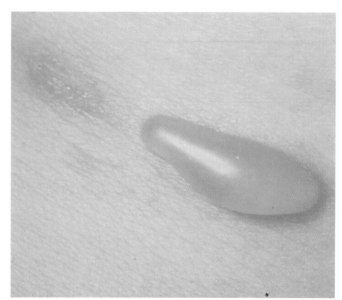

23.102

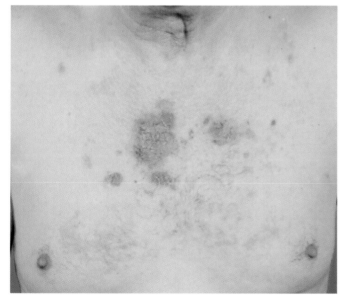

23.103

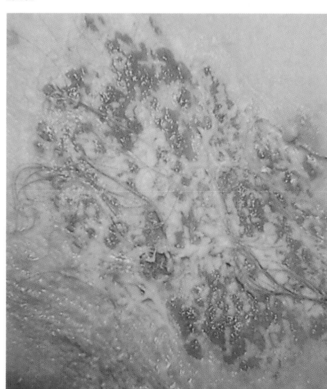

23.104

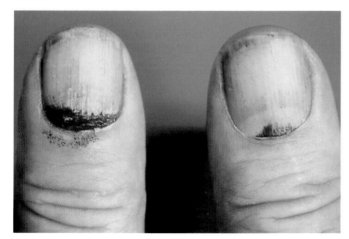

23.105

Pemphigus vegetans of either type often presents initially in the mouth and, even in those with initial skin lesions, the mouth is usually eventually involved. White serpiginous lesions, pustules or sometimes vegetations (**Fig. 23.106**) are the main manifestations. The commissures are the sites most commonly affected and the tongue may be affected and sometimes described as a 'cerebriform tongue' (see **Fig. 23.107**).

- *Paraneoplastic pemphigus* typically presents first on the lips but may result in oral erosions or lichenoid lesions (**Figs 23.108, 23.109**).
- *Intra-epidermal IgA pustulosis* may manifest with oral blisters and erosions described in the few patients with this disease. There is acantholysis with intercellular IgA deposits.
- *Benign pemphigus* (Hailey–Hailey disease) only rarely presents with oral lesions and these are indistinguishable clinically from those of pemphigus vulgaris.

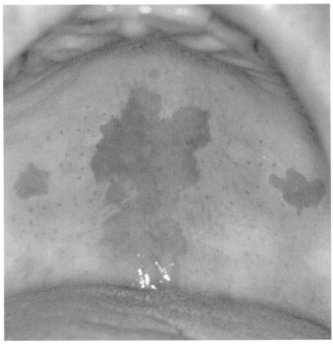

23.107

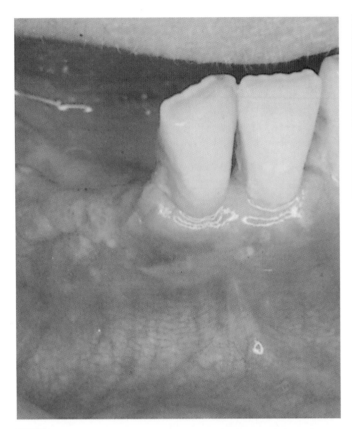

23.106

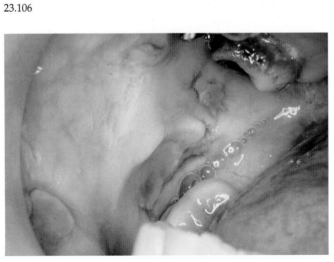

23.108

23.109

PIGMENTED PURPURIC STOMATITIS

The pigmented purpuric dermatoses are a group of disorders in which there is chronic capillaritis, with pigmented purpuric lesions predominantly on the lower limbs. Chronic oral lesions in keeping with the purpuric lichenoid dermatitis of Gougerot and Blum disease are rarely seen (**Fig. 23.110**).

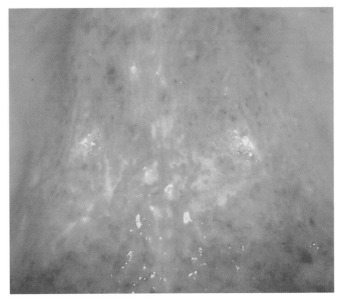

23.110

PSORIASIS

Classical psoriasis affects the elbows, knees, scalp and nails, it may cause an arthropathy and in rare cases may result in oral white lesions or ulcers (**Figs 23.111–23.113**) or temporomandibular arthropathy.

Erythema migrans is regarded by some as a *forme fruste* of psoriasis. Pustular psoriasis may occasionally involve the mouth with pustules in the palate or elsewhere. Skin and nail changes of psoriasis are shown in **Figs 23.114–23.116**.

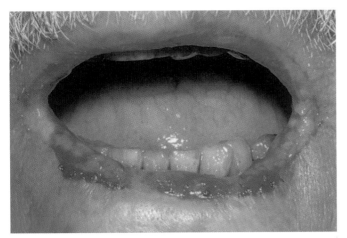

23.111

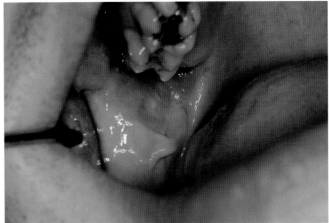

23.112

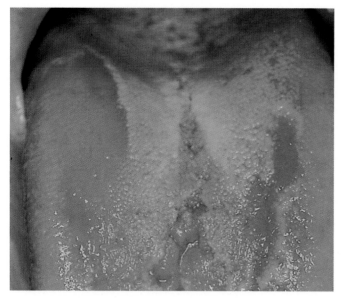

23.113

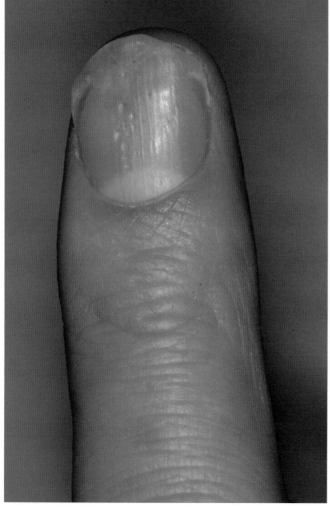

23.115

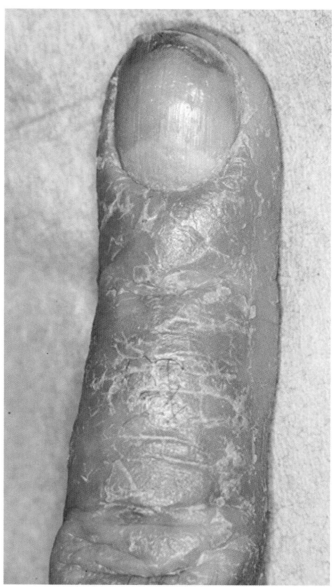

23.114

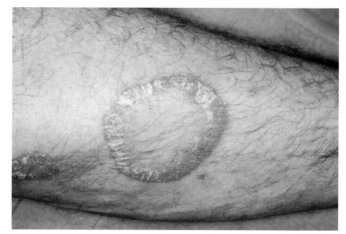

23.116

STEVENS–JOHNSON SYNDROME *(erythema multiforme exudativum)*

This syndrome is major erythema multiforme: conjunctivitis, stomatitis, genital lesions, fever and rash constitute the main manifestations (**Figs 23.117–23.121**).

The oral changes are those of erythema multiforme. The ocular changes of Stevens–Johnson syndrome resemble those of mucous membrane pemphigoid: dry eyes and symblepharon may result. **Figure 23.119** shows the patient shown in **Fig. 23.118** upon recovery.

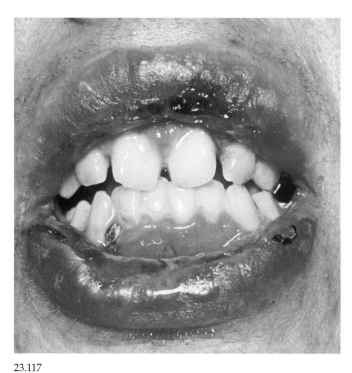

23.117

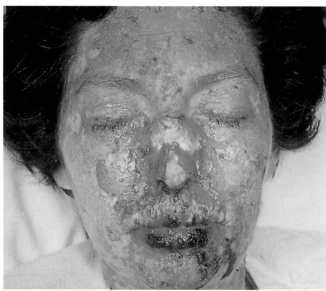

23.118

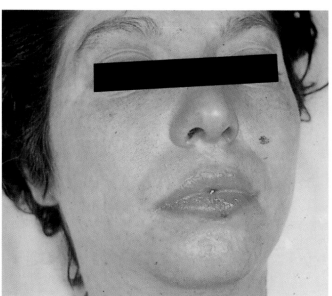

23.119

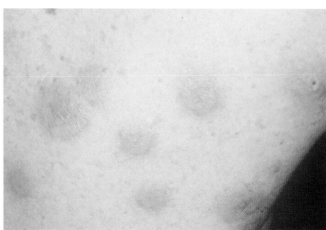

23.120

The typical genital lesions include balanitis (see **Fig. 23.121**), urethritis and vulval ulcers. Bronchopulmonary and renal involvement may also be seen.

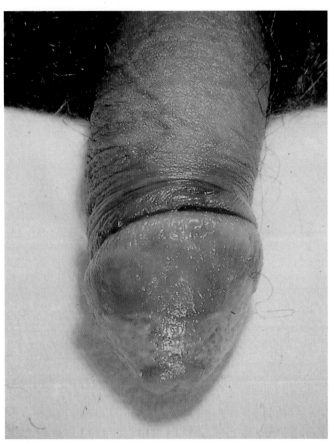

23.121

TOXIC EPIDERMAL NECROLYSIS

Toxic epidermal necrolysis (TEN) is a variant of erythema multiforme that may also produce oral ulceration, in children it is sometimes known as staphylococcal scalded skin syndrome (or Lyell's disease). Toxic epidermolysis may be associated with antimicrobials (sulfonamides, thiacetazone), analgesics (phenazones), antiepileptics, allopurinol, chlormezanone, rifampicin, fluconazole and vancomycin, and can be an occasional feature of HIV disease or graft-versus-host disease.

VITILIGO

Vitiligo may occasionally affect the lip (**Fig. 23.122**) and occurs in the lip–tip syndrome or the penis.

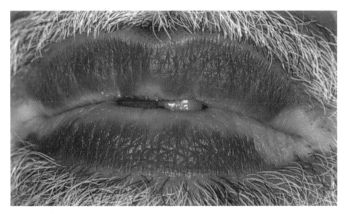

23.122

FURTHER READING

Bagan J, Eisen D, Scully C. The diagnosis and management of oral lichen planus. Oral Biosciences Med 2004; 1: 21–8).

Bez C, Hallet R, Carrozzo M, *et al*. Lack of association between hepatotropic transfusion transmitted virus infection and oral lichen planus in British and Italian populations. Br J Dermat 2001; 145: 990–3.

Burton J, Scully C. The lips. In Champion RH, Burton J and Ebling FJG (eds) Textbook of Dermatology, 6th edn, Oxford, Blackwell, 1998.

Carbone M, Conrotto D, Carrozzo M, Broccoletti R, Gandolfo S, Scully C. Topical corticosteroids in association with miconazole and chlorhexidine in the long-term management of atrophic-erosive lichen planus; a placebo-controlled and comparative study between clobetasol and fluocinonide. Oral Dis 1999; 5: 44–9.

Carrozzo M, Gandolfo S, Lodi G, *et al*. Oral lichen planus patients infected or non-infected with hepatitis C virus; the role of autoimmunity. J Oral Path Med 1999; 28: 16–19.

Challacombe SJ, Setterfield J, Shirlaw P, Harman K, Scully C, Black MM. Immunodiagnosis of pemphigus and mucous membrane pemphigoid. Acta Odontologica Scandinavica 2001; 59: 226–34.

Chorzelski TP, Olszewska M, Jarzabek-Chorzelska M, Jablonska S. Is chronic ulcerative stomatitis an entity? Clinical and immunological findings in 18 cases. Euro J Dermat 1998: 8, 261–5.

Cohen DM, Bhattacharyya I, Zunt SL, Tomich CE. Linear IgA disease histopathologically and clinically masquerading as lichen planus. Oral Surg Oral Med Oral Pathol Oral Radiol Endod 1999; 88: 196–201.

Dabelsteen E. Molecular biological aspects of acquired bullous diseases. Crit Rev Oral Biol Med 1998; 9: 162–78.

Dahn KA, Glode MP, Chan KH. Periodic fever and pharyngitis in young children: a new disease for the otolaryngologist? Arch Otolaryngol Head Neck Surg 2000; 126(9): 1146–9.

DiAlberti L, Porter SR, Speight PM, *et al*. Presence of human herpesvirus-8 variants in the oral ulcer tissues of HIV-infected individuals. J Infect Dis 1997; 175: 703–7.

Epstein JB, Wan LS, Gorsky M, Zhang L. Oral lichen planus: progress in understanding its malignant potential and the implications for clinical management. Oral Surg Oral Med Oral Pathol Oral Radiol Endod 2003; 96: 32–7.

Feder HM Jr. Periodic fever, aphthous stomatitis, pharyngitis, adenitis: a clinical review of a new syndrome. Curr Opin Pediatr 2000; 12(3): 253–6.

Femiano F, Gombos F, Scully C. Oral erosive/ulcerative lichen planus: preliminary findings in an open trial of sulodexide compared with cyclosporine (ciclosporin) therapy. Intern J Dermatol 2001; 42: 308–11.

Femiano F, Gombos F, Scully C. Pemphigus vulgaris with oral involvement; evaluation of two different systemic corticosteroid therapeutic protocols. J Euro Acad Dermat Venereol 2002; 16: 353–6.

Femiano F, Scully C, Gombos F. Linear IgA dermatosis induced by a new angiotensin-converting enzyme inhibitor. Oral Surg Oral Med Oral Pathol Oral Radiol Endod 2003; 95: 169–73.

Herranz P, Arribas JR, Navarro A, Pena JM, Gonzalez J, Rubio FA, Casado M. Successful treatment of aphthous ulcerations in AIDS patients using topical granulocyte-macrophage colony-stimulating factor. Br J Dermatol 2000; 142(1): 171–6.

Hodgson TA, Malik F, Hegarty AM, Porter SR. Topical tacrolimus: a novel therapeutic intervention for recalcitrant labial pemphigus vulgaris. Eur J Dermatol 2003; 13: 142–4.

Ingafou M, Porter SR, Scully C, Teo CG. No evidence for HCV infection or liver disease in British patients with lichen planus. Int J Oral Maxillofacial Surg 1998; 27: 65–66.

Jimenez Y, Bagan JV, Milian MA, Gavalda C, Scully C. Lichen sclerosus et atrophicus manifesting with localized loss of periodontal attachment. Oral Dis 2002; 8(6): 310–13.

Lodi G, Carrozzo M, Harris K, et al. Hepatitis G virus-associated oral lichen planus; no influence from hepatitis G virus co-infection. J Oral Pathol Med 2000; 29: 39–42.

Longman LP, Higham SM, Rai K, Edgar WM, Field EA. Salivary gland hypofunction in elderly patients attending a xerostomia clinic. Gerodontology 1995; 12(12): 67–72.

Longman LP, Higham SM, Bucknall R, Kaye SB, Edgar WM, Field EA. Signs and symptoms in patients with salivary gland hypofunction. Postgrad Med J 1997; 73(856): 93–7.

Mattsson U, Jontell M, Holmstrup P. Oral lichen planus and malignant transformation: is a recall of patients justified? Crit Rev Oral Biol Med 2002; 13: 390–6.

McBride DR. Management of aphthous ulcers. Am Fam Physician 2000; 62(1): 149–54, 160.

Nisengard RJ. Periodontal implications: mucocutaneous disorders. Ann Periodontol 1996; 1(1): 401–38.

Ouellet B, Agha-Amiri M, Dube-Baril C, Mascres C. Ectodermal dysplasia: multiple manifestations of a hereditary disease. J Can Dent Assoc 1997; 63(5): 377–81.

Porter SR, Scully C, Midda M, Eveson JW. Adult linear immunoglobulin A disease manifesting as desquamative gingivitis. Oral Surg Oral Med Oral Pathol 1990; 70: 450–3.

Porter SR, Kirby A, Olsen I, Barrett W. Immunologic aspects of dermal and oral lichen planus: a review. Oral Surg Oral Med Oral Pathol Oral Radiol Endod 1997; 83: 358–66.

Ramon-Fluixa, Bagan JV, Milian MA, Scully C. Periodontal status in patients with oral lichen planus; a study of 90 cases. Oral Dis 1999; 5: 303–6.

Rishiraj B, Epstein JB. Basal cell carcinoma: what dentists need to know. J Am Dent Assoc 1999; 130(3): 375–80.

Robinson CM, DiBiase AT, Leigh IM, et al. Oral psoriasis. Br J Dermatol 1996; 134: 347–9.

Roujeau JC, Kelly JP, Naldi L, et al. Medication use and the risk of Stevens–Johnson syndrome or toxic epidermal necrolysis. N Engl J Med 1995; 333: 1600–7.

Scully C. Prevention of oral mucosal disease. In Murray JJ (ed.) Prevention of Oral and Dental Disease, 3rd edn, Oxford, Oxford University Press, 1995, pp. 160–72.

Scully C. The mouth in dermatological disorders. Practitioner 2001; 245: 942–52.

Scully C. The oral cavity. In Champion RH, Burton J and Ebling FJG (eds) Textbook of Dermatology, 6th edn, Oxford, Blackwell 2004.

Scully C, Challacombe SJ. Pemphigus vulgaris: update on etiopathogenesis, oral manifestations, and management. Crit Rev Oral Biol Med 2002; 13: 397–408.

Scully C, Porter SR. The clinical spectrum of desquamative gingivitis. In Eisen D (ed.) Seminars in Cutaneous Medicine and Surgery 1997; 16: 308–13.

Scully C, Beyli M, Ferreiro MC, et al. Update on oral lichen planus: etiopathogenesis and management. Crit Rev Oral Biol Med 1998; 9: 86–122.

Scully C, Paes De Almeida O, Porter SR, Gilkes JJ. Pemphigus vulgaris: the manifestations and long-term management of 55 patients with oral lesions. Br J Dermatol 1999; 140: 84–9.

Scully C, Eisen D, Carrozzo M. Management of oral lichen planus. Am J Clin Dermatol 2000; 1: 287–306.

Scully C, Carrozzo M, Gandolfo S, Puiatti P, Monteil R. Update on mucous membrane pemphigoid (an immune mediated sub-epithelial blistering disease); a heterogeneous entity. Oral Surg Oral Med Oral Pathol Oral Radiol Endod 1999; 88: 56–68.

Scully C, Gorsky M, Lozada-Nur F. Aphthous ulcerations. In Camisa C (ed.) Diagnosis and Treatment of Oral Lesions. Dermatologic Therapy 2002; 15: 185–205.

Shotts R, Scully C. How to identify and deal with tongue problems. Pulse 2002; 62: 73–6.

Sugerman PB, Savage NW, Walsh LJ, et al. The pathogenesis of oral lichen planus. Crit Rev Oral Biol Med 2002; 13: 350–65.

Zhu JF, Kaminski MJ, Pulitzer DR, et al. Psoriasis; pathophysiology and oral manifestations. Oral Dis 1996; 2: 135–44.

24 DISEASES OF CONNECTIVE TISSUE

- dermatomyositis
- Felty's syndrome
- mixed connective-tissue disease
- Raynaud's phenomenon
- rheumatoid arthritis
- scleroderma
- Sjögren's syndrome
- systemic lupus erythematosus.

438

DERMATOMYOSITIS

Dermatomyositis and polymyositis are part of a group of immuno-logically mediated inflammatory disorders of skeletal muscle. All have symmetric weakness of proximal muscles. Primary idiopathic dermatomyositis presents mainly in the middle-aged or elderly, with difficulty in climbing stairs, getting out of a chair or raising the head from the pillow.

Oral lesions may resemble lichen planus (**Fig. 24.1**) or may show a dark red or bluish colour, and there may be oedema of the gingiva.

Sjögren's syndrome, or other connective tissue disorders such as systemic lupus erythematosus (SLE), may be seen in some patients with dermatomyositis.

Dermatomyositis is characterized by localized or diffuse erythema of the skin, maculopapular rash, eczematoid dermatitis or an almost pathognomonic lilac-coloured (heliotrope) change, especially over the eyelids, midface, around the nails and over the knuckles, the elbow or the knee (**Figs 24.2–24.5**). Skin changes precede, accompany or follow a proximal muscle weakness resembling polymyositis.

Dermatomyositis is occasionally (up to 20%) associated with internal malignancy (lung; ovary; breast; stomach) or may be induced by drugs such as penicillamine or by Coxsackieviruses.

Childhood dermatomyositis is distinguished by vasculitis, arthritis, Raynaud's phenomenon and calcinosis.

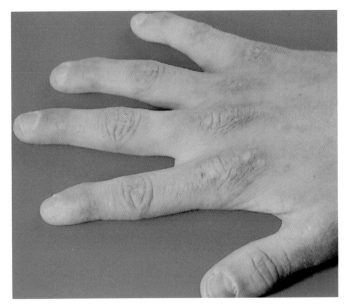

24.2

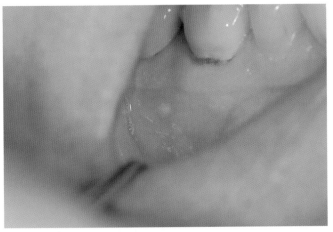

24.1

24.3

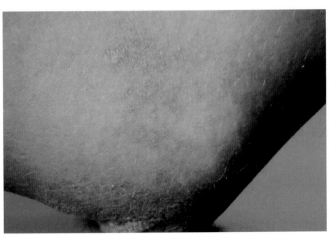

24.4

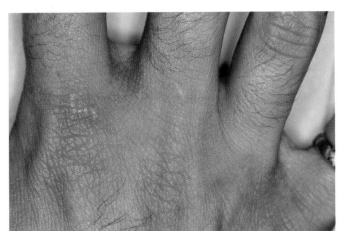

24.5

FELTY'S SYNDROME

Felty's syndrome is the association of rheumatoid arthritis with splenomegaly and neutropenia, manifesting with recurrent infections. Patients have a higher incidence of episcleritis, leg ulcers, pleurisy and neuropathy than do those with classical rheumatoid arthritis. Oral ulceration may be seen, either herpetic or nonspecific (**Fig. 24.6**).

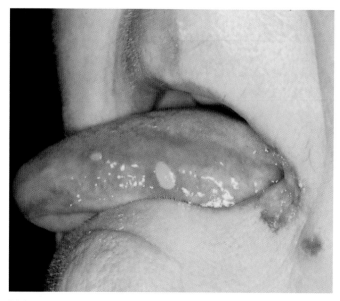

24.6

MIXED CONNECTIVE-TISSUE DISEASE

Mixed connective-tissue disease (MCTD) is an uncommon multisystem disorder with two or more of the following: SLE, scleroderma or polymyositis. Sjögren's syndrome is the main complication of oral interest.

Presenting features include polyarthropathy, sclerodactyly, myositis, oesophageal hypomotility and Raynaud's phenomenon. Patients have antibodies to nuclear ribonucleoprotein (URNP).

Oral features, apart from Sjögren's syndrome, include weakness of the tongue and occasionally petechiae and gingival lesions, as well as ulceration, neuralgia, neuropathy and lymphadenopathy (**Figs 24.7–24.9**).

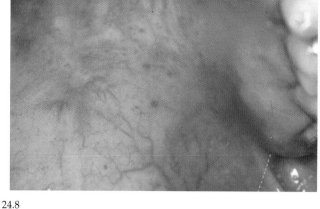

24.8

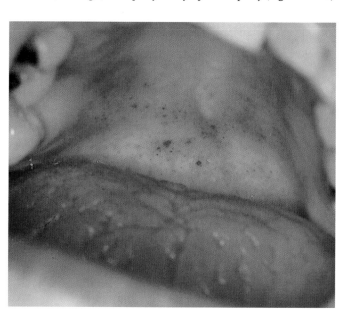

24.7

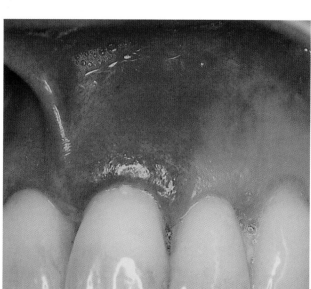

24.9

RAYNAUD'S PHENOMENON

Raynaud's phenomenon, in which there is exceptional vasoconstriction in the digits in response to cold (**Fig. 24.10**), is common in many of the connective-tissue disorders. Rarely, Raynaud's of the tongue can be a feature of scleroderma.

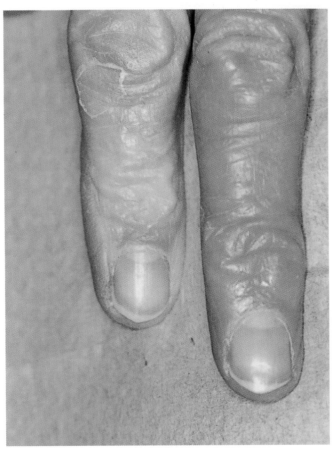

24.10

RHEUMATOID ARTHRITIS

Rheumatoid arthritis (RA) is a chronic relapsing inflammatory arthritis. It usually affects many diathrodial joints and is characterized by morning stiffness of the joints which, in advanced disease, become severely deformed (arthritis mutilans: **Fig. 24.11**).

Involvement of the temporomandibular joint is common but symptoms are rare.

Osteoporosis, flattening of the mandibular condyle, marginal irregularities and limited movement may be seen; there may be restricted oral opening. The condyle may necrose in a patient on corticosteroids, leading to a slight anterior open bite (**Fig. 24.12**).

Extra-articular features of RA include subcutaneous nodules (**Fig. 24.13**), nailbed vascular loops, pleurisy, pulmonary fibrosis, pericarditis, scleritis and episcleritis, nerve entrapment syndromes and vasculitic skin ulcers.

Juvenile rheumatoid arthritis (20% of which is Still's syndrome, with systemic disease) may interfere with mandibular growth (**Figs 24.14–24.17**) and cause ankylosis. Sjögren's syndrome, however, is the most common oral complication of rheumatoid arthritis.

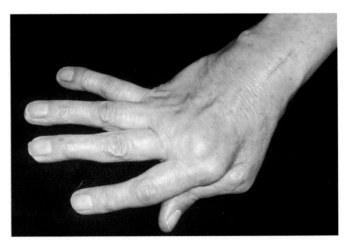

24.11

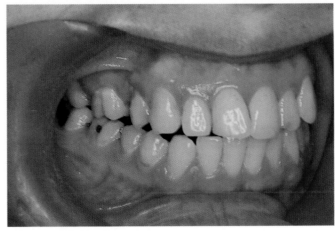

24.12

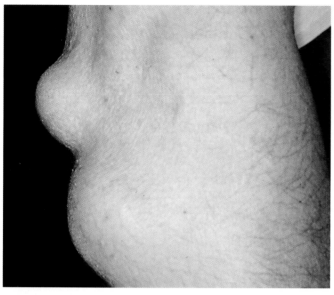

24.13

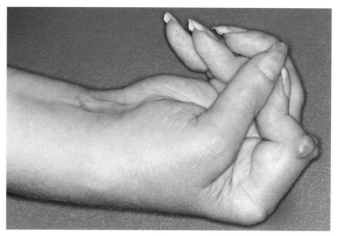

24.14

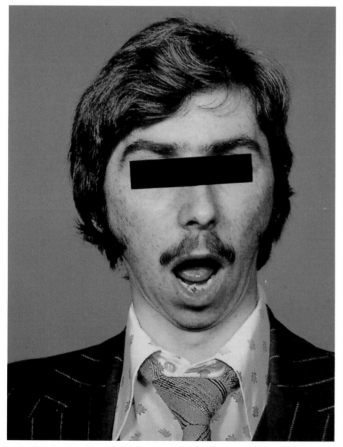

24.15

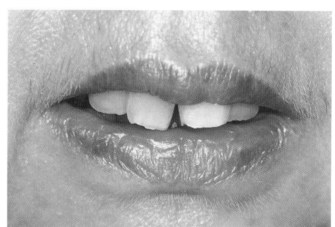

24.16

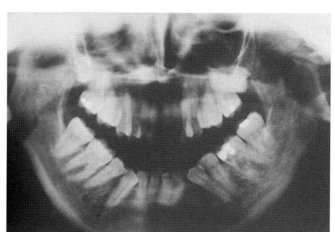

24.17

SCLERODERMA

Scleroderma is an immunologically mediated multisystem disorder. The most common manifestation is Raynaud's phenomenon. The skin becomes tight, waxy and eventually hidebound, and the face smooth with a 'Mona Lisa' appearance (**Fig. 24.18**). Skin pigmentation may also be increased. The lips tighten with radiating furrows — the so-called 'tobacco pouch' mouth (**Figs 24.19–24.22**) — and oral opening is restricted not only by the tight skin but also by pseudoankylosis of the temporomandibular joint. The mandibular condyles, coronoids or zygomatic arches are, rarely, resorbed.

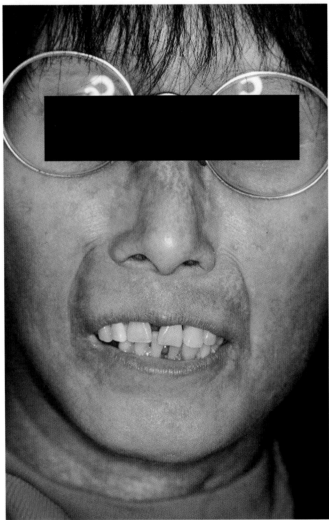

24.18

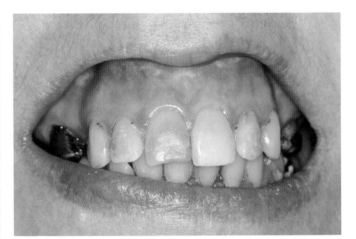

24.19

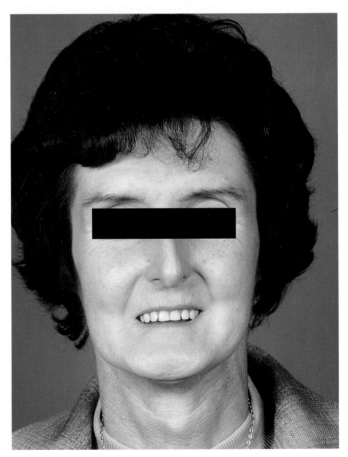

24.20

Telangiectasia may appear in the mouth and periorally, especially in the CRST variant (**Fig. 24.23**). Widening of the periodontal ligament is seen radiographically in some patients and Sjögren's syndrome may be associated.

Raynaud's phenomenon is common in systemic sclerosis and can lead to digital wasting and necrosis (**Figs 24.24, 24.25**), or ulceration (**Fig. 24.26**).

Systemic manifestations of scleroderma include pulmonary fibrosis in most patients, hypomobile gastrointestinal tract, pulmonary hypertension, pleurisy and pericarditis. Rare cases are drug induced (bleomycin; tryptophan; carbidopa), associated with graft-versus-host disease or occupational (polyvinyl chloride; silicosis).

CRST or CREST syndrome is the association of calcinosis with Raynaud's phenomenon, scleroderma, oesophageal immobility and telangiectasia (see **Fig. 24.27**). The calcific deposits are most evident in the fingers (**Figs 24.27 and 24.28**) but there may also be widespread calcification of internal organs.

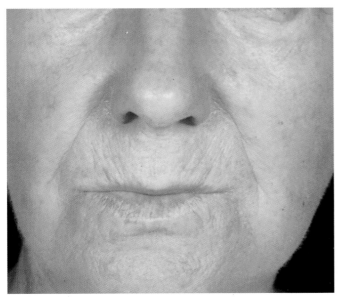

24.21

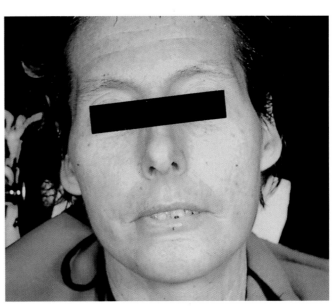

24.22

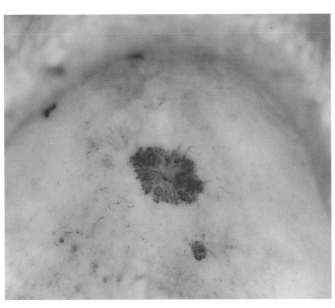

24.23

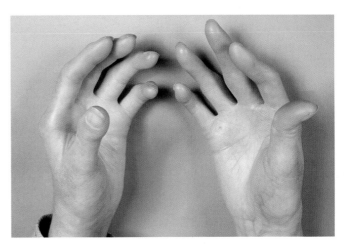

24.24

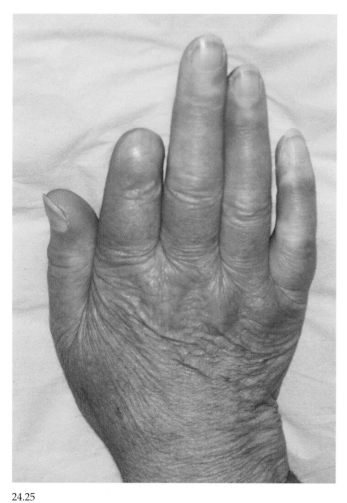

24.25

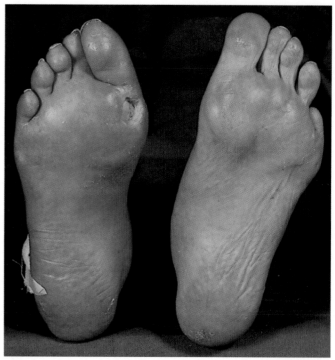

24.26

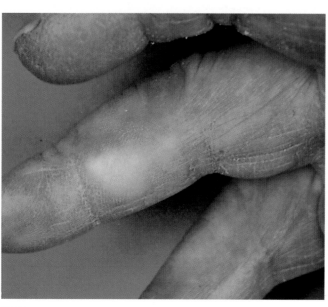

24.28

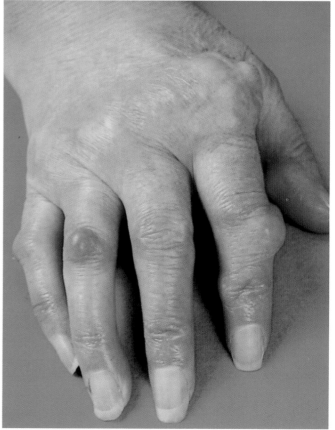

24.27

Localized scleroderma (morphoea) presents with lesions, typically a perpendicular groove paramedially running from the forehead to the hairline, or on the chin and intraorally (**Fig. 24.29**) giving a 'coup de sabre' appearance (**Fig. 24.30**).

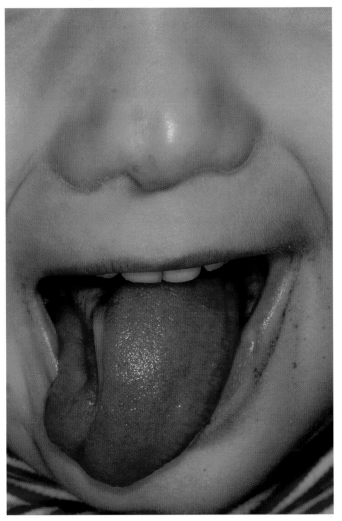

24.29

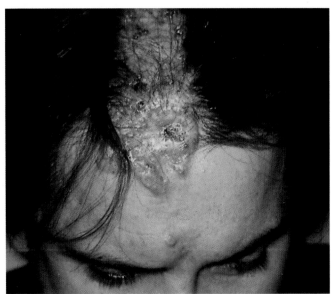

24.30

SJÖGREN'S SYNDROME

Sjögren's syndrome (dry eyes and dry mouth) is an inflammatory autoimmune exocrinopathy, common in many of the connective-tissue disorders. The salivary glands, particularly the parotid glands, may enlarge (**Fig 24.31**). This syndrome is the association of dry eyes

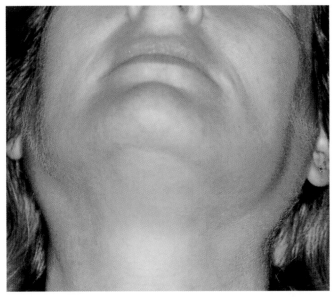

24.31

(keratoconjunctivitis sicca: **Figs 24.32, 24.33**) with dry mouth (xerostomia; **Figs 24.34–24.37**). Alone these are termed primary Sjögren's syndrome (SS-1) but if a connective tissue disorder such as RA is present, the condition is termed secondary Sjögren's syndrome (SS-2).

Rheumatoid arthritis (see **Fig. 24.38**) is a most common feature.

There are also frequent associations with primary biliary cirrhosis, SLE, systemic sclerosis and other disorders.

Dry mouth predisposes to oral infections, especially candidosis and caries (see **Figs 24.40–24.41**; incidentally, the black lesion in the lower vestibule is an amalgam tattoo after a previous apicectomy).

The salivary glands swell in up to one-third of patients with Sjögren's syndrome and the parotid glands most commonly enlarge (see **Fig. 24.31**). The enlargement may be due to the inflammatory infiltrate of Sjögren's syndrome itself, acute bacterial sialadenitis or, if persistent,

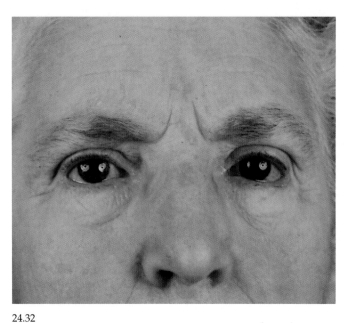

24.32

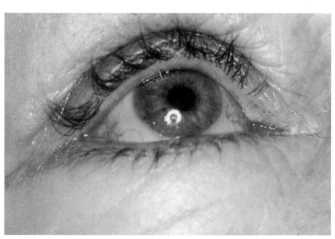

24.33

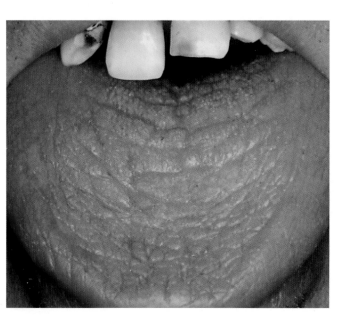

24.34

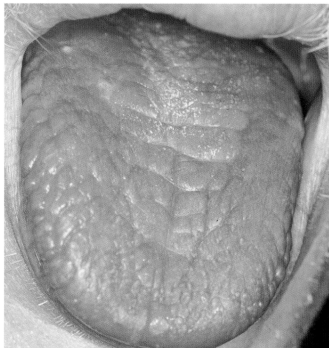

24.35

can reflect an underlying mucosa-associated lymphoid tissue (MALT) neoplasm. Complications include caries (**Figs 24.40–24.41**) and candidosis (**Figs 24.42–24.43**). Acute bacterial sialadenitis may be a complication in Sjögren's syndrome (see **Fig. 24.44**) as this syndrome is a multisystem disorder affecting many exocrine glands.

Respiratory, vaginal and gastrointestinal secretions are impaired. There may also be neuropathy, renal tubular acidosis and interstitial pneumonitis. Rare complications of Sjögren's syndrome include lymphomas (usually the non-Hodgkin's type — MALT) and other lymphoproliferative disorders.

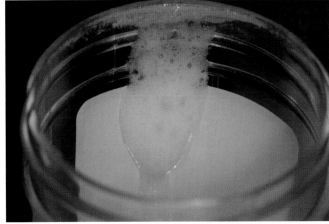

24.37

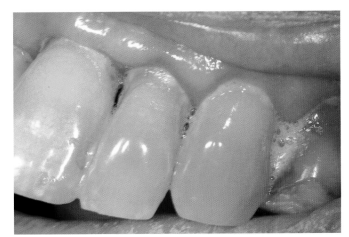

24.36

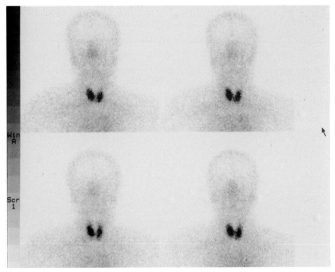

24.39

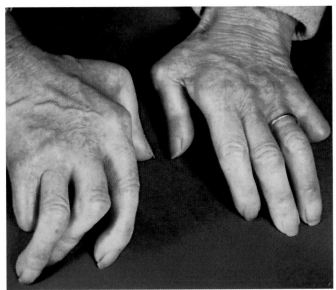

24.38

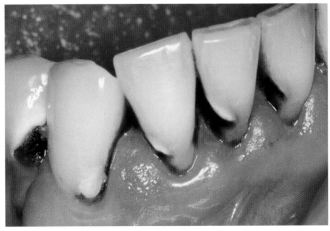

24.40

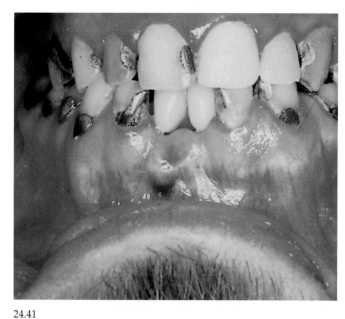

24.41

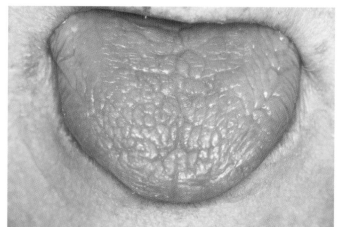

24.42

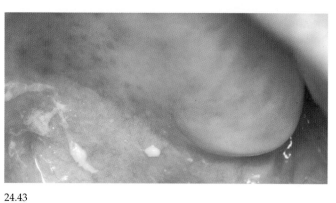

24.43

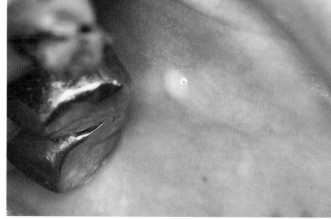

24.44

SYSTEMIC LUPUS ERYTHEMATOSUS

Systemic lupus erythematosus (SLE) is a multisystem immune complex-mediated disorder particularly affecting the skin, blood and kidneys. The classic rash is over the bridge of the nose and cheeks ('butterfly' or 'malar' rash; **Figs 24.45, 24.46**). SLE is also associated with photosensitivity, arthritis, serositis, anaemia, leukopenia and multiple autoantibodies, especially antibodies to double-stranded DNA, as well as nonspecific features such as malaise or fever.

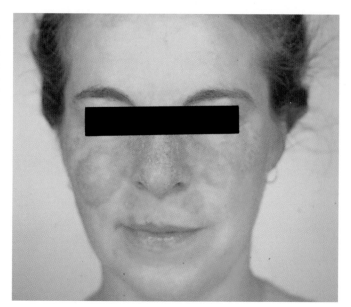

24.45

Oral lesions include ulceration secondary to autoimmune neutropenia (**Fig. 24.47**), petechiae and persistent irregular red lesions, sometimes with keratosis (**Figs 24.47–24.54**), desquamative gingivitis (**Fig. 24.49**) and petechiae (**Fig. 24.50**). The palate is a common site (**Figs. 24.51–24.53**) and the lip may be affected (**Fig. 24.54**) and Sjögren's syndrome may be associated. Hydroxychloroquine treatment may give rise to lichen planus or occasionally oral hyperpigmentation.

Nail lesions are shown in **Fig. 24.55**.

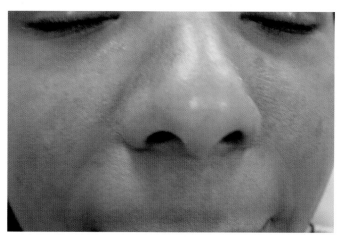

24.46

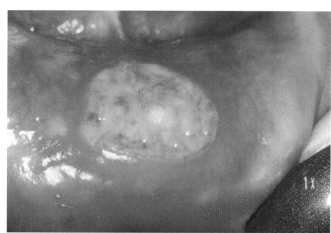

24.47

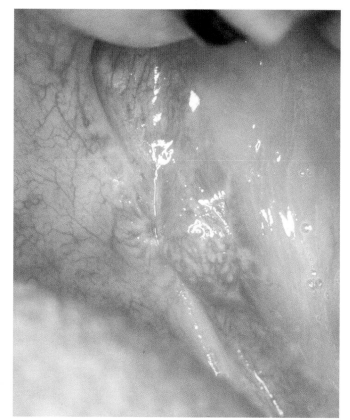

24.48

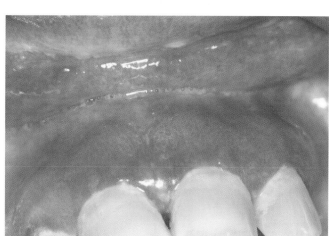

24.49

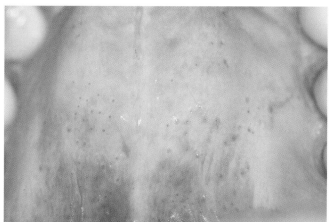

24.50

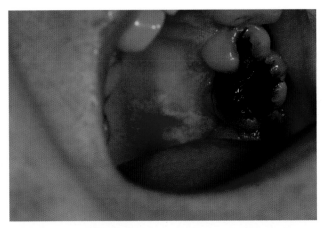

24.51

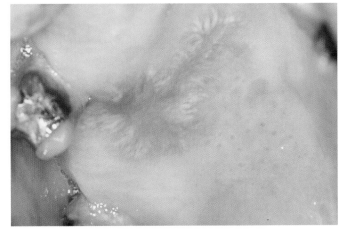

24.52

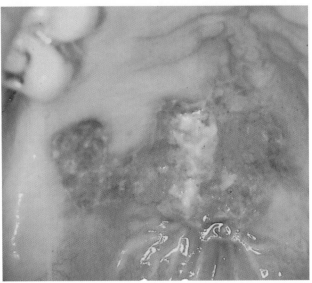

24.53

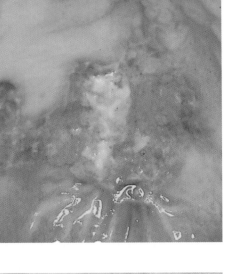

24.54

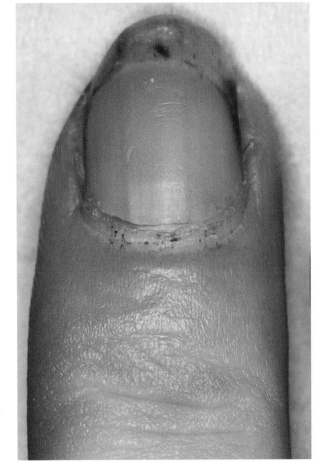

24.55

FURTHER READING

Antonen JA, Markula KP, Pertovaara MI, Pasternack AI. Adverse drug reactions in Sjogren's syndrome. Scand J Rheumatol 1999; 28: 157–9.

Bernstein ML, Neal DC. Oral lesion in a patient with calcinosis and arthritis: case report and differential diagnosis. J Oral Pathol 1985; 14(1): 8–14.

Callen JP. Oral manifestations of collagen vascular disease. Semin Cutan Med Surg 1997; 16(4): 323–7.

Chaffee NR. CREST syndrome: clinical manifestations and dental management. J Prosthodont 1998; 7(3): 155–60.

Cunningham JD Jr, Lowry LD. Head and neck manifestations of dermatomyositis-polymyositis. Otolaryngol Head Neck Surg 1985; 93(5): 673–7.

De Rossi SS, Glick M. Lupus erythematosus: considerations for dentistry. J Am Dent Assoc 1998; 129(3): 330–9.

Di Pietro G, Riccio E, Valentino C, Di Pietro A. Collagen diseases and the involvement of the mouth in childhood. Pediatr Med Chir 1998; 20(4): 275–6.

Fox RI. Sjogren's syndrome: current therapies remain inadequate for a common disease. Expert Opin Investig Drugs 2000; 9(9): 2007–16.

Fox RI, Stern M. Sjogren's syndrome: evolving therapies. Expert Opin Investig Drugs 2003; 12: 247–54.

Fox RI, Michelson P, Casiano CA, Hayashi J, Stern M. Sjogren's syndrome. Clin Dermatol 2000; 18: 589–600.

Fridrich KL, Taylor RW, Olson RA. Dermatomyositis presenting with Ludwig's angina. Oral Surg Oral Med Oral Pathol 1987; 63(1): 21–4.

Gobetti JP, Froeschle ML. Sjogren's syndrome: a challenge for dentistry. Gen Dent 1997; 45(3): 268–72.

Gonzales TS, Coleman GC. Lupus erythematosus in an orthodontic patient. J Clin Orthod 1999; 33(8): 451–2.

Hughes CT, Downey MC, Winkley GP. Systemic lupus erythematosus: a review for dental professionals. J Dent Hyg 1998; 72(2): 35–40.

Jackowski J, Johren P, Muller AM, Kruse A, Dirschka T. Imaging of fibrosis of the oral mucosa by 20 MHz sonography. Dentomaxillofac Radiol 1999; 28(5): 290–4.

Jonsson R, Moen K, Vestrheim D, Szodoray P. Current issues in Sjogren's syndrome. Oral Dis 2002; 8(3): 130–40.

Mahoney EJ, Spiegel JH. Sjogren's disease. Otolaryngol Clin North Am 2003; 36(4): 733–45.

Mandel L, Sunwoo J. Primary Sjogren's syndrome. NY State Dent J 2003; 69(7): 34–6.

Miller CS, Egan RM, Falace DA, Rayens MK, Moore CR. Periodontal manifestations of collagen vascular disorders. Periodontol 2000 1999; 21: 94–105.

Nagy G, Kovacs J, Zeher M, Czirjak L. Analysis of the oral manifestations of systemic sclerosis. Oral Surg Oral Med Oral Pathol 1994; 77: 141–6.

Paquette DL, Falanga V. Cutaneous concerns of scleroderma patients. J Dermatol 2003; 30(6): 438–43.

Pizzo G, Scardina GA, Messina P. Effects of a nonsurgical exercise program on the decreased mouth opening in patients with systemic scleroderma. Clin Oral Investig 2003; 7(3): 175–8.

Price CJ, Frankel JP, Hammans SR. Palatal palsy in dermatomyositis. Eur J Neurol 2001; 8(2): 197–8.

Romanides N, Marulli RD, Novo E, Garcia-MacGregor E, Viera N, Chaparro N, Crozzoli Y. Periodontitis and anti-neutrophil cytoplasmic antibodies in systemic lupus erythematosus and rheumatoid arthritis: a comparative study. J Periodontol 1999; 70(2): 185–8.

Rout PG, Hamburger J, Potts AJ. Orofacial radiological manifestations of systemic sclerosis. Dentomaxillofac Radiol 1996; 25(4): 193–6.

Saito T, Sato J, Kondo K, Horikawa M, Ohmori K, Fukuda H. Low prevalence of clinicopathologic and sialographic changes in salivary glands of men with Sjogren's syndrome. J Oral Pathol Med 1999; 28(7): 312–16.

Sanger RG, Kirby JW. The oral and facial manifestations of dermatomyositis with calcinosis: a case. Oral Surg Oral Med Oral Pathol 1973; 35(4): 476–88.

Shah NM, Balakrishnan C, Mangat GK, Joshi VR. Pulmonary nocardial infection and pseudomonas infection of the tongue in a patient with dermatomyositis. J Assoc Physicians India 2001; 49: 850–1.

Spackman GK. Scleroderma: what the general dentist should know. Gen Dent 1999; 47(6): 576–9.

Sreebny L, Zhu WX. Whole saliva and the diagnosis of Sjogren's syndrome: an evaluation of patients who complain of dry mouth and dry eyes. Part 2: Immunologic findings. Gerodontology 1996; 13(1): 44–8.

Vitali C, Bombardieri S, Moutsopoulos H, Scully C, European Study Group on Diagnostic Criteria for Sjogren's Syndrome. Assessment of the European classification criteria for Sjogren's syndrome in a series of clinically defined cases: results of a prospective multicentre study. Ann Rheum Dis 1996; 55: 116–21.

Vitali C, Bombardieri S, Jonsson R, et al. European Study Group on Classification Criteria for Sjogren's Syndrome. Classification criteria for Sjogren's syndrome: a revised version of the European criteria proposed by the American-European Consensus Group. Ann Rheum Dis 2002; 61(6): 554–8.

Yamamoto K. Pathogenesis of Sjögren's syndrome. Autoimmun Rev 2003; 2: 13–18.

25 ODONTOGENIC CYSTS AND NEOPLASMS

- adenomatoid odontogenic tumour (adenoameloblastoma)
- ameloblastoma (adamantinoma)
- calcifying odontogenic cyst
- calcifying odontogenic tumour (Pindborg tumour)
- dentigerous cyst (follicular cyst)
- eruption cyst
- globulomaxillary cyst
- lateral periodontal cyst
- nasopalatine duct cyst (incisive canal cyst)
- odontogenic fibromyxoma
- odontogenic keratocyst (primordial cyst).

Dental (periapical) residual cysts are discussed in Chapter 15.

ADENOMATOID ODONTOGENIC TUMOUR
(adenoameloblastoma)

This benign odontogenic tumour is most common in the maxillary canine region (**Figs 25.1, 25.2**), although **Fig. 25.1** shows a lesion in the mandible.

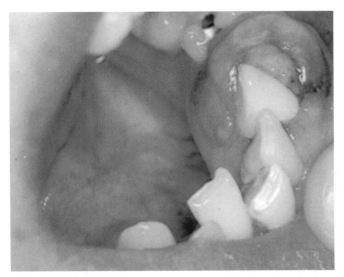

25.1

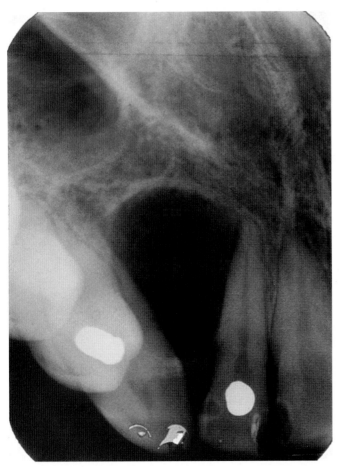

25.2

AMELOBLASTOMA *(adamantinoma)*

This locally invasive odontogenic tumour affects the mandible four times more frequently than the maxilla, and 75% of mandibular lesions are at the angle. Although the lesion may appear at any age, it usually presents in middle age. It grows insidiously and rarely causes neuropathy or mucosal breakdown. Swelling and ulceration (**Fig. 25.3**) may be caused by trauma from a denture. The plain radiographic appearance of ameloblastoma is generally of a cystic multilocular radiolucency (**Fig. 25.4**) though this is not always readily apparent (**Fig. 25.5**). Bony expansion may be seen, especially lingually (**Fig. 25.6**). Excision is sometimes followed by recurrence and even by metastases, mainly to the lung (**Fig. 25.7**).

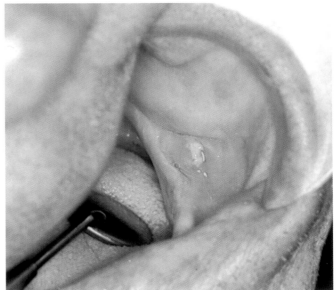

25.3

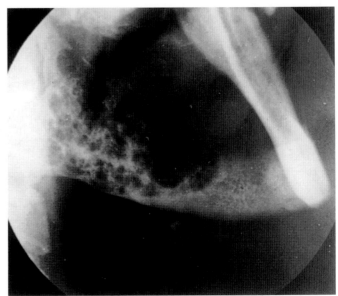

25.4

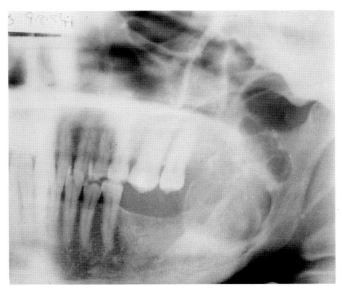

25.5

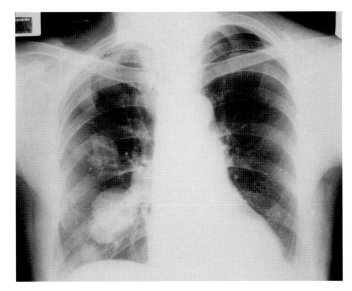

25.7

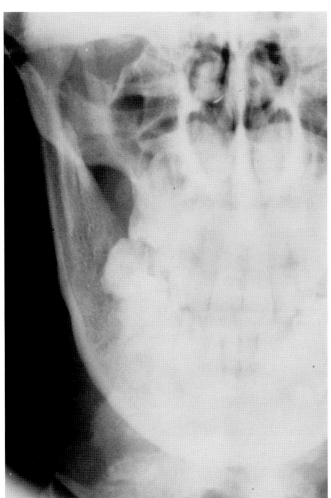

25.6

CALCIFYING ODONTOGENIC CYST

Calcifying odontogenic cyst is an uncommon odontogenic tumour that tends to manifest as a painless swelling with bony expansion in the second and third decades of life. There may be displacement or external root resorption of adjacent teeth and the cysts arise equally in the mandible or maxilla. Maxillary lesions have a predilection for the anterior jaw (**Fig. 26.8**), while mandibular lesions can arise at any site. They usually manifest radiographically as well-circumscribed unilocular radiolucencies or mixed radiolucencies and radioopacities although occasionally they may be multilocular (**Fig. 25.9**). Enucleation is usually effective as recurrence is rare, nevertheless long-term clinical and radiological follow-up is advisable.

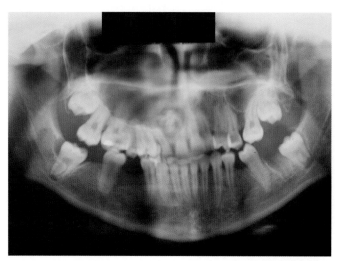

25.8

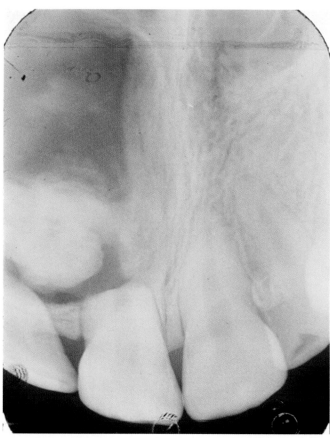

25.9

CALCIFYING ODONTOGENIC TUMOUR
(Pindborg tumour)

A Pindborg tumour is a rare odontogenic tumour manifesting as a slow-growing, bony swelling, usually of the mandible and sometimes associated with unerupted teeth. The tumour manifests radiologically as a unilocular, multilocular or honeycomb-like radiolucency with diffuse radiopacities within the lesion, sometimes with a 'driven snow' appearance (**Fig. 25.10**). The tumour is invasive and thus wide excision is required. Recurrence is possible but this depends upon the exact type of tumour and the extent of excision.

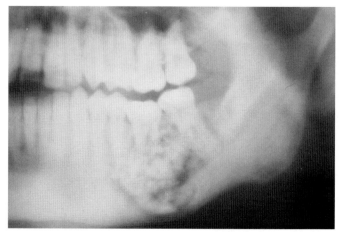

25.10

DENTIGEROUS CYST *(follicular cyst)*

A dentigerous cyst envelops the crown of a tooth and is attached to its neck (**Fig. 25.11**); most dentigerous cysts involve third molars or canine teeth (**Figs 25.12, 25.13**). In **Figure 25.12** there is an ectopic mandibular third molar on the right side.

Multiple dentigerous cysts can be a feature of cleidocranial dysplasia (see Chapter 28).

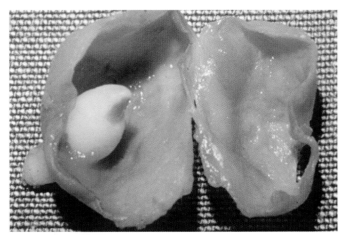

25.11

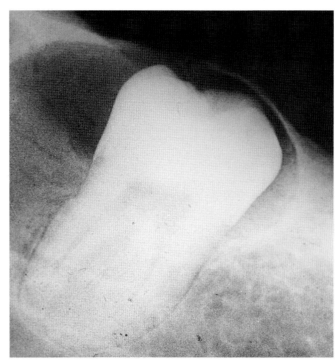

25.13

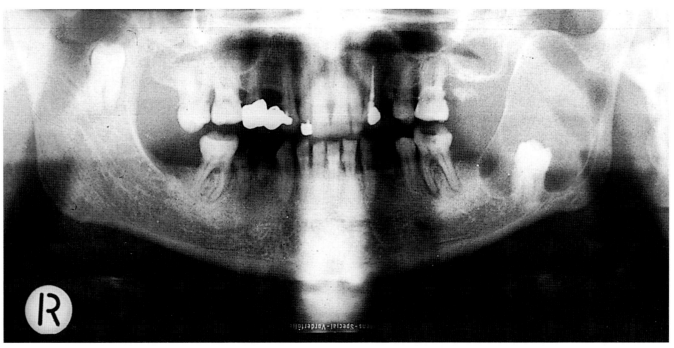

25.12

ERUPTION CYST

A cyst often presents clinically as a smooth, rounded swelling with a bluish appearance if there is no overlying bone (**Fig. 25.14**). Eruption cysts often break down spontaneously as the tooth erupts. The eruption cyst is a type of dentigerous cyst, i.e., it surrounds the crown of the tooth.

Removal of the operculum (and incidental papilloma) from the cyst in **Fig. 25.15** reveals an erupting upper first molar (**Fig. 25.16**).

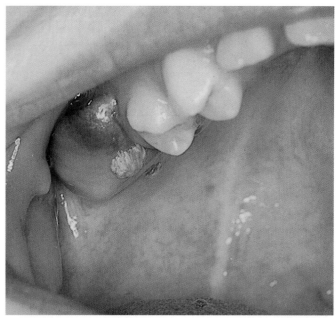

25.15

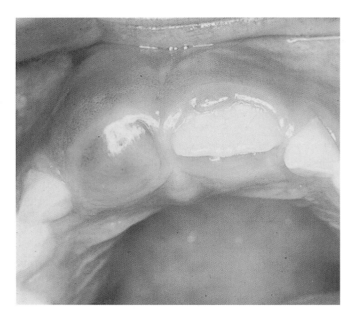

25.14

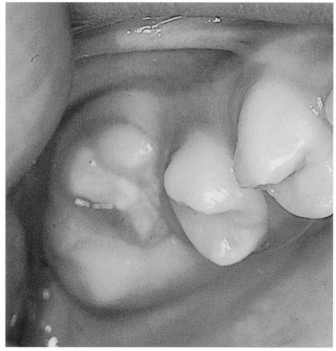

25.16

GLOBULOMAXILLARY CYST

A probable misnomer, most cysts in the upper lateral incisor canine region (**Fig. 25.17**) prove to be odontogenic rather than developmental (nonodontogenic, fissural) cysts. This cyst has displaced the maxillary right canine and lateral incisor teeth.

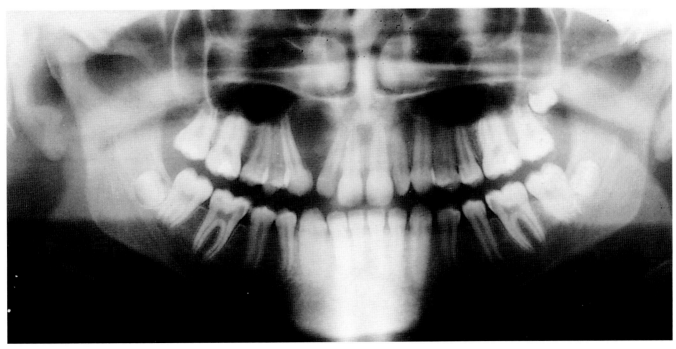

25.17

LATERAL PERIODONTAL CYST

A lateral periodontal cyst may be follicular in origin; it may arise from remnants of the dental lamina or it may be associated with a lateral pulp canal in a nonvital tooth. The cyst in **Fig. 25.18** closely resembles a dentigerous cyst.

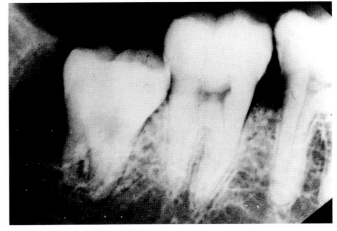

25.18

NASOPALATINE DUCT CYST
(incisive canal cyst)

Epithelial remnants related to the nasopalatine canal may give rise to a cyst. Most nasopalatine cysts are seen in adult males from the age of 40 years. If large, the cyst may produce a swelling beneath the upper lip and anterior nares (**Fig. 25.19**).

The swelling may extend to the nasal floor and palatal vault (**Fig. 25.20**), and it may discharge a salty fluid. Sometimes simply a bluish tinge is seen (**Fig. 25.21**).

Dental cysts related to nonvital incisors can be confused with the nasopalatine cyst. Furthermore, the normal incisive canal can be difficult to distinguish radiographically from a cyst, although it is generally accepted that a radiolucency greater than 6 mm in diameter is probably a cyst (**Fig. 25.22**). As the cyst expands round the nasal spine it assumes a heart-shaped configuration on radiography.

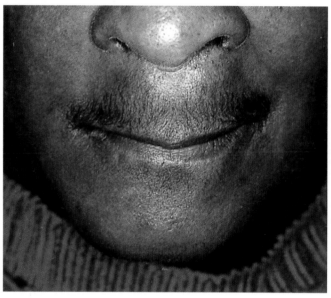

25.19

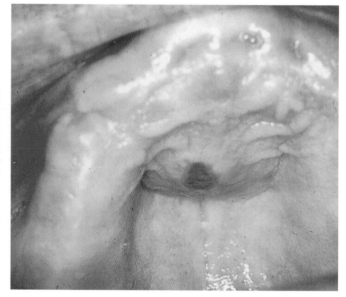

25.20

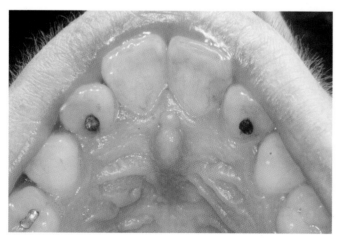

25.21

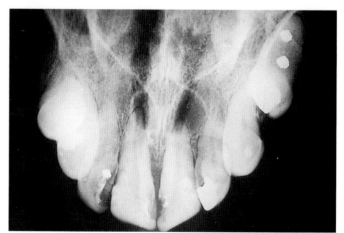

25.22

ODONTOGENIC FIBROMYXOMA

Odontogenic fibromyxoma is a variant of odontogenic myxoma — a rare odontogenic tumour seen mainly in young adult females, and manifests as a painless swelling of either jaw. Plain radiology demonstrates a unilocular or multilocular radiolucency with bone expansion (**Fig. 25.23**). Although benign, the tumour can infiltrate widely and despite wide excision, recurrence is possible. Hence long-term clinical and radiological follow-up is required.

ODONTOGENIC KERATOCYST
(primordial cyst)

Odontogenic cysts are often asymptomatic but may produce an intraoral swelling and occasionally an extraoral swelling (**Figs 25.24, 25.25**). Odontogenic keratocysts are typically seen in young persons and especially in the mandibular molar region (**Fig. 25.26**).

The odontogenic keratocyst has a tendency to recur after removal. Usually seen in isolation, multiple cysts are one feature of Gorlin's syndrome (see Chapter 28).

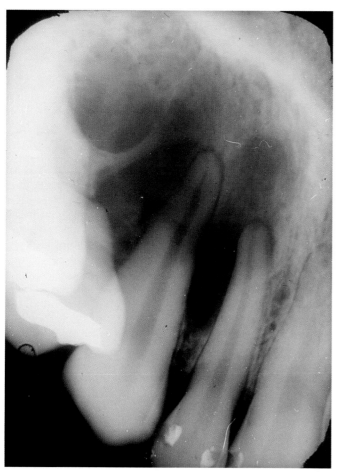

25.23

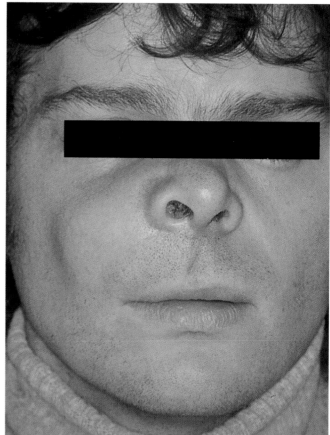

25.24

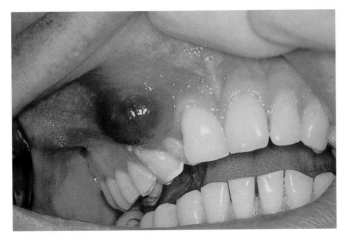

25.25

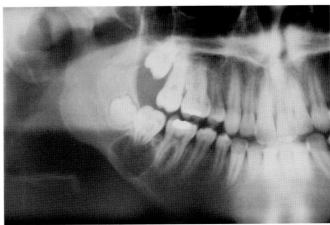

25.26

FURTHER READING

Aithal D, Reddy BS, Mahajan S, Boaz K, Kamboj M. Ameloblastomatous calcifying odontogenic cyst: a rare histologic variant. J Oral Pathol Med 2003; 32(6): 376–8.

Ali M, Baughman RA. Maxillary odontogenic keratocyst: a common and serious clinical misdiagnosis. J Am Dent Assoc 2003; 134(7): 877–83.

Amado-Cuesta S, Gargallo-Albiol J, Berini-Aytes L, Gay-Escoda C. Review of 61 cases of odontoma. Presentation of an erupted complex odontoma. Med Oral 2003; 8(5): 366–73.

Amlashi SF, Riffaud L, Brassier G, Morandi X. Nevoid basal cell carcinoma syndrome: relation with desmoplastic medulloblastoma in infancy. A population-based study and review of the literature. Cancer 2003; 98(3): 618–24.

Anavi Y, Kaplan I, Citir M, Calderon S. Clear-cell variant of calcifying epithelial odontogenic tumor: clinical and radiographic characteristics. Oral Surg Oral Med Oral Pathol Oral Radiol Endod 2003; 95(3): 332–9.

August M, Faquin W, Troulis M, Kaban L. Clear cell odontogenic carcinoma: evaluation of reported cases. J Oral Maxillofac Surg 2003; 61(5): 580–6.

Baughman R, Storoe W, Stuart K. Testing your diagnostic skills. Case no. 1. Odontogenic keratocyst. Todays FDA 2003; 15(5): 16, 18.

Braunshtein E, Vered M, Taicher S, Buchner A. Clear cell odontogenic carcinoma and clear cell ameloblastoma: a single clinicopathologic entity? A new case and comparative analysis of the literature. J Oral Maxillofac Surg 2003; 61(9): 1004–10.

Campbell D, Jeffrey RR, Wallis F, Hulks G, Kerr KM. Metastatic pulmonary ameloblastoma. An unusual case. Br J Oral Maxillofac Surg 2003; 41(3): 194–6.

Carinci F, Francioso F, Piattelli A, Rubini C, Fioroni M, Evangelisti R, Arcelli D, Tosi L, Pezzetti F, Carinci P, Volinia S. Genetic expression profiling of six odontogenic tumors. J Dent Res 2003; 82(7): 551–7.

Carinci F, Volinia S, Rubini C, Fioroni M, Francioso F, Arcelli D, Pezzetti F, Piattelli A. Genetic profile of clear cell odontogenic carcinoma. J Craniofac Surg 2003; 14(3): 356–62.

Cleveland DB, Rinaggio J, Schneider L. Oral pathology quiz #38. Case 4. Odontogenic keratocysts. JNJ Dent Assoc 2003; 74(1): 23, 37.

Dhir K, Sciubba J, Tufano RP. Ameloblastic carcinoma of the maxilla. Oral Oncol 2003; 39(7): 736–41.

Dunsche A, Babendererde O, Luttges J, Springer IN. Dentigerous cyst versus unicystic ameloblastoma – differential diagnosis in routine histology. J Oral Pathol Med 2003; 32(8): 486–91.

Edgin W, Simmons R, Terezhalmy GT, Moore WS. Ameloblastoma. Quintessence Int 2003; 34(5): 394–5.

Ertas U, Yavuz MS. Interesting eruption of 4 teeth associated with a large dentigerous cyst in mandible by only marsupialization. J Oral Maxillofac Surg 2003; 61(6): 728–30.

Fenton S, Slootweg PJ, Dunnebier EA, Mourits MP. Odontogenic myxoma in a 17-month-old child: a case report. J Oral Maxillofac Surg 2003; 61(6): 734–6.

Fregnani ER, Fillipi RZ, Oliveira CR, Vargas PA, Almeida OP. Odontomas and ameloblastomas: variable prevalences around the world? Oral Oncol 2002; 38(8): 807–8.

Gruica B, Stauffer E, Buser D, Bornstein M. Meloblastoma of the follicular, plexiform, and acanthomatous type in the maxillary sinus: a case report. Quintessence Int 2003; 34(4): 311–14.

Ide F, Saito I. Many faces of odontogenic keratocyst. Oral Oncol 2003; 39(2): 204–5.

Kumar M, Fasanmade A, Barrett AW, Mack G, Newman L, Hyde NC. Metastasising clear cell odontogenic carcinoma: a case report and review of the literature. Oral Oncol 2003; 39(2): 190–4.

Levin MP, Kratochvil FJ, Nolan J. Ameloblastoma of the mandible: a case report. J Periodontol 2003; 74(6): 883–6.

Liapatas S, Nakou M, Rontogianni D. Inflammatory infiltrate of chronic periradicular lesions: an immunohistochemical study. Int Endod J 2003; 36(7): 464–71.

McGuff HS, Alderson GL, Jones AC. Oral and maxillofacial pathology case of the month. Gingival cyst of the adult. Tex Dent J 2003; 120(1): 108, 112.

Mosqueda-Taylor A, Carlos-Bregni R, Ramirez-Amador V, Palma-Guzman JM, Esquivel-Bonilla D, Hernandez-Rojase LA. Odontoameloblastoma. Clinico-pathologic study of three cases and critical review of the literature. Oral Oncol 2002; 38(8): 800–5.

Ng KH, Siar CH. Odontogenic keratocyst with dentinoid formation. Oral Surg Oral Med Oral Pathol Oral Radiol Endod 2003; 95(5): 601–6.

Olasoji HO, Enwere ON. Treatment of ameloblastoma — a review. Niger J Med 2003; 12(1): 7–11.

Oliver RJ, Coulthard P, Carre C, Sloan P. Solitary adult myofibroma of the mandible simulating an odontogenic cyst. Oral Oncol 2003; 39(6): 626–9.

Reichart PA, Philipsen HP. Odontogenic tumors and allied lesions. Quintessence Books, London 2004: 1–387.

Reichart PA, Philipsen HP. Revision of the 1992 edition of the WHO histological typing of odontogenic tumors. A suggestion. Mund Kiefer Gesichtschir 2003; 7(2): 88–93.

Robledo J, Alderson GL, Jones AC, McGuff HS, Peterson T, Potter M. Oral and maxillofacial pathology case of the month. Odontogenic myxoma. Tex Dent J 2003; 120(7): 616, 621.

Simon D, Somanathan T, Ramdas K, Pandey M. Central mucoepidermoid carcinoma of mandible — a case report and review of the literature. World J Surg Oncol 2003; 1(1): 1.

Ustuner E, Fitoz S, Atasoy C, Erden I, Akyar S. Bilateral maxillary dentigerous cysts: a case report. Oral Surg Oral Med Oral Pathol Oral Radiol Endod 2003; 95(5): 632–5.

White DK, Street CC, Jenkins WS, Clark AR, Ford JE. Panoramic radiograph in pathology. Atlas Oral Maxillofac Surg Clin North Am 2003; 11(1): 1–53.

Yamazaki M, Cheng J, Nomura T, Saito C, Hayashi T, Saku T. Maxillary odontogenic keratocyst with respiratory epithelium: a case report. J Oral Pathol Med 2003; 32(8): 496–8.

26 DISORDERS OF BONE

- Albright's syndrome (McCune–Albright syndrome)
- alveolar atrophy
- aneurysmal bone cyst
- cemento-ossifying fibroma (cementifying fibroma)
- cherubism (familial fibrous dysplasia)
- dry socket (alveolar osteitis)
- exostoses
- fibrous dysplasia

- giant cell granuloma (central giant cell granuloma)
- haemorrhagic bone cyst (simple bone cyst)
- ossifying fibroma
- osteomyelitis
- Paget's disease (osteitis deformans)
- Stafne bone cavity (latent bone cyst)
- torus mandibularis
- torus palatinus.

ALBRIGHT'S SYNDROME *(McCune–Albright syndrome)*

Albright's syndrome is the association of polyostotic fibrous dysplasia with cutaneous hyperpigmentation (**Figs 26.1–26.3**), precocious puberty and occasionally other endocrine disorders. Oral hyperpigmentation is occasionally a feature of Albright's syndrome (**Fig. 26.4**).

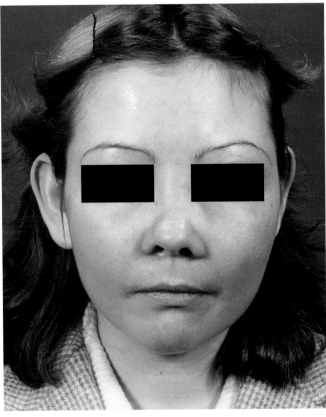

26.1

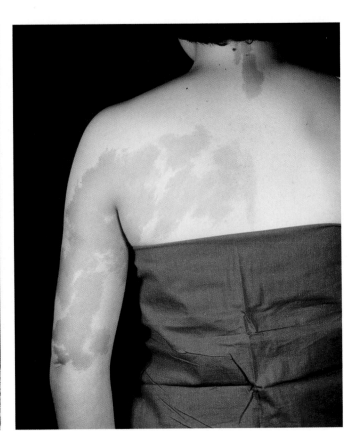

26.2

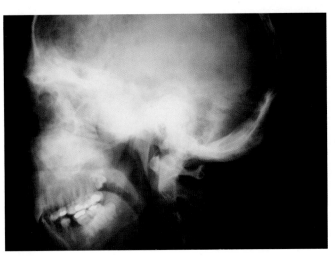

26.3

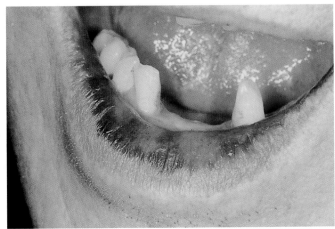

26.4

ALVEOLAR ATROPHY

The alveolar bone of the jaw normally bears the teeth. When teeth are removed, or exfoliate in periodontitis, the alveolar bone atrophies and the jaw occasionally becomes so thin (**Fig. 26.5**) that denture retention is difficult and implants need bone augmentation to place; in extreme cases the mandible fractures under relatively little stress.

Osteoporosis may affect the jaws as with other bones and is seen particularly in postmenopausal women and patients taking systemic corticosteroids. It is also seen in short-bowel syndrome.

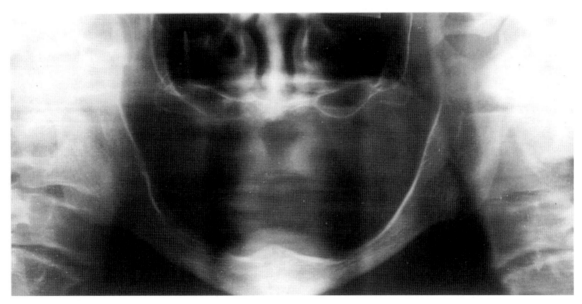

26.5

ANEURYSMAL BONE CYST

Aneurysmal bone cysts present as painless swellings of the posterior mandible or maxilla, usually in early adulthood. The lesions manifest radiologically as unilocular, and less commonly multilocular, radiolucencies with bony expansion and displacement and external resorption of adjacent teeth (**Figs 26.6–26.8**). Of note they are characterized histopathologically by the absence of an epithelial lining having instead, areas of sinusoidal blood spaces lined by connective tissue. Wide surgical excision is required.

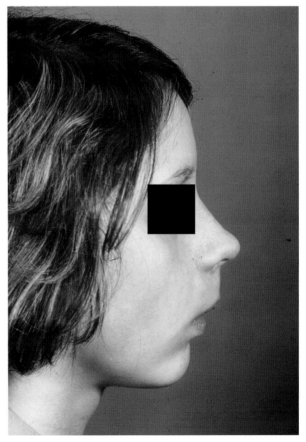

26.6

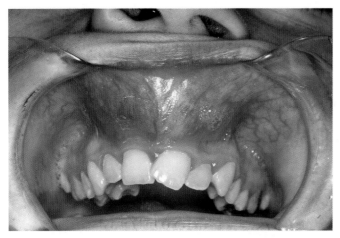

26.7

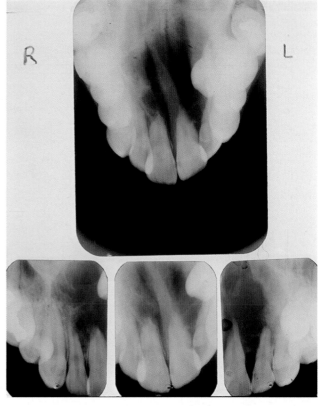

26.8

CEMENTO-OSSIFYING FIBROMA
(cementifying fibroma)

Cemento-ossifying fibroma is an uncommon odontogenic tumour manifesting as a painless swelling of the jaws. Radiologically it appears as a well-defined radiolucency with varying amounts of calcification (Figs 26.9, 26.10). Enucleation is often effective as the lesion is usually encapsulated and recurrence rare.

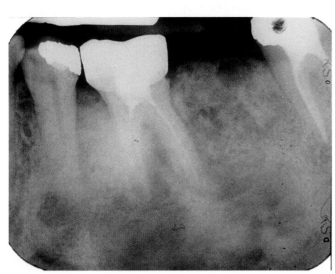

26.10

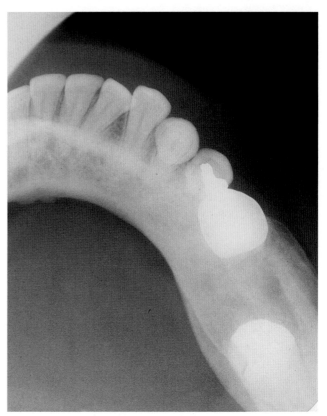

26.9

CHERUBISM *(familial fibrous dysplasia)*

Cherubism is the term given to a familial type of fibrous dysplasia which typically affects the angles of the mandible to produce a cherubic appearance (**Fig. 26.11**).

This is an autosomal dominant trait (**Fig. 26.12** is the brother of the patient in **Fig. 26.11**). Cherubism is seen especially in males and presents usually after the age of 4–5 years.

The radiograph shows multilocular mandibular radiolucencies, expansion of the mandible and absent second molar (**Fig. 26.13**), features common to cherubism. The swellings increase in size and then at puberty usually regress, at least partially. Occasionally the maxillae are involved.

Rarely, cherubism may be associated with Noonan's syndrome (short stature, neck webbing, cubitus valgus and often cardiac anomalies) (**Fig. 26.14**).

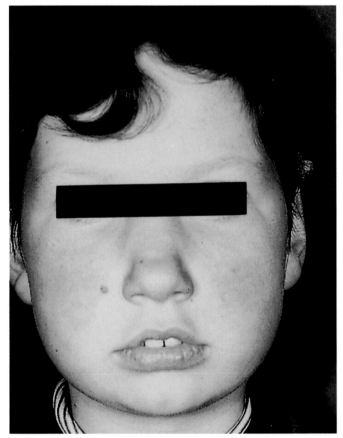

26.11

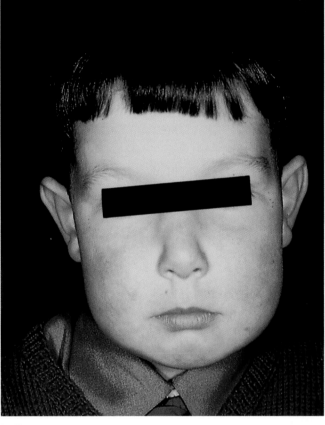

26.12

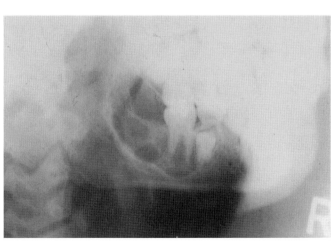

26.13

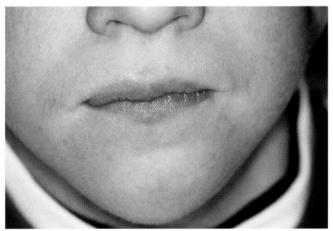

26.14

DRY SOCKET *(alveolar osteitis)*

If the blood clot in an extraction socket breaks down, presumably from the action of fibrinolysins, then the socket is said to be 'dry'.

Dry socket manifests with the onset of fairly severe pain 2–4 days after extraction, a bad taste in the mouth and halitosis. The socket has no clot and the surrounding mucosa is inflamed (**Figs 26.15–26.17**).

Dry socket is typically seen after extractions in young persons, in the mandible, in the molar region, after extractions under local anaesthesia and after traumatic extractions. Oral contraceptive use and smoking predispose to dry socket as do any immunocompromising conditions or bone disorders such as Paget's disease. Healing is aided if debris (such as the pea in **Fig. 26.17**) is irrigated away and the socket dressed.

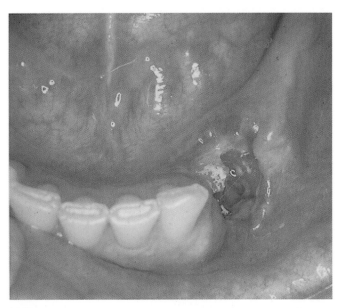

26.15

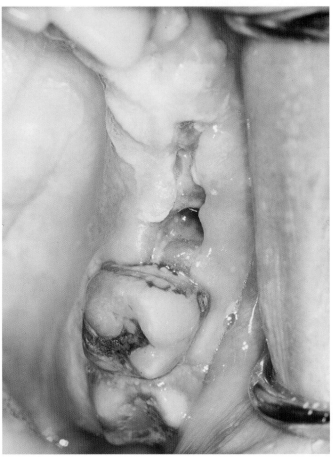

26.16

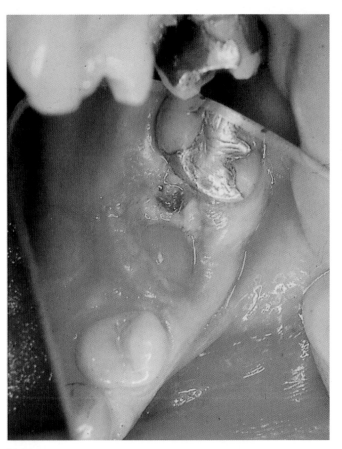

26.17

EXOSTOSES

Exostoses buccal to the maxillary posterior teeth are fairly common (**Fig. 26.18**) but the possibility of osteomas and Gardner's syndrome should be considered (Chapter 28).

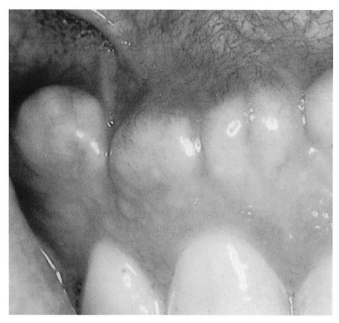

26.18

FIBROUS DYSPLASIA

Fibrous dysplasia is an uncommon benign fibro-osseous lesion, of unknown aetiology and often affecting one bone (**Fig. 26.19**). The swelling may cause facial swelling (**Figs 26.20, 26.21** are the same patient) and/or swelling intraorally (**Figs 26.22, 26.23** are the same patient) but it is painless and typically ceases to grow at the time of skeletal maturity.

Four subgroups of fibrous dysplasia have been described:

- monostotic (Jaffe–Lichtenstein syndrome)
- polyostotic
- polyostotic fibrous dysplasia of Albright's syndrome
- a form confined to the craniofacial complex (craniofacial fibrous dysplasia).

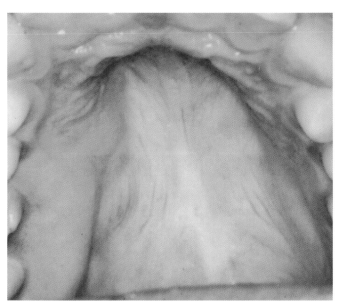

26.19

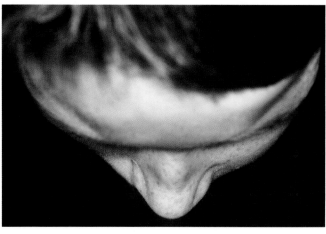

26.20

The typical appearance on radiography is of a 'ground glass' pattern (**Figs 26.24–26.26**). Scans confirm the lesion (**Fig. 26.27**) and bone scan using technetium diphosphonate shows an increased uptake of radionuclide in fibrous dysplasia (**Fig. 26.28**).

Several bones may be affected (**Fig. 26.29**; here the humerus is involved).

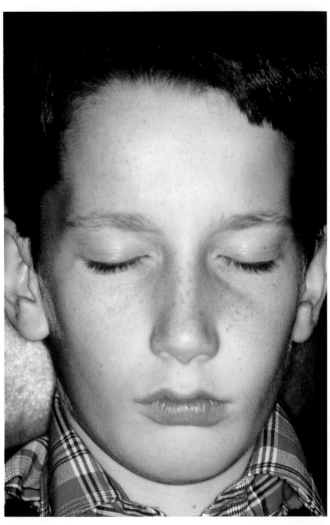

26.21

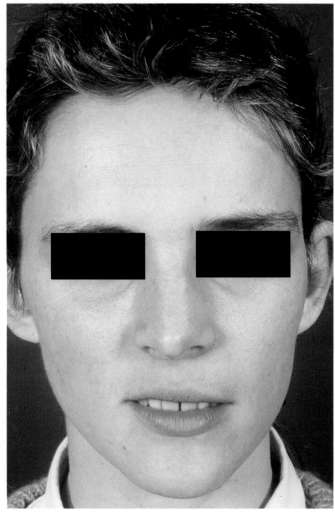

26.22

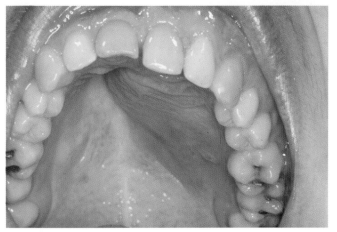

26.23

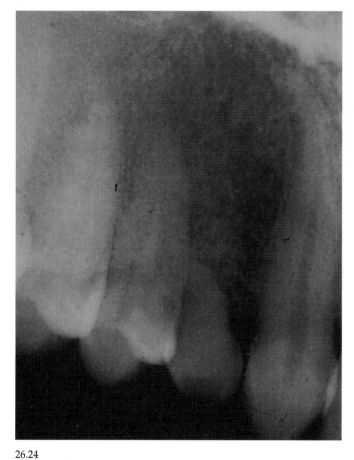

26.24

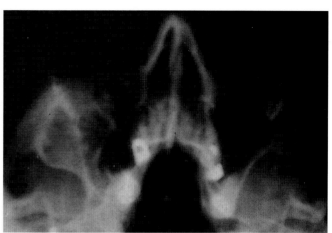

26.25

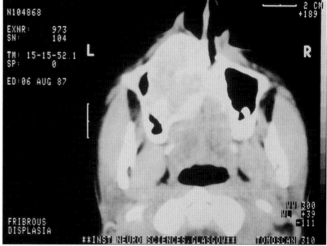

26.27

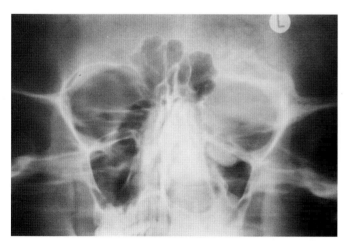

26.26

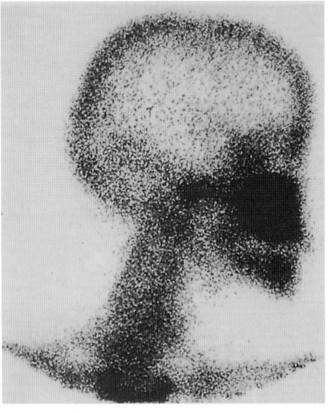

26.28

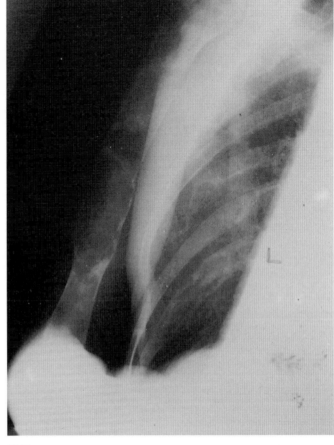

26.29

GIANT CELL GRANULOMA *(central giant cell granuloma or giant cell reparative granuloma)*

Central giant cell granuloma is an uncommon lesion that tends to arise in the anterior mandible as a painless swelling, and radiologically gives rise to a well-defined unilocular or multilocular radiolucency (Fig. 26.30). Despite the title, these lesions do not contain granulomas but instead comprise vascular connective tissue with many giant cells. The histopathological features are identical to those of the bony lesions of hyperparathyroidism although patients with central giant cell granuloma do not have such disease. Curettage is the typical treatment.

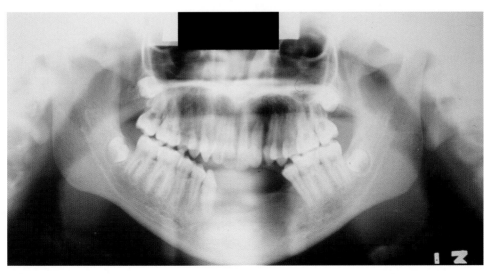

26.30

HAEMORRHAGIC BONE CYST
(simple bone cyst)

The simple bone cyst almost always occurs in the mandible, rarely affecting the maxilla, and is almost identical to the solitary or unicameral bone cyst, it is frequently located in the metaphyses of the upper extremity of the humerus or the femur in teenagers. Haemorrhagic bone cysts occur mainly in patients, between 20 and 40 years old, most of whom are diagnosed in the second decade of life (**Fig. 26.31**).

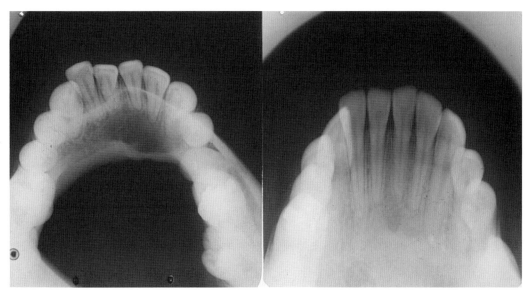

26.31

OSSIFYING FIBROMA

This is now regarded as a cemento-ossifying fibroma: see above (**Figs 26.32–26.35**).

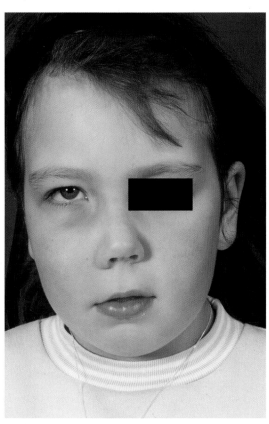

26.32

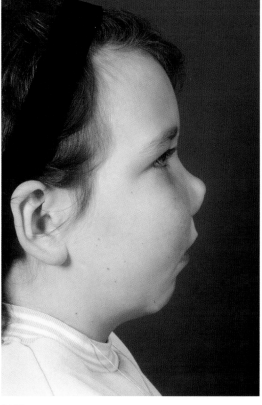

26.33

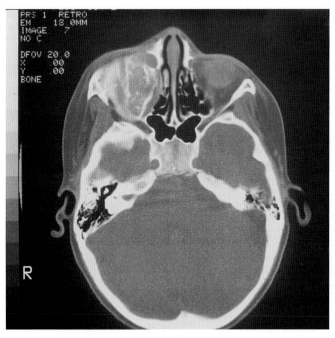

26.34

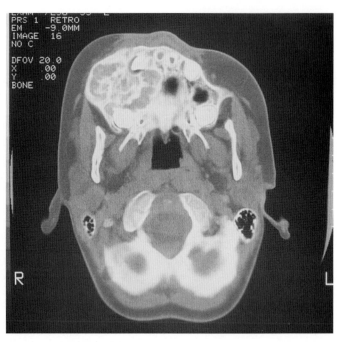

26.35

OSTEOMYELITIS

Osteomyelitis is an infection of the bone, rare in the jaws. It is predisposed by various immune defects, diabetes mellitus, Paget's disease, osteopetrosis, irradiation or local factors such as foreign bodies.

Acute osteomyelitis is mainly seen in the mandible, the infection usually originating from odontogenic infection or trauma. Extreme pain, swelling (**Fig. 26.36**), labial anaesthesia, tenderness on biting and eventual discharge of pus (**Fig. 26.37**) are the main features.

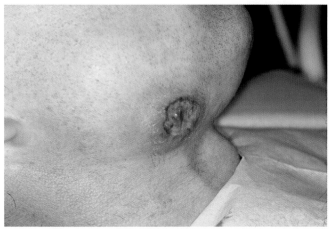

26.36

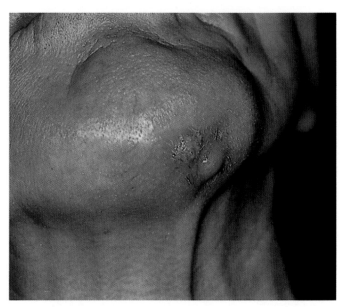

26.37

Figures **26.38–26.40** show a sequence from a patient with rare maxillary osteomyelitis. At the early stage (see **Fig. 26.38**) there was pain and swelling by the upper second premolar and first molar, which were then extracted. Two months later, a sequestrum appeared (see **Fig. 26.39**).

After a further 2 weeks the necrotic bone sequestrates (see **Fig. 26.40**). The sequestrum is shown in **Fig. 26.41**. Sequestration may occur intra- or extra-orally.

Radiological signs of osteomyelitis take some weeks to develop but the bone eventually becomes 'moth-eaten' (**Fig. 26.42**).

Acute osteomyelitis is rare in the maxilla and, when seen, is usually in neonates (**Fig. 26.43**). It is possible that *Staphylococcus aureus* infects the maxilla, either haematogenously or entering via an oral wound.

Proliferative periostitis is an uncommon, chronic, low-grade infection, seen usually in the lower molar region (**Fig. 26.44**). There are several clinical patterns of chronic osteomyelitis.

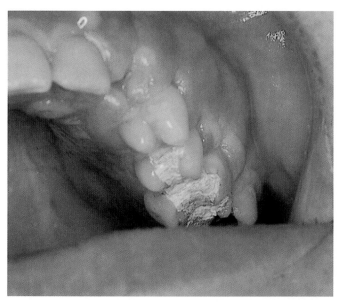

26.38

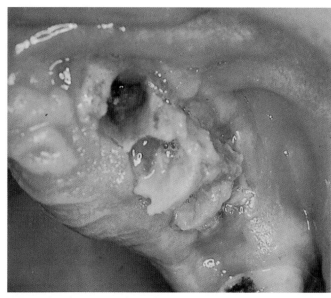

26.39

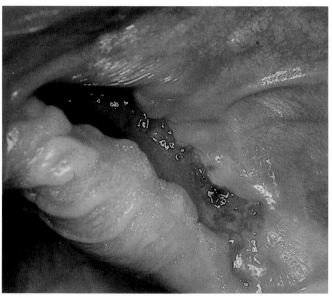

26.40

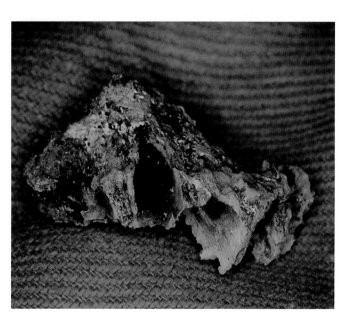

26.41

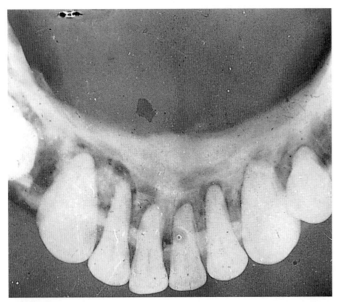

26.42

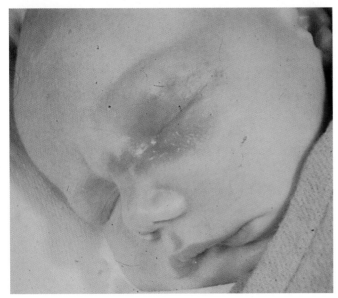

26.43

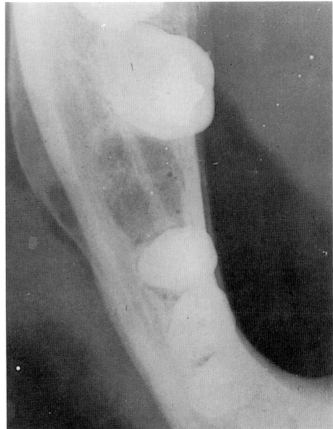

26.44

PAGET'S DISEASE *(osteitis deformans)*

Paget's disease of bone is common in Western countries, particularly the UK and in males aged over 50 years. It is of unknown aetiology, possibly viral, and usually presents with swelling, often of the skull bones. The calvarium thickens in about half of the patients with clinical Paget's disease.

Swelling of the maxilla (leontiasis ossea) may be seen in Paget's disease (**Fig. 26.45**; the same patient after 4 years shows an increase in maxillary swelling in **Fig. 26.46**).

Apart from the maxillary swelling, the teeth may become spaced (**Fig. 26.47**).

The skull bones thicken (**Fig. 26.48**) and show a 'cotton wool' appearance on radiography (**Figs 26.49–26.52**). There may be overgrowth at the skull base.

The radiolucent lesions (**Figs 26.50, 26.51**) are termed osteitis crani circumscripta. **Figure 26.52** shows chronic osteomyelitis with seqeustra following third molar removal. Hypercementosis is a common feature, affecting the jaws (**Fig. 26.53**). It can complicate tooth extraction, which is sometimes accompanied by profuse haemorrhage.

The sacral and lumbar vertebrae, pelvis, tibiae and femur are commonly involved. The affected bones soften and bend (**Fig. 26.54**).

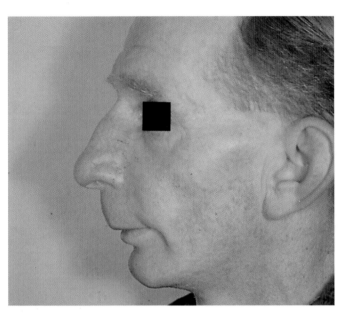

26.45

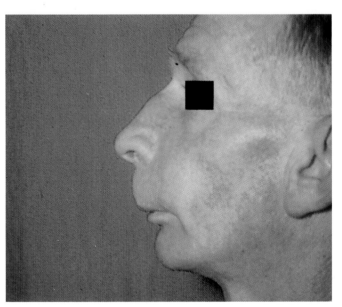

26.46

26.47

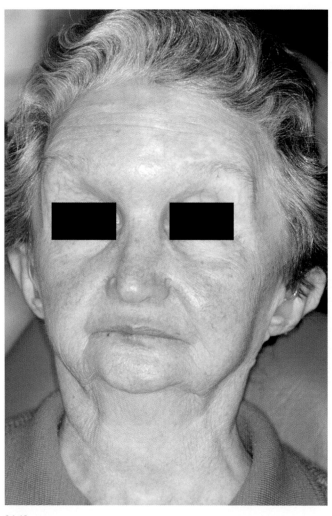

26.48

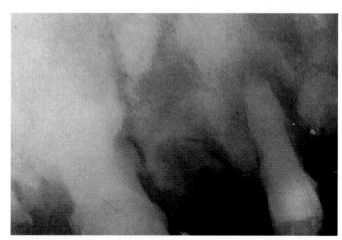

26.49

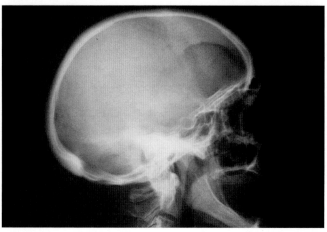

26.50

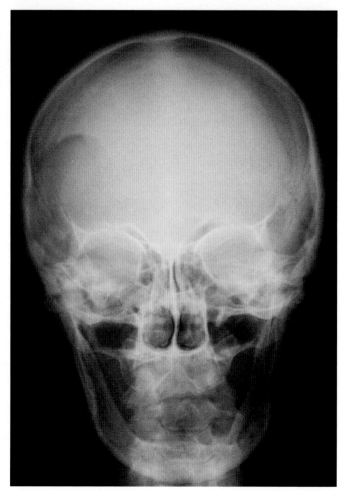

26.51

Lytic areas are seen in long bones in the early phase of Paget's disease (**Fig. 26.55**). The bone shows an irregularly widened cortex and sometimes perpendicular radiolucent lines (cortical infractions) or fractures.

Pelvic changes include bone resorption, new bone formation and a thickening of the pelvic brim (**Fig. 26.56**; here there is mainly innominate and ilial involvement).

Osteosarcoma (**Fig. 26.57**) is a rare complication of Paget's disease and is particularly unusual in the jaws.

Other complications include pathological fractures, spinal compression, arteriovenous shunts that may lead to high-output cardiac failure, calcific aortic valve disease, cranial nerve palsies and postextraction haemorrhage or infection.

Hyperostosis corticalis deformans juvenilis is a rare disorder that may be a juvenile form of Paget's disease with skull and maxillary enlargement and bowing of the legs.

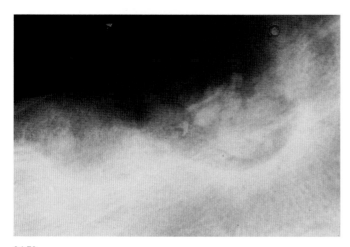

26.52

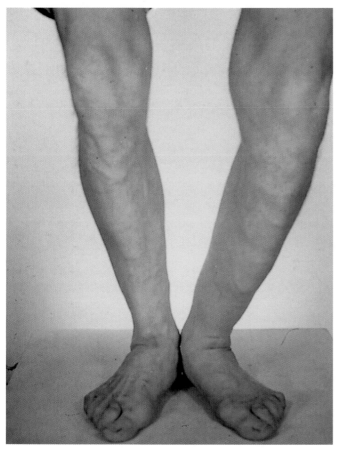

26.54

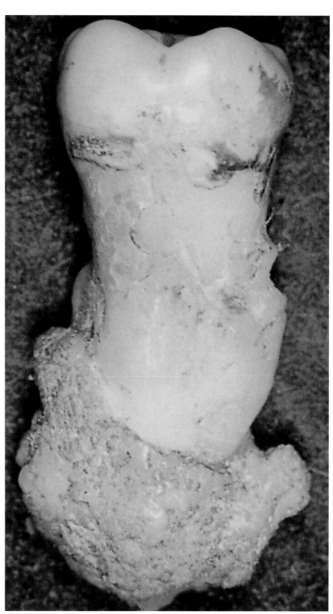

26.53

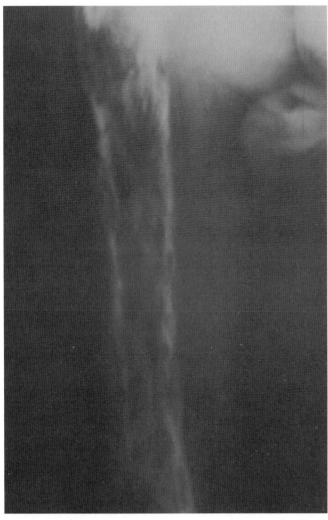

26.55

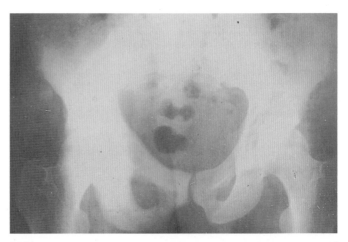

26.56

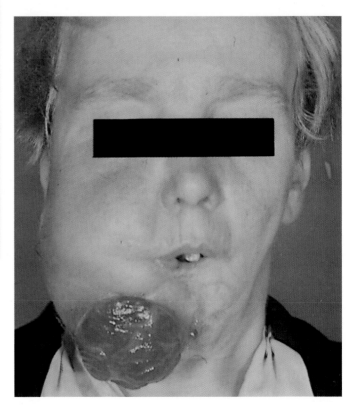

26.57

STAFNE BONE CAVITY
(latent bone cyst)

A Stafne 'cyst' is not a cyst at all but a well-demarcated radiolucency at the lower border of the mandible, always below the inferior alveolar canal (**Fig. 26.58**). It contains some normal submandibular salivary gland tissue and is a developmental defect.

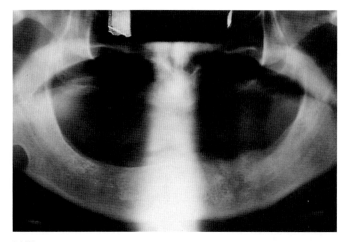

26.58

TORUS MANDIBULARIS

Mandibular tori are uni- or bilateral bony lumps lingual to the lower premolars (**Figs 26.59–26.61**). They are of developmental origin and benign. Tori are fairly common (found in about 60% of the population of the UK) but are especially seen in mongoloid races. They are said to be more common in parafunctional states.

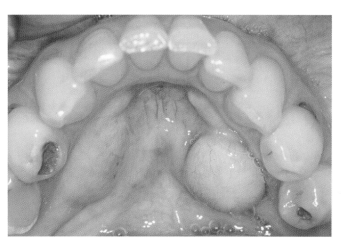

26.59

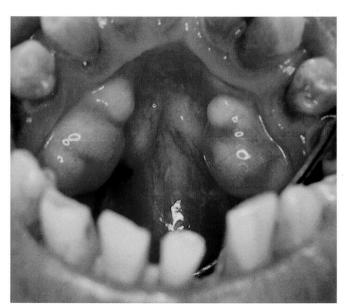

26.60

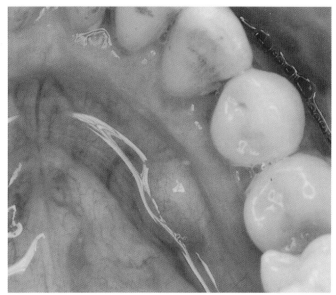

26.61

TORUS PALATINUS

Palatal tori are common bony lumps (seen in up to 20% of the population of the UK) and typically in the midline vault of the palate (**Figs 26.62–26.64**).

Palatal tori are most common in mongoloid races and can sometimes be quite protrusive. Again, they are benign.

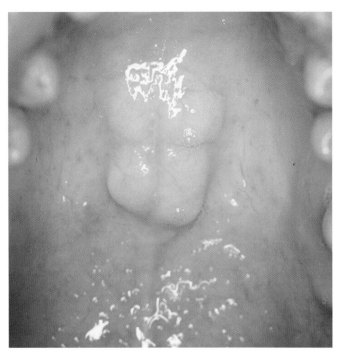

26.62

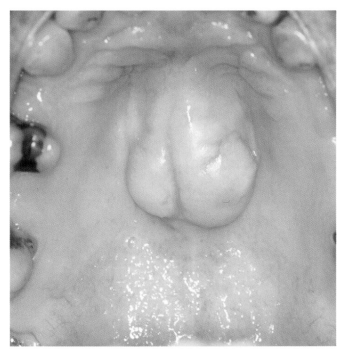

26.63

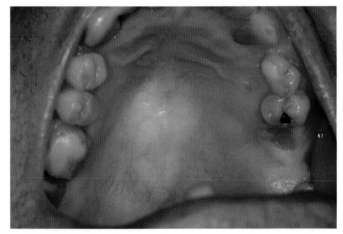

26.64

FURTHER READING

Adeyemo WL. Re: critical review on dry socket. Int J Oral Maxillofac Surg 2003; 32(1): 111.

Akintoye SO, Lee JS, Feimster T, *et al.* Dental characteristics of fibrous dysplasia and McCune–Albright syndrome. Oral Surg Oral Med Oral Pathol Oral Radiol Endod 2003; 96(3): 275–82.

Alawi F. Benign fibro-osseous diseases of the maxillofacial bones. A review and differential diagnosis. Am J Clin Pathol 2002; 118 Suppl: S50–70.

Belsky JL, Hamer JS, Hubert JE, Insogna K, Johns W. Torus palatinus: a new anatomical correlation with bone density in postmenopausal women. J Clin Endocrinol Metab 2003; 88(5): 2081–6.

Blum IR. Contemporary views on dry socket (alveolar osteitis): a clinical appraisal of standardization, aetiopathogenesis and management: a critical review. Int J Oral Maxillofac Surg 2002; 31(3): 309–17.

Chohayeb AA, Volpe AR. Occurrence of torus palatinus and mandibularis among women of different ethnic groups. Am J Dent 2001; 14(5): 278–80.

Hosking D, Meunier PJ, Ringe JD, *et al.* Paget's disease of bone: diagnosis and management. Br Med J 1996; 312: 491–4.

Houston JP, McCollum J, Pietz D, Schneck D. Alveolar osteitis: a review of its etiology, prevention, and treatment modalities. Gen Dent 2002; 50(5): 457–63.

Kozakiewicz M, Perczynska-Partyka W, Kobos J. Cherubism — clinical picture and treatment. Oral Dis 2001; 7: 123–30.

Lindholm TS. Bone Morphogenetic Proteins: Biology, Biochemistry and Reconstructive Surgery. San Diego, Academic Press, 1996.

Paganini-Hill A. The benefits of estrogen replacement therapy on oral health. Arch Intern Med 1996; 155: 2325–9.

Reuther T, Schuster T, Mende U, Kubler A. Osteoradionecrosis of the jaws as a side effect of radiotherapy of head and neck tumour patients — a report of a thirty year retrospective review. Int J Oral Maxillofac Surg 2003; 32(3): 289–95.

Schultze-Mosgau S, Holbach LM, Wiltfang J. Cherubism: clinical evidence and therapy. J Craniofac Surg 2003; 14: 201–6.

Scully C, Watt-Smith P, Dios RD, Giangrande PL. Complications in HIV-infected and non-HIV-infected haemophiliacs and other patients after oral surgery. Int J Oral Maxillofac Surg 2002; 31(6): 634–40.

Stephen LX, Hamersma H, Gardner J, Beighton P. Dental and oral manifestations of sclerosteosis. Int Dent J 2001; 51(4): 287–90.

Talbott JF, Gorti GK, Koch RJ. Midfacial osteomyelitis in a chronic cocaine abuser: a case report. Ear Nose Throat J 2001; 80(10): 738–40.

Von Wowern N. General and oral aspects of osteoporosis: a review. Clin Oral Invest 2001; 5: 71–82.

Wheeler TT, Alberts MA, Dolan TA, McGorray SP. Dental, visual, auditory and olfactory complications in Paget's disease of bone. J Am Geriatr Soc 1995; 43(12): 1384–91.

27 JOINT DISORDERS

- condylar anklosis
- polyvinyl chloride acro-osteolysis
- temporomandibular joint arthritides
- temporomandibular joint subluxation
- temporomandibular joint pain-dysfunction syndrome.

CONDYLAR ANKYLOSIS

Condylar ankylosis can result from infection, arthritis, or trauma and leads to deviation of the chin towards the affected side (**Figs 27.1, 27.2**)—the right in these figures.

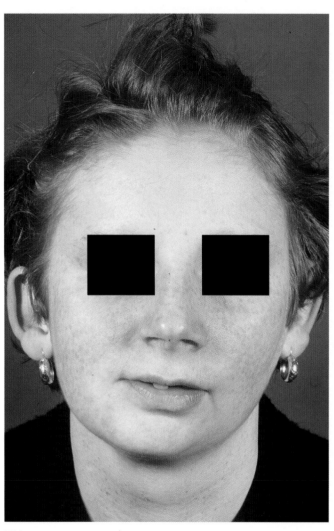

27.1

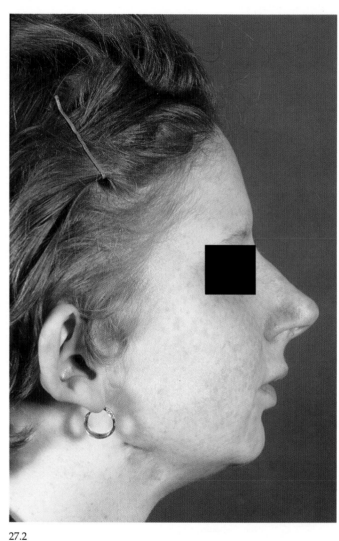

27.2

POLYVINYL CHLORIDE ACRO-OSTEOLYSIS

Occupational exposure to polyvinyl chloride may rarely cause a scleroderma-like disorder, sometimes with destruction of the mandibular condyle (**Fig. 27.3**) or resorption of the zygomatic arches.

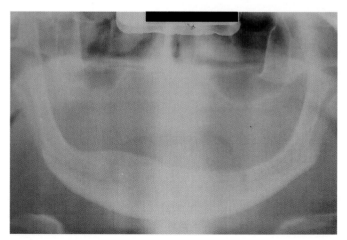

27.3

TEMPOROMANDIBULAR JOINT ARTHRITIDES

Apart from rheumatoid arthritis and osteoarthritis, psoriatic arthritis and, rarely, infective arthritis may be encountered. Rheumatoid arthritis may result in limited opening or anterior open bite, and is often associated with Sjögren's syndrome.

Osteoarthrosis may also affect the TMJ but, unlike rheumatoid arthritis, virtually never causes ankylosis.

Pyogenic arthritis of the temporomandibular joint (TMJ) is rare but may follow a penetrating injury. It may result from contiguous infection, especially from the middle ear or it may be haematogenous, for example, gonococcal, tuberculous, salmonella or from other infective arthritides (**Fig. 27.4**). Infection may result in micrognathia and ankylosis.

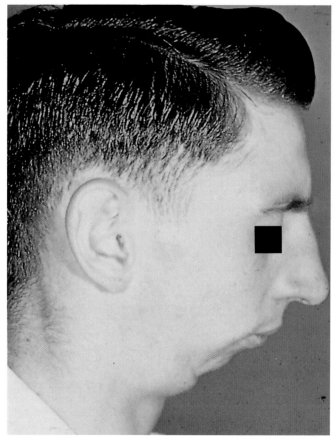

27.4

TEMPOROMANDIBULAR JOINT SUBLUXATION

Some patients are able to sublux their TMJ deliberately (**Fig. 27.5**). Subluxation is especially liable to occur in hypermobility conditions, such as Ehlers–Danlos syndrome (**Figs 27.6, 27.7**).

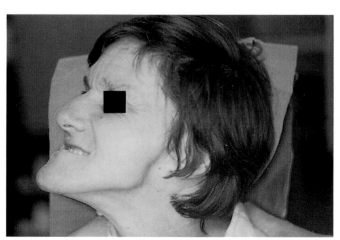

27.5

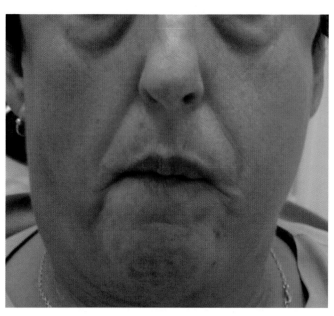

27.6

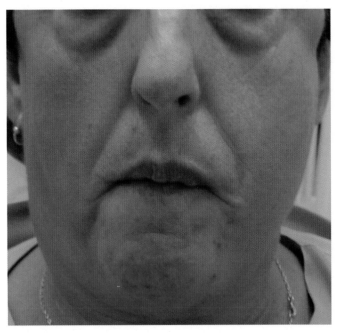

27.7

TEMPOROMANDIBULAR PAIN-DYSFUNCTION SYNDROME

A common complaint is of discomfort and/or clicking and/or locking of the TMJ. Seen predominantly in young adult females the aetiology is unclear but may include psychogenic and/or occlusal factors. Clinical features include normal radiographic findings or sometimes narrowing of the joint space, but there is discomfort on palpation of the TMJ and masticatory muscles, sometimes crepitus, and limitation of mandibular movements. **Figure 27.8** shows a girl who has caused erythema on the face by repeatedly rubbing the painful area. Pain-dysfunction syndrome of the TMJ may be associated with other disorders which have a psychogenic element.

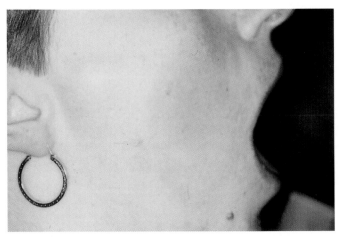

27.8

FURTHER READING

Bonjardim LR, Gaviao MB, Carmagnani FG, Pereira LJ, Castelo PM. Signs and symptoms of temporomandibular joint dysfunction in children with primary dentition. J Clin Pediatr Dent 2003; 28(1): 53–8.

Church CA, Rowe M, Llaurado R, Liwnicz BH, Martin PA. Pigmented villonodular synovitis of the temporomandibular joint: a report of two cases. Ear Nose Throat J 2003; 82(9): 692–5.

Conti A, Freitas M, Conti P, Henriques J, Janson G. Relationship between signs and symptoms of temporomandibular disorders and orthodontic treatment: a cross-sectional study. Angle Orthod 2003; 73(4): 411–17.

Defabianis P. Post-traumatic TMJ internal derangement: impact on facial growth (findings in a pediatric age group). J Clin Pediatr Dent 2003; 27(4): 297–303.

Donaldson KW. Rheumatoid diseases and the temporomandibular joint: a review. Cranio 1995; 13(4): 264–9.

Goulet JP. Contemporary approach to the nonsurgical management of temporomandibular disorders. Alpha Omegan 2003; 96(2): 47–56.

Heo MS, An BM, Lee SS, Choi SC. Use of advanced imaging modalities for the differential diagnosis of pathoses mimicking temporomandibular disorders. Oral Surg Oral Med Oral Pathol Oral Radiol Endod 2003; 96(5): 630–8.

Kapur N, Kamel IR, Herlich A. Oral and craniofacial pain: diagnosis, pathophysiology, and treatment. Int Anesthesiol Clin 2003; 41(3): 115–50.

Kent JN, Carlton DM, Zide MF. Rheumatoid disease and related arthropathies. Oral Surg Oral Med Oral Pathol 1986; 61: 432–9.

Macfarlane TV, Gray RJM, Kincey J, Worthington HV. Factors associated with the temporomandibular disorder, pain dysfunction syndrome (PDS): Manchester case-control study. Oral Dis 2001; 7: 321–30.

Manganello-Souza LC, Mariani PB. Temporomandibular joint ankylosis: report of 14 cases. Int J Oral Maxillofac Surg 2003; 32(1): 24–9.

Nitzan DW. Rationale and indications for arthrocentesis of the temporomandibular joint. Alpha Omegan 2003; 96(2): 57–63.

Pereira FJ. Disorders of the temporomandibular joint. What comes next? Oral Dis 2002; 8(1): 1–2.

Rhodus NL, Fricton J, Carlson P, Messner R. Oral symptoms associated with fibromyalgia syndrome. J Rheumatol 2003; 30(8): 1841–5.

Sieber M, Grubenmann E, Ruggia GM, Palla S. Relation between stress and symptoms of craniomandibular disorders in adolescents. Schweiz Monatsschr Zahnmed 2003; 113(6): 648–54.

Suvinen TI, Reade PC, Kononen M, Kemppainen P. Vertical jaw separation and masseter muscle electromyographic activity: a comparative study between asymptomatic controls and patients with temporomandibular pain and dysfunction. J Oral Rehabil 2003; 30(8): 765–72.

28 CONGENITAL AND DEVELOPMENTAL DISORDERS

- abnormal labial fraenum
- absent uvula
- ankyloglossia (tongue-tie)
- Apert's syndrome (acrocephalosyndactyly)
- Ascher's syndrome
- bifid uvula (cleft uvula)
- blue rubber-bleb naevus syndrome (Bean's syndrome)
- branchial cyst
- Caffey's disease (infantile cortical hyperostosis)
- Carney's syndrome
- Chievitz's organ
- chondroectodermal dysplasia (Ellis–van Creveld syndrome)
- cleft lip and palate
- cleidocranial dysplasia (cleidocranial dysostosis)
- Cowden's syndrome (multiple hamartoma and neoplasia syndrome)
- craniofacial microsomia
- craniometaphyseal dysplasia
- cri du chat syndrome
- Crouzon's syndrome (craniofacial dysostosis)
- cystic hygroma
- Darier's disease (dyskeratosis follicularis)
- de Lange's syndrome (Amsterdam dwarf)
- Down's syndrome
- dyskeratosis congenita
- ectodermal dysplasia
- Ehlers–Danlos syndrome
- epidermolysis bullosa
- epiloia (tuberous sclerosis; Bourneville–Pringle disease)
- familial gingival fibromatosis
- fissured tongue (scrotal or plicated tongue)
- Fordyce's spots
- fragile X syndrome (Martin–Bell syndrome)
- Gardner's syndrome
- Gorlin's syndrome (Gorlin–Goltz syndrome; multiple basal cell naevi syndrome)
- Hallermann–Streiff syndrome
- hemifacial hypertrophy
- hereditary haemorrhagic telangiectasia
- hereditary palmoplantar keratoses
- ichthyosis
- incontinentia pigmenti (Bloch–Sulzberger disease)
- Klippel–Trenaunay–Weber syndrome
- Laband's syndrome
- leukoedema
- lip pit
- Maffucci's syndrome
- Marfan's syndrome
- mucinosis
- myotonic dystrophy (Steinert's syndrome)
- naevi
- Olmsted's syndrome
- orofaciodigital syndrome
- osteogenesis imperfecta (fragilitas ossium)
- osteopetrosis (Albers–Schönberg syndrome)
- pachyonychia congenita
- Patau's syndrome
- Peutz–Jegher's syndrome (lentigo polyposis)
- Pierre Robin sequence syndrome
- racial pigmentation
- Romberg's syndrome (Parry–Romberg syndrome; progressive hemifacial atrophy)
- Smith–Lemli–Opitz syndrome
- Sturge–Weber syndrome (encephalofacial angiomatosis)
- tetralogy of Fallot
- thyroid (lingual)
- tori
- Treacher Collins' syndrome (mandibulofacial dysostosis)
- Van der Woude syndrome
- Von Recklinghausen's disease (generalized neurofibromatosis)
- white sponge naevus (familial white folded gingivostomatosis).

ABNORMAL LABIAL FRAENUM

A labial maxillary fraenum may occasionally be associated with spacing between the central incisors — a maxillary median diastema (**Fig. 28.1**). **Figure 28.2**, which is the same patient as in **Fig. 28.1**, shows the palatal attachment of the fraenum.

ABSENT UVULA

The uvula is rarely absent (**Fig. 28.3**) and then usually as a result of trauma or surgery. The uvula may be hypoplastic in Cowden's syndrome.

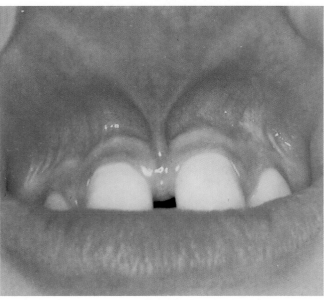

28.1

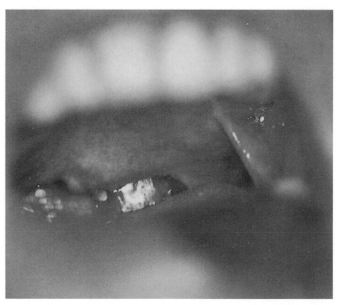

28.3

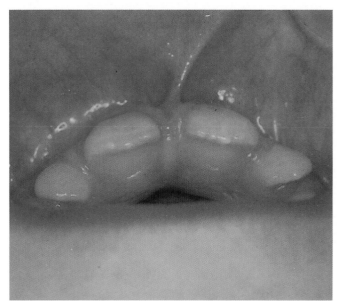

28.2

ANKYLOGLOSSIA *(tongue-tie)*

Ankyloglossia (**Fig. 28.4**) is usually a congenital anomaly. There is no evidence that it seriously interferes with speech but it can result in difficulty in using the tongue to cleanse food away from the teeth and vestibules (**Fig. 28.5**).

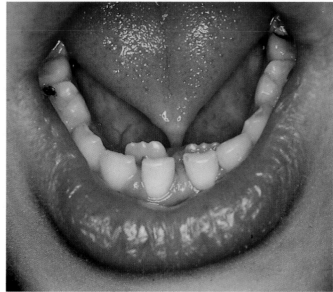

28.4

Associations have been reported of ankyloglossia with maternal cocaine use, and with deviation of the epiglottis and larynx but these remain to be confirmed.

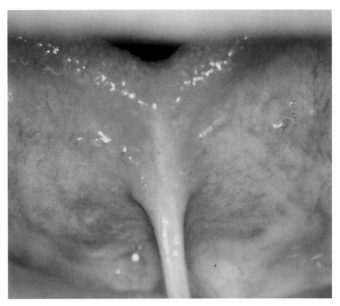

28.5

APERT'S SYNDROME *(acrocephalo-syndactyly)*

Apert's syndrome is an acrocephalosyndactyly syndrome characterized by craniosynostosis, severe syndactyly of the hands and feet, and dysmorphic facial features. The coronal sutures most commonly involved produce acrocephaly (cone-shaped head), brachycephaly (shortened A–P diameter), a flat occiput and a high prominent forehead. Craniosynostosis, a high steep forehead, ocular hypertelorism and antimongoloid slope to the eyes are characteristics of Apert's (**Figs 28.6, 28.7**) and Crouzon's syndromes.

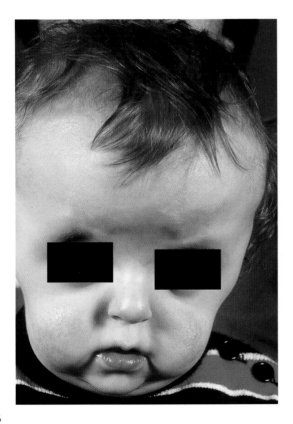

28.6

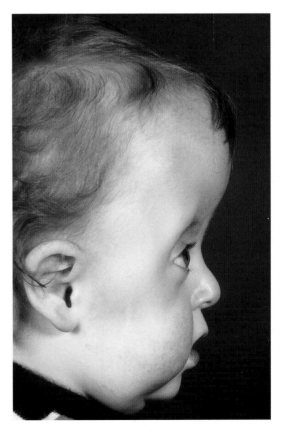

28.7

Apert's syndrome involves progressive synostosis of bones in the hands (**Fig. 28.8**), feet and vertebrae as well as ankylosis of the joints. Syndactyly may involve the hands and feet giving a spoon-like deformity which ranges from partial to complete fusion of the digits, involving mainly digits 2, 3 and 4.

Palatal anomalies are common (**Fig. 28.9**), and one-third of patients have cleft palate. Maxillary hypoplasia is also seen.

There are several variants of this condition, namely:

- Type I. Apert's syndrome
- Type II. Apert–Crouzon syndrome
- Type III. Chotzen's syndrome (Saethre–Chotzen syndrome)
- Type IV. Pfeiffer syndrome

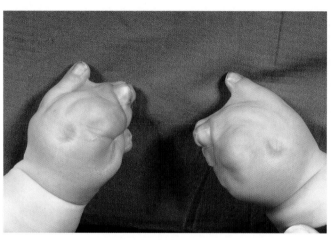

28.8

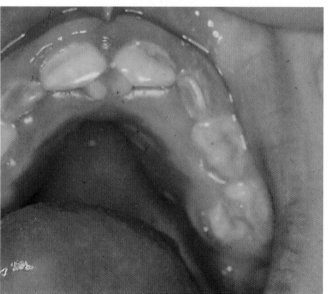

28.9

ASCHER'S SYNDROME

The combination of double lip (**Fig. 28.10**) with sagging eyelids (blepharochalasis) and nontoxic thyroid enlargement is termed Ascher's syndrome.

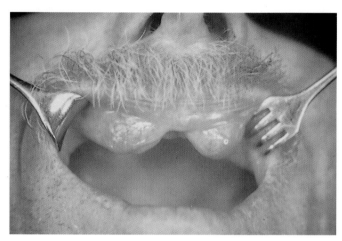

28.10

BIFID UVULA (cleft uvula)

Bifid or cleft uvula (**Fig. 28.11**) is a fairly common minor manifestation of cleft palate but of little consequence apart from sometimes signifying a submucous cleft palate.

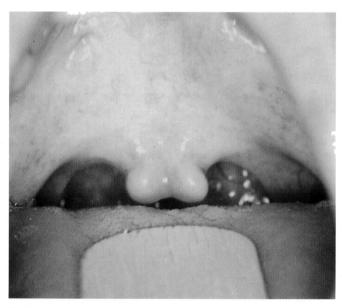

28.11

BLUE RUBBER-BLEB NAEVUS SYNDROME (Bean's syndrome)

Blue rubber-bleb naevus syndrome is a rare autosomal dominant disorder comprising multiple venous malformations of the skin and gastrointestinal tract, liver and lungs. The fragile vessels bleed causing anaemia. Intraoral and lip haemangiomas are blue and rubber-like (**Fig. 28.12**).

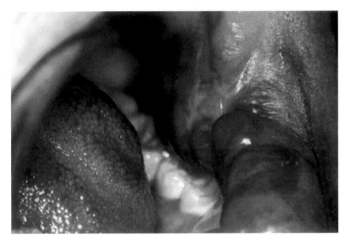

28.12

BRANCHIAL CYST

A branchial (cleft) cyst is a painless, developmental fluctuant swelling on the lateral aspect of the neck (**Fig. 28.13**). Located at the junction of the upper and middle thirds of the sternomastoid muscle on either side, the cyst originates from the vestigial remnants of the branchial clefts. A fibrous track of tissue leads upwards from the deep surface of the cyst between the external and internal carotid arteries, to finish on the wall of the pharynx in the region of the tonsil. The branchial cleft cyst is usually a smooth, round, nontender mass located along the anterior border of the sternocleidomastoid muscle at any position between the tragus and the clavicle. It may be first noticed at any age but it is most commonly noticed in the second to fourth decades of life; males and females are equally affected. It may enlarge with or without tenderness during periods of upper respiratory tract infection. An inflamed cyst may progress to abscess formation with the possibility that rupture will lead to permanent sinus formation.

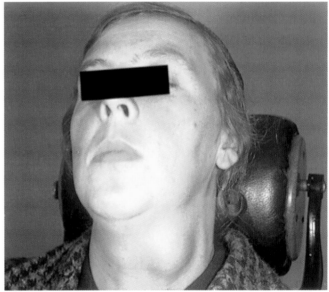

28.13

CAFFEY'S DISEASE (infantile cortical hyperostosis)

This is a rare, possibly autosomal dominant condition, which often presents with swellings around the eyes or over the mandible (**Fig. 28.14**). The condition resembles cherubism but appears at 2–4 months of age. The teeth are neither hypoplastic nor delayed in eruption.

There are also tender, soft tissue swellings over the tibiae (**Fig. 28.15**) with fever, anaemia and irritability. Radiographs show periosteal new bone formation (**Fig. 28.16**). Note that these features are extremely similar to those seen in child abuse or osteomyelitis.

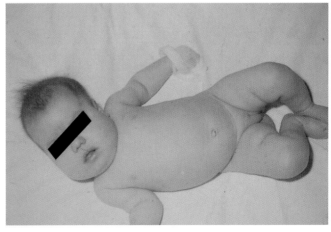

28.14

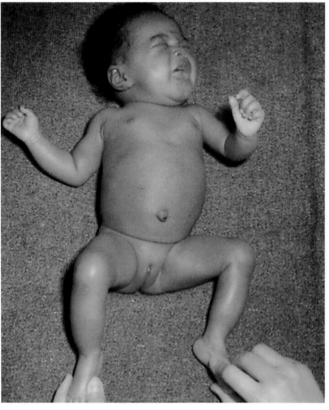

28.15

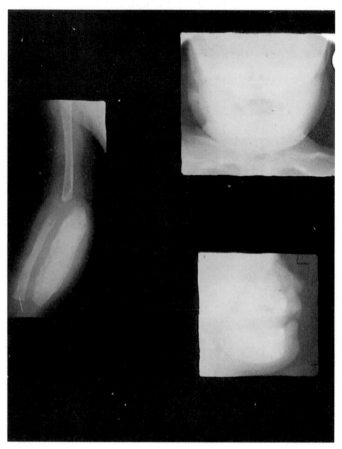

28.16

CARNEY'S SYNDROME

Carney's syndrome (or complex) is an autosomal dominant complex of myxomas, spotty pigmentation and endocrine overactivity. Mucocutaneous pigmentation on the lips develops in the first decade of life (**Figs 28.17, 28.18**) and clinically resembles Peutz–Jegher's syndrome. However, Carney's complex is more involved, with familial multiple neoplasia, primary pigmented nodular adrenocortical disease and a pituitary-independent, primary adrenal form of hypercortisolism. There are also lentigines, ephelides and blue naevi of the skin and mucosae with a variety of nonendocrine and endocrine tumours. The latter include myxomas of the skin, heart, breast (and other sites), psammomatous melanotic schwannoma, growth hormone-producing

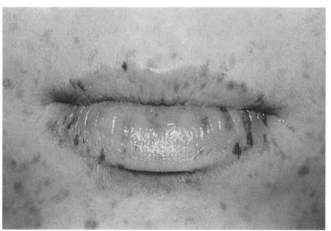

28.17

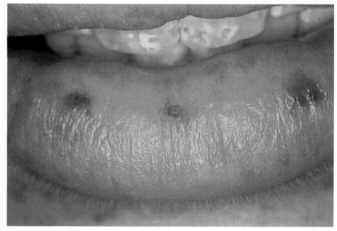

28.18

pituitary adenoma, testicular Sertoli-cell tumour and, possibly, other benign and malignant neoplasms and conditions, including tumours of the thyroid gland and ductal adenoma of the breast, and acromegaly due to somatomammotroph hyperplasia and adenoma not dependent on growth hormone-releasing hormone. Cardiac myxomas cause death or serious disability in a quarter of affected patients.

CHIEVITZ'S ORGAN

The juxtaoral organ described by Chievitz is considered to be a vestigial organ, perhaps of the developing parotid gland, or to be epithelium entrapped during the embryonic development of the interface between the maxillary and mandibular processes. A neuroendocrine receptor function has been suggested.

It is present in almost all individuals, located bilaterally in buccotemporal fascia on the medial surface of the mandible, near the angle (**Fig. 28.19**). Rarely, a proliferative mass of the lingual aspect of the posterior mandible has been reported.

CHONDROECTODERMAL DYSPLASIA
(*Ellis–van Creveld syndrome*)

Dwarfism, polydactyly, ectodermal dysplasia affecting the nails and teeth (**Fig. 28.20**; lateral incisors are missing), multiple fraenae, oligodontia, hypoplastic teeth and polydactyly (**Fig. 28.21**) characterize this syndrome. Typically, the lower incisors are absent.

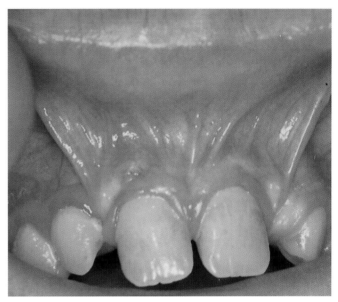

28.20

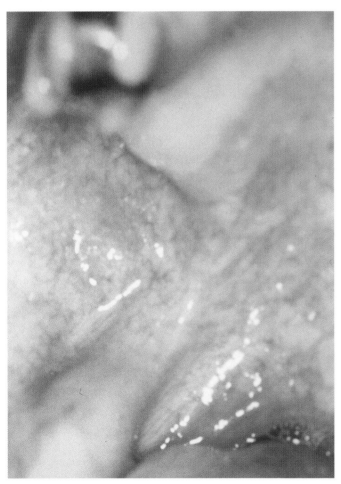

28.19

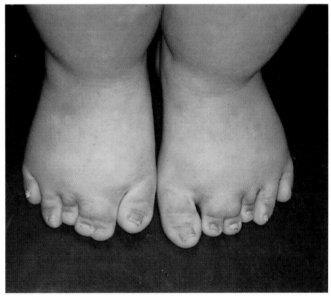

28.21

CLEFT LIP AND PALATE

Cleft lip and palate are more common together than is cleft lip alone. **Figure 28.22** shows a patient with a submucous cleft while **Fig. 28.23** shows a complete unilateral cleft palate and lip after repair.

The cleft is on the left in over 60% of patients and there is a familial tendency in this condition. When one parent is affected, the risk to a child is about 1 in 10 live births.

Cleft lip and palate are, in about 20% of cases, associated with anomalies of the head and neck, extremities, genitalia or heart. There are occasional associations with conditions such as orofaciodigital syndromes.

Isolated cleft palate is especially associated with Down's syndrome, Pierre Robin sequence, Treacher Collins' syndrome and Klippel–Feil syndrome.

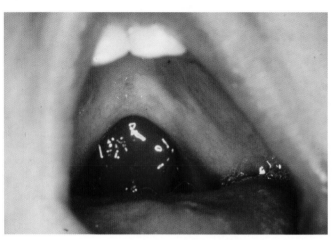

28.22

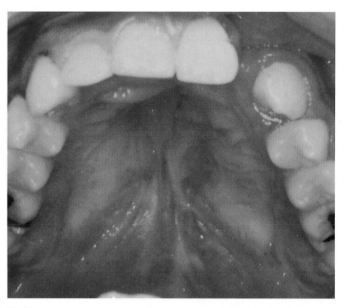

28.23

CLEIDOCRANIAL DYSPLASIA (*cleidocranial dysostosis*)

Cleidocranial dysplasia is an inherited defect of membrane bones, often an autosomal dominant trait, characterized by generalized dysplasia of osseous and dental tissue commonly resulting in defects in the skull, clavicles and teeth.

Defects mainly involve the skull and clavicles. Persistence of the metopic suture gives rise to a vertical midline furrow in the forehead with frontal bossing (**Fig. 28.24**).The sutures are still open and multiple wormian bones are evident in the metopic (**Fig. 28.25**) and occipitoparietal sutures (**Fig. 28.26**). The midface is hypoplastic.

The clavicles are hypoplastic or aplastic (**Fig. 28.27**). In **Fig. 28.28** the right clavicle is aplastic, the left hypoplastic. The clavicular defects

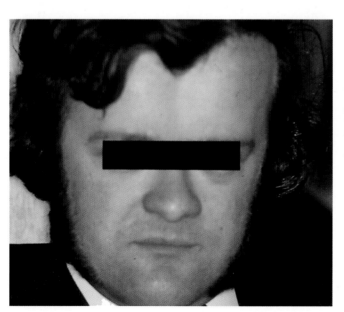

28.24

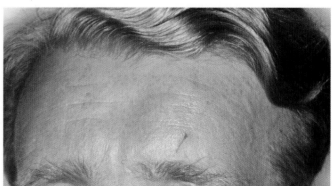

28.25

mean that when patients attempt to bring the shoulders forward and together, they can almost approximate them (**Fig. 28.29**). Radiography shows absence of the clavicles (**Fig. 28.30**).

Pelvic anomalies may also be seen in cleidocranial dysplasia (**Fig. 28.31**) and kyphoscoliosis is common. The dentition may be disrupted because of multiple supernumerary teeth and impactions (**Fig. 28.32**). Radiography shows multiple unerupted and impacted teeth (**Fig. 28.33**) and dentigerous cysts (**Fig. 28.34**).

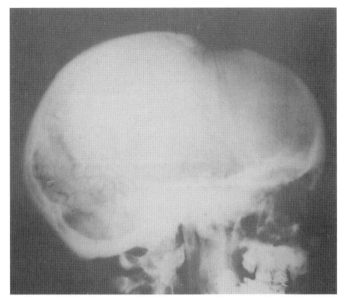

28.26

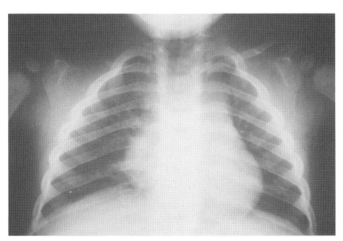

28.27

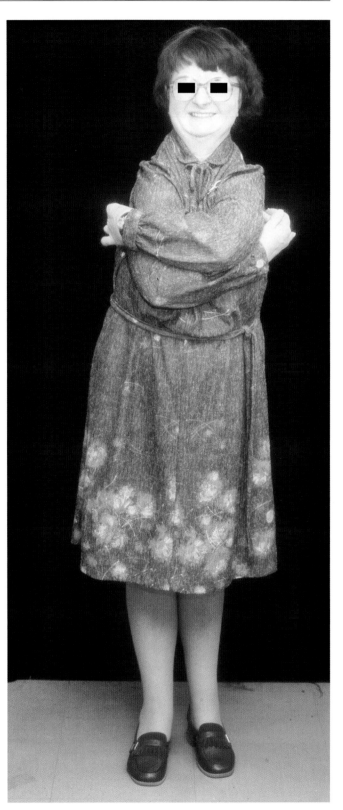

28.28

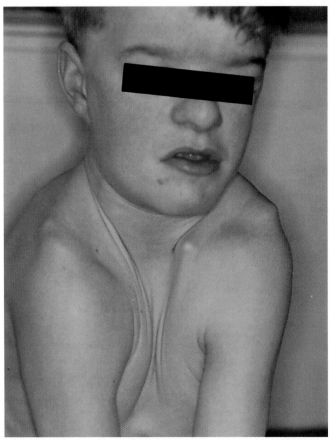

28.29

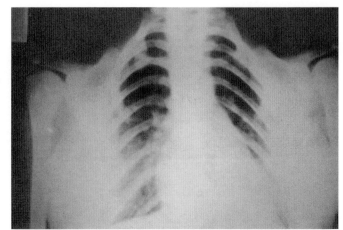

28.30

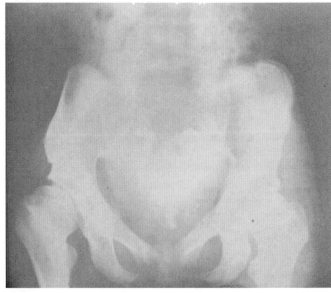

28.31

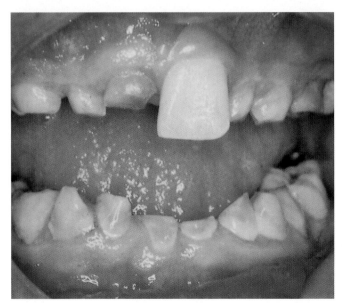

28.32

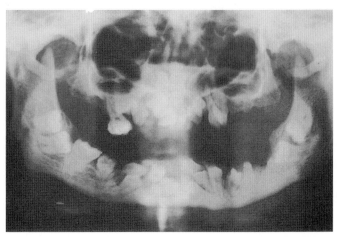

28.33

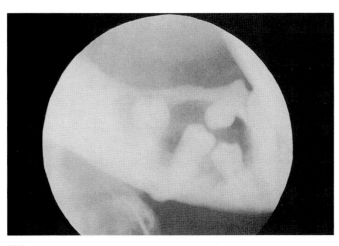

28.34

COWDEN'S SYNDROME *(multiple hamartoma and neoplasia syndrome)*

This is an autosomal dominant condition of multiple hamartomas, with a predisposition to tumours, particularly carcinomas of the breast, thyroid and colon. Papular oral lesions are common (**Figs 28.35–28.38**).

Other oral lesions may include fissured tongue, hypoplasia of the uvula, and maxillary and mandibular hypoplasia.

Large numbers of papillomatous lesions are seen on the skin, especially over the neck, nose, and ear and axilla (see **Fig. 28.39**).

Mucocutaneous lesions often precede the appearance of malignant disease elsewhere. Other manifestations of Cowden's syndrome may include small keratoses on the palms and soles, learning disability and motor incoordination.

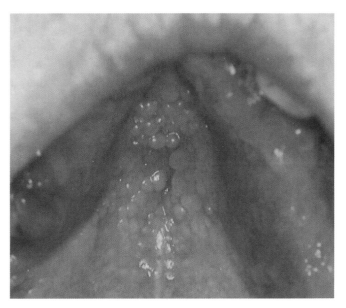

28.36

28.35

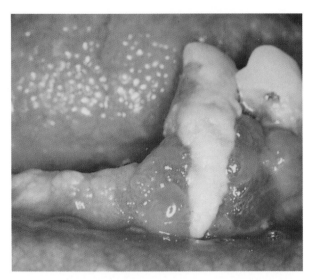

28.37

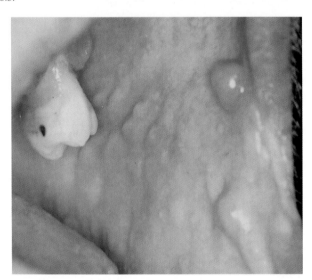

28.38

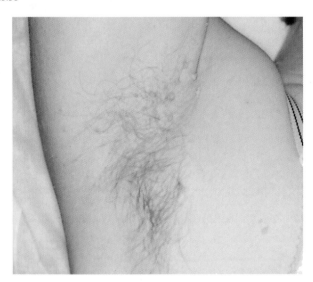

28.39

CRANIOFACIAL MICROSOMIA

Craniofacial microsomia is the second most common facial birth defect after cleft lip and palate. It is a spectrum of morphogenetic abnormalities involving structures derived from the first and second branchial arches, including first and second branchial arch syndrome, hemifacial microsomia and Goldenhar–Gorlin syndrome. Most cases are sporadic with stapedial artery disruption being considered the most likely aetiology.

The parotid salivary gland can be malformed or missing, and auricular and facial nerve abnormalities have been reported in up to 50% of affected persons.

Isolated microtia is now considered a microform of craniofacial microsomia.

Current classification is based on skeletal abnormalities:

- *Type 1* patients have small mandibles with normal shape, a normal glenoid fossa and a short mandibular ramus.
- *Type 2* findings include anteriorly and medially displaced temporomandibular joints and an abnormally contoured TMJ cavity, with a short and abnormally shaped ramus.
- *Type 3* patients have complete absence of the mandibular ramus and glenoid fossa, no TMJ and the body of the mandible ending at the molar region (**Figs 28.40–28.43**).

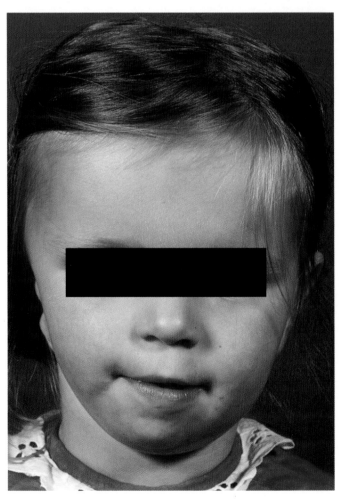

28.40

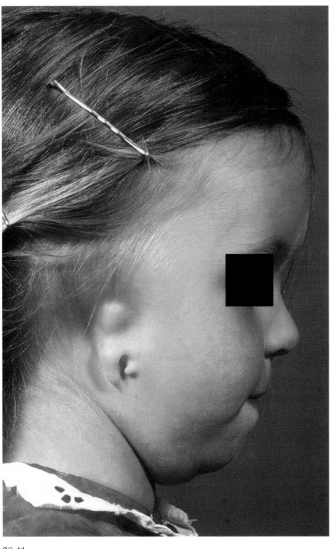

28.41

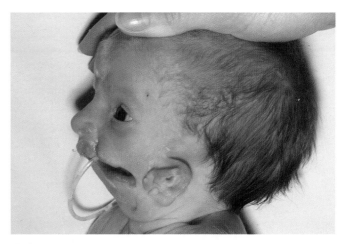

28.42

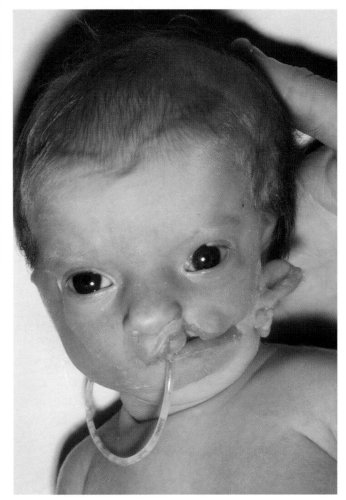

28.43

CRANIOMETAPHYSEAL DYSPLASIA

Craniometaphyseal dysplasia (CMD) is characterized by increased bone deposition and mineralization of bone, which leads to thickening of the craniofacial bones (**Figs 28.44–28.46**) and to an hourglass-shaped widening of the metaphyses of long bones. Other features are hyperplastic supraorbital ridges, hyperteleorism, macrocephaly, osteosclerosis or osteopetrosis, prominent eyes (proptosis), a prominent mandible, sclerosis of the skull and thick calvarium.

The hyperostosis frequently leads to neuronal compression due to closure of the cranial nerve foramina, cranial nerve palsies (including facial palsy, blindness and hearing loss) and, in severe cases, even to death (due to reduction of the foramen magnum). Autosomal dominant CMD is caused by mutations in the transmembrane protein ANK.

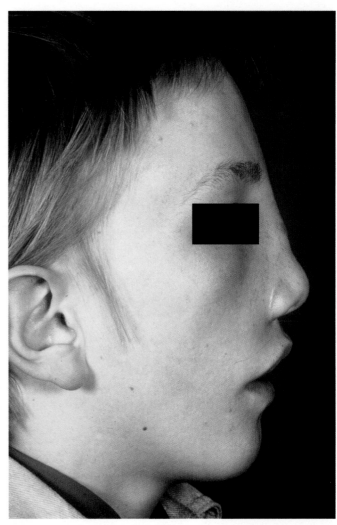

28.45

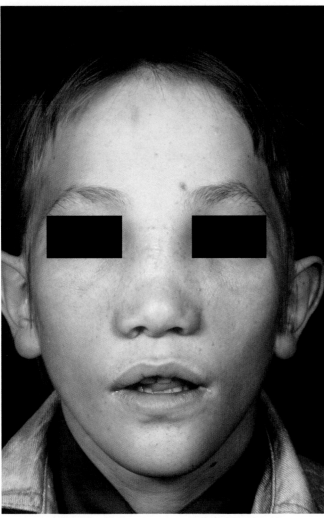

28.44

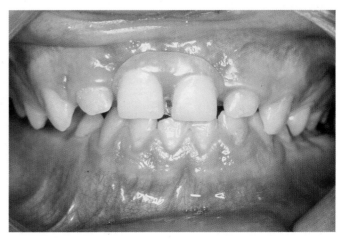

28.46

CRI DU CHAT SYNDROME

Deletion of the short arm of chromosome 5 is a rare disorder characterized by a cry like a cat in infancy, and facial dysmorphogenesis (**Fig. 28.47**). Most patients are of short stature, with learning disability and often have cardiac and skeletal anomalies.

Micrognathia, high-arched palate, enamel hypoplasia and a poorly defined mandibular angle are the main features. Microcephaly (**Fig. 28.48**), small pituitary fossa and large frontal sinuses may be seen on radiography.

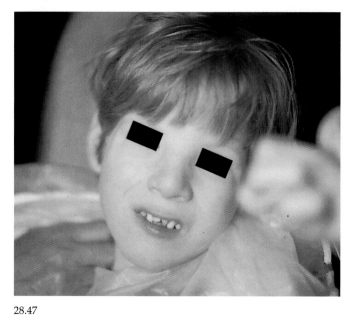

28.47

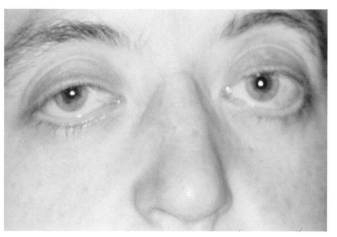

28.48

CROUZON'S SYNDROME *(craniofacial dysostosis)*

Craniosynostosis, ocular hypertelorism and proptosis are characteristics of Crouzon's syndrome (**Figs 28.49–28.53**). Teeth may be missing, peg shaped or enlarged.

Radiography shows craniosynostosis and abnormal skull morphology with pronounced digital impressions ('copper-beaten skull'; see **Fig. 28.53**).

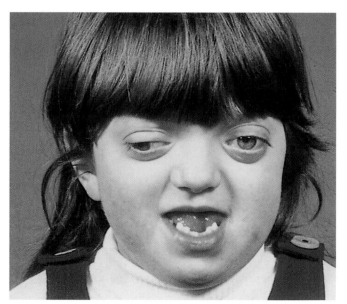

28.49

28.50

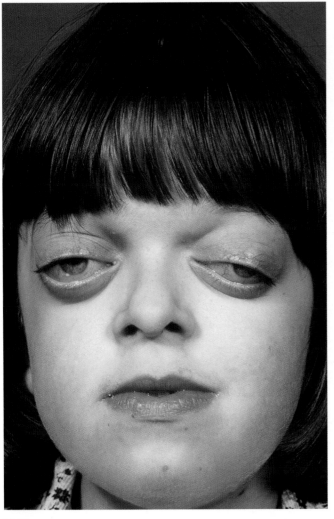

28.51

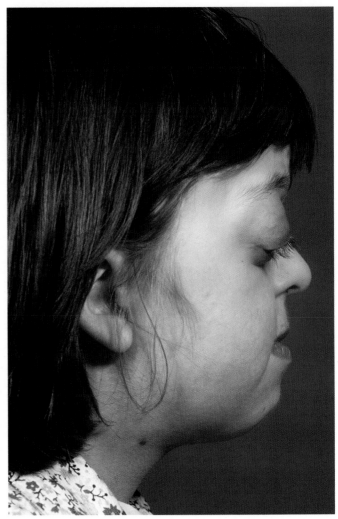

28.52

28.53

CYSTIC HYGROMA

Cervical cystic hygroma is a lymphangioma extending from the tongue down into the neck (**Fig. 28.54**). A developmental anomaly, cystic hygroma usually presents at birth and virtually always in the first 2 years of life; some patients have dysphagia or respiratory embarrassment. A minority extend into the base of the tongue and some extend into the mediastinum. This hamartoma transilluminates brightly.

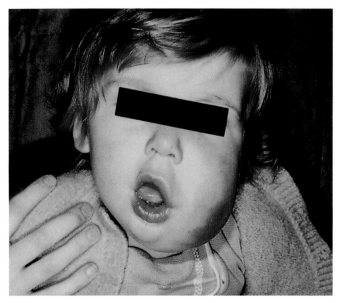

28.54

DARIER'S DISEASE *(dyskeratosis follicularis)*

Darier's disease is a rare autosomal dominant skin disorder. Papules over the shoulders, upper arms, back and knees are seen, with nail defects that include longitudinal splits and fragility such that the nails tend to be wider than they are long (**Figs 28.55–28.57**). Oral lesions are seen in up to 40%, starting as red papules that turn to white pebbly lesions seen especially in the palate, gingiva and dorsum of the tongue (**Fig. 28.58**).

Warty dyskeratoma is a *forme fruste* of Darier's disease in which similar oral lesions are seen in the absence of skin lesions.

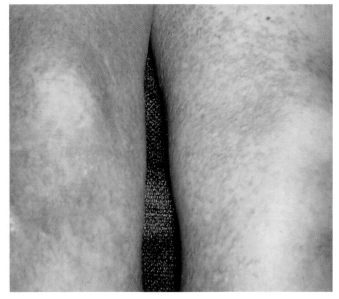

28.55

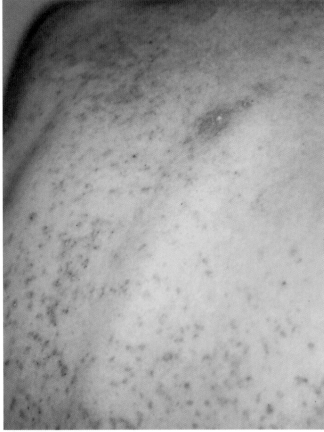

28.56

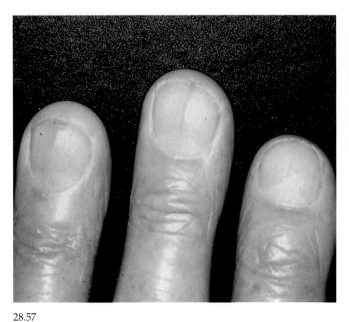

28.57

28.58

DE LANGE'S SYNDROME *(Amsterdam dwarf)*

De Lange's syndrome is a rare congenital disorder of 'fish mouth' with a long philtrum (**Fig. 28.59**), eyebrows that meet (synophrys), dwarfism and learning disability. Hands and feet are small and there is often syndactyly or oligodactyly (**Fig. 28.60**).The mandible is hypoplastic and the palate is small and may be cleft (**Fig. 28.61**). Teeth are often small and delayed in eruption.

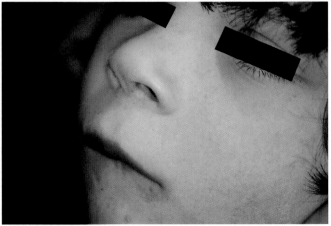

28.59

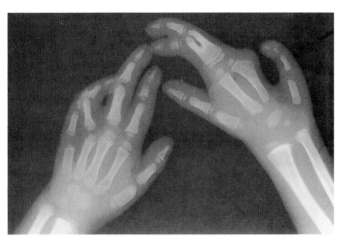

28.60

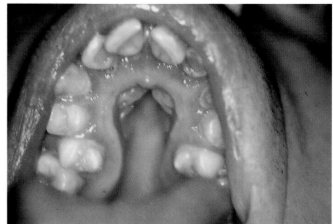

28.61

DOWN'S SYNDROME

Down's syndrome is a trisomic chromosome anomaly, in most instances affecting children of elderly mothers. There is a typical mongoloid appearance (**Fig. 28.62**) with brachycephaly (**Fig. 28.63**) and short stature. There are anomalies of many organs and virtually all patients have learning disabilities.

A fairly characteristic, though not pathognomonic feature, is the presence of white spots (Brushfield's spots) around the iris (**Fig. 28.64**). Another feature is a single palmar crease (the simian crease) and clinodactyly of the fifth finger (**Fig. 28.65**).

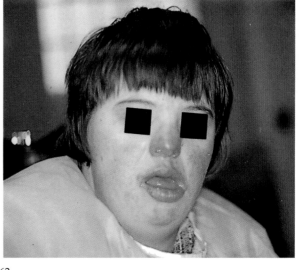

28.62

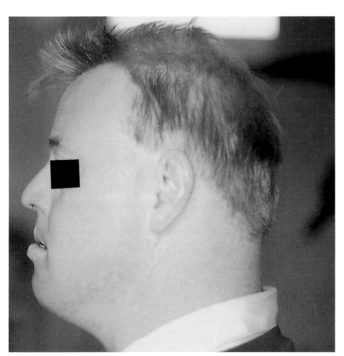

28.63

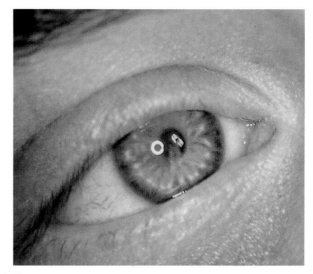

28.64

Patients with Down's syndrome have multiple immune defects. Blepharitis and keratitis are common (**Fig. 28.66**), as are hepatitis and upper respiratory infections (**Fig. 28.67**). There may be a dry mouth as a consequence of mouth breathing because of nasal obstruction. Cheilitis and cracking of the lips are common, possibly because of mouth breathing (**Fig. 28.68**). Macroglossia and a fissured tongue are often seen (**Fig. 28.69**).

The midface is hypoplastic and palatal anomalies are common (**Fig. 28.70**). Cleft lip and palate are more prevalent in Down's syndrome than in the general population (**Fig. 28.71**).

Early loss of teeth is a feature, not only because of poor oral hygiene in many patients but because the teeth have short roots and there may be rapidly destructive periodontal disease (**Figs 28.72, 28.73**).

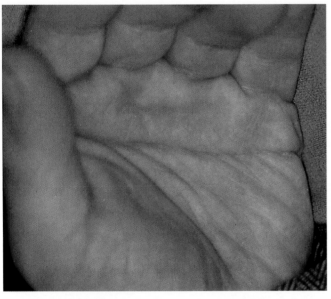

28.65

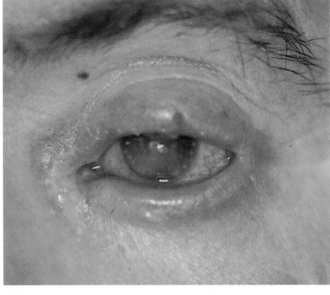

28.66

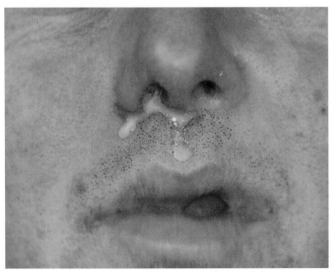

28.67

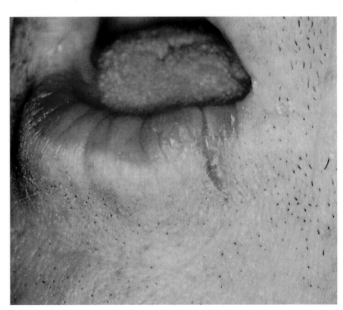

28.68

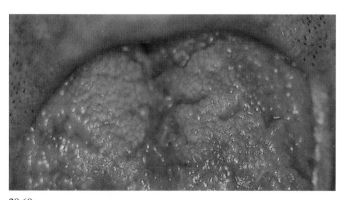

28.69

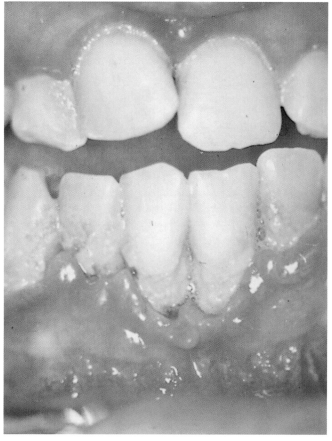

28.70

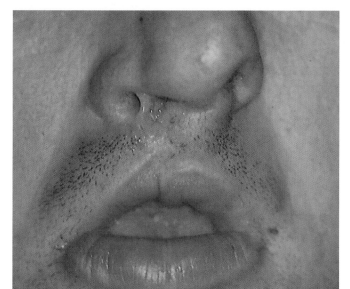

28.71

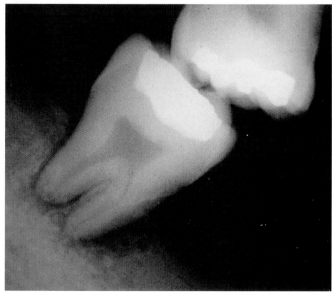

28.73

28.72

DYSKERATOSIS CONGENITA

Dyskeratosis congenita is an inherited bone-marrow failure syndrome usually, but not always, following a sex-linked recessive pattern of inheritance. It is clinically characterized by a triad of skin pigmentation, nail dystrophy and leukoplakia of mucous membranes, although a range of other features can arise. These include mild learning disability, poor growth, sparse hair, hepatomegaly, splenomegaly, skin atrophy, hyperkeratinization, hyperhidrosis, lacrimal duct stenosis, dysphagia, and bone, ear and oral defects. The oral manifestions include hypodontia, short blunted roots, enamel defects, accelerated periodontitis and early tooth loss, mucosal erosions and leukoplakia (**Figs 28.74, 28.75**). The leukoplakia reflects underlying oral epithelial dysplasia, and affected patients may therefore be at increased risk of oral squamous cell carcinoma.

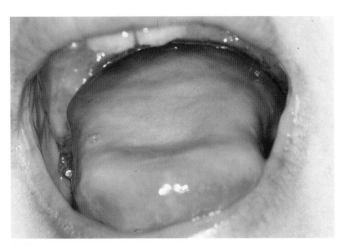

28.74

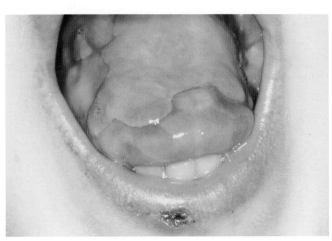

28.75

ECTODERMAL DYSPLASIA

Hypohidrotic ectodermal dysplasia is a genetic disorder, usually sex linked, characterized by sparse hair (hypotrichosis; **Figs 28.76–28.78**), high forehead and sometimes frontal bossing, absent sweat glands (hypohidrosis) and consequent fever, with respiratory infections. Patients are otherwise well.

There is usually oligodontia (hypodontia **Fig. 28.79**) rather than anodontia, and the few teeth that are present are often of simple conical shape, small, taurodont and erupt late (**Figs 28.79–28.82**). Dry mouth from reduced salivation predisposes to caries.

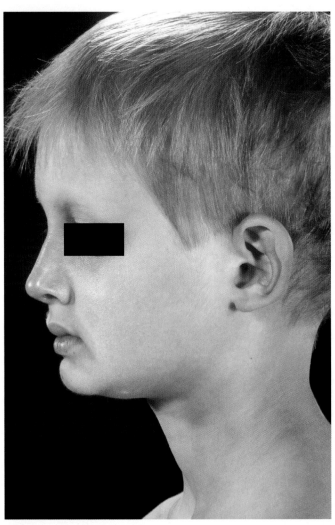

28.76

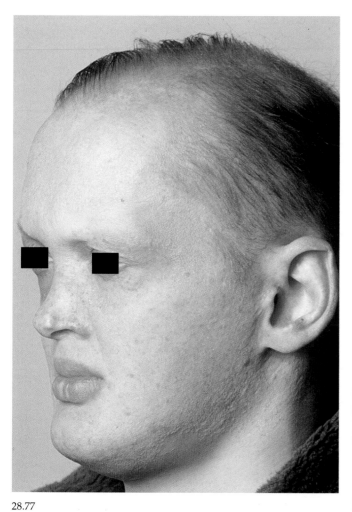

28.77

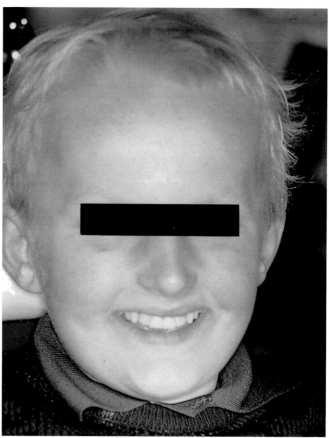

28.78

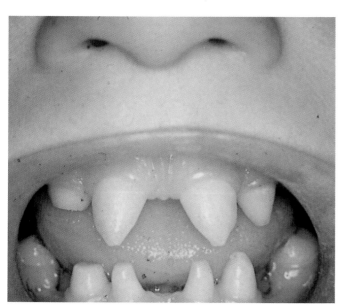

28.79

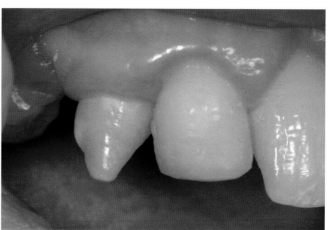

28.80

Rare varieties include an autosomal dominant variety (the 'tooth-and-nail' type), characterized by hypodontia and hypoplastic nails, and a subtype in which the teeth are normal (hypohidrotic ectodermal dysplasia with hypothyroidism).

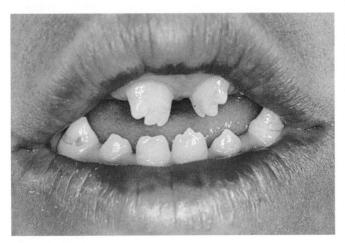

28.81

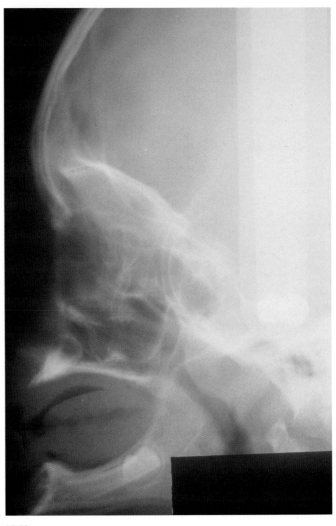

28.82

EHLERS–DANLOS SYNDROME

Ehlers–Danlos syndrome is a group of inherited disorders of collagen. Most types are inherited as autosomal dominant traits and involve abnormal collagen type III.

Hypermobility of joints is common, the skin is soft, extensible and fragile (**Figs 28.83–28.86**), purpura is common and there may be other defects, such as mitral valve prolapse. Patients may be able to touch the tip of their nose with their tongue. The teeth may be small with abnormally shaped roots and multiple pulp stones (**Fig. 28.87**). Temporomandibular joint subluxation is common (**Figs 27.4, 27.5**).

Types VIII or IX Ehlers–Danlos syndrome may be associated with early-onset periodontal disease.

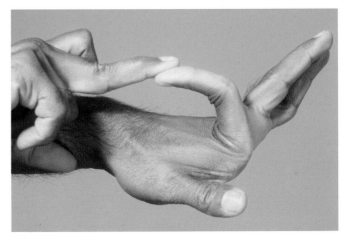

28.83

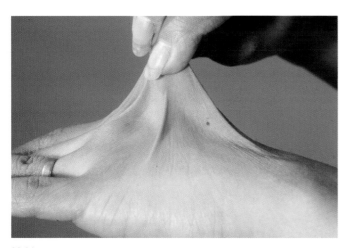

28.84

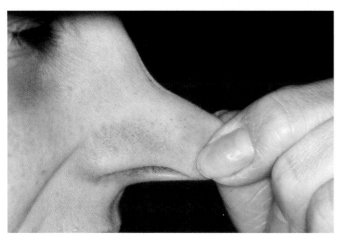

28.86

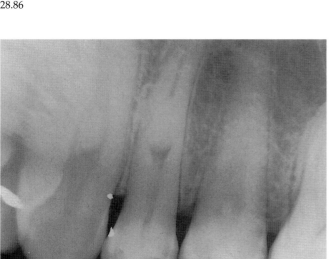

28.87

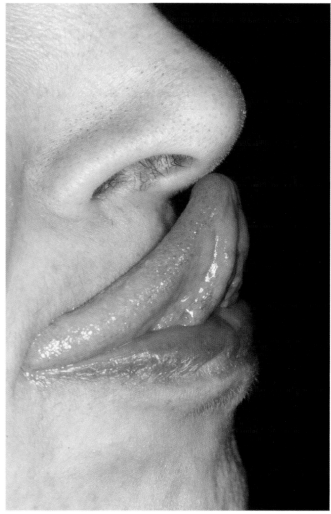

28.85

EPIDERMOLYSIS BULLOSA

Epidermolysis bullosa (EB) is a group of rare mainly inherited disorders of skin and mucosa often due to defects in the epithelial basement membrane zone, mostly characterized by vesiculation zone in response to minor trauma, and often consequent scarring (**Figs 28.88–28.90**). The dystrophic form is due to collagen VII defects and affects the extremities including the nails with scarring (**Fig. 28.88**).

The nonscarring simplex type of EB, in which the vesiculation is intraepithelial and due to keratin 5 and 14 defects, rarely affects the mouth but in most other forms bullae may be seen in the mouth and scar formation may distort the lower lip (**Figs 28.91–28.93**) and restrict oral opening. These forms include junctional EB (which affects laminin) and hemidesmosomal EB (which affects plectin or integrins). Bullae in EB appear early in life, often precipitated by suckling, and break down to persistent ulcers which eventually heal with scarring. The tongue may become ulcerated (see **Fig. 28.91**), depapillated and scarred, the gingiva desquamated and caries is common (**Fig 28.92**). The teeth are often hypoplastic and squamous cell carcinoma is a rare complication.

An acquired form of EB (epidermolysis bullosa acquisita) is a chronic blistering disease of skin and mucosa with autoantibodies to type VII procollagen of epithelial basement membrane.

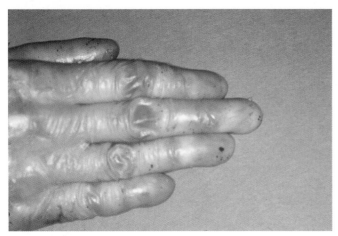

28.88

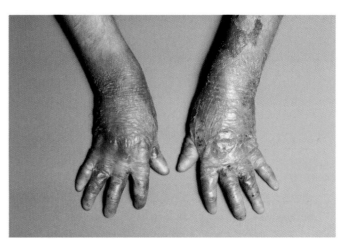

28.89

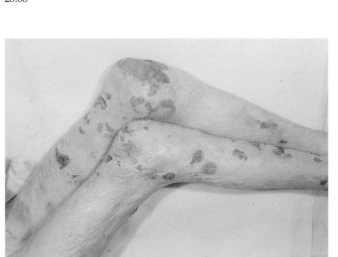

28.90

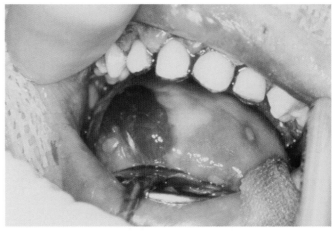

28.91

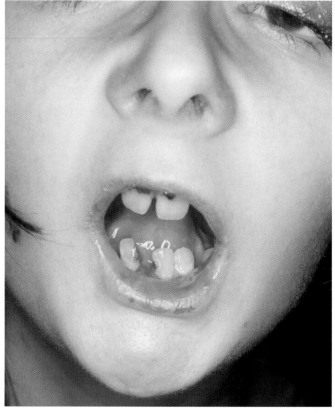

28.92

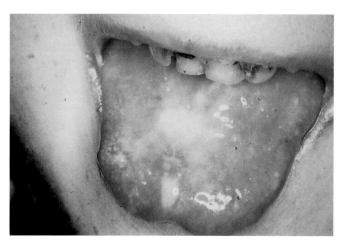

28.93

EPILOIA *(tuberous sclerosis; Bourneville–Pringle disease)*

Tuberous sclerosis is an autosomal dominant condition of learning disability, epilepsy and skin lesions. The development of tuberous sclerosis is associated with alterations within a gene on chromosome 9q34 (TSC1) and a gene on chromosome 16p13 (TSC2).

Adenoma sebaceum is the pathognomonic feature and is typically seen in the nasolabial fold (**Figs 28.95–28.101**). This is an angiofibroma that can be severely disfiguring and may involve other sites, such as the chin. Fibrous plaques on the forehead and shagreen patches elsewhere are other cutaneous features.

Cerebral calcifications are seen (**Fig. 28.96**). Ocular lesions (phakomas) and neurological complications (astrocytomas) may be

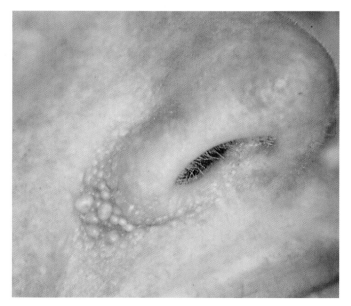

28.94

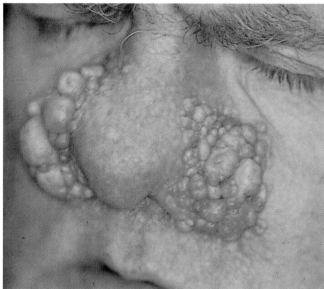

28.95

seen. Patients may also have cardiac rhabdomyoma or renal hamartomas (cysts or angiomyolipomas).

Subungual fibromas (Koenen's tumours) are another pathognomonic feature (**Figs 28.97, 28.98**) and may be seen with longitudinal ridging of the nails. Depigmented 'ash leaf' naevi may be seen on the trunk (**Fig. 28.99**).

Papilliferous oral mucosa lesions may be seen (**Fig. 28.100**) in 10% of cases (angiofibromas).

Pit-shaped enamel defects are a feature and there may be phenytoin-induced gingival hyperplasia (**Fig. 28.101**).

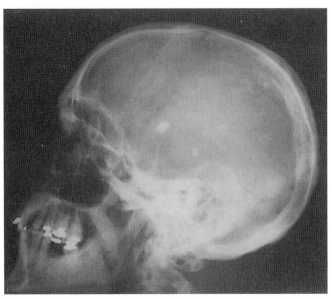

28.96

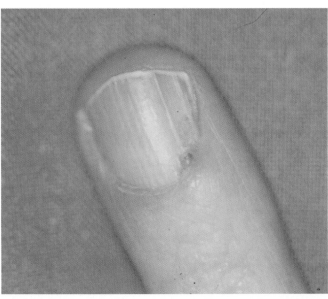

28.97

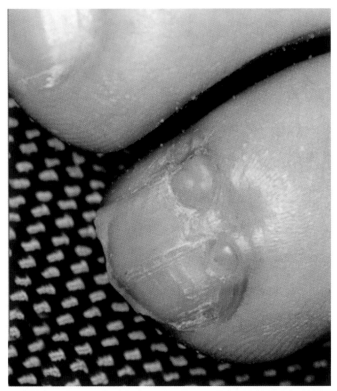

28.98

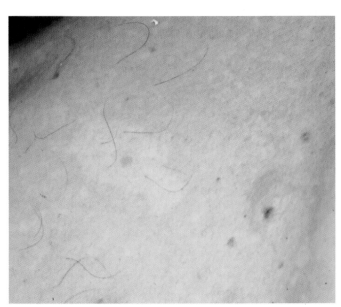

28.99

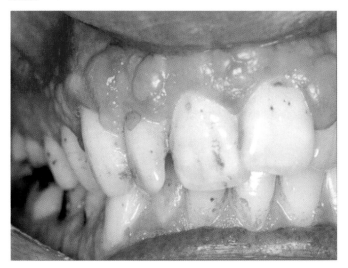

28.100

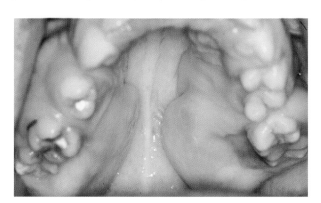

28.101

FAMILIAL GINGIVAL FIBROMATOSIS

Hereditary gingival fibromatosis (**Fig. 28.102**) is frequently an isolated condition of little consequence apart from a cosmetic problem and occasional associations with hypertrichosis and/or epilepsy but it may be part of a wider syndrome (see Laband's syndrome).

FISSURED TONGUE *(scrotal or plicated tongue)*

Fissured tongue (**Fig. 28.103**) is a common developmental anomaly (affecting up to 15% of the population) that may appear after puberty. It is of little significance, though it is often (20% of cases) associated with erythema migrans. Fissured tongue is one feature of Melkersson–Rosenthal syndrome and is found more frequently than normal in Down's syndrome and psoriasis.

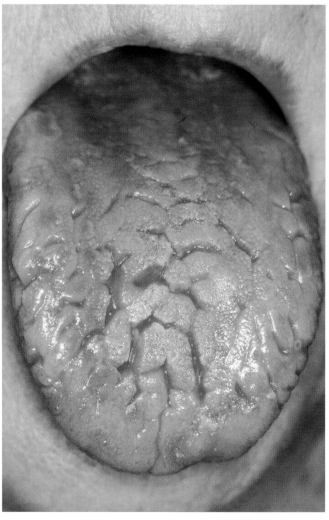

28.103

28.102

FORDYCE'S SPOTS

Fordyce's spots are sebaceous glands in the vermilion of the lip (mainly the upper lip) and in the oral mucosa, especially in the anterior buccal mucosa and retromolar region (**Figs 28.104–28.106**).

Often few in number, Fordyce's spots are rare in children but found in about 80% of the adult population and become increasingly obvious with age.

Fordyce's spots may cause the patient to complain because of their appearance. They are of no medical consequence but appear to be increased in patients with rheumatic disorders, especially Reiter's syndrome.

Intraoral sebaceous hyperplasia occurs when a lesion, judged to require biopsy has histologic features of one or more well-differentiated sebaceous glands that exhibit no fewer than 15 lobules per gland. Sebaceous glands with fewer than 15 lobules, forming an apparently distinct clinical lesion on the buccal mucosa, are considered normal, whereas similar lesions of other intraoral sites are considered ectopic sebaceous glands.

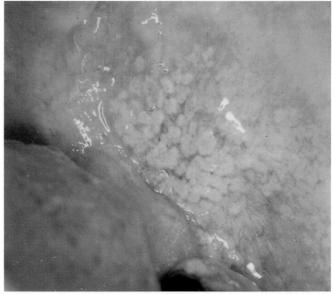

28.105

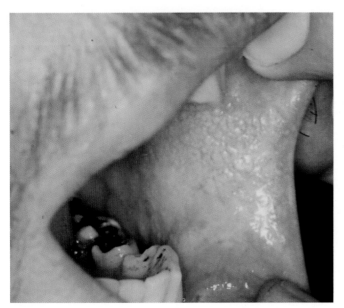

28.104

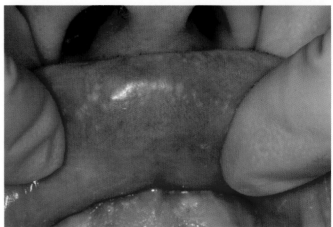

28.106

FRAGILE X SYNDROME
(Martin–Bell syndrome)

Fragile X syndrome (FraX) is a neurodevelopmental disorder which results from a single gene mutation on the X chromosome; it is the most common genetic cause of learning disability. FraX is characterized phenotypically mainly by a long coarse face, unusual lip morphology (**Fig. 28.107**), prominent ears and macro-orchidism. Affected individuals are also typically mentally challenged and may have mitral valve prolapse and seizures.

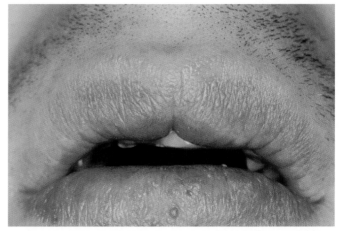

28.107

GARDNER'S SYNDROME

Multiple jaw osteomas are occasionally a feature of Gardner's syndrome (an autosomal dominant trait due to a defect within a gene on chromosome 5), which is characterized by epidermoid cysts (**Figs 28.108 and 28.109**), impacted supernumerary teeth (**Figs 28.110–28.112**), colonic polyps which may be premalignant (**Fig. 28.113**), Osteomas (**Figs 28.114 and 28.115**) and desmoid tumours (**Fig. 28.116**).

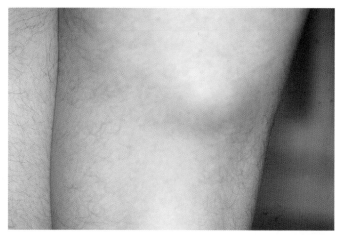

28.108

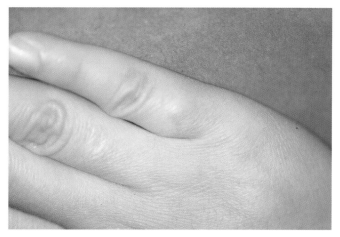

28.109

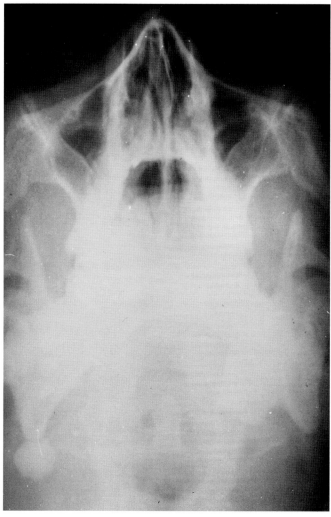

28.110

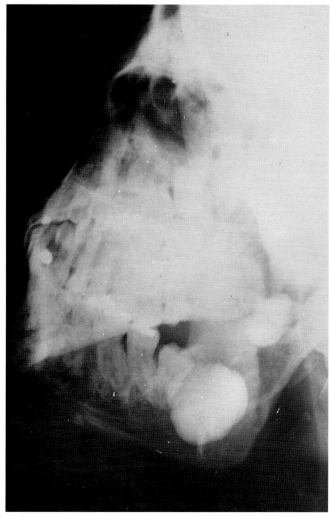

28.111

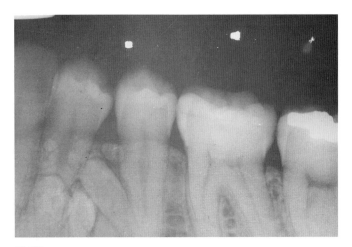

28.112

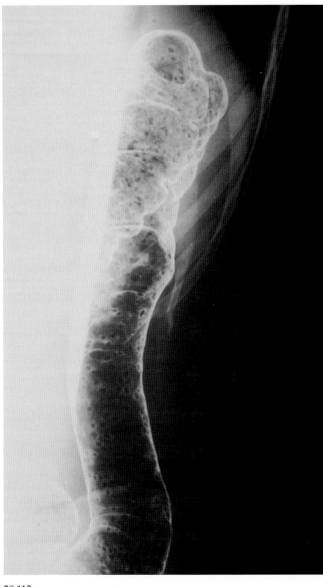

28.113

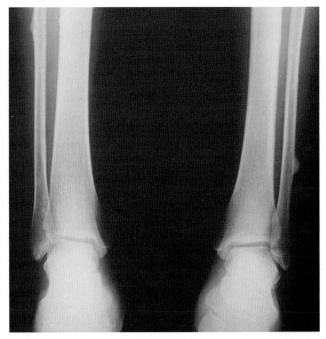

28.114

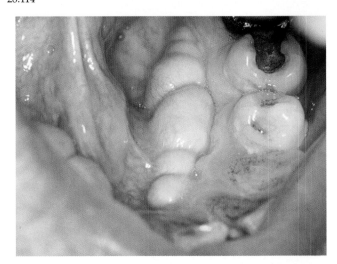

28.115

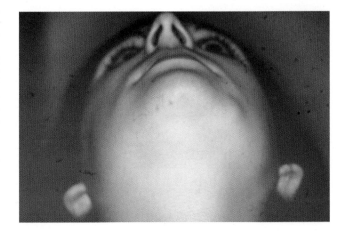

28.116

GORLIN'S SYNDROME (Gorlin–Goltz syndrome; multiple basal cell naevi syndrome)

Gorlin's syndrome is an autosomal dominant condition of multiple basal cell naevi (Figs 28.117–28.119), with odontogenic keratocysts, especially in the mandible (Fig. 28.120), and other features. Frontal and parietal bossing and a broad nasal root give the typical facial appearance.

Multiple basal cell naevi, often with milia, appear in childhood or adolescence, mainly over the nose, eyelids and cheeks (see Figs 28.117 and 28.118). The abdomen or extremities are rarely affected.

Figure 28.119 shows a close-up of a naevus that is developing into a basal cell carcinoma. Only about 50% of adult patients have significant numbers of naevoid basal cell carcinomas and only rarely are the lesions aggressive.

Keratocysts develop mainly in the mandible as shown by radiography (see Fig. 28.120). These develop during the first 30 years of life. Cleft lip and/or palate are seen in about 5% of cases. Calcification of the falx cerebri (see Fig. 28.121) is a common feature, seen in over 80% of patients.

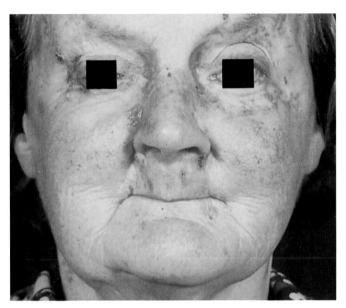

28.117

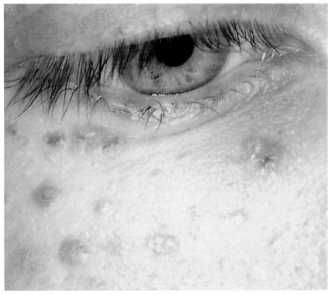

28.118

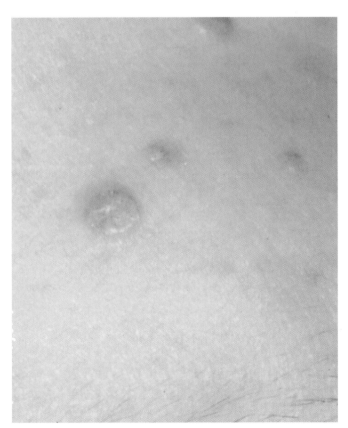

28.119

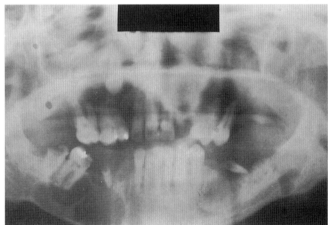

28.120

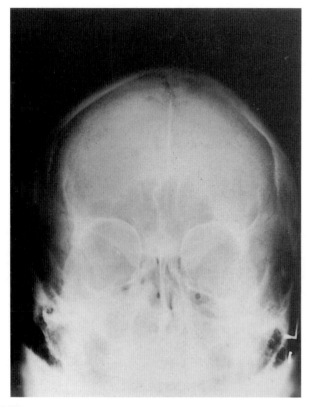

28.121

Medulloblastomas and other brain tumours have been reported in up to 5% of patients, as have a range of neoplasms of other tissues, especially cardiac fibromas. There are many skeletal anomalies but bifid ribs are a common feature (see **Fig. 28.122**). Kyphoscoliosis is often seen in Gorlin's syndrome (see **Fig. 28.123**) and vertebral defects are common. Other occasional associations include pseudohypoparathyroidism and diabetes mellitus. Pits may be seen in the soles or palms (see **Fig. 28.124**) and occasionally basal cell carcinomas arise in these pits.

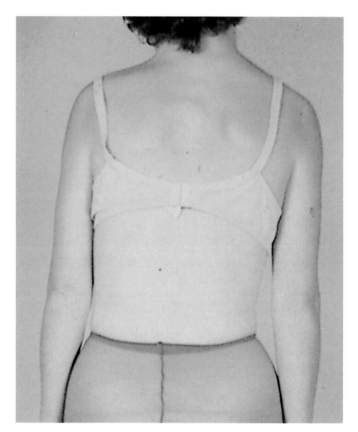

28.123

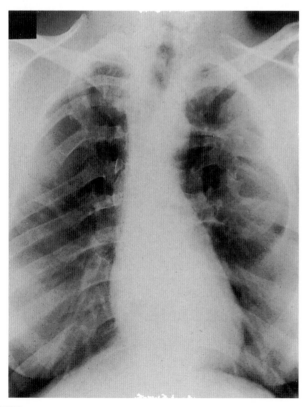

28.122

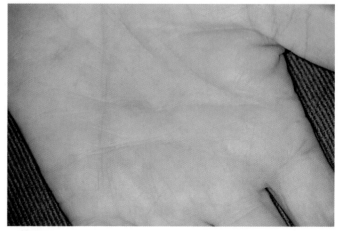

28.124

HALLERMANN–STREIFF SYNDROME

The Hallermann–Streiff syndrome is characterized by dyscephaly, hypotrichosis, microphthalmia, cataracts, a beaked nose, micrognathia (**Fig. 28.125**) and proportionate short stature. Radiological findings can include a large, poorly ossified skull with decreased ossification in the sutural areas, an increase in the number of wormian bones, severe midfacial hypoplasia, a prominent nasal bone and obtuse or nearly straight gonial angles. Potential complications are related to the narrow upper airway.

Teeth may be supernumerary (**Fig. 28.126** which also shows ankylog lossia), malformed or absent. Natal teeth may sometimes be seen in affected infants.

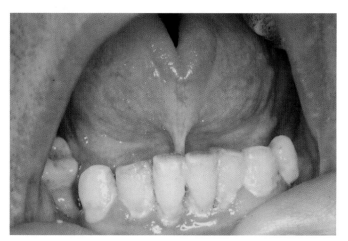

28.126

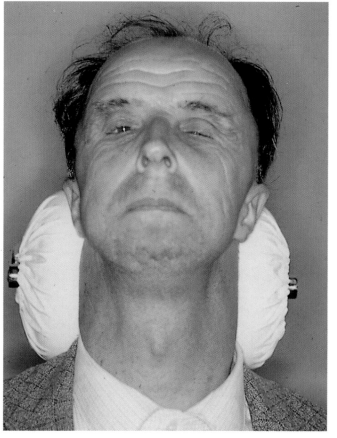

28.125

HEMIFACIAL HYPERTROPHY

Hemifacial hypertrophy usually involves the cheek and is limited rostally by the orbits and caudally by the jaw. It may occur either isolated or associated with one of several syndromes. Syndromes associated with facial hemihypertrophy are proteus syndrome, Klippel–Trenaunay–Weber syndrome and other neurocutaneous diseases. Hemifacial hypertrophy may be accompanied by hemimegalencephaly.

HEREDITARY HAEMORRHAGIC TELANGIECTASIA

Hereditary haemorrhagic telangiectasia is characterized by multiple telangiectasia.

HEREDITARY PALMOPLANTAR KERATOSES

This heterogeneous group of disorders may occasionally be associated with oral disease. Oral mucosal hyperkeratosis is seen in the focal palmoplantar and oral mucosa hyperkeratosis syndrome. Dental dysplasia has been seen in other variants. In particular, this is so in Papillon–Lefèvre syndrome, a rare, genetically linked disorder of prepubertal periodontitis due to cathepsin C deficiency, in association with palmar-plantar hyperkeratosis (**Figs 28.127–28.130**). Virtually all

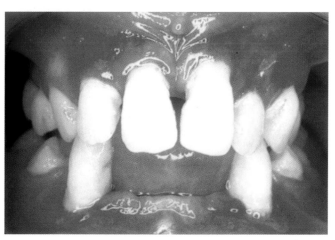

28.127

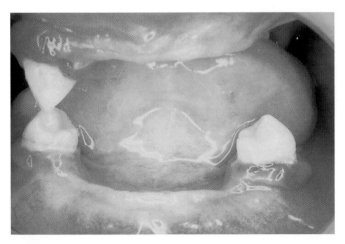

28.128

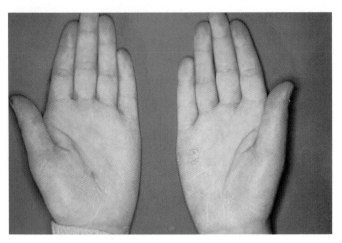

28.130

deciduous teeth are involved and the permanent dentition is usually also affected.

Most of the deciduous teeth are lost by the age of 4 years, and the permanent teeth by age 16 years (see **Fig. 28.128**). Skin lesions tend to appear between the ages of 2 and 4 years; the soles are usually affected more severely than the palms (see **Figs 28.129 and 28.130**). The dura mater may be calcified as may the tentorium or choroid.

A rare variant of the Papillon–Lefèvre syndrome includes arachnodactyly and tapered phalanges as well as the above features.

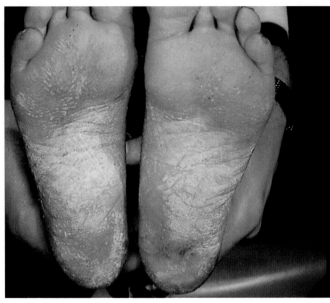

28.129

ICHTHYOSIS

The disorders of cornification (ichthyoses) comprise acquired and inherited disorders characterized clinically by generalized scaling and histologically by hyperkeratosis. They may arise through defects in the production or maintenance of a normal cornified cell compartment.

Perioral involvement is not uncommon (**Fig. 28.131**) and there may be enamel hypoplasia, delayed tooth eruption, periodontal disease and caries. Hyperkeratotic plaques have also been described on the tongue.

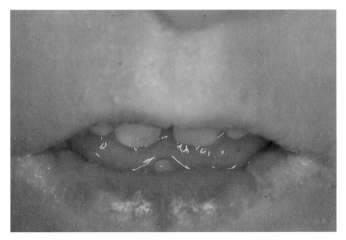

28.131

Scales may involve many sites (see **Fig. 28.132**), depending on the type of ichthyosis. The most common is ichthyosis vulgaris, which is an autosomal dominant condition affecting the extremities in particular, including the nails (see **Fig. 28.133**) and rarely the mouth.

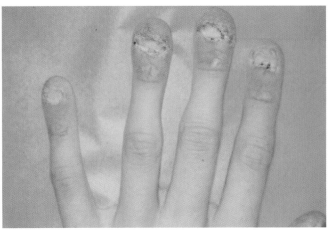

28.133

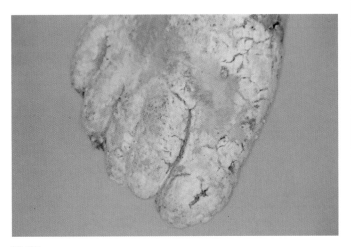

28.132

INCONTINENTIA PIGMENTI *(Bloch–Sulzberger disease)*

Incontinentia pigmenti is a type of ectodermal dysplasia. It is a rare dominant disorder that is either sex linked or lethal to males; virtually all surviving patients are female.

Pigmented, vesicular or verrucous skin lesions are seen (**Fig. 28.134**) often with learning and visual disabilities and hypoplastic nipples.

Most patients have dental anomalies and both dentitions may exhibit anomalies. Hypodontia, conical teeth and delayed eruption are the usual features (**Figs 28.135, 28.136**).

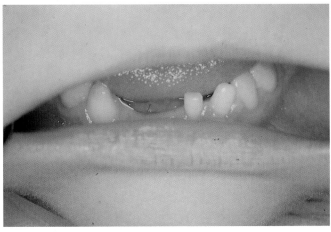

28.135

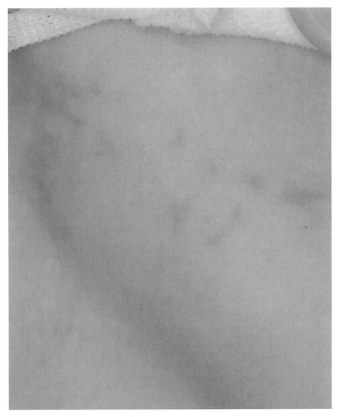

28.134

528

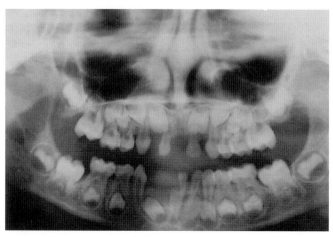

28.136

KLIPPEL–TRENAUNAY–WEBER SYNDROME

Haemangiomas of the buccal mucosa and tongue, macroglossia, maxillary hyperplasia and an anterior open bite have been recorded in this syndrome of bone and soft tissue hypertrophy and varicose veins (**Figs 28.137–28.139**).

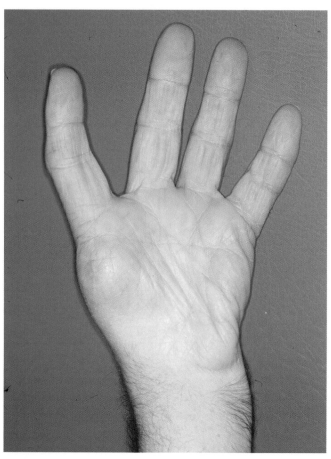

28.137

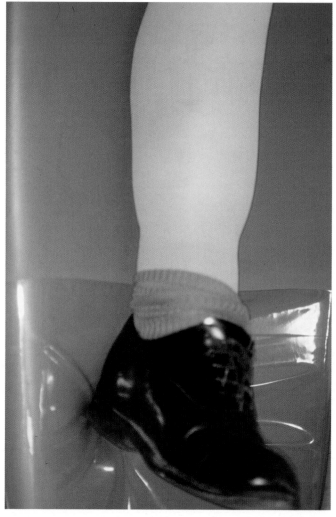

28.138

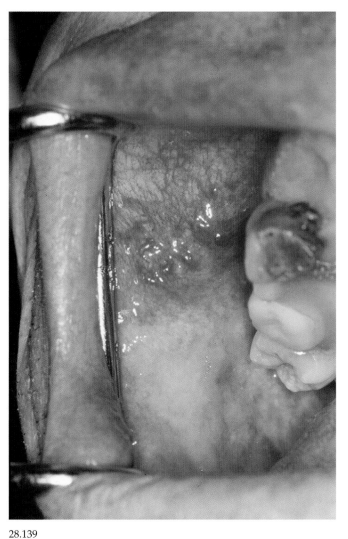

28.139

LABAND'S SYNDROME (*Zimmermann–Laband Syndrome*)

Hereditary gingival fibromatosis is frequently an isolated condition of little consequence apart from a cosmetic problem and occasional associations with hypertrichosis and/or epilepsy. There are, however, several uncommon or rare eponymous syndromes described in which gingival fibromatosis can be a feature. These also include Murray–Puretic–Drescher, Rutherfurd's, Cowden's and Cross's syndromes (see **Table 28.1**).

The Laband's syndrome consists of gingival hyperplasia (**Fig. 28.140**) together with hypoplastic terminal phalanges (**Fig. 28.141**) and other skeletal defects.

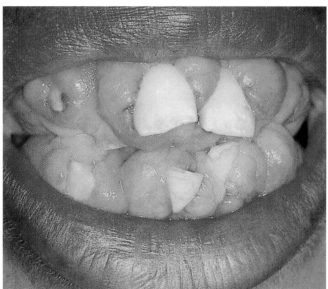

28.140

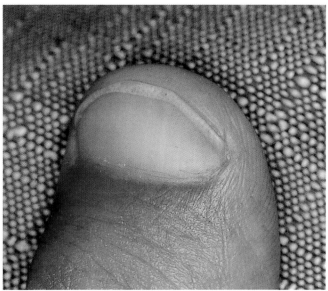

28.141

Table 28.1 SYNDROMES ASSOCIATED WITH GINGIVAL FIBROMATOSIS

Syndrome	Inheritance	Main features apart from gingival fibromatosis
Zimmermann–Laband	AD	Ears and nose thickened and enlarged Nail dysplasia Terminal phalanges hypoplastic Joint hyperextensibility Hepatosplenomegaly
Murray–Puretic–Drescher	AR	Hyaline fibrous tumours over scalp, neck and limbs Osteolysis of terminal phalanges Recurrent infections
Rutherfurd's	AD	Retarded tooth eruption Corneal opacities
Cowden's	AD	Giant fibroadenoma of breast Hypertrichosis Multiple hamartomas
Cross's	AR	Hypopigmentation Microphthalmia with cloudy corneas Learning disability Athetoid cerebral palsy
Gingival fibromatosis	AD	Hypertrichosis Epilepsy Learning disability
Gingival fibromatosis with progressive deafness	AD	Progressive sensorineural deafness

AD = autosomal dominant, AR = autosomal recessive.

LEUKOEDEMA

This is not a mucosal disease but simply the description of very faint whitish lines in some normal buccal mucosae, often prominent in black patients. The whitish lines disappear if the mucosa is stretched, which is a diagnostic test (**Figs 28.142, 28.143**).

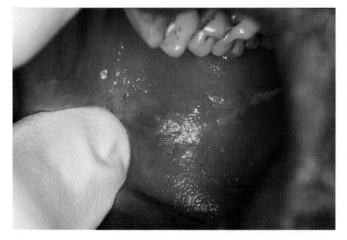

28.142

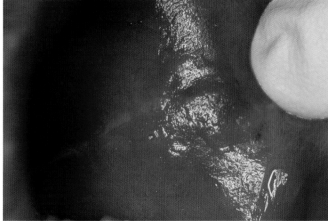

28.143

LIP PIT

Commissural lip pits are blind epithelial-lined developmental anomalies of no medical consequence (**Fig. 28.144**). They may be part of van der Woude syndrome (p. 545). Pits may also be paramedian on the vermilion and may exude mucus (**Figs 28.145, 28.146**).

MAFFUCCI'S SYNDROME

Haemangiomas are typically in the tongue in Maffucci's syndrome, when they are associated with multiple enchondromas elsewhere, particularly in cartilage bones such as in the hands and feet. Haemangiomas can also involve skin, other mucosae and the viscera (**Figs 28.147, 28.148**).

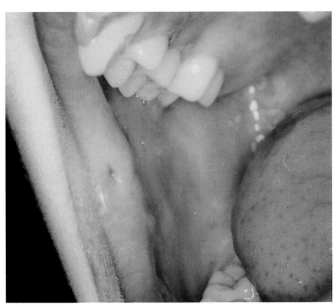

28.144

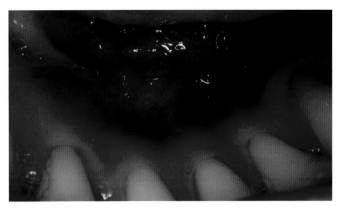

28.147

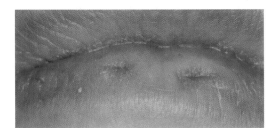

28.145

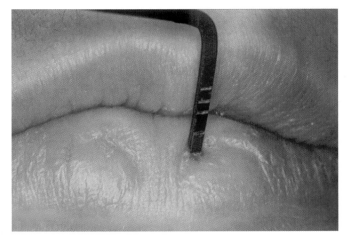

28.146

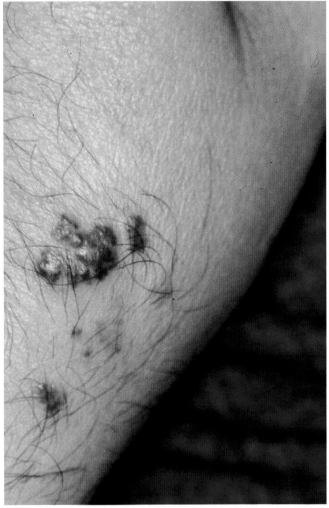

28.148

MARFAN'S SYNDROME

Marfan's syndrome is an autosomal dominant disorder of connective tissue, a defect in fibrillin, with skeletal, cardiovascular and ocular manifestations. Marfan's syndrome shares the features of loose-jointedness, cardiac valvular defects and ocular lesions with various subtypes of the Ehlers–Danlos syndrome. However, the most obvious distinguishing feature of Marfan's syndrome is the long thin body habitus and long slender fingers and toes. The palatal vault is high and temporomandibular joint dysfunction or recurrent subluxation may be troublesome (**Figs 28.149–28.152**).

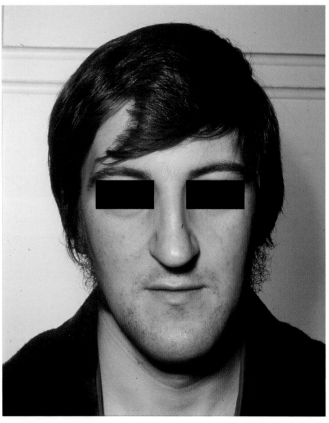

28.149

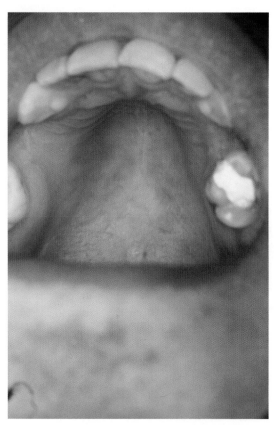

28.150

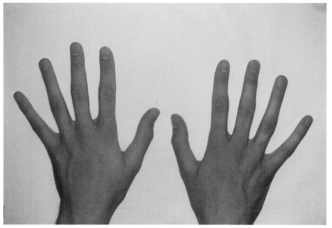

28.151

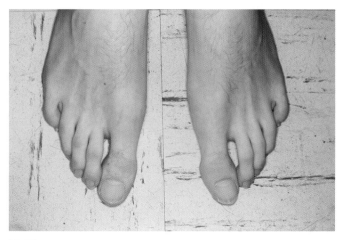

28.152

MUCINOSIS

Focal mucinosis is a term used to describe a group of diseases or conditions in which the accumulation of mucin in the skin or mucosa is a prominent feature. The mucinoses include myxoedema (both diffuse and localized), lichen myxoedematosus (papular mucinosis), lipoid proteinosis, follicular mucinosis, cutaneous focal mucinosis (**Fig. 28.153**), cutaneous myxoid cyst and others.

Oral focal mucinosis is an uncommon clinicopathological entity, which is considered to be the oral counterpart of cutaneous focal mucinosis and/or cutaneous myxoid cyst. The nature of the lesion is unclear and it is suggested that the mucinous accumulation is the result of fibroblastic overproduction of hyaluronic acid. Most of the lesions affect the gingiva and alveolar mucosa.

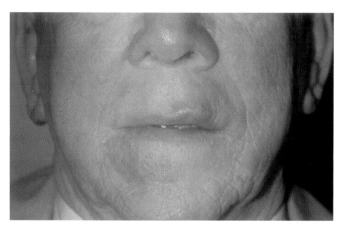

28.153

MYOTONIC DYSTROPHY *(Steinert's syndrome)*

Myotonic dystrophy (dystrophia myotonica) is the most disabling form of myotonia and can lead to ptosis (**Fig. 28.154**), facial weakness, cataracts, testicular atrophy and frontal baldness. Other complications include cardiac conduction defects, respiratory impairment, mild endocrinopathies, intellectual deterioration and personality changes.

There is atrophy of the temporalis, masseter and sternomastoid muscles, and distal limb weakness and wasting (**Fig. 28.155**).

Atrophy of the masticatory muscles leads to an open mouth posture (myopathic facies; **Fig. 28.156**) and myotonia in the tongue causes difficulty in speaking (dysarthria). There may also be dysphagia and increased caries.

There are pronounced changes in dental arch form with open occlusal relationships, expanded arches and labially or buccally displaced teeth, often with diastemas, and a high arched palate (**Fig. 28.157**).

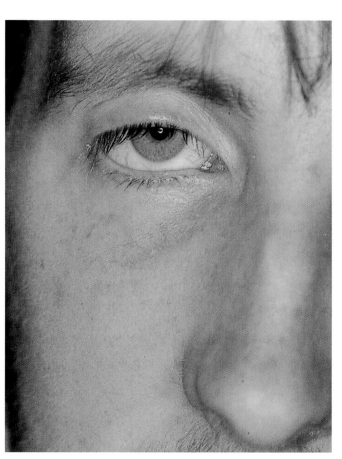

28.154

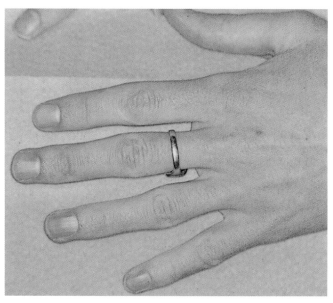

28.155

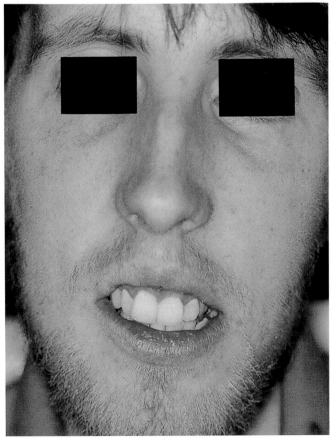

28.156

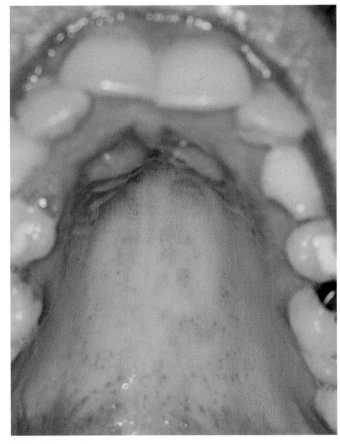

28.157

NAEVI

Most intraoral melanotic naevi are seen on the hard palate (**Figs 28.158, 28.159**) or in the buccal mucosa (**Figs 28.160, 28.161**). Most are circumscribed, small, greyish or brownish macules and are benign.

The most common are intramucosal naevi (see **Fig. 28.159**), which are typically seen in the palate or buccal mucosa as brown macules or papules. Less common are oral melanotic macules and compound, junctional and blue naevi.

Naevus unius lateris is a warty proliferation (verrucous naevus) of unknown aetiology (**Fig. 28.162**).

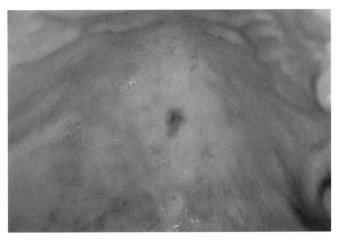

28.158

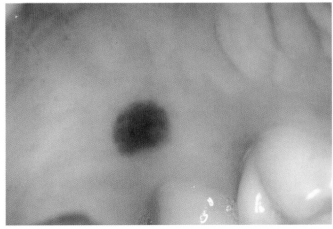

28.159

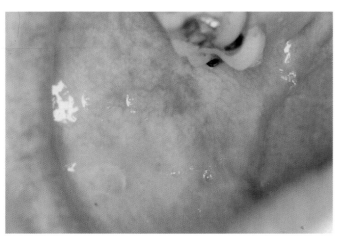

28.160

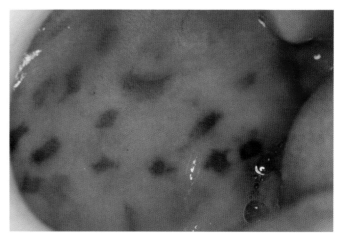

28.161

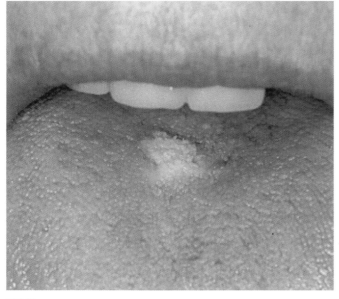

28.162

OLMSTED'S SYNDROME

This is a rare autosomal dominant disorder characterized by mutilating palmoplantar and periorofacial hyperkeratosis. Contraction of fingers and deep fissuring of the feet are common complications.

Symmetrical, yellow-brown hyperkeratotic plaques and papules are seen around the mouth (**Fig. 28.163**) and other body orifices such as the nares, inguinal region, and perianal and gluteal areas. Other manifestations include oral keratosis and large axillary verrucous plaques.

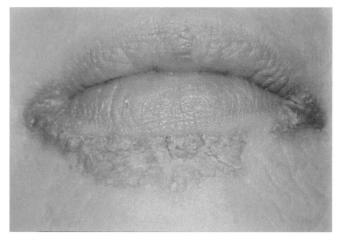

28.163

OROFACIODIGITAL SYNDROME

Multiple fibrous bands may be associated with cleft or lobulated tongue, polydactyly and often a midline cleft of the upper lip in Mohr's syndrome: orofaciodigital syndrome (OFD) type II (**Figs 28.164–28.166**).

In OFD type I, the tongue may be bifid or lobed, with cleft lip or palate and hypodontia or supernumerary teeth; fraenae and fraenulae are short and there is hyperteleorism, mental changes and brachy-, syn-, or clinodactyly.

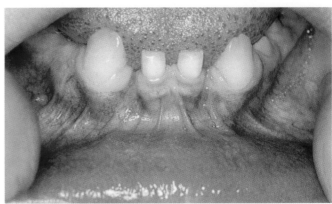

28.165

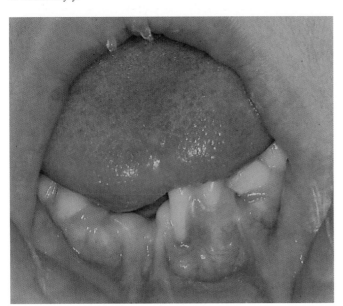

28.164

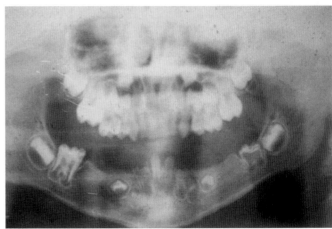

28.166

OSTEOGENESIS IMPERFECTA *(fragilitas ossium)*

Osteogenesis imperfecta is a group of rare disorders in which a defect in type I collagen leads to fragile bones that fracture with minimal trauma. Autosomal dominant and recessive types have been described. There are several subtypes varying in severity and in features such as otosclerosis, blue sclerae (**Figs 28.167, 28.168**; see also **Fig. 15.37**). hypermobile joints, cardiac valve defects (mitral valve prolapse or aortic incompetence) and dentinogenesis imperfecta.

The primary dentition may be affected by dentinogenesis imperfecta in some types of osteogenesis imperfecta (**Fig. 28.169**). The permanent dentition may be unaffected.

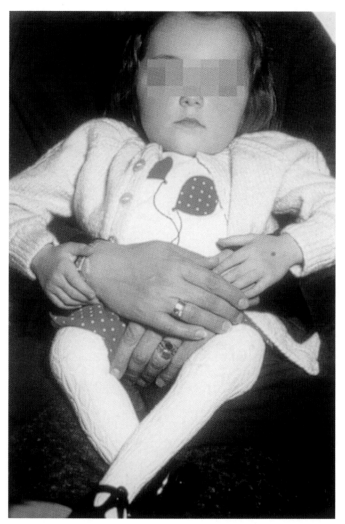

28.167

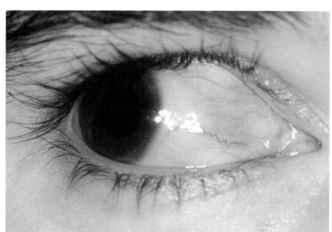

28.168

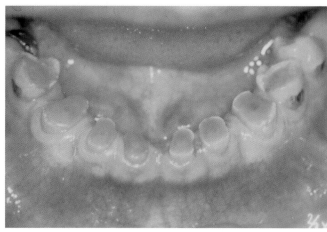

28.169

OSTEOPETROSIS *(Albers-Schönberg syndrome)*

Osteopetrosis is a rare inherited disorder of bone. The autosomal recessive malignant type is lethal in early life but the autosomal dominant type is compatible with life. The maxilla is hypoplastic (**Fig. 28.170**) and sinuses obliterated.

The bones are extremely dense (**Fig. 28.171**) and teeth often have short roots and may erupt late or not at all; the dense bone causes a predisposition to osteomyelitis. Bone-marrow transplantation as therapy can lead to graft-versus-host disease.

Van Buchem's disease (sclerosteosis) consists of generalized osteosclerosis with hyperostosis of the calvaria, mandible and clavicles, syndactyly and facial palsy.

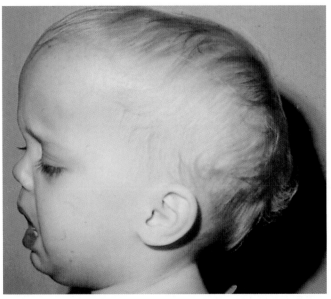

28.170

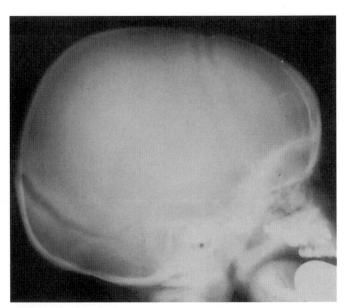

28.171

PACHYONYCHIA CONGENITA

In this autosomal dominant condition, there is palmar and plantar hyperhidrosis and hyperkeratosis with oral white lesions, which typically clinically resemble those of white sponge naevus, though they are occasionally isolated, and the nails become thickened, hard and yellow (**Figs 28.172–28.175**). The dorsum of tongue is the common site, although other sites may be affected. Natal teeth may be seen in affected neonates.

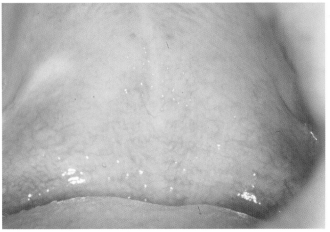

28.172

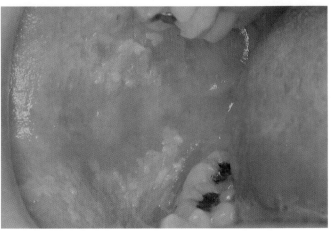

28.173

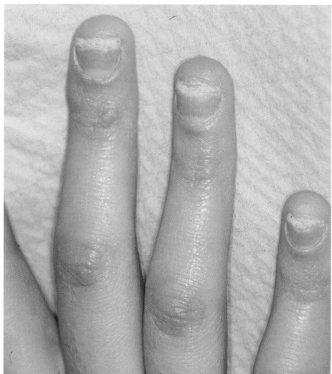

28.174

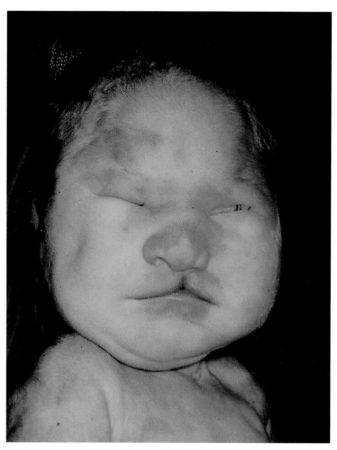

28.176

28.175

PATAU'S SYNDROME

Cleft lip (often bilateral) and cleft palate with micrognathia are orofacial features of trisomy 13 (**Fig. 28.176**).

PEUTZ–JEGHER'S SYNDROME *(lentigo polyposis)*

Peutz–Jeghers syndrome is an autosomal dominant disorder (the causative gene lying within chromosome 19p13.3) consisting of circumoral melanosis with intestinal polyposis (**Figs 28.177, 28.178**). Polyps are mainly in the small intestine. Brown or black small macules are seen around the mouth, nose and sometimes the eyes, and intraorally at any site, although rarely on the tongue or floor of the mouth. The pigmentation is typically spray like and brown and precedes detection of the polyps.

Peutz–Jeghers syndrome may occasionally be associated with malignant neoplasms of the gastrointestinal tract, ovary, cervix, testis and breast, and must be differentiated from the Carney complex.

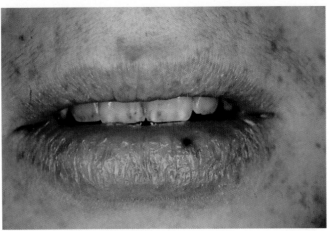
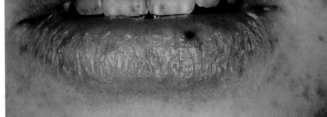

28.177

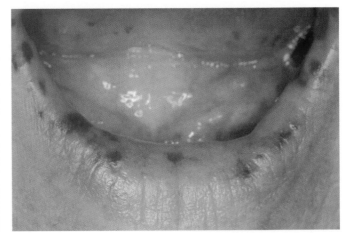

28.178

PIERRE ROBIN SEQUENCE SYNDROME

In this condition of severe congenital micrognathia with a cleft palate there may be glossoptosis and respiratory embarrassment. Periodic dyspnoea is often evident from birth. There may also be congenital cardiac anomalies and learning disability (**Fig. 28.179**).

RACIAL PIGMENTATION

Brown pigmentation is common, especially on the gingival in persons of Asian, African or Mediterranean origin (**Figs 28.180–28.182**).

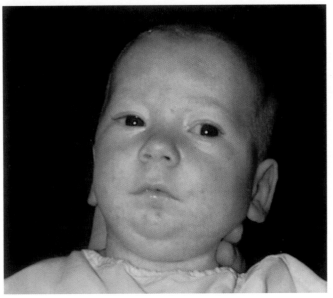

28.179

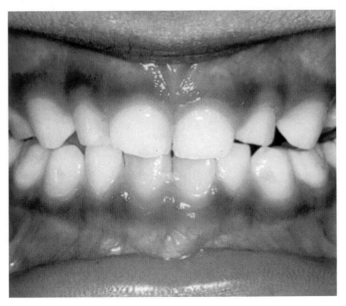

28.180

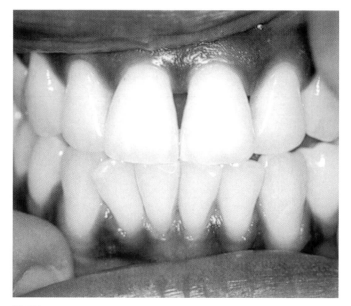

28.181

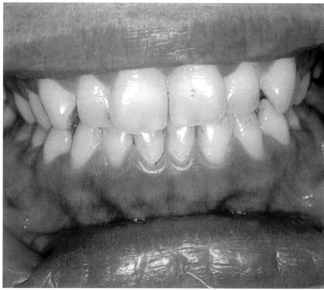

28.182

ROMBERG'S SYNDROME *(Parry–Romberg syndrome; progressive hemifacial atrophy)*

This syndrome consists of slowly progressive atrophy of the soft tissues of essentially half the face, accompanied usually by contralateral jacksonian epilepsy, trigeminal neuralgia, and changes in the eyes and hair.

SMITH–LEMLI–OPITZ SYNDROME

This is a rare autosomal recessive syndrome consisting of ptosis, broad nose and anteverted nostrils, low-set ears and micrognathia (**Figs 28.183, 28.184**). Most patients have some syndactyly, growth retardation and learning disability.

The maxillary alveolar ridges are broad and the palate high arched or cleft (see **Fig. 28.184**).

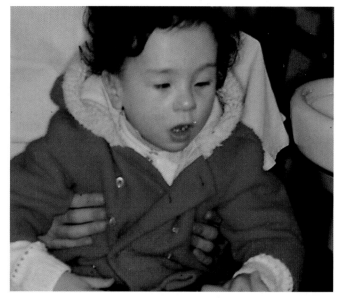

28.183

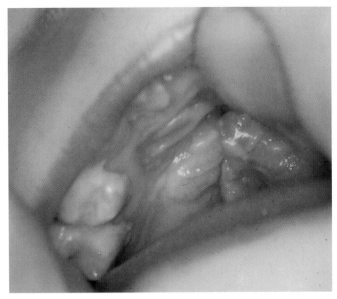

28.184

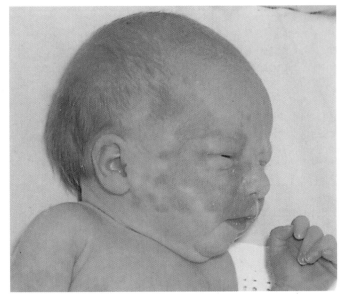

28.185

STURGE–WEBER SYNDROME (encephalofacial angiomatosis)

In this syndrome an angioma affects the upper face (**Figs 28.185–28.187**) and usually extends into the occipital lobe of the brain, producing epilepsy and often glaucoma, hemiplegia and learning disability.

The haemangioma often appears to be limited to the area of distribution of one or more of the divisions of the trigeminal nerve.

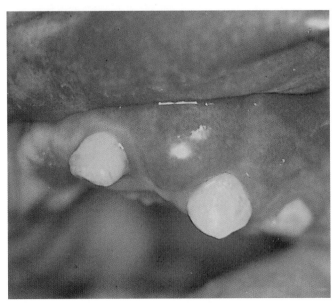

28.187

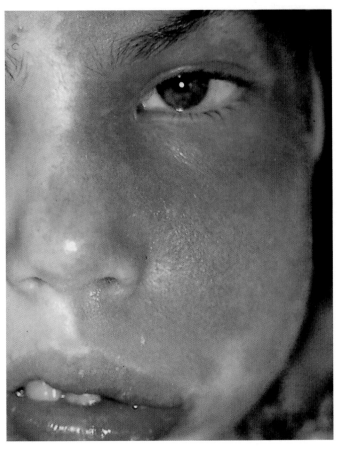

28.186

There may be neuralgia and the affected area is somewhat swollen and hypertrophic.

Radiography shows calcification intracranially in the angioma (see **Fig. 28.188**).

The haemangioma may extend intraorally and be associated with hypertrophy of the affected jaw, macrodontia, and accelerated tooth eruption. Since the patients are often treated with phenytoin there is frequently also gingival swelling.

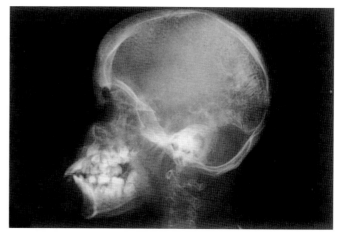

28.188

TETRALOGY OF FALLOT

Tetralogy of Fallot is one of the most frequent of the cyanotic congenital heart diseases. Ventricular septal defect, pulmonary stenosis, right ventricular hypertrophy and an aorta that overrides both ventricles are the features of the tetralogy. Central cyanosis is seen in the lips, tongue and other mucosae and the teeth are milky white in contrast (**Figs 28.189, 28.190**). There is an increased prevalence of fissured and geographic tongue in children with cyanotic heart disease.

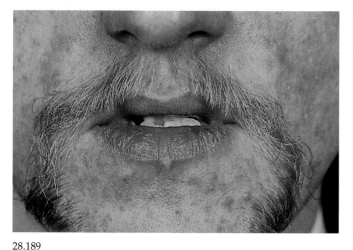

28.189

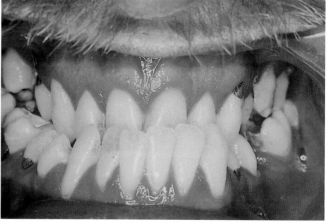

28.190

THYROID *(lingual)*

The thyroid arises embryonically from an invagination of lingual mucosa but occasionally thyroid tissue remains in the tongue (**Fig. 28.191**). Complications may include hypothyroidism in up to 20% of patients, dysplasia, dysarthria or dyspnoea. A radionuclide scan will define exactly what thyroid tissue is present, and where, since in about two-thirds of cases no thyroid tissue is present in the neck.

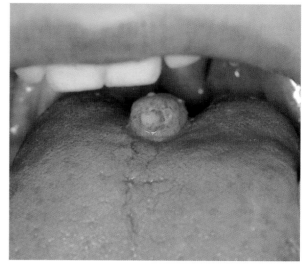

28.191

TORI

Tori, which are discussed in Chapter 26, present as bony lumps.

TREACHER COLLINS' SYNDROME
(mandibulofacial dysostosis)

Treacher Collins' syndrome is an autosomal dominant condition, caused by a first branchial arch anomaly. The face is characteristic, with pronounced antimongoloid slanting of the eyes and lower lid colobomas, defective orbital rims, zygomatic and mandibular hypoplasia (defective ramus, coronoid and condylar processes) and low-set malformed ears, often with deafness (**Figs 28.192–28.195**).

Malocclusion is common (see **Fig. 28.197**) and there may be parotid hypoplasia. Cleft palate is seen in about one-third of patients.

The association of this first arch anomaly with absent thumbs is Nager's syndrome.

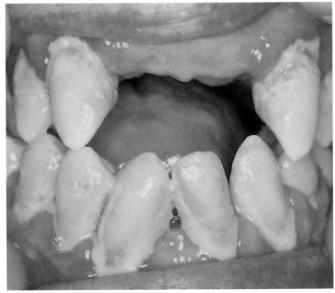

28.193

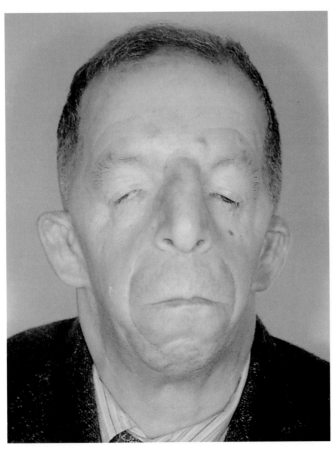

28.192

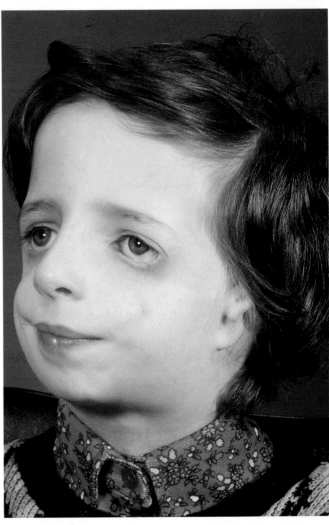

28.194

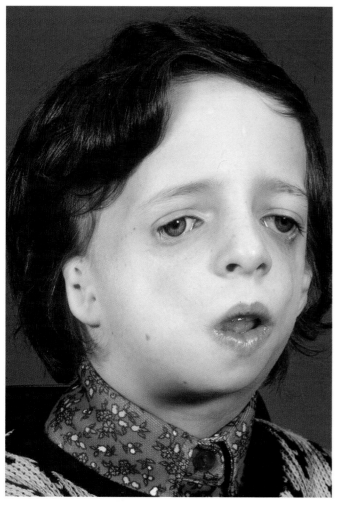

28.195

VAN DER WOUDE SYNDROME

Lower lip pits are often (75–80%) associated with a cleft lip and/or palate in the Van der Woude syndrome. This is a rare autosomal dominant syndrome, sometimes seen with syndactyly or talipes equinovarus (**Fig. 28.196**).

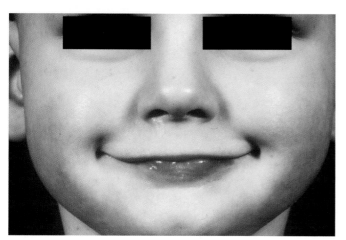

28.196

VON RECKLINGHAUSEN'S DISEASE
(generalized neurofibromatosis)

The disease known as neurofibromatosis is now recognized to consist of distinct variants that differ from each other genetically, microscopically, and clinically. Neurofibromatosis type I (NF-I) is often referred to as von Recklinghausen's disease of the skin.

Neurofibromatosis type II (NF-II) is a much more uncommon manifestation, which probably results from a structural defect in chromosome 22, as opposed to NF-I, which is related to chromosome 17. Although neurofibromas occur in NF-II, neurilemmomas and acoustic neuromas are the predominant neural tumours; bilateral acoustic neuromas are the hallmark of the disease. NF-II largely afflicts the central nervous system and has a more gradual onset than, and different clinical features from, NF-I. One of the most feared complications of NF-I is the development of cancer, which is estimated to occur in about 5% of cases. The most common associated malignancy is the neurofibrosarcoma but this is rare in the mouth.

Cutaneous and subcutaneous neurofibromas (**Figs 28.197–28.203**), with skin hyperpigmentation are the features of von Recklinghausen's disease (NF-I). This is an autosomal dominant condition but many cases are new mutations.

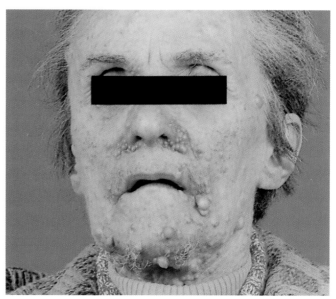

28.197

Café-au-lait hyperpigmented patches are seen, especially in the axillary region (see **Figs 28.198, 28.200**; **Fig. 28.199** also shows an adjacent neurofibroma).

Dystrophic kyphoscoliosis is common (see **Fig. 28.202**) and there may sometimes be learning disability and epilepsy, or rarely renal artery stenosis or phaeochromocytoma.

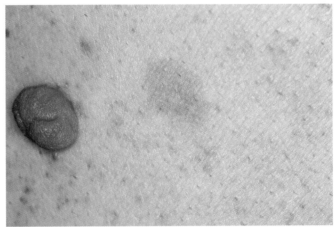

28.199

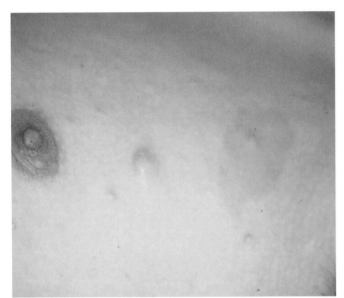

28.198

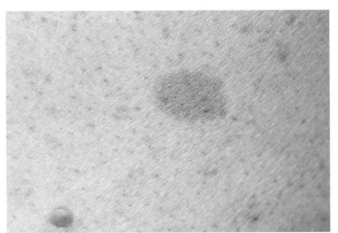

28.200

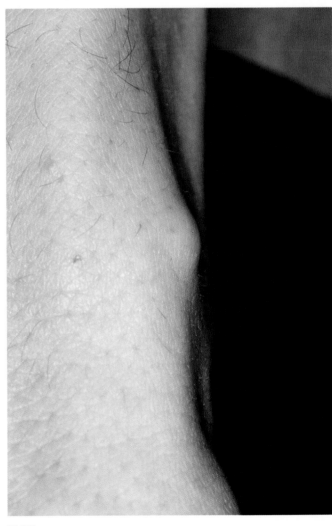

28.201

Acoustic neuromas are not common — many earlier reports were of a distinct condition of bilateral acoustic neurofibromatosis (NF-II). However, optic nerve or optic chiasmal gliomas may be present.

Neurofibromas may affect any part of the body, including the oral cavity, and typically the tongue or palate (see **Fig. 28.203**).

Most patients also have small dome-shaped brown hamartomas (Lisch nodules) on the front of the iris (on slit-lamp examination).

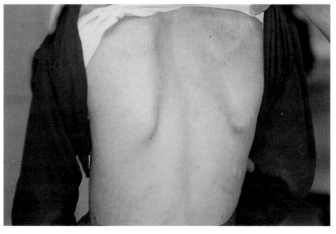

28.202

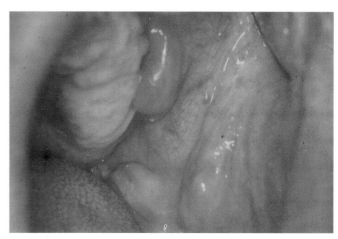

28.203

WHITE SPONGE NAEVUS *(familial white folded gingivostomatosis)*

White sponge naevus is a symptomless inconsequential autosomal dominant condition, which manifests from infancy. The oral mucosa is thickened, folded, spongy and white or grey (**Figs 28.204, 28.205**).

Lesions are bilateral in the oral mucosa and can affect the oesophageal, nasal, vaginal or anal mucosa. Rare cases have iris coloboma.

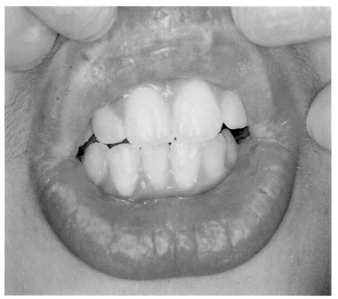

28.204

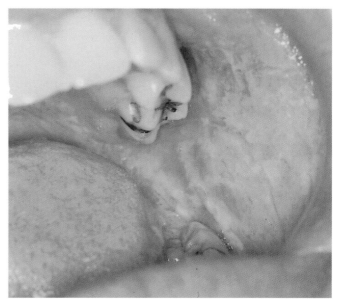

28.205

FURTHER READING

Aggarwal VR, Sloan P, Horner K, et al. Dento-osseous changes as diagnostic markers in familial adenomatous polyposis families. Oral Dis 2003; 9(1): 29–33.

Auyeung J, Mohanty K, Tayton K. Maffucci lymphangioma syndrome: an unusual variant of Ollier's disease, a case report and a review of the literature. J Pediatr Orthop B 2003; 12(2): 147–50.

Bazopoulou-Kyrkanidou E, Tosios KI, Zebelis G, Charalampopoulou S, Papanicolau SI. Hyalinosis cutis et mucosae: gingival involvement. J Oral Pathol Med 1998; 27: 233–7.

Becelli R, Renzi G, Cerulli G, Saltarel A, Perugini M. Von Recklinghausen neurofibromatosis with palatal localization. Diagnostic and surgical problems in two clinical cases. Minerva Stomatol 2002; 51(9): 391–7.

Chao SC, Tsai YM, Yang MH, Lee JY. A novel mutation in the keratin 4 gene causing white sponge naevus. Br J Dermatol 2003; 148(6): 1125–8.

Chaudhary SJ, Dayal PK. Hyalinosis cutis et mucosae. Review with a case report. Oral Surg Oral Med Oral Pathol 1995; 80: 168–71.

Chaudhry SI, Shirlaw PJ, Morgan PR, Challacombe SJ. Cowden's syndrome (multiple hamartoma and neoplasia syndrome): diagnostic dilemmas in three cases. Oral Dis 2000; 6: 248–52.

Cicek Y, Ertas U. The normal and pathological pigmentation of oral mucous membrane: a review. J Contemp Dent Pract 2003; 4(3): 76–86.

Cohen MM Jr. Asymmetry: molecular, biologic, embryopathic, and clinical perspectives. Am J Med Genet 2001; 101: 292–314.

Cohen MM Jr. Craniofacial anomalies: Clinical and molecular perspectives. Ann Acad Med Singapore 2003; 32(2): 244–51.

Czarny-Ratajczak M, Latos-Bielenska A. Collagens, the basic proteins of the human body. J Appl Genet 2000; 41(4): 317–30.

De Coster PJ, Malfait F, Martens LC, De Paepe A. Unusual oral findings in dermatosparaxis (Ehlers–Danlos syndrome type VIIC). J Oral Pathol Med 2003; 32(9): 568–70.

Eng C. PTEN: one gene, many syndromes. Hum Mutat 2003; 22(3): 183–98.

Flores-Sarnat L. New insights into craniosynostosis. Semin Pediatr Neurol 2002; 9(4): 274–91.

Francis-West PH, Robson L, Evans DJ. Craniofacial development: the tissue and molecular interactions that control development of the head. Adv Anat Embryol Cell Biol 2003; 169: III–VI, 1–138.

Frohberg U, Tiner BD. Surgical correction of facial deformities in a patient with cleidocranial dysplasia. J Craniofac Surg 1995; 6: 49–53.

Hamada T. Lipoid proteinosis. Clin Exp Dermatol 2002; 27: 624–9.

Hand JL, Rogers RS 3rd. Oral manifestations of genodermatoses. Dermatol Clin 2003; 21: 183–94.

Happle R. A fresh look at incontinentia pigmenti. Arch Dermatol 2003; 139(9): 1206–8.

Hewitt C, McCormick D, Linden G, et al. The role of cathepsin C in Papillon-Lefevre syndrome, prepubertal periodontitis, and aggressive periodontitis. Hum Mutat 2004; 23(3): 222–8.

Holzhausen M, Goncalves D, Correa F de O, Spolidorio LC, Rodrigues VC, Orrico SR. A case of Zimmermann-Laband syndrome with supernumerary teeth. J Periodontol 2003; 74(8): 1225–30.

Hunt JA, Hobar PC. Common craniofacial anomalies: the facial dysostoses. Plast Reconstr Surg 2002; 110(7): 1714–25.

Israel H. Gingival lesions in lipoid proteinosis. J Periodontol 1992; 62: 561–4.

Kahler SG, Fahey MC. Metabolic disorders and mental retardation. Am J Med Genet 2003; 17C(1): 31–41.

Katz J, Guelmann M, Barak S. Hereditary gingival fibromatosis with distinct dental, skeletal and developmental abnormalities. Pediatr Dent 2002; 24(3): 253–6.

Lalakea ML, Messner AH. Ankyloglossia: does it matter? Pediatr Clin North Am 2003; 50(2): 381–97.

Lim W, Hearle N, Shah B, et al. Tuberous sclerosis: presentation of a clinical case with oral manifestations. Med Oral 2003; 8: 122–8.

Makhoul EN, Ayoub NM, Helou JF, Abadjian GA. Familial Laugier–Hunziker syndrome. J Am Acad Dermatol 2003; 49(2 Suppl Case Reports): S143–5.

Mirowski GW, Liu AA, Stone ML, Caldemeyer KS. Sturge–Weber syndrome. J Am Acad Dermatol 1999; 41: 772–3.

Moko SB, Mistry Y, Blandin de Chalain TM. Parry–Romberg syndrome: intracranial MRI appearances. J Craniomaxillofac Surg 2003; 31(5): 321–4.

Morava E, Karteszi J, Weisenbach J, Caliebe A, Mundlos S, Mehes K. Cleidocranial dysplasia with decreased bone density and biochemical findings of hypophosphatasia. Eur J Pediatr 2002; 161(11): 619–22.

Patrono C, Dionisi-Vici C, Giannotti A, et al. Two novel mutations of the human delta7-sterol reductase (DHCR7) gene in children with Smith–Lemli–Opitz syndrome. Mol Cell Probes 2002; 16(4): 315–18.

Porter S, Cawson R, Scully C, Eveson J. Multiple hamartoma syndrome presenting with oral lesions. Oral Surg Oral Med Oral Pathol Oral Radiol Endod 1996; 82: 295–301.

Reifenberger J, Rauch L, Beckmann MW, Megahed M, Ruzicka T, Reifenberger G. Cowden's disease: clinical and molecular genetic findings in a patient with a novel PTEN germline mutation. Br J Dermatol 2003; 148(5): 1040–6.

Sabry MA, Farag TI, Shaltout AA, et al. Kenny–Caffey syndrome: an Arab variant? Clin Genet 1999; 55(1): 44–9.

Sandrini F, Stratakis C. Clinical and molecular genetics of Carney complex. Mol Genet Metab 2003; 78(2): 83–92.

Shibuya Y, Zhang J, Yokoo S, Umeda M, Komori T. Constitutional mutation of keratin 13 gene in familial white sponge nevus. Oral Surg Oral Med Oral Pathol Oral Radiol Endod 2003; 96(5): 561–5.

Smith F. The molecular genetics of keratin disorders. Am J Clin Dermatol 2003; 4(5): 347–64.

Smith D, Porter SR, Scully C. Gingival and other oral manifestations in tuberous sclerosis — a case report. Periodontal Clinical Investigations 1994; 15: 13–16.

Straub AM, Grahame R, Scully C, Tonetti MS. Severe periodontitis in Marfan's syndrome. J Periodontol 2002; 73: 823–6.

Terezhalmy GT, Riley CK, Moore WS. Progressive facial hemiatrophy (Parry–Romberg syndrome). Quintessence Int 2001; 32(10): 820–1.

Thomas D, Rapley J, Strathman R, Parker R. Tuberous sclerosis with gingival overgrowth. J Periodontol 1992; 63: 713–17.

29 CHEMICAL AGENTS

- acrodynia
- allergic reactions
- amalgam tattoo
- angioedema
- betel nut staining
- body art
- burns
- candidosis
- cheilitis
- drug-induced gingival swelling
- drug-induced hyperpigmentation
- drug-induced mucositis and ulceration
- drug-induced xerostomia
- erosions
- facial palsy
- herpesvirus infections
- human papillomavirus infections
- leukoplakia
- lichenoid lesions
- neoplasms and potentially malignant lesions
- orofacial granulomatosis
- osteonecrosis
- stomatitis nicotina
- tooth erosion
- tooth staining.

ACRODYNIA

Chronic mercury exposure, from mercuric oxide (calomel) in teething powders, was a common cause of acrodynia up until the early 1950s. Now rare, acrodynia may still be caused by mercury from paints, ointments, broken fluorescent light bulbs, or metallic mercury. Most cases are in children up to the age of 8 years and present with profuse sweating, rashes, photophobia, alopecia, and puffiness and pink colour of the face (**Fig. 29.1**), hands and feet (Pink disease).

Oral ulcers, disturbed tooth development and tooth exfoliation may be seen in severe acrodynia (**Fig. 29.2**).

Acrodynia in many ways resembles Kawasaki's disease (mucocutaneous lymph node syndromes.

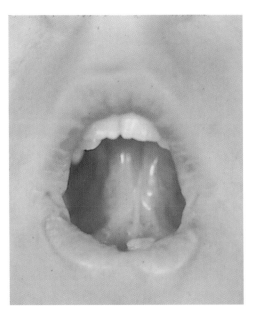

29.1

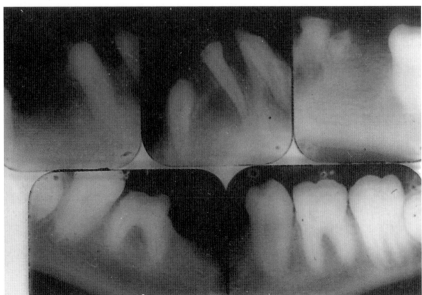

29.2

ALLERGIC REACTIONS

Latex, and other rubber products, such as dental dams (**Fig. 29.3**), eugenol and other essential oils (**Fig. 29.4**), various dentifrices (**Fig. 29.5**), mouthwashes and cosmetics occasionally induce allergic reactions. Rarely, drugs may induce a fixed drug eruption (**Fig. 29.6**).

Orofacial granulomatosis may have a background in hypersensitivity to components of some food and drinks (see Chapter 19).

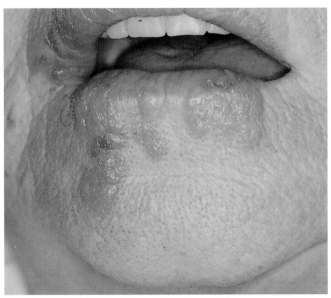

29.4

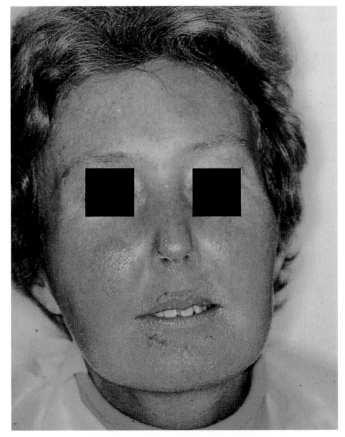

29.3

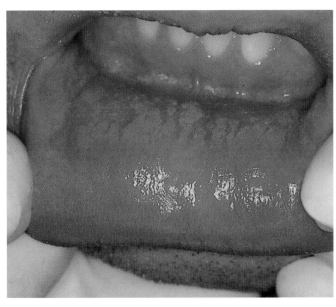

29.5

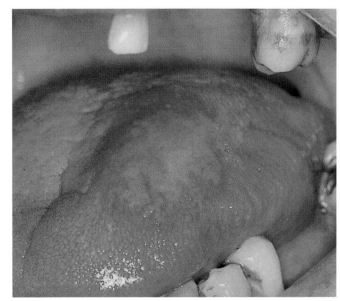

29.6

AMALGAM TATTOO

Dental amalgam is a common cause of acquired oral hyper-pigmentation (**Fig. 29.7**). Amalgam used as a retrograde root-filling material may cause discoloration high on the alveolar mucosa towards the vestibule (**Figs 29.7–29.10**).

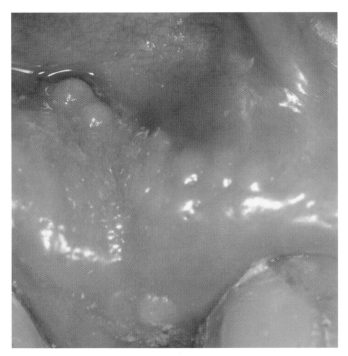

29.9

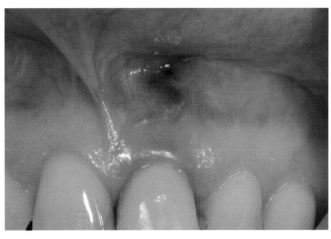

29.7

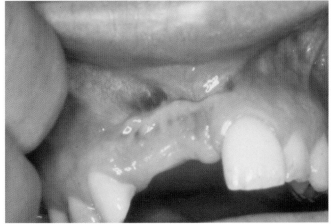

29.8

Amalgam can also be incorporated into the tissues accidentally during conservative dentistry procedures. A bluish-black macule is usually seen in the gingiva or vestibule, especially in the mandible in the premolar–molar region (**Fig. 29.10**).

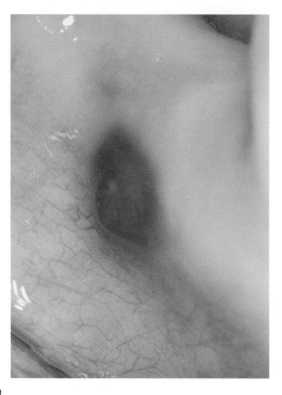

29.10

BETEL NUT STAINING

Betel use, typically in a quid with tobacco, not only causes discoloration of the mucosa (**Fig. 29.12**) and teeth (**Fig. 29.13**), but can predispose to oral submucous fibrosis, leukoplakia and carcinoma.

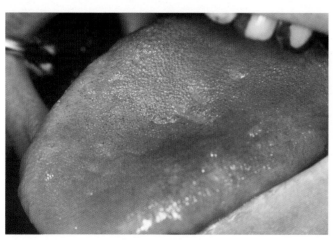

29.12

ANGIOEDEMA

Allergic angioedema is a type 1 response mediated by leukotrienes and vasoactive amines released from mast cells and basophils in an IgE-mediated response to an allergen. Labial swelling is a common presentation (**Fig. 29.11**).

Allergens can be as varied as systemically administered drugs (such as penicillin) or topically contacted allergens in foodstuffs (such as benzoic and sorbic acids) (see also Section 1.5).

Nonallergic angioedema can arise in patients receiving angiotensin-converting enzyme (ACE) inhibitors. Hereditary angioedema is discussed elsewhere.

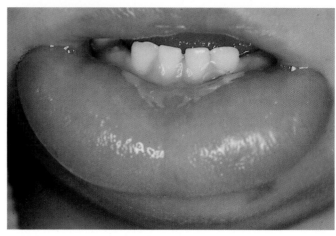

29.11

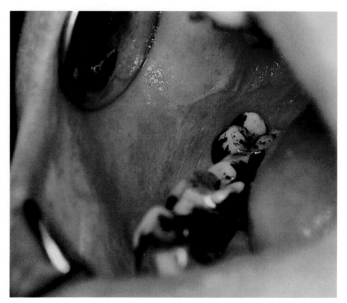

29.13

BODY ART

Tattoos may be seen as part of a cultural behaviour in both the developing and developed world (**Figs 29.14, 29.15**).

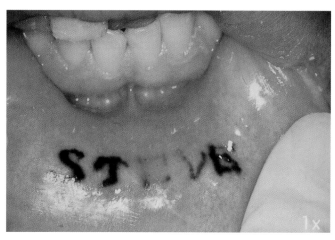

29.15

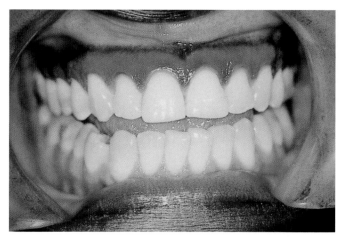

29.14

BURNS

Some patients burn their mucosa by attempts to relieve oral pain by holding an analgesic such as aspirin, or applying eugenol (**Figs 29.16, 29.17**) at the site of pain. Sometimes relatively severe oral burns can result.

Overenthusiastic or undiluted use of concentrated solutions of aqueous chlorhexidine may rarely produce burns (**Fig. 29.18**) and often produces superficial tooth and mucosal discoloration. Taste disturbances and salivary gland swelling are rare sequelae of chlorhexidine use.

Natural products such as cannabis (**Fig. 29.19**) and cocaine (**Figs 29.20, 29.21**) are sometimes deliberately rubbed into the gingivae or vestibule when gingival ulceration and necrosis, accompanied by a brief 'high', can occur. Oral neglect with caries and gingivitis are seen in **Figs 29.20** and **29.21** in juveniles who applied cocaine and amfetamine (mixed with sugar) to the maxillary gingiva, consequently with

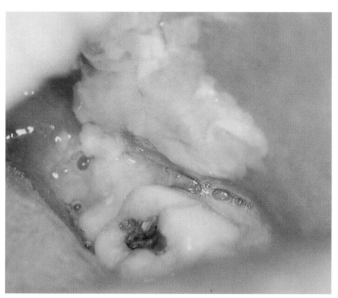

29.16

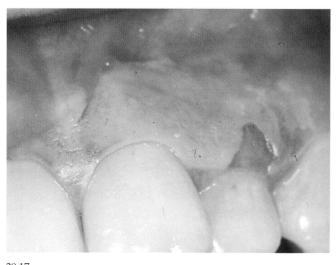

29.17

vestibular burns and caries. The powerful vasoconstrictive effects are probably responsible for some of the local destruction. Tissue damage can develop within a few days of the regular application of cocaine causing both soft- and hard-tissue destruction, although lesions usually heal when there is a cessation of the cocaine abuse. Crack cocaine (smoked) can cause ulceration of the palate and rarely oronasal fistulae. Ecstasy can cause bruxism.

The houseplant *Dieffenbachia*, or the enzyme bromelin in pineapple, may occasionally cause burns.

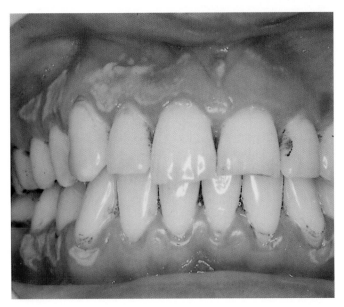

29.18

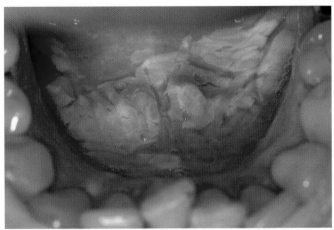

29.19

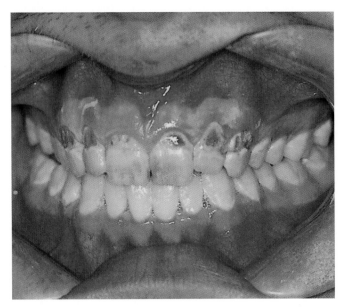

29.20

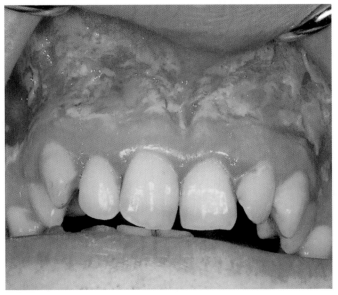

29.21

CANDIDOSIS

Many systemic immunosuppressants predispose to candidosis. Some forms of candidosis such as erythematous candidosis (**Fig. 29.22**) are predisposed by smoking.

Oral thrush can be induced by use of a corticosteroid inhaler (**Figs 29.23, 29.24**). Lesions are typically seen in the fauces.

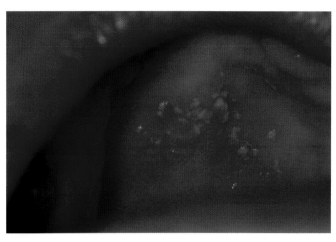

29.23

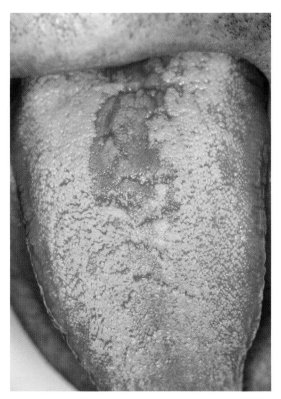

29.22

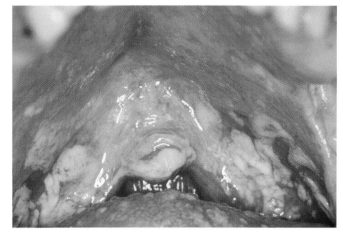

29.24

CHEILITIS

Inflammation of the lips can result from contact reactions to various substances, including cosmetics, lip salves, dentifrices and mouthwashes, dental materials and even some food and drink (**Fig. 29.25**).

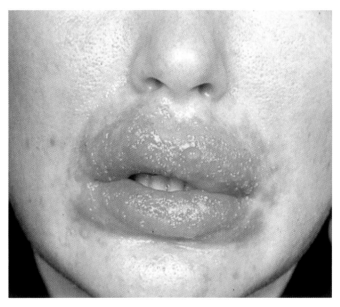

29.25

DRUG-INDUCED GINGIVAL SWELLING

Gingival enlargement may occur in patients receiving phenytoin, ciclosporin and calcium channel blocker therapy (**Figs 29.26–29.29**; see also Section 1.5), particularly nifedipine, but also diltiazem, felodipine, amlodipine and others. It is suggested that the gingival overgrowth is due to impaired collagen resorption secondary to defective fibroblast function.

The anticonvulsant phenytoin is the drug which classically can produce gingival hyperplasia. Poor oral hygiene exacerbates the swelling, which appears interdentally 2–3 months after treatment is started. The papillae enlarge to a variable extent, with relatively little tendency to bleed.

Ciclosporin is a commonly used immunosuppressive drug that can cause gingival hyperplasia closely resembling that induced by phenytoin. It is seen mainly anteriorly and labially and is exacerbated

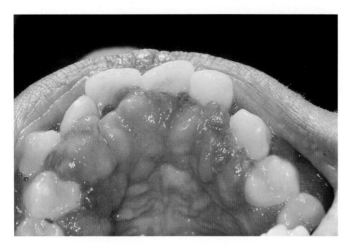

29.26

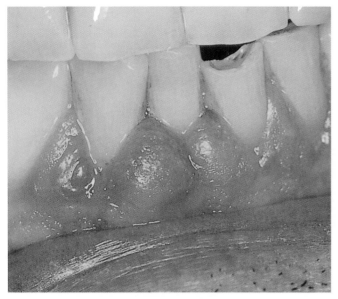

29.28

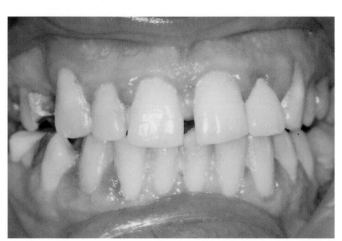

29.27

29.29

by poor oral hygiene and concurrent administration of nifedipine. Tacrolimus does not cause this adverse oral side-effect but has been associated with ulceration.

Drugs that produce gingival hyperplasia may also induce hirsutism (**Fig. 23.30**).

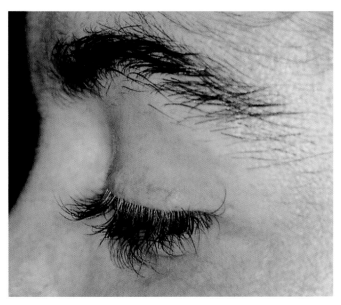

29.30

DRUG-INDUCED HYPERPIGMENTATION

Facial and/or oral hyperpigmentation may be caused in particular by phenothiazines (**Figs 29.31, 29.32**), but also by phenytoin (**Fig. 29.33**), minocycline, antimalarials (**Figs 29.34, 29.35**), zidovudine (**Fig. 29.36**), ACTH, clofazimine, ketoconazole, busulfan and other drugs (see Section 1.5). Long-term use of tranquillizers, such as chlorpromazine, may also produce xerostomia and facial dyskinesias. Heavy metal poisoning is fortunately now rare. Bismuth and lead caused a line at the gingival margin where sulphides were deposited in areas of poor oral hygiene (**Figs 29.37, 29.38**).

Arsenic poisoning is also now rare and usually follows the ingestion of pesticides containing arsenates. Arsenic binds to keratins and chronic intoxication leads to mucositis, pigmentation and facial oedema (**Figs 29.39, 29.40**). This poisoning causes 'rain-drop' hyperpigmentation of the skin with hyperkeratosis of the palms and soles, and white transverse striae on the nails (Mees' lines).

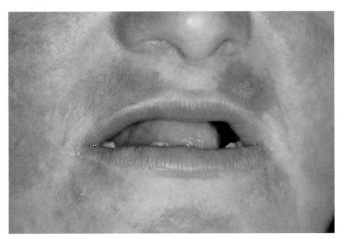

29.31

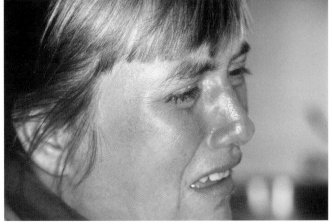

29.32

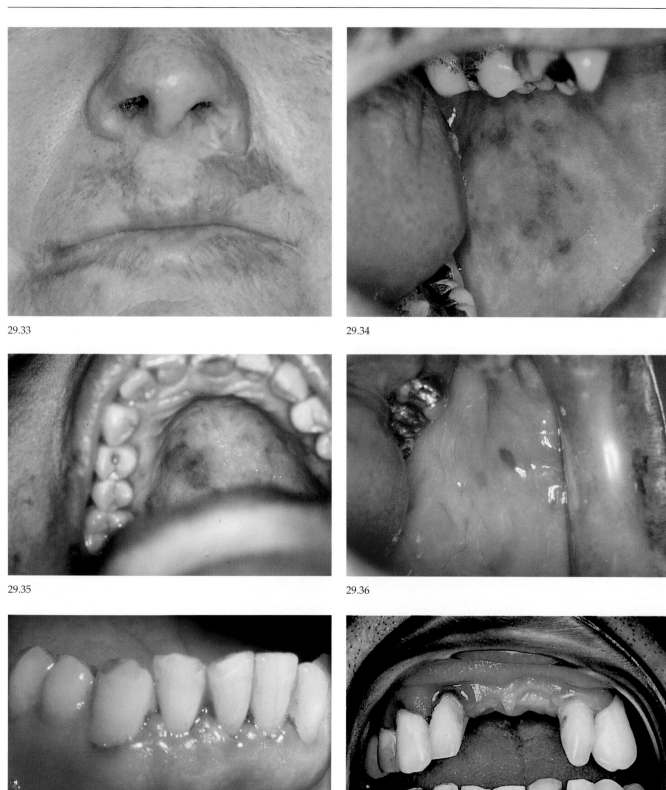

29.33

29.34

29.35

29.36

29.37

29.38

A wide range of other poisons can cause oral problems. These may include a burning mouth, ulceration, oedema, changes in salivation, changes in taste, hyperpigmentation or changes in sensation (see Section 1.5).

Various chemicals that may produce a photosensitive dermatitis and pigmentation include furocumarine, bergamot oil and eugenol, which may be found in perfumes, sprays, creams, mouthwashes and breath fresheners.

Chloasma (perioral hyperpigmentation) may arise during pregnancy or in patients using the oral contraceptive (**Fig. 29.41**) or various other products (see Section 1.5). Superficial mucosal and tooth staining may be caused particularly by chlorhexidine (**Figs 29.42, 29.43**), betel and tobacco use and also iron, bismuth subsalicylate, some antimicrobial agents and various other substances. Black hairy tongue may occasionally be a consequence of antimicrobial use

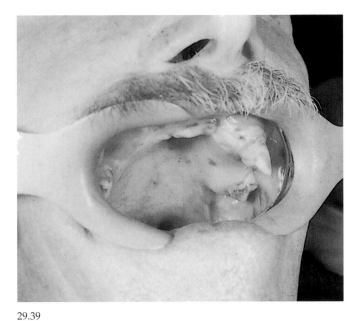

29.39

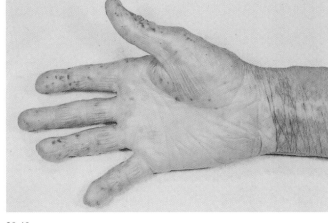

29.40

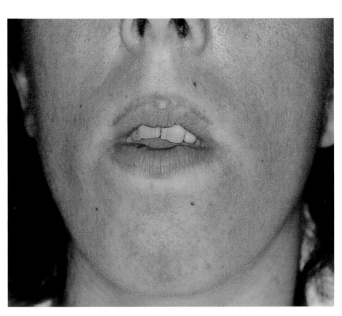

29.41

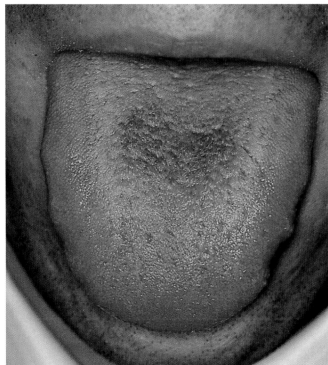

29.42

(**Fig. 29.44**) or lanzoprasole (**Fig. 29.45**), or through sucking lozenges. Even hormone replacement therapy may transiently stain the tongue (**Fig. 29.46**).

Toluidine blue is sometimes used to highlight for biopsy areas of potentially malignant lesions (**Fig. 29.47**); accidental injection can result in the permanent tattooing of the tongue (**Figs 29.48, 29.49**).

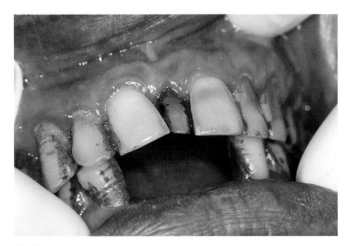

29.43

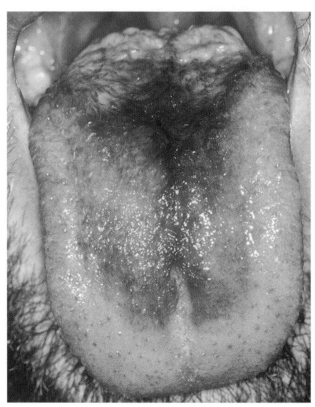

29.44

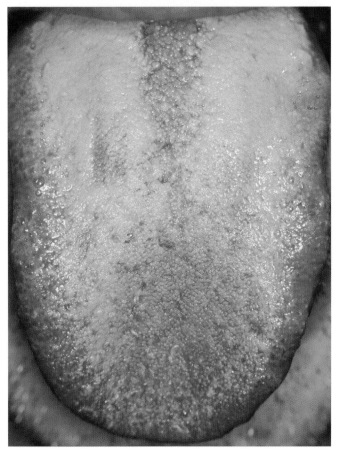

29.45

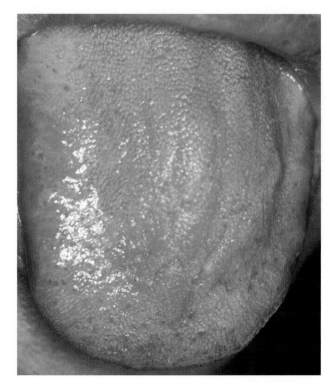

29.46

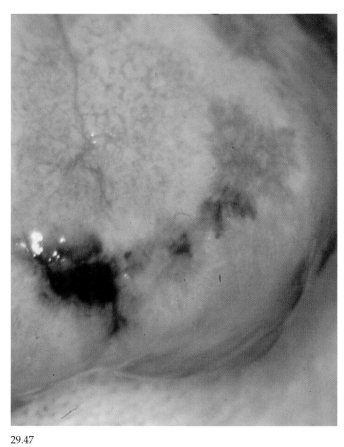

29.47

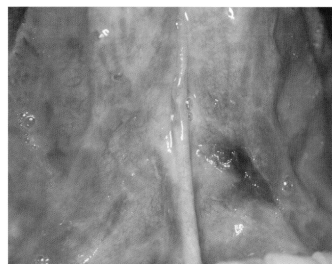

29.48

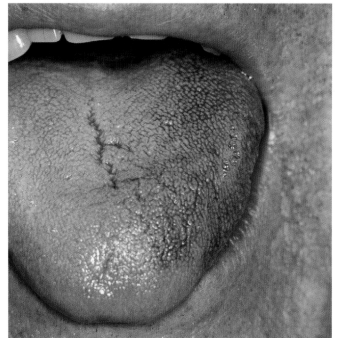

29.49

DRUG-INDUCED MUCOSITIS AND ULCERATION

A range of drugs may produce mucositis and/or oral ulceration (see Section 1.5). The most consistent association of mucositis is with cytotoxic chemotherapeutic agents (**Fig. 29.50**). Ulceration may also be caused by nonsteroidal anti-inflammatory drugs (NSAIDs), nicorandil (a cardiac drug with potassium channel blocking action; **Fig. 29.51**), alendronate (**Fig. 29.52**), some of the drugs causing lichenoid reactions, and many others.

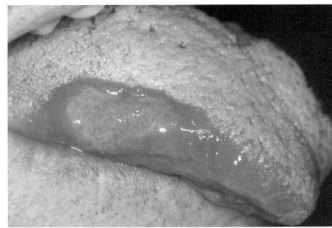

29.51

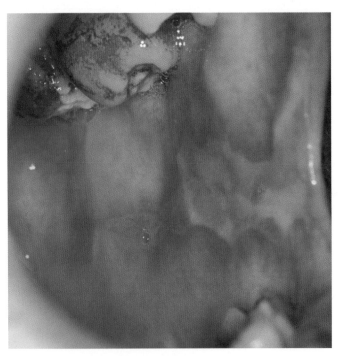

29.50

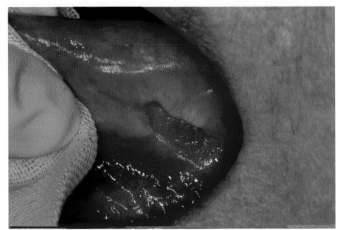

29.52

DRUG-INDUCED XEROSTOMIA

Various drugs may produce xerostomia (**Fig. 29.53**). Atropinics or sympathomimetics are usually responsible, especially some tranquillizers, antihypertensives, antidepressants and agents used to control a overactive bladder (see Section 1.5 and **Table 29.1**).

Table 29.1 DRUGS CAUSING DRY MOUTH

Anticholinergic drugs
Tricyclic antidepressants
Muscarinic receptor antagonists for treatment of overactive bladder
Alpha-receptor antagonists for treatment of urinary retention
Antipsychotics, such as phenothiazines
Diuretics
Antihistamines

Sympathomimetic drugs
Antihypertensive agents
Antidepressants (serotonin agonists, or noradrenaline (norepinephrine) and/or serotonin re-uptake blockers)
Appetite suppressants
Decongestants and 'cold cures'
Bronchodilators

Skeletal muscle relaxants

Antimigraine agents

Benzodiazepines, hypnotics, opioids and drugs of abuse

H_2 antagonists and proton pump inhibitors

Cytotoxic drugs

Retinoids

Anti-HIV drugs
E.g. dideoxyinosine (DDI) and protease inhibitors

Cytokines

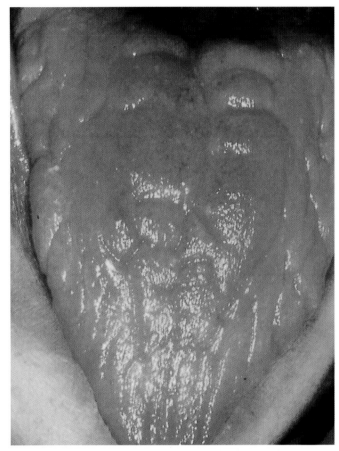

29.53

EROSIONS

Chemicals such as acids (chromic; trichloracetic; phosphoric) may be used during dental procedures and can cause ulcers. Self-curing resins, especially epoxy resins for oral use may also produce mucosal erosions (**Fig. 29.54**), as may various mouthwashes. Rubber or silicone-based impression materials occasionally produce an erosive reaction (**Fig. 29.55**).

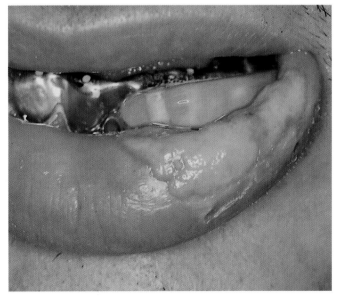

29.54

Lesions of erythema multiforme, toxic epidermal necrolysis or resembling lichen planus, lupus erythematosus, leukoplakia, pemphigoid or pemphigus may be drug induced.

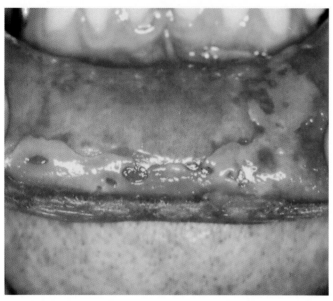

29.55

FACIAL PALSY

Inferior dental (alveolar) regional nerve local analgesic injections, if misplaced, may track through the parotid gland to reach the facial nerve and cause transient facial palsy (**Fig. 29.56**).

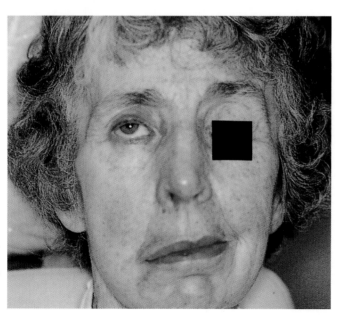

29.56

HERPESVIRUS INFECTIONS

Many systemic immunosuppressants predispose to herpesvirus infections.

HUMAN PAPILLOMAVIRUS INFECTIONS

Many systemic immunosuppressants predispose to HPV infections.

LEUKOPLAKIA

Sanguinaria may cause white mucosal lesions.

LICHENOID LESIONS

NSAIDs, antidiabetic, antihypertensive and antimalarial drugs are causes of lichenoid lesions. **Figs 29.57 and 29.58** were reactions to antihypertensive drugs (**Fig. 29.59** was to metronidazole; see also Section 1.5). Also responsible are some restorative materials, occasionally chronic graft-versus-host disease and possibly hepatitis C virus infection.

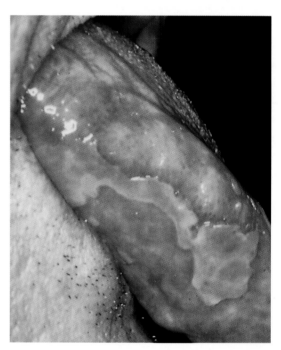

29.57

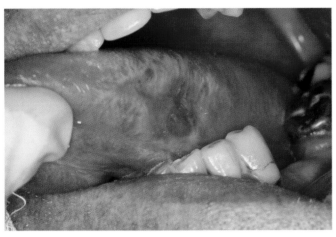

29.58

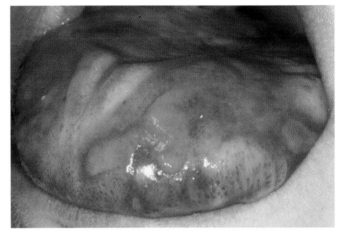

29.59

NEOPLASMS AND POTENTIALLY MALIGNANT LESIONS

Iatrogenic Kaposi's sarcoma, non-Hodgkin's lymphoma, leukoplakias and carcinoma — at least of the lip — may arise in the mouth as a consequence of long-term immunosuppressive therapy.

OROFACIAL GRANULOMATOSIS

Orofacial granulomatosis (see Chapter 19) may be caused by allergens or other materials in foods or drinks, such as cinnamonaldehyde or bezoates (**Fig. 29.60**).

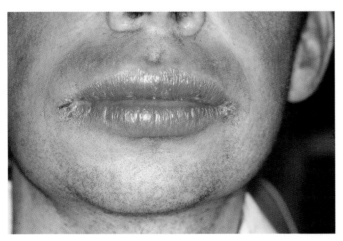

29.60

OSTEONECROSIS

Bisphosphonates may induce jaw osteonecrosis (**Fig. 29.61**).

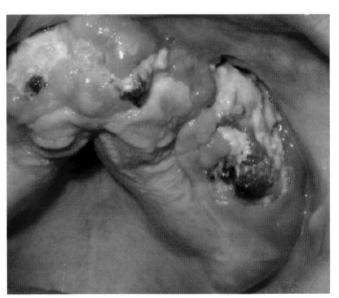

29.61

STOMATITIS NICOTINA

Pipe smoking is the main cause of keratosis in the palate, shown well here, where keratosis does not affect the mucosa protected by the denture (**Figs 29.62, 29.63**).

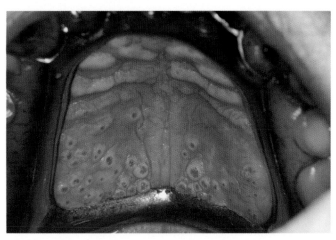

29.62

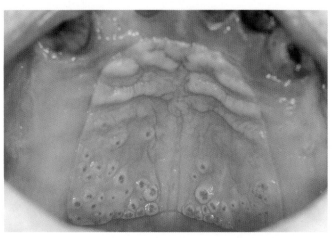

29.63

TOOTH EROSION

Teeth can be eroded by gastric acid, carbonated beverages, swimming-pool water and other solutions (see Chapter 15).

TOOTH STAINING

This may be extrinsic, e.g. caused by nicotine, betelnut, cannabis or other drugs (**Fig. 29.64**), or intrinsic, e.g. caused by tetracyclines (**Fig. 29.65**).

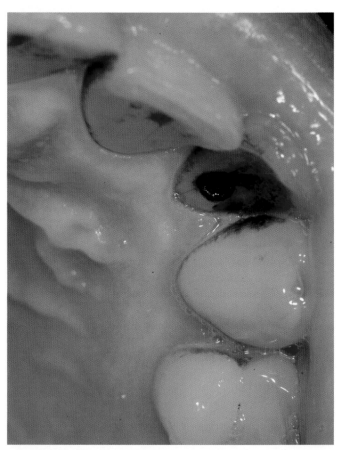

29.64

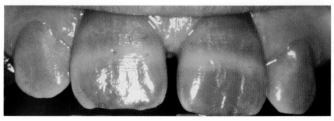

29.65

FURTHER READING

Abdollahi M, Radfar M. A review of drug-induced oral reactions. J Contemp Dent Pract 2003; 4(1): 10–31.

Ayangco L, Sheridan PJ. Minocycline-induced staining of torus palatinus and alveolar bone. J Periodontol 2003; 74(5): 669–71.

Brazier WJ, Dhariwal DK, Patton DW, Bishop K. Ecstasy related periodontitis and mucosal ulceration — a case report. Brit Dent J 2003; 194: 197–9.

Bullock K. Dental care of patients with substance misuse. Dent Clin North Am 1999; 43(3): 513–26.

Cicardi M, Agostoni A. Hereditary angioedema. N Engl J Med 1996; 334: 1666–7.

Condemi JJ. Update in allergy and immunology. Ann Intern Med 1996; 125: 744–50.

Glick M. Intravenous drug users: a consideration for infective endocarditis in dentistry? Oral Surg Oral Med Oral Pathol 1995; 80: 125.

Hollander J, Todd K, Green G, et al. Chest pain associated with cocaine: an assessment of prevalence in suburban and urban emergency departments. Ann Emerg Med 1995; 26: 671–6.

Horst G, Molendijk B, Brouwer E, Verhey HG. Differences in dental treatment plan and planning for drug-addicted and non-drug-addicted patients. Community Dent Oral Epidemiol 1996; 24(2): 120–3.

Johnson CD, Lewis VA, Faught KS, Brown RS. The relationship between chronic cocaine or alcohol use and blood pressure in black men during uncomplicated tooth extraction. J Oral Maxillofac Surg 1998; 56(3): 323–9.

Krall EA, Garvey AJ, Garcia RI. Alveolar bone loss and tooth loss in male cigar and pipe smokers. J Am Dent Assoc 1999; 130(1): 57–64.

Kuttan NA, Narayana N, Moghadam BK. Desquamative stomatitis associated with routine use of oral health care products. Gen Dent 2001; 49(6): 596–602.

Lane JE, Buckthal J, Davis LS. Fixed drug eruption due to fluconazole. Oral Surg Oral Med Oral Pathol Oral Radiol Endod 2003; 95(2): 129–30.

Liccardi G, D'Amato G. Oral allergy syndrome after ingestion of salami in a subject with monosensitisation to mite allergens. J Allergy Clin Immunol 1996; 98: 850–2.

Liede KE, Haukka JK, Hietanen JH, Mattila MH, Ronka H, Sorsa T. The association between smoking cessation and periodontal status and salivary proteinase levels. J Periodontol 1999; 70(11): 1361–8.

McDiarmid M. Dental treatment and the alcoholic. NZ Dent J 1996; 92(409): 83–5.

Moghadam BK, Gier R, Thurlow T. Extensive oral mucosal ulcerations caused by misuse of a commercial mouthwash. Cutis 1999; 64(2): 131–4.

Molendijk B, Ter Horst G, Kasbergen M, Truin GJ, Mulder J. Dental health in Dutch drug addicts. Community Dent Oral Epidemiol 1996; 24(2): 117–19.

Nainar SMH. Dental management of children with latex allergy. Int J Paediatr Dent 2001; 11: 322–6.

Ostrowski DJ, DeNelsky GY. Pharmacologic management of patients using smoking cessation aids. Dent Clin North Am 1996; 40(3): 779–801.

Parry J, Porter SR, Scully C, Flint SF, Parry MG. Mucosal lesions due to oral cocaine use. Br Dent J 1996; 180: 462–4.

Porter SR, Scully C. Adverse drug reactions in the mouth. Clin Dermatol 2000; 18: 525–32.

Robb ND, Smith BG. Chronic alcoholism: an important condition in the dentist–patient relationship. J Dent 1996; 24(1–2): 17–24.

Ross Kerr Karlis V, Glickman RS, Stern R, Kinney L. Hereditary angioedema: case report and review of management. Oral Surg Oral Med Oral Pathol Oral Radiol Endod 1997; 83(4): 462–4.

Roy A, Epstein J, Onno E. Latex allergies in dentistry: recognition and recommendations. J Canad Den Assoc 1997; 63: 297–300.

Sainsbury D. Drug addiction and dental care. NZ Dent J 1999; 95(420): 58–61.

Sandler NA. Patients who misuse drugs. Oral Surg 2001; 91: 12–14.

Sapir S, Bimstein E. Cholinesalicylate gel induced oral lesion: report of case. J Clin Pediatr Dent 2000; 24(2): 103–6.

Schreiber A. Alcoholism. Oral Surg 2001; 92: 127–31.

Scully C, Bagan JV. Drug adverse effects. Crit Rev Oral Biol Med (in press).

Seyer BA, Grist W, Muller S. Aggressive destructive midfacial lesion from cocaine abuse. Oral Surg Oral Med Oral Pathol Oral Radiol Endod 2002; 94: 465–70.

Spina AM, Levine HJ. Latex allergy: a review for the dental professional. Oral Surg Oral Med Oral Pathol Oral Radiol Endod 1999; 87: 5–11.

Talbott JF, Gorti GK, Koch RJ. Midfacial osteomyelitis in a chronic cocaine abuser: a case report. Ear Nose Throat J 2001; 80: 738–40, 742–3.

Taybos G. Oral changes associated with tobacco use. Am J Med Sci 2003; 326(4): 179–82.

Terezhalmy GT, Esposito SJ, Safadi GS. Immunopharmacology. Dent Clin North Am 1996; 40(3): 685–707.

Underwood B, Fox K. A survey of alcohol and drug use among UK based dental undergraduates. BDJ Launchpad 2001; 8: 26–29.

Vilela RJ, Langford C, McCullagh L, Kass ES. Cocaine-induced oronasal fistulas with external nasal erosion but without palate involvement. Ear Nose Throat J 2002; 81: 562–3.

Wesson DR, Ling W. Addiction medicine. J Am Med Assoc 1996; 275: 1792–3.

Wynn RL. Dental considerations of patients taking appetite suppressants. Gen Dent 1997; 45(4): 324–8, 330–1.

30 PHYSICAL AGENTS

- body art
- burns
- cicatrization
- foreign bodies
- Frey's syndrome (gustatory sweating)
- frictional keratosis
- grafts
- iatrogenic injury
- oroantral fistula
- oronasal fistula
- surgical emphysema
- trauma to dentition
- traumatic hyperplasia
- traumatic ulcers and haematomas.

BODY ART

Oral piercing may involve a variety of objects and may be seen particularly in persons with other forms of body art (see also **Figs 29.15, 29.16**). The placing of so-called jewellery, usually stainless-steel studs, rings or barbells, has sexual connotations and in the oral region is typically seen in the lower lip and tongue but may be seen virtually anywhere on the head and neck. The labrette piercing is usually a central piercing of the lip below the vermilion carrying a stud or ring (**Figs 30.1–30.3**).

The practice of tongue piercing is a cause of some concern since bleeding or oedema can occasionally be pronounced, widespread and a hazard to the airway. Thereafter, the permanent jewellery is placed and worn constantly, to avoid the perforation closing over spontaneously (**Figs 30.4–30.7**). Speech can be impaired and the teeth and gingiva may be damaged by the jewellery. Body art also includes the placement of gold or other crowns or inserts in intact teeth (**Fig. 30.8**).

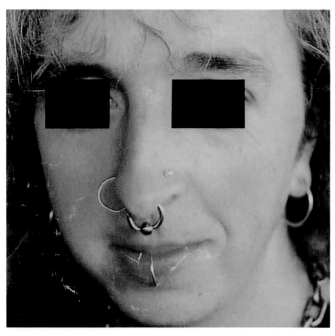

30.1

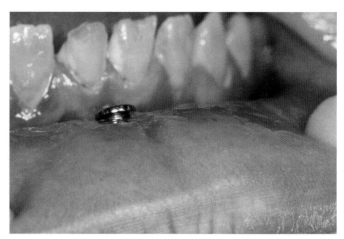

30.2

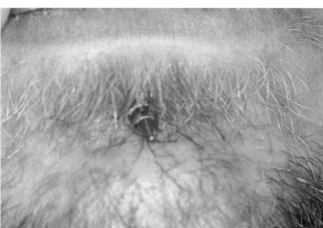

30.3

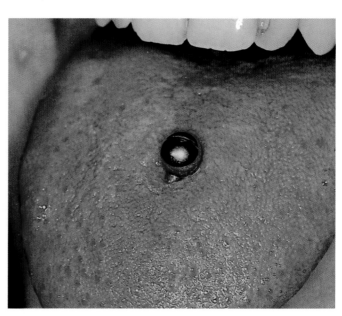

30.4

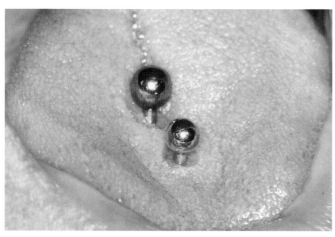

30.5

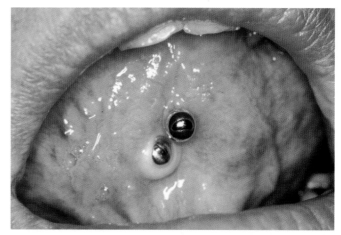

30.6

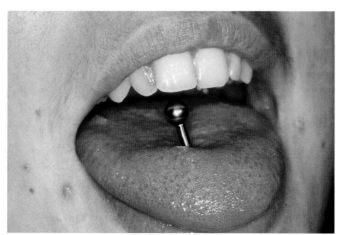

30.7

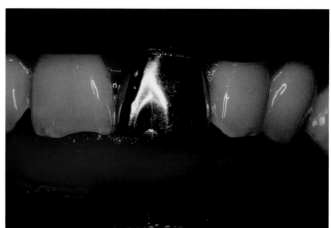

30.8

BURNS

Burns are most common after the ingestion of hot foods and are seen especially on the palate or tongue, for example 'pizza-palate' (**Figs 30.9–30.11**). Chronic ingestion of hot foods or liquids may produce an appearance resembling stomatitis nicotina (**Fig. 30.12**).

Cold injury is uncommon, but follows cryosurgery.

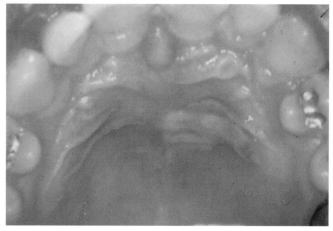

30.9

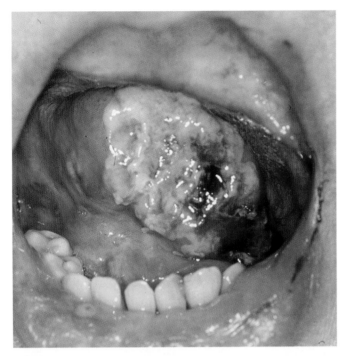

30.10

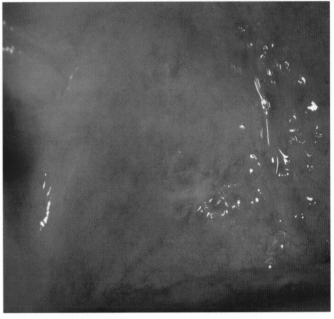

30.11

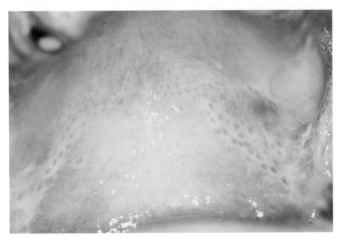

30.12

CICATRIZATION

Scarring and some deformity is unavoidable in cancer surgery (**Figs 30.13, 30.14**) although intraoral scarring is usually minimal except in severe tissue loss, self-mutilation (**Fig. 30.15**) or some types of epidermolysis bullosa and mucous membrane pemphigoid. Keloids are rare intraorally.

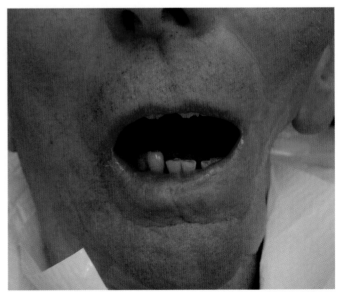

30.13

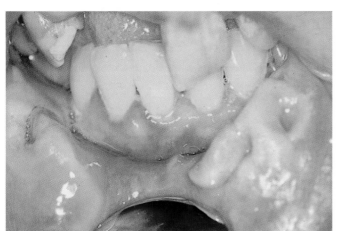

30.14

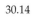
30.15

FOREIGN BODIES

Foreign bodies may result from facial trauma and may even enter the maxillary antrum; foreign bodies in soft tissues often lead to hyperpigmented lesions (**Fig. 30.16**). Palatal pigmentation from a foreign body (a pencil lead) is shown in **Fig. 30.17**.

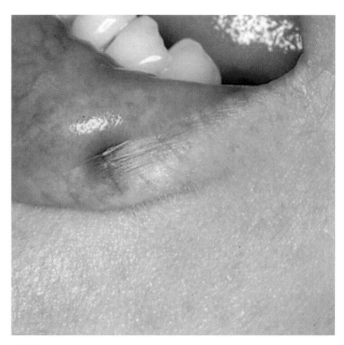

30.16

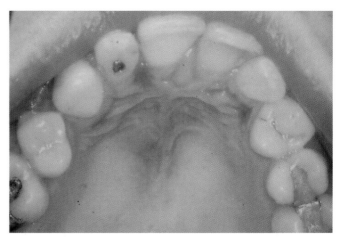

30.17

FREY'S SYNDROME *(gustatory sweating)*

Gustatory sweating is a rare clinical problem characterized by sweating, flushing, a sense of warmth, and occasional mild pain over an area of skin of the face while eating foods that produce a strong salivary stimulus. The disorder usually involves the area of skin innervated by the auriculotemporal nerve (Frey's syndrome) and is often termed the auriculotemporal syndrome.

Sweating of the skin over the area of innervation can easily be induced by the patient sucking on a piece of orange (**Fig. 30.18**). A starch-iodine test confirms the precise areas of sweating (**Fig. 30.19**).

Gustatory sweating is usually a consequence of interruption and alteration in the neural supply to sweat glands and blood vessels in an area of skin of the face and is usually a result of surgery or candylar

fracture. The syndrome follows between 6% and 60% of parotidectomies but has also been recorded after submandibular salivary gland surgery and orthognathic surgery.

Less commonly, gustatory sweating follows facial injury or infection. Diabetes mellitus is a rare cause.

During subsequent nerve regeneration, parasympathetic fibres are misdirected down previously sympathetic pathways, such that normal parasympathetic stimulation results in a sympathetic-driven vasomotor effect of sweating and flushing of the skin. The typical lag time of months to years between neural damage and the onset of clinical signs suggests that altered regeneration is the likely pathogenesis of most instances of this condition but other theories of the cause have been postulated. Gustatory lacrimation, rhinorrhoea and otorrhoea have also been described.

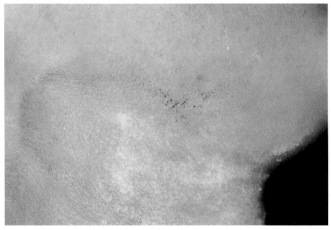

30.18

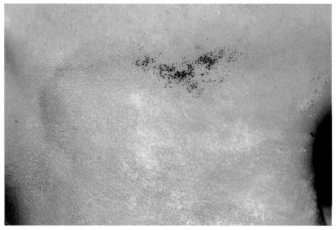

30.19

FRICTIONAL KERATOSIS

Repeated friction can result in keratosis, and this is typically seen on edentulous ridges or surrounding chronic traumatic ulcers (**Figs 30.20, 30.21**).

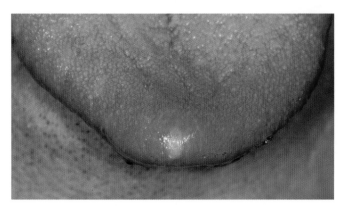

30.20

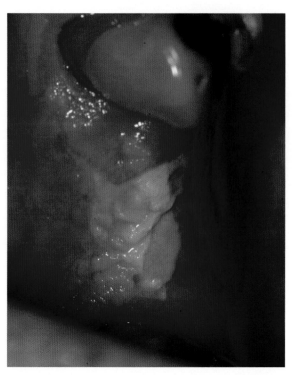

30.21

GRAFTS

A skin graft of a defect following excision of a carcinoma remains paler than the mucosa, becomes wrinkled and white and may grow hairs (**Figs 30.22, 30.23**).

Mucosal grafts from the palate for periodontal treatment are less white than skin grafts (**Fig. 30.24**).

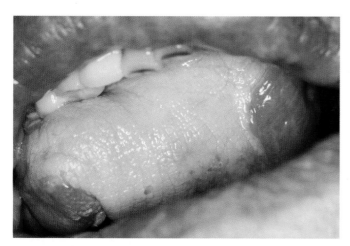

30.22

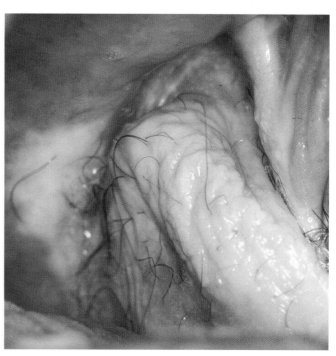

30.23

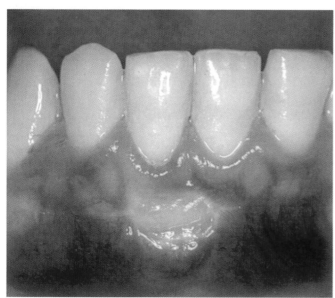

30.24

IATROGENIC INJURY

Dental local analgesic injections may produce temporary local pallor because of the contained vasoconstrictor but this is of no consequence. Dental local analgesic injections, especially regional blocks, also not uncommonly produce a small haematoma (**Fig. 30.25**) which is usually inconsequential unless it is intramuscular (in which case it can cause trismus) or if it is infected or the blood tracks extraorally (**Fig. 30.26**).

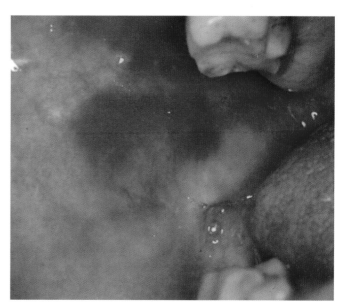

30.25

Extraoral discoloration and/or swelling may be produced by a haematoma after surgery, especially in the mandibular molar region (**Fig. 30.27**). Blood may track through fascial planes of the neck to cause extensive bruising, even down to the chest wall.

Postoperative oedema is particularly common after poor surgical technique — **Fig. 30.28** shows bruising from careless handling of the tissues. However, in persons with a bleeding tendency, haematomas can easily arise even with good technique (**Fig. 30.29**).

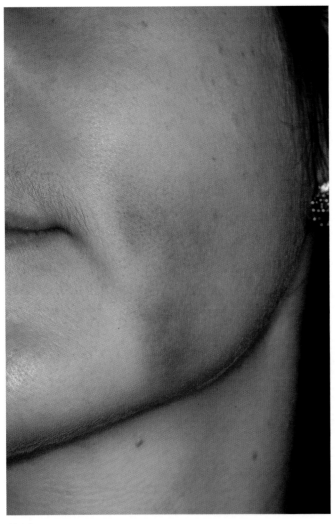

30.26

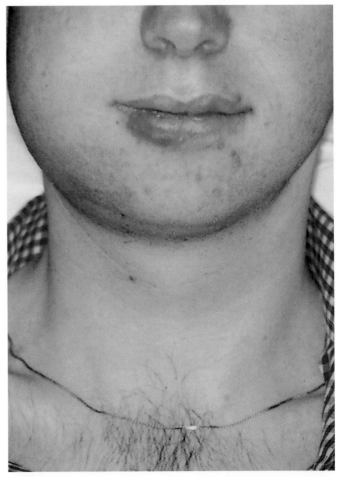

30.27

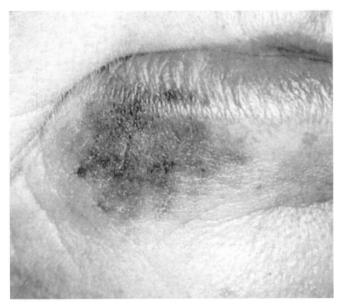

30.28

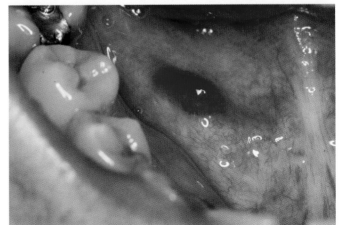

30.29

Damage to nerves during surgery may produce paraesthesiae or permanent neurological deficit. Lingual nerve damage causes a loss of sensation and taste; inferior alveolar nerve or mental nerve damage can produce mental nerve sensory changes and facial nerve damage can lead to facial palsy or Frey's syndrome.

OROANTRAL FISTULA

Oroantral fistula (OAF) is almost invariably traumatic in aetiology, usually following the extraction of an upper molar or premolar tooth (**Fig. 30.30**). Fluid passes from the mouth into the sinus, which may become infected. Occasionally, the antral lining prolapses through an OAF (**Fig. 30.31**).

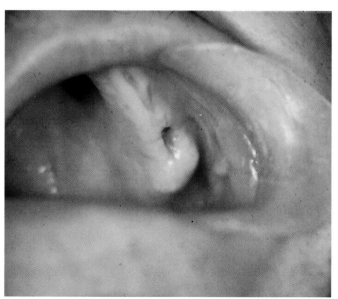

30.30

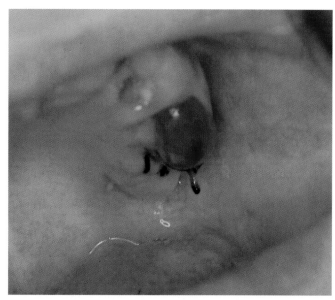

30.31

ORONASAL FISTULA

Surgery, such as the removal of a palatal neoplasm, may produce this defect (**Fig. 30.32**).

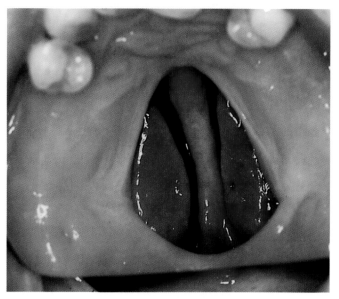

30.32

SURGICAL EMPHYSEMA

Dental instrumentation using air-turbine handpieces or air syringes occasionally introduces air into the tissues, producing surgical emphysema (**Fig. 30.33**), which is recognized by acute swelling with crackling on palpation. Early recognition is essential to prevent such life-threatening complications as airway obstruction, deep neck infection or mediastinitis.

TRAUMA TO DENTITION

Teeth can be devitalized, fractured, subluxed or lost from assaults, and domestic, sport and road and other accidents, or in epilepsy.

TRAUMATIC HYPERPLASIA

Suction discs formerly used to help denture retention may produce hyperplasia in the palatal vault, as seen in **Fig. 30.34**. Such a suction disc is shown in **Fig. 30.35**.

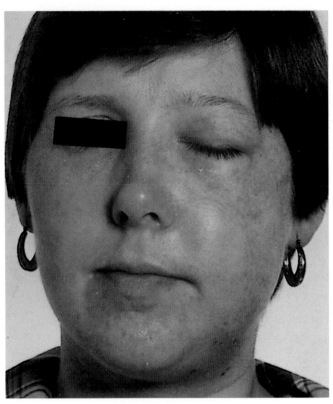

30.33

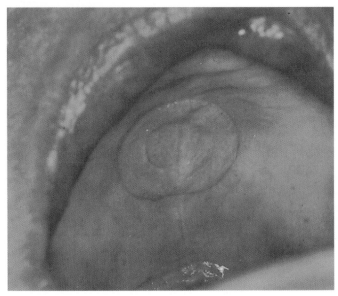

30.34

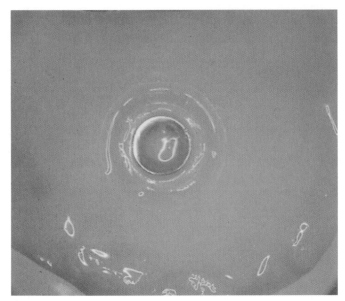

30.35

TRAUMATIC ULCERS AND HAEMATOMAS

Acute trauma may result in haematoma or ulcer formation, and some of these are produced by orogenital sexual habits (**Figs 30.36–30.37**) but they are seen more commonly as a consequence of biting (**Fig. 30.38**), aggressive flossing (**Fig. 30.38**), trauma in an epileptic fit (**Figs 30.40 and 30.41**) or chronic trauma such as from a sharp tooth cusp (**Figs 30.42–30.44**). Trauma to teeth may cause fractures, attrition or abrasion (**Fig. 30.47**).

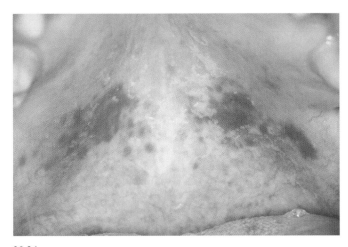

30.36

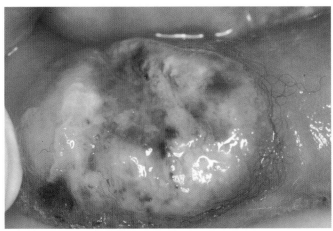

30.38

30.37

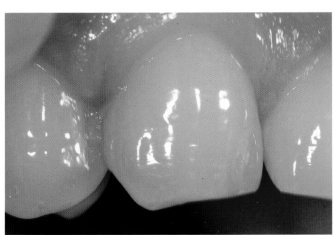

30.39

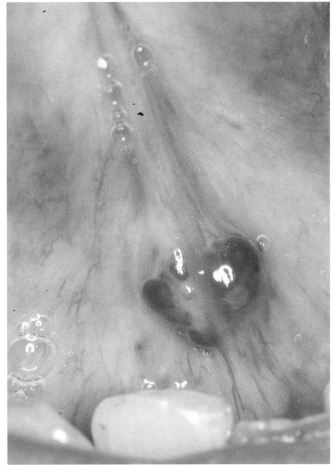

30.40

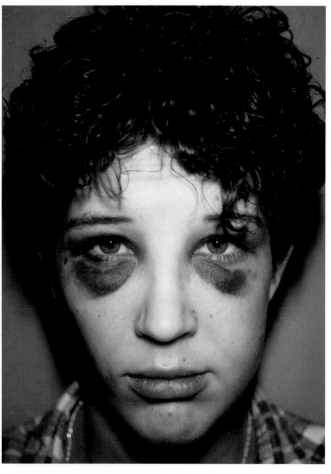

30.41

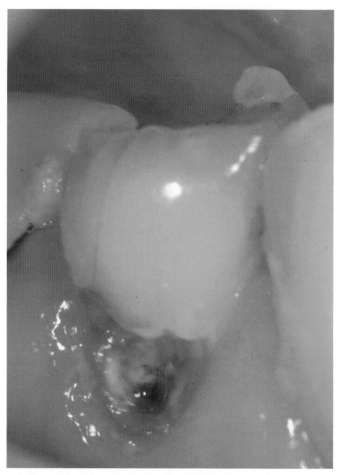

30.42

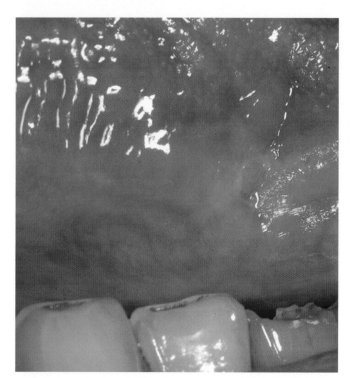

30.43

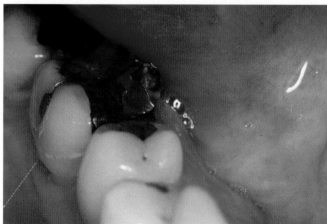

30.44

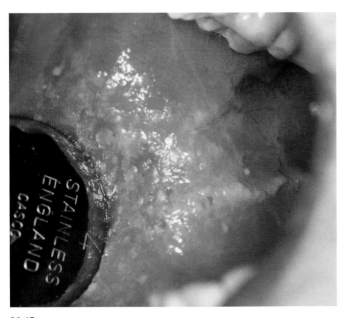

30.45

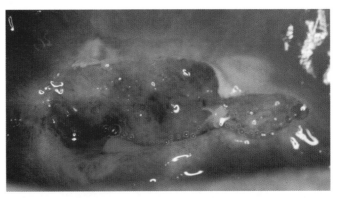

30.46

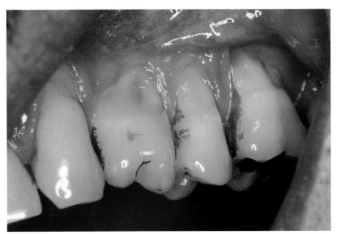

30.47

FURTHER READING

Boardman R, Smith RA. Dental implications of oral piercing. J Calif Dent Assoc 1997; 25: 200–7.

Eckardt A, Kuettner C. Treatment of gustatory sweating (Frey's syndrome) with botulinum toxin A. Head Neck 2003; 25: 624–8.

Haddock A, Porter SR, Scully C, Smith I. Submandibular gustatory sweating. Oral Surg Oral Med Oral Pathol 1994; 77: 317.

Kerekhanjanarong V, Supiyaphun P, Saengpanich S. Upper aerodigestive tract burn: a case report of firework injury. J Med Assoc Thai 2001; 84(2): 294–8.

Kuspis DA, Krenzelok EP. Oral frostbite injury from intentional abuse of a fluorinated hydrocarbon. J Toxicol Clin Toxicol 1999; 37(7): 873–5.

Malatskey S, Rabinovich I, Fradis M, Peled M. Frey syndrome — delayed clinical onset: a case report. Oral Surg Oral Med Oral Pathol Oral Radiol Endod 2002; 94: 338–40.

Nahlieli O, Eliav E, Shapira Y, Baruchin AM. Central palatal burns associated with the eating of microwaved pizzas. Burns 1999; 25(5): 465–6.

Nahlieli O, Shapira Y, Yoffe B, Baruchin AM. An unusual iatrogenic burn from a heated dental instrument. Burns 2000; 26(7): 676–8.

Oginni FO, Fagade OO, Akinwande JA, Arole GF, Odusanya SA. Pattern of soft tissue injuries to the oro-facial region in Nigerian children attending a teaching hospital. Int J Paediatr Dent 2002; 12(3): 201–6.

Scully C. Oral piercing in adolescents. CPD Dentistry 2001; 2: 79–81.

Scully C, Chen M. Tongue piercing (oral body art). Br J Oral Maxillofac Surg 1994; 32(1): 37–8.

Shacham R, Zaguri A, Librus HZ, Bar T, Eliav E, Nahlieli O. Tongue piercing and its adverse effects. Oral Surg Oral Med Oral Pathol Oral Radiol Endod 2003; 95(3): 274–6.

Shimoyama T, Kaneko T, Nasu D, Suzuki T, Horie N. A case of an electrical burn in the oral cavity of an adult. J Oral Sci 1999; 41(3): 127–8.

Simon PA. Recognizing and reporting the orofacial trauma of child abuse/neglect. Tex Dent J 2000; 117(10): 21–32.

31 RADIATION EFFECTS

- actinic cheilitis
- actinic prurigo
- ionizing radiation-induced epithelial changes
- ionizing radiation-induced hard-tissue damage
- ionizing radiation-induced xerostomia
- radiation accidents.

ACTINIC CHEILITIS

Sunlight can be damaging to the lips and skin, particularly to the vermilion of the lower lip. Acute cheilitis due to acute sunburn is common and clinically resembles 'chapping'. Actinic cheilitis is seen mainly on the lower lip, with sparing of the oral commissures. In the early stages there may be redness and oedema (**Figs 31.1, 31.2**), but later the lip becomes dry and scaly and wrinkled with grey to white changes in pigmentation.

Chronic actinic cheilitis is a premalignant keratosis of the lip caused by chronic exposure to solar irradiation. The epithelium becomes palpably thickened with small greyish white plaques of keratosis and eventually one or more may undergo malignant change.

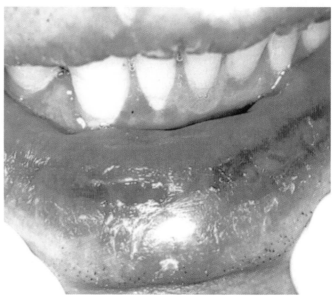

31.2

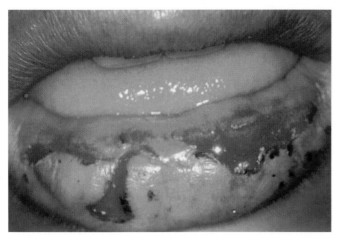

31.1

ACTINIC PRURIGO

Actinic prurigo is a rare photodermatitis affecting children (Hutchinson's summer prurigo) but a rare familial form also affects adults and is seen mainly in native Americans living at high altitude, especially in Latin America. Pruritic cheilitis affecting the lower lip (**Fig. 31.3**) may be associated with conjunctivitis, eyebrow alopecia and the formation of pterygia.

IONIZING RADIATION-INDUCED EPITHELIAL CHANGES

Radiotherapy involving the mouth and salivary glands invariably produces ionizing radiation-induced mucositis (**Figs 31.4, 31.5**). This is dose-dependent.

The skin in the path of teletherapy becomes erythematous but then tends to lose hair and pigment, and it may scar with telangiectasia

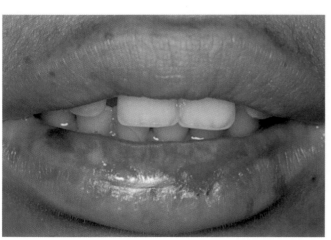

31.3

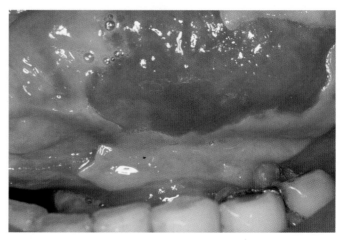

31.4

developing on the skin and mucosa (**Figs 31.6–31.9**). Endarteritis obliterans produces mucosal scarring (**Fig. 31.10**) and, if involving muscle, produces trismus.

Previous irradiation predisposes to subsequent neoplasia, for example, radiotherapy to oropharyngeal neoplasms predisposes to subsequent salivary neoplasms.

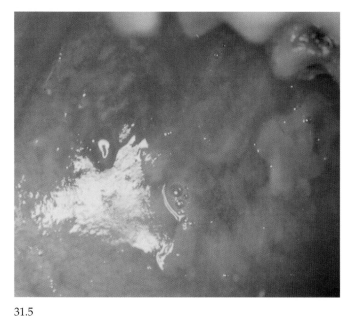

31.5

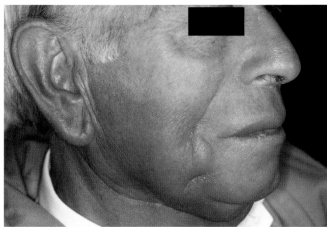

31.6

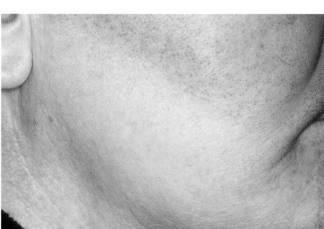

31.7

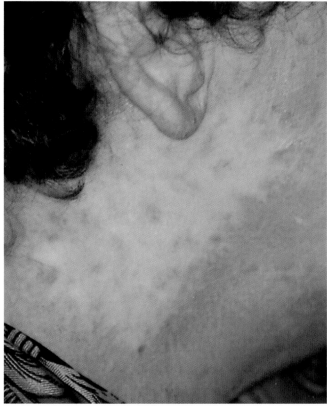

31.8

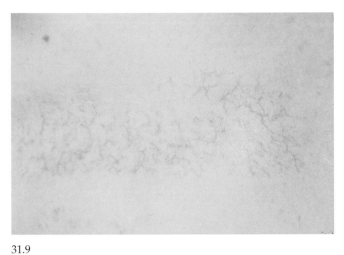

31.9

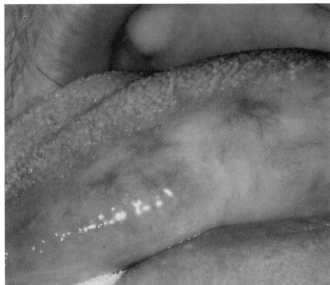

31.10

IONIZING RADIATION-INDUCED HARD-TISSUE DAMAGE

Xerostomia predisposes to caries (see below). Irradiation of developing teeth can cause hypoplasia, stunted root formation and retarded eruption (**Fig. 31.11**). Irradiation of the mandibular condyle, or other growth areas, can result in facial deformity.

Endarteritis obliterans, following irradiation of the jaws, predisposes to infection after tooth extraction and osteoradionecrosis (**Figs 31.12–13.15**). This was not an uncommon problem in the past but —

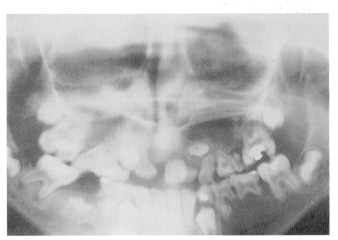

31.11

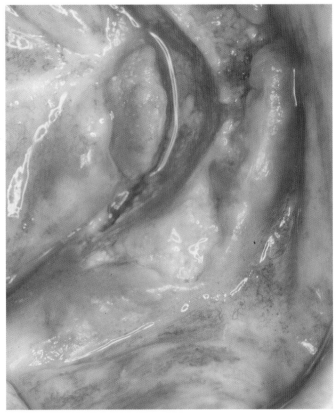

31.12

with the advent of plesiotherapy and other improved radiotherapeutic techniques and a better understanding by dental surgeons — it is now less common.

Jaw necrosis was also caused in the past by occupational exposure to red phosphorus or heavy metals, and still occasionally follows the use of toxic endodontic materials, or the development of severe herpes zoster or other infections, particularly in patients who have been irradiated in the head and neck or who are immunocompromised.

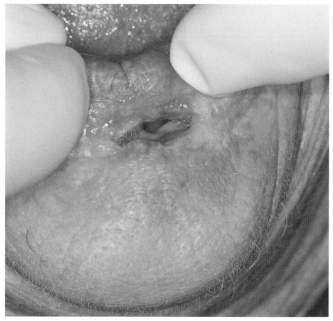

31.14

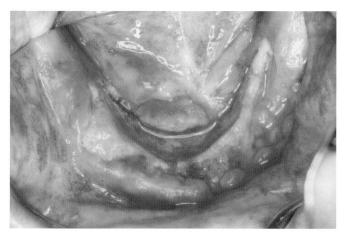

31.13

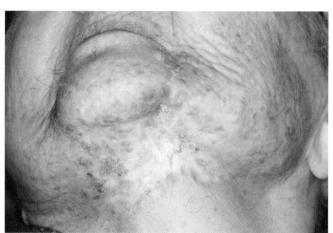

31.15

IONIZING RADIATION-INDUCED XEROSTOMIA

Radiotherapy involving the mouth and salivary glands invariably produces xerostomia; this is dose dependent. Xerostomia predisposes to dental caries (**Figs 31.16, 31.17**), candidosis and sialadenitis.

Pseudomembranous and erythematous candidosis are common, especially where xerostomia is pronounced (**Fig. 31.18**). Irradiation of the tongue, together with the xerostomia, often produces taste loss.

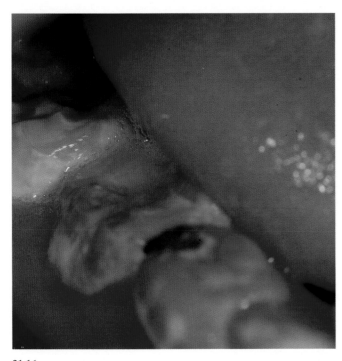

31.16

31.17

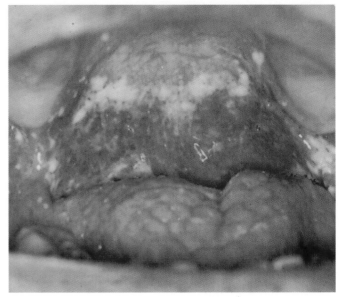

31.18

RADIATION ACCIDENTS

Figures 31.19 and **31.20** show cutaneous seaming and oral hyperpigmentation respectively, following the burns resulting from the accidental handling of radioactive caesium.

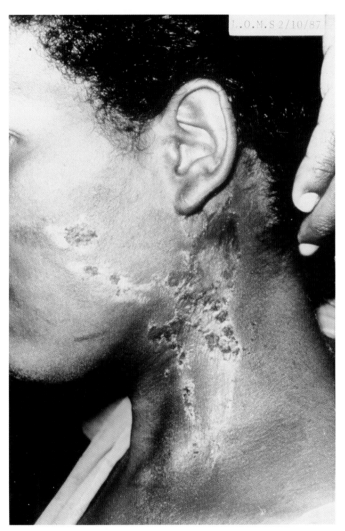

31.19

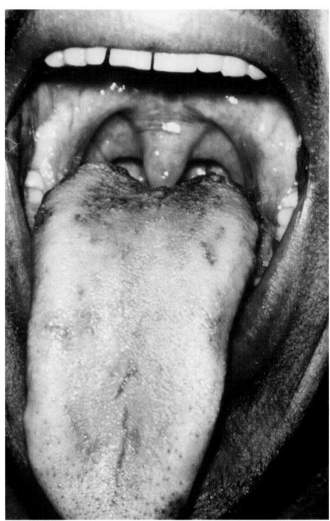

31.20

FURTHER READING

Bentley JM, Barankin B, Lauzon GJ. Paying more than lip service to lip lesions. Can Fam Physician 2003; 49: 1111–16.

Chin EA. A brief overview of the oral complications in pediatric oncology patients and suggested management strategies. ASDC J Dent Child 1998; 65(6): 468–73.

Clarkson JE, Eden OB. Dental health in children with cancer. Arch Dis Child 1998; 78(6): 560–1.

de Sevaux RG, Smit JV, de Jong EM, van de Kerkhof PC, Hoitsma AJ. Acitretin treatment of premalignant and malignant skin disorders in renal transplant recipients: clinical effects of a randomized trial comparing two doses of acitretin. J Am Acad Dermatol 2003; 49(3): 407–12.

Epstein JB, Ransier A, Lunn R, Chin E, Jacobson JJ, Le N, Reece D. Prophylaxis of candidiasis in patients with leukemia and bone marrow transplants. Oral Surg Oral Med Oral Pathol Oral Radiol Endod 1996; 81(3): 291–6.

Epstein JB, Emerton S, Lunn R, Le N, Wong FL. Pretreatment assessment and dental management of patients with nasopharyngeal carcinoma. Oral Oncol 1999; 35(1): 33–9.

Jensen SB, Pedersen AM, Reibel J, Nauntofte B. Xerostomia and hypofunction of the salivary glands in cancer therapy. Support Care Cancer 2003; 11: 207–25.

Kaugars GE, Pillion T, Svirsky JA, Page DG, Burns JC, Abbey LM. Actinic cheilitis: a review of 152 cases. Oral Surg Oral Med Oral Pathol Oral Radiol Endod 1999; 88: 181–6.

Kinirons MJ, Fleming P, Boyd D. Dental caries experience of children in remission from acute lymphoblastic leukaemia in relation to the duration of treatment and the period of time in remission. Int J Paediatr Dent 1995; 5: 169–72.

Laws RA, Wilde JL, Grabski WJ. Comparison of electrodessication with CO_2 laser for the treatment of actinic cheilitis. Dermatol Surg 2000; 26: 349–53.

Lunn R. Oral management of the cancer patient. Part I: Overview of cancer and oral cancer. Probe 1997; 31(4): 137–41.

Maire F, Borowski B, Collangettes D, Farsi F, Guichard M, Gourmet R, Kreher P. Standards, Options and Recommendations (SOR) for good practices in dentistry for head and neck cancer patients. Bull Cancer 1999; 86(7–8): 640–65.

Martinez A, Morales R, Brethauer U, Jimenez M, Alarcon R. Porphyria cutanea tarda affecting lower lip. Oral Surg Oral Med Oral Pathol Oral Radiol Endod 2000; 90(6): 705–8.

Ochsenius G, Ormeno A, Godoy L, Rojas R. A retrospective study of 232 cases of lip cancer and pre cancer in Chilean patients. Clinical-histological correlation. Rev Med Chil 2003; 131(1): 60–6.

Redding SW. Oral complications of cancer therapy. Tex Med 2003; 99(5): 54–7.

Satorres Nieto M, Gargallo Albiol J, Gay Escoda C. Surgical management of actinic cheilitis. Med Oral 2001; 6(3): 205–17.

Scully C. Management of the sore mouth: other causes of oral soreness. Eur J Palliative Care 1995; 2 (Suppl 1): 13–15.

Scully C, Epstein J, Sonis S. Oral mucositis: a challenging complication of radiotherapy, chemotherapy, and radiochemotherapy. Part 2: diagnosis and management of mucositis. Head Neck 2004; 26(1): 77–84.

Scully C, Epstein J, Sonis S. Oral mucositis: a challenging complication of radiotherapy, chemotherapy, and radiochemotherapy: Part 1, pathogenesis and prophylaxis of mucositis. Head Neck 2003; 25(12): 1057–70.

Singh N, Scully C, Joyston-Bechal S. Oral complications of cancer therapies: prevention and management. Clin Oncol 1996; 8: 15–24.

Smith KJ, Germain M, Yeager J, Skelton H. Topical 5% imiquimod for the therapy of actinic cheilitis. J Am Acad Dermatol 2002; 47(4): 497–501.

Toljanic JA, Bedard JF, Larson RA, Fox JP. A prospective pilot study to evaluate a new dental assessment and treatment paradigm for patients scheduled to undergo intensive chemotherapy for cancer. Cancer 1999; 85(8): 1843–8.

Vega-Memije ME, Mosqueda-Taylor A, Irigoyen-Camacho ME, Hojyo-Tomoka MT, Dominguez-Soto L. Actinic prurigo cheilitis: clinicopathologic analysis and therapeutic results in 116 cases. Oral Surg Oral Med Oral Pathol Oral Radiol Endod 2002; 94(1): 83–91.

Vissink A, Burlage FR, Spijkervet FK, Jansma J, Coppes RP. Prevention and treatment of the consequences of head and neck radiotherapy. Crit Rev Oral Biol Med 2003; 14(3): 213–25.

Vissink A, Jansma J, Spijkervet FK, Burlage FR, Coppes RP. Oral sequelae of head and neck radiotherapy. Crit Rev Oral Biol Med 2003; 14(3): 199–212.

INDEX

abducent nerve lesion, 250
abfraction of teeth, 276
abrasion of teeth, 276
Abrikosov's tumour *see*
    granular cell tumour
abscesses
    dental (periapical,
        odontogenic), 20,
        301–4, 318
    gingival, 318
    lateral periodontal
        (parodontal), 38, 318
    lingual, 362
    peritonsillar, 273
    submandibular, 405
acanthosis nigricans, 20, 381, 404
    benign/malignant, 404
acetoaminophen (paracetamol),
    46
acquired immune deficiency
    syndrome *see* AIDS/HIV
acquired immune deficiency
    syndrome (AIDS)
    see also human
        immunodeficiency virus
acro-osteolysis, polyvinyl
    chloride, 488
acrocephalosyndactyly, 493–4
acrodermatitis enteropathica, 180
acrodynia, 550
acromegaly, 20, 181
actinic cheilitis *see* cheilitis,
    actinic
actinic prurigo, 584
actinomycosis, 20, 96
acute bacterial sialadenitis, 20,
    332–3
    in Sjögren's syndrome, 447
acute necrotizing ulcerative
    gingivitis, 20, 97
adamantinoma, 454
Addison's disease, 20, 183
adenoameloblastoma, 454
adenoid cystic carcinoma, 20, 161
adenomas
    MENS, 44, 194
    monomorphic salivary, 162
    pleomorphic salivary, 40,
        158–61, 338
    sebaceum, 517
adenomatoid hyperplasia, 333
adenomatoid odontogenic
    tumour, 454
agammaglobulinaemia, 20, 200
AIDS/HIV, 20, 203–18
Albers–Schönberg syndrome
    (osteopetrosis), 38, 537
Albright's syndrome, 20, 466
alcoholism, 388
allergic reactions, 550, 552
    food additive 'allergy', 378

see also coeliac disease;
    dermatitis, photosensitive
alveolar atrophy, 467
alveolar osteitis (dry socket),
    20, 470
alveolar ridge carcinoma, 168
alveolar soft part sarcoma, 162
amalgam tattoo, 11, 20, 327, 371,
    551–2
ameloblastoma, 20, 454
    see also adenoameloblastoma
amelogenesis imperfecta, 276–8
E-amino caproic acid, 57
amitriptyline, 56
amoxicillin, 49
amphoteracin, 48
ampicillin, 49
Amsterdam dwarf, 508
amyloidosis
    primary, 198
    secondary, 199
anaemias
    aplastic, 222
    in chronic renal failure, 394
    Fanconi's, 225
    iron deficiency, 229
    pernicious, 185, 232
anaesthesia, 2, 257
analgesic/anaesthetic injection
    facial palsy, 564
    haematoma, 575
analgesics, 46–7
aneurysmal bone cysts, 467
angina, 235, 265
    bullosa haemorrhagica *see*
        localized oral purpura
    Ludwig's, 271
angio-osteohypertrophy
    syndrome, 174
angioedema, 22
    allergic, 552
    drug-related, 58
    hereditary (HANE), 30, 199
    non-allergic, 552
angiofibroma, 518
angiomatosis, encephalofacial,
    542–3
angiosarcoma, 162
angular cheilitis (stomatitis), 24,
    118–19, 229, 378, 379
ankyloglossia (tongue-tie), 492
ankylosis, 279
    condylar, 488
anodontia, 293
anorexia nervosa, 240, 289
anterior open bite, 296–7
anthrax, cutaneous, 98
antibacterials, 49–53
antibiotic sore tongue, 116
antidepressants, 56
    interactions/cautions, 56–7

antifibrinolytics, 57
antifungals, 48
antivirals, 48
antral carcinoma, 270
Apert's syndrome, 493–4
aphthae, 22, 342–4
    herpetiform, 344
        pinpoint (Cooke's), 344
    major, 343–4
    minor (Mikulicz's), 342
aplastic anaemia, 222
'apple-jelly' nodules, 107, 108
arsenic poisoning, 557
artefactual lesions, 247
arteritis
    giant cell/cranial/temporal,
        263
    lingual, 263
arthritis
    mutilans, 440
    pyogenic, 40
        of TMJ, 489
    rheumatoid, 42, 440, 446
        juvenile, 440
arthromyalgia, facial, 26
Ascher's syndrome, 494
aspergillosis, 112
aspirin, 46
asthma, 271
atrophy
    alveolar, 467
    central papillary, 22
    of tongue, 28, 104, 184
attrition, tooth, 281, 285, 303
atypical facial pain, 10, 22, 241
augmentin (co-amoxiclav), 49
azathioprine, 54

bacterial infections, 95–110
    actinomycosis, 20, 96
    acute necrotizing ulcerative
        gingivitis, 20, 97
    anthrax, cutaneous, 98
    cancrum oris, 22, 98
    cat-scratch disease, 99
    epithelioid angiomatosis, 99
    leprosy, 32, 100
    in leukaemia, 138, 140
    Ludwig's angina, 271
    pericoronitis, 325
    pinta, 108
    Reiter's syndrome, 40, 101
    syphilis, 102–6, 108, 215, 362
    tuberculosis, 44, 107–8
    yaws, 108
basal cell carcinoma, 134
Bean's syndrome, 495
beclometasone, 53
Bednar's ulcer, 373
Behçet's syndrome, 22, 343, 345–6
Bell's palsy, 22, 250–1

Bell's sign, 251
benethamine penicillin
    (triplopen), 50
benign migratory glossitis *see*
    erythema, migrans
benzylpenicillin, 49
betamethasone, 53, 54
betel nut staining, 552
bile pigment staining of
    teeth, 312
biliary atresia, 327, 388
biliary cirrhosis, 389–90
bismuth poisoning, 557
black hairy tongue, 22, 347, 559
black staining of teeth, 311
blastomycoses, 38, 42, 112
blisters, 2
Bloch–Sulzberger disease *see*
    incontinentia pigmenti
blood/blood-forming organ
    disease, 221–38
blue rubber-bleb naevus
    syndrome, 495
body art
    piercing, 570
    tattoos, 553
Boeck's sarcoid *see* sarcoidosis
Bohn's nodules, 322
bone cysts, latent, 483
bone disorders, 465–85
bone-marrow transplantation,
    222–4
Bournville–Pringle disease, 22,
    517–18
branchial cysts, 495
brown staining of teeth, 311
Brunsting–Perry disease, 426
Brushfield's spots, 509
Bruton's syndrome, 22, 200
bruxism, 22, 245
buccal mucosa, carcinoma of,
    169–70
bulbar palsy, 253
bulimia nervosa, 22, 240, 289
bullosa haemorrhagica, 235
buprenorphine, 47
Burkitt's lymphoma
    African, 143
    non-African, 145
burning mouth/tongue, 2, 22,
    242, 357
burns
    chemical, 553–4
    from hot food, 571
'butterfly' rash, 448

cacogeusia, 4
café-au-lait spots, 546
Caffey's disease, 495
calcifying odontogenic
    cysts, 456

calcifying odontogenic tumour, 456
calculus/calculi
  dental, 320
  salivary glands, 22, 335–6
calibre-persistent arteries, 262
cancrum oris, 22, 98
candidal leukoplakia, 120
candidosis, 22, 114–22
  acute, 114–16, 588
    atrophic (antibiotic sore tongue), 116
  in cardiac transplantation, 262
  and cell-mediated immunodeficiency, 200
  chronic
    atrophic (denture-related stomatitis), 116–18
    mucocutaneous, 24, 120–2
    multifocal, 120
  drug-related, 58, 555
  erythematous, 116, 203–4, 555, 588
  in HIV, 203
  in leukaemia, 138–9
  pseudomembranous, 114–16, 588
  in Sjögren's syndrome, 447
candidosis–endocrinopathy syndrome, 121, 122, 189
carbamazepine, 55
carbuncles, 406
carcinoid syndrome, 183
carcinomas, 22
  adenoid cystic, 20, 161
  of alveolar ridge, 168
  of antrum, 270
  basal cell, 134
  of buccal mucosa, 169–70
  of gingiva, 167–8
  gingival, 329
  of lip, 165, 565
  of lung, 272
  of palate, 169–70
  of tongue (lingual), 166–7, 254
cardiac transplantation, 262–3
Carney's syndrome, 496–7
cat-scratch disease, 99
cell-mediated immunodeficiency, 200
cemento-ossifying fibroma, 468
central giant cell granuloma, 474
central papillary atrophy, 22
cephalosporins/cephamycins, 51–2
cerebral palsy, 252
cerebrovascular accident, 252
cervical lymphadenitis, 405
chancres, 22, 102
cheek-chewing, 22, 348
cheilitis, 349–50
  actinic, 24, 584

angular, 24, 118–19, 229, 378, 379
  chemical-induced, 555
  in Down's syndrome, 510
  drug-related, 58
  exfoliative, 349
  glandularis, 350
  in HIV, 217
  Miescher's, 383
  pruritic, 584
chemical agents, 549–67
cherubism (familial fibrous dysplasia), 24, 469
chickenpox (varicella) see herpes, varicella
Chievitz's organ, 497
child abuse syndrome, 24, 372
chloasma, 400, 559
chlordiazepoxide, 55
chlormethiazole, 57
chloromas (leukaemic deposits), 137, 140
chlorpromazine, 55
chondroectodermal dysplasia, 497
chorioretinitis, 129
Christmas disease (haemophilia B), 227
chronic bullous dermatosis of childhood, 422
chronic granulomatous disease, 24, 225
chronic hyperplastic gingivitis, 319
chronic mucocutaneous candidosis, 24, 120–2
cicatricial pemphigoid see mucous membrane pemphigoid
cicatrization, 572
cinnamon exposure, 328, 378, 383
circulatory system, diseases of, 261–8
cirrhosis
  of liver, 388
  primary biliary, 389–90
clavicular hypoplasia, 498–9
'claw hand', 192
cleft cysts, 495
cleft lip/palate, 497
cleidocranial dysplasia/dysostosis, 24, 291, 498–9
clomipramine, 56
co-trimoxazole, 50
'cobblestone' mucosa, 379, 383
codeine phosphate, 46
coeliac disease (gluten sensitivity), 24, 382
colchicine, 54
cold injury, 571

complex/compound odontomes, 301
condylar ankylosis, 488
condyloma acuminata, 24, 83
congenital/developmental disorders, 491–548
connective tissue diseases, 437–51
Cooke's aphthae, 344
'copper-beaten' skull, 505
cornification, 526–7
corticosteroids
  intra-articular, 53
  intralesional, 53
  topical, 53
'coup de sabre', 445
Cowden's syndrome, 492, 501, 530
Coxsackie viruses
  hand foot and mouth disease, 30, 66
  herpangina, 30, 67
  lymphonodular pharyngitis, 272
  in mumps, 36, 89
cranial arteritis, 263
craniofacial dysostosis (Crouzon's syndrome), 493, 505
craniofacial microsomia, 502
craniometaphyseal dysplasia, 504
CREST syndrome, 24, 390, 443
cri du chat syndrome, 505
Crohn's disease, 24, 378–9
Cross's syndrome, 530
Crouzon's syndrome (craniofacial dysostosis), 493, 505
CRST syndrome, 390, 443
cunnilingus tongue, 372
Cushing's syndrome, 183
cusp of Carabelli, 307
cyanosis, 265
cyclic neutropenia, 24, 231
cystic fibrosis, 271, 337
cystic hygroma, 507
cysts
  aneurysmal bone, 467
  bone
    haemorrhagic (simple), 475
    latent (Stafne), 483
  branchial (cleft), 495
  calcifying odontogenic, 456
  dentigerous (follicular), 457, 458
  dermoid, 26, 351
  eruption, 458
  follicular, 457, 458
  gingival, 322
  globulo-maxillary, 459
  lateral periodontal, 459
  nasopalatine duct (incisive canal), 460

  odontogenic keratocyst, 307
  periapical/radicular/dental, 307
  primordial, 461
  residual, 307
cytomegalovirus, 205

dapsone, 54
Darier's disease, 507
De Gugliemo's disease, 138
de Lange's syndrome, 508
deficiency states, 184–5
dens evaginatus, 300
dens-in-dente, 299–300
dental abscesses, 301–4
dental bacterial plaque, 320
dental calculus, 320
dental caries, 282–4, 314
  arrested, 283
  in Sjögren's syndrome, 447
dentigerous cysts, 457, 458
dentinogenesis imperfecta, 537
  type I, 284–5
  types II-IV, 285
denture sore mouth, 116–18
dermatitis
  acrodermatitis enteropathica, 180
  herpetiformis, 24, 382, 407
  multiforme, 3
  photosensitive, 559, 584
dermatomyositis, 24, 438
dermatosis, chronic bullous, of childhood, 422
dermoid cysts, 26, 351
desquamative gingivitis, 321
developmental/congenital disorders, 491–548
dexamethasone, 54
dextropropoxyphene, 46
diabetes mellitus, 26, 187
diagnosis
  differential
    by site, 14–19
    by symptoms/signs, 2–13
  guide to diseases, 20–45
diamorphine, 47
diazepam, 55, 57
dichloralphenazone, 57
diclofenac, 46
differential diagnosis
  by site, 14–19
  by symptoms/signs, 2–13
diflunisal, 46
dihydrocodeine tartrate, 46
dilated odontomes, 299–300
discharges, differential diagnosis of, 4
discoid lupus erythematosus (DLE), 26, 408
dosulepin, 56

double teeth, 299
Down's syndrome, 509–10, 519
doxycycline, 50
drug abuse, 553–4
drug-induced/related conditions
  acanthosis nigricans, 404
  candidosis, 58, 555
  chloasma cosmeticum, 400
  discoid lupus erythematosus,
    408
  erythema multiforme, 59, 215,
    409, 564
  facial palsy, 564
  gingival swelling, 60,
    262–3, 321, 556–7
  herpes, viral infections
    in, 564
  human papillomavirus
    infections, 564
  hyperpigmentation, 60, 64,
    557–60
  Kaposi's sarcoma, 565
  leukoplakia, 564, 565
  lichenoid lesions, 34, 61, 217,
    421, 564
  linear IgA disease, 422
  mucositis, 562
  neoplasms, 565
  non-Hodgkin's lymphoma, 565
  orofacial granulomatosis, 565
  osteonecrosis, 61, 565
  papillary hyperplasia, 368
  tooth discolouration, 63,
    559, 566
  toxic epidermal necrolysis
    (TEN), 564
  ulcers, 63, 562
  xerostomia (dry mouth),
    58–9, 563
  see also under drugs
drugs
  causing dry mouth, 563
  for oral disease management,
    46–57
  oral/perioral side-effects,
    58–64
dry mouth see xerostomia
dry socket (alveolar osteitis),
  20, 470
Duhring's disease see
  dermatitis, herpetiformis
dysarthria, 5, 533
dysautonomia, familial see
  Riley–Day
  syndrome
dyskeratosis
  congenita, 512;
  follicularis, 507
dysphagia, 6
dysplasias
  chondroectodermal, 497
  cleidocranial, 24, 291, 498–9

craniometaphyseal, 504
ectodermal, 26, 293, 512–14
  familial fibrous (cherubism),
    24, 469
  fibrous, 471–2
  hypohidrotic ectodermal see
    ectodermal
    dysplasia
  myelodysplastic syndrome,
    36, 230
dystrophic kyphoscoliosis, 546

ecchymoses, 235
ectodermal dysplasia, 26, 293,
  512–14;
  'tooth and nail' type, 514
eczema herpeticum, 74
Ehlers–Danlos syndrome,
  489, 514
Elllis–van Creveld syndrome, 497
emphysema, surgical, 44, 578
enamel, cleft, 287
enamel hypocalcification,
  hereditary, 278
enamel hypoplasia, 185, 225,
  287–8, 388
  hereditary, 277
enamel nodules/pearls, 288
enameloma, 288–9
encephalofacial angiomatosis,
  542–3
endarteritis obliterans, 585, 586
eosinophilic granuloma, 135
ephelides (freckles), 28, 351
epidermolysis bullosa, 26, 516
  acquisita, 409, 516
  junctional, 516
epilepsy, 253
epiloia see Bournville–Pringle
  disease
epithelioid angiomatosis, 99
Epstein–Barr virus
  and infectious mononucleosis,
    83, 86
  and lymphomas, 143, 145
Epstein's pearls, 322
epulis
  congenital, 26, 153
  fibrous, 26, 322
  fissuratum (denture-induced
    hyperplasia), 24, 26, 350
  giant cell, 26, 322
  pregnancy, 26, 400
erosion(s)
  mucosal, 563–4
  tooth, 289, 566
eruption cysts, 458
erythema
  in denture-related
    stomatitis, 118
  linear gingival, 214
  migrans, 26, 352–4

persistans, 353
  multiforme, 3, 26, 409–12
  drug-induced, 564
  drug-related, 59, 215
  exudativum, 433–4
  major/minor, 409
  'target'/'iris' lesions,
    410, 412
  nodosum, 26, 346
erythroleukaemia, 138
erythromycin, 52
erythroplakia (erythroplasia),
  26, 355
espundia see leishmaniasis
etretinate, 55
evaginated odontomes, 300
exfoliative cheilitis, 349
exostoses, 471
extravasion mucoceles, 334

facial arthromyalgia, 26, 490
facial flushing, 59–60
facial hirsutism, 59
facial movements, 60
facial oedema, 60
facial pain, atypical, 10, 22, 241
facial palsy, 6
  drug-induced, 564
  infectious mononucleosis, 86
  lower motor neurone, 250–1,
    255, 382
facial swelling, 6–7
  Crohn's disease, 378
  periapical abscesses, 302–3, 304
  tooth attrition, 303
factitious lesions, 247
  see also self-mutilation/
    habit-induced lesions
familial dysautonomia see
  Riley–Day syndrome
familial fibrous dysplasia
  (cherubism), 24, 469
familial gingival fibromatosis,
  323, 519
familial white folded
  gingivostomatitis see white
  sponge naevus
Fanconi's anaemia, 225
fascial space infections, 271
fellatio palate, 373
Felty's syndrome, 26, 439
Ferguson–Smith syndrome, 135
fibroepithelial polyps, 28, 355
fibromas
  cemento-ossifying, 468, 475
  leaf, 28, 355
  ossifying, 475
  subungual, 518
fibromatosis, gingival, 28,
  323, 530
  associated syndromes, 530
  hereditary, 323, 519

fibrous dysplasia, 471–2
  familial, 24, 469
fibrous lumps see fibroepithelial
  polyps
finger clubbing, 271
fissured (scrotal, plicated)
  tongue, 7, 519
flucloxacillin, 49
fluconazole, 48
fluorosis, 290
fluoxetine, 56
flupentixol, 56
flushing, facial, 59–60
focal epithelial hyperplasia
  (Heck's disease), 30, 83
folate deficiency, 225
foliate papillitis, 28, 357
follicular cysts, 457, 458
food additive 'allergy', 378
Fordyce spots, 28, 520
foreign bodies, 573
fragile X syndrome, 520
fragilitas ossium, 28, 537
freckles (ephelides), 28, 351
Frey's syndrome, 28, 574
fungal infections see mycoses
furred tongue, 357

ganglioneuroblastoma, 152
ganglioneuroma, 152
gangrene, 231
  labial, 263
  progressive bacterial
    synergistic, 424
gangrenous cellulitis, 424
Gardner's syndrome, 28, 291,
  382, 521
gargoylism, 192
gastric regurgitation, 381
gastrointestinal diseases, 377–86
gastrointestinal neoplasms, 381
gentamicin, 52
geographic stomatitis, 353
geographic tongue see erythema
  migrans
geometric herpetic stomatitis, 74
German measles (rubella), 28, 91
germination/germinated
  odontomes, 299
Gilchrist's disease see North
  American blastomycosis
Gilles de la Tourette syndrome,
  247
gingival carcinoma, 167–8, 329
gingival cysts, 322
gingival fibromatosis, 28,
  323, 530
  associated syndromes, 530
  hereditary, 323, 519
gingival hyperplasia, 556–7
gingival lesions, differential
  diagnosis of, 15–16

gingival/periodontal disease,
317–30;
traumatic occlusion, 329
gingival pigmentation changes,
327
gingival recession, 324
gingival swelling, 378
drug-related, 60, 262–3, 321
gingival tumours, 329
gingivitis
acute necrotizing ulcerative,
20, 97
in HIV, 212
chronic hyperplastic, 319
chronic marginal, 319
desquamative, 26, 321, 384, 407
linear IgA disease, 422
pemphigoid, 425
pemphigus, 427
during menstruation, 400
phenytoin-induced, 253
plasma cell, 328
pregnancy, 401
glandular fever (infectious
mononucleosis), 28
facial palsy, 86
Paul–Bunnell positive, 85
globulo-maxillary cysts, 459
glossitis, 229, 357
atrophic, 28, 104, 184
benign migratory see
erythema, migrans
drug-related, 60
in iron deficiency, 28
median rhomboid, 28, 36, 120
Moeller's, 28, 184
glossodynia (glossopyrosis) see
burning mouth/tongue
glossopharyngeal nerve
palsy, 253
glucagonoma, 187
gluten-sensitive enteropathy
(coeliac disease), 24, 382
'golden' tongue, 347
Good's sign, 122
Gorlin–Goltz syndrome, 28,
523–4
graft-versus-host disease
(GVHD), 222
grafts, 575
granular cell
tumour/myoblastoma, 134
granulomas, 122
eosinophilic, of oral
mucosa, 351
giant cell, 188, 322, 474
midline, 265
pregnancy, 400
pyogenic, 40, 328, 370, 400
granulomatous disease, chronic,
24, 225
green staining of teeth, 312, 388

'ground glass' radiographs, 472
gummas, 104, 108
gustatory sweating see Frey's
syndrome

Hapsburg chin, 296
haemangiomas, 28, 174–6, 531
Sturge–Weber syndrome, 542
haemarthrosis, 227
haematomas
iatrogenic, 575–6
lingual, 364
traumatic, 579
haematopoietic stem cell
transplantation, 222–4
haemoglobinopathies, 226
haemophilia, 30, 226–7
Christmas disease
(haemophilia B), 227
classic (haemophilia A), 227
haemorrhagic bone cysts, 475
Hailey–Hailey disease, 430
hairy leukoplakia, 30
in HIV, 205, 208
halitosis (oral malodour), 30, 270
differential diagnosis, 7
drug-related, 60
Hallermann–Streiff syndrome,
525
haloperidol, 55
hamartomas, 173–8
Cowden's syndrome, 501
haemangiomas, 28, 174–6,
531, 542
lymphangiomas, 34, 176, 507
neurofibromatosis, 547
hand foot and mouth disease,
30, 66
Hand–Schüller–Christian
disease, 135
haylinosis cutis et mucosae, 192
heart diseases, 265
heavy metal poisoning,
557, 587
Heck's disease, 30, 83
Heerfordt's syndrome, 30, 128
hemifacial hypertrophy, 525
progressive, 541
hepatitis
chronic active, 388
viral, 390
hereditary angioedema, 30
hereditary angioedema
(HANE), 199
hereditary enamel
hypocalcification, 278
hereditary enamel
hypoplasia, 277
hereditary gingival fibromatosis,
323, 519
hereditary haemorrhagic
telangiectasia, 30, 264, 525

hereditary opalescent dentine,
285
hereditary palmoplantar
keratoses, 525–6
herpangina, 30, 67
herpes
drug-related infections, 564
labialis, 30, 70, 73, 200
in HIV, 204
in leukaemia, 139
simplex, 48, 68–9
and Bell's palsy, 250
in cardiac transplantation,
262
in HIV, 204–5
in leukaemia, 139
in liver transplantation, 389
recurrent infection, 70, 74
varicella, 48, 76
in HIV, 208
zoster, 42, 48, 77–81
in HIV, 208
and immunodeficiency, 77
and jaw necrosis, 587
in leukaemia, 140
mandibular/maxillary, 78, 80
ophthalmic, 79, 80
Ramsay Hunt syndrome,
81, 251
herpetic stomatitis, 30
highly active antiretroviral
therapy (HAART), 203, 215
hilar adenopathy with erythema
nodosum see sarcoidosis
hirsutism, 8
facial, 59
histiocytosis, 30, 135–6
histoplasmosis, 30, 122, 214–15
HIV see AIDS/HIV
Hodgkin's lymphoma, 30
Horner's syndrome, 30
human immunodeficiency virus
see AIDS/HIV
human papillomavirus infections,
30, 82–4, 208
drug-related, 564
Hurler's syndrome, 192–3
Hutchinson's incisors, 105
Hutchinson's summer
prurigo, 584
hydrocortisone, 53, 54
hypercementosis, 290, 479
hyperdontia, 291
hyperglycaemia, 187
hyperkeratosis, 324, 358, 407
hyperostosis corticalis deformans
juvenilis, 481, 495
hyperparathyroidism, 30, 188
hyperpigmentation
Addison's disease, 183
Albright's syndrome, 466
drug-related, 60, 557–60

different colours, 64
gingival, 327
in HIV, 218
radiation-induced, 589
'rain-drop', 557
hyperplasia, 373
adenomatoid, 333
denture-induced (epulis
fissuratum), 24, 26, 350
focal epithelial, 30, 83
gingival, drug-induced, 556–7
papillary, 38, 368
traumatic, 578
verrucous, 373
hyperplastic pulpitis, 292
hypersalivation (sialorrhoea),
12, 42
drug-related, 60–1
hypnotics, 57
hypo-adrenocorticism see
Addison's disease
hypodontia, 292–3
hypoglossal palsy, 254
hypohidrotic ectodermal
dysplasia see ectodermal
dysplasia
hypoparathyroidism, 189
congenital, 32
hypophosphataemia, 395
hypophosphatasia, 32, 189
hypoplasminogenaemia, 228
hypothyroidism, 191

iatrogenic injury, 575–7
ichthyosis, 526–7
vulgaris, 527
idiopathic midfacial granuloma
syndrome, 32, 265
idiopathic trigeminal
neuralgia, 10
IgA disorders
linear IgA disease, 3, 34
pustilosis, intra-epidermal, 430
selective IgA deficiency, 201–2
immune disorders, 197–220
genetically based, 200–2
immunomodulators, 54
impacted teeth, 294, 297
impetigo, 32, 412
and herpes simplex, 73
with zoster, 80–1
incisive canal cysts, 460
incontinentia pigmenti, 293, 527
infantile cortical hyperostosis,
481, 495
infectious mononucleosis see
glandular fever
infestations, 126, 127
influenza, 271
intraoral sebaceous
hyperplasia, 520
invaginated odontomes, 299–300

ionizing radiation damage, 584–9
'iris' lesions, 412
iron-deficiency anaemia, 229
iron staining of teeth, 312
ischaemic diseases, 265
isolated hypoplasia, 288

Jaffe–Lichtenstein syndrome, 471–2
jaundice, 388
jaw necrosis, 587
Job syndrome, 201
joint disorders, 487–90
juvenile rheumatoid arthritis, 440

Kaposi's sarcoma, 32, 329
    drug-related, 565
    in HIV, 208–9
Kawasaki disease, 32, 126
keratoacanthoma, 135
keratoconjunctivitis sicca   see Sjögren's syndrome
keratosis, 324, 358–62
    diffuse, 383
    frictional, 32, 362, 574
    hereditary palmoplantar, 525–6
    homogenous, 358
    in SLE, 449
    smoker's, 32
    speckled, 359
    sublingual, 32, 359
    and syphilis, 362
    verrucous (nodular), 32, 358
        proliferative, 83, 359
    see also leukoplakia
ketoconazole, 48
Klippel–Trenaunay–Weber syndrome, 174, 528
Koenen's tumours, 518
koilonychia, 229
Koplik's spots, 87

Laband's syndrome, 529, 530
labial fraenum, abnormal, 492
labial gangrene, 263
laceration, lingual, 364
Langerhan's cell histiocytosis, 30, 135–6
larva migrans, 126
latent bone cysts, 483
lateral medullary syndrome, 254
lateral periodontal cysts, 459
lateral periodontal (parodontal) abscesses, 38, 318
lead poisoning, 557
leaf fibroma, 28, 355
learning disabilities, 241, 245
leiomyoma, 136
leishmaniasis, 32, 127
lentigo polyposis   see Peutz–Jeghers syndrome
leontiasis ossea, 479

leprosy, 32, 100
Lesch–Nyhan syndrome, 191, 247
Letterer–Siwe disease, 32, 135
leukaemias, 32, 137–41
leukaemic deposits (chloromas), 137, 140
leukoedema, 362, 530
leukopenia, 32, 73, 231
leukoplakia, 104, 324
    candidal, 120
    drug-induced, 564, 565
    in dyskeratosis congenita, 512
    hairy, 30
        in HIV, 205, 208
    proliferative verrucous, 83, 359
    see also keratosis
lichen
    planus, 34, 369, 388, 413–22
        atrophic, 415
        cutaneous lesions, 419
        erosive, 415
        malignancy, 416
        nail involvement, 421
        papular, 413
        plaque type, 413
        striated (reticular), 413
    sclerosis et atrophicus, 422
lichenoid lesions, drug-induced, 34, 61, 421, 564
    in HIV, 217
linea alba, 362
linear gingival erythema, 214
linear IgA disease, 3, 34, 422
lingual arteritis, 263
lingual carcinoma, 166–7, 254
lingual haematoma, 364
lingual hemihypertrophy, 365
lingual laceration, 364
lingual necrosis, 263
lingual thyroid, 543
lingual tonsils, inflammation of, 357
lip disorders
    carcinoma, 165, 565
    chapping, 365
    fissures, 365–6
    lesions, differential diagnosis of, 14–15
    lip chewing/biting (morsicatio buccarum), 36, 246, 348
    lip horn, 366
    lip licking, 247, 349
    lip pits, 531
    swelling, 378
    see also cheilitis
lipid proteinosis, 192
lipomas, 141
liver
    diseases, 387–91
    transplantation, 389
local analgesic injury, 564, 575

localized oral purpura, 34, 235, 423
    differential diagnosis, 3
lower motor neurone facial palsy, 382
    Bell's palsy, 22, 250–1
    congenital (Möbius syndrome), 251, 255
Ludwig's angina, 34, 271
lung cancer, 272
lupoid reactions, drug-related, 61
lupus
    erythematosus, 34
        discoid, 26, 408
        systemic, 448–9
    pernio, 129
    vulgaris, 107
Lutz's disease   see South American blastomycosis
Lyme disease, 34
lymphadenitis
    acute, 34, 405
    chronic, 34
    Staphylococcus aureus, 44
lymphadenopathy, cervical, 58
lymphangioma, 34, 176
    cystic hygroma, 507
lymphomas, 34, 142–5
    gingival, 329
    in HIV, 209
lymphonodular pharyngitis, 272
lymphosarcoma   see lymphomas

Maffucci's syndrome, 531
MAGIC syndrome, 34, 346
"la maladie du petit papiers", 241
'malar' rash, 448
malignant melanoma, 146
malocclusion, 296–7
    see also occlusion, traumatic
management of disease
    drugs used, 46–57
    guide to diseases, 20–45
mandibular retrusion, 296
mandibulofacial dysostosis, 544
Marfan's syndrome, 532
Martin–Bell syndrome, 520
masseteric hypertrophy, 34, 245
materia alba, 325
maxillary sinusitis, 272
McCune–Albright's syndrome, 20, 466
measles (rubeola), 36, 87
median rhomboid glossitis, 28, 36, 120
Mees' lines, 557
mefanamic acid, 46
melanoacanthoma, 147
melanoma, 36
    malignant, 146
melanotic macules, 11, 36, 367

Melkersson–Rosenthal syndrome, 36, 382, 519
MENS, 44
    type IIb, 194
menstruation/menopause, 400–1
mental disorders, 239–48
    see also psychogenic conditions
meptazinol, 47
mercury exposure, 550
metal staining, 314
metastases, 147–8
methylprednisolone, 53, 54
metronidazole, 52–3
miconazole, 48
microtia, isolated, 502
migraine, 10
migrainous neuralgia, 36
Mikulicz's aphthae, 342
minocycline, 51
    staining of bone, 327
mixed connective-tissue disease, 439
Möbius syndrome, 251, 255
Moeller's glossitis, 28, 184
Mohr's syndrome, 536
molluscum contagiosum, 36, 88, 209
moniliasis   see candidosis, acute
monomorphic salivary adenoma, 162
Moon's molars, 105
morphine, 47
morphoea, 445
morsicatio buccarum   see under lip disorders
'moth-eaten' radiographs, 477
mucinoses, 533
mucoceles, 36, 333–4
mucoepidermoid tumour, 36, 161
mucopolysaccharidoses, 192–3
mucormycosis, 36, 123
mucosal disorders, 341–75
mucosal staining, 559
mucosal tags, 378–9
mucositis
    after BMT, 222
    drug-induced, 562
    radiation-induced, 584
mucous membrane pemphigoid, 3, 36, 424–6
mulberry molars, 105
multiple basal cell naevus syndrome   see Gorlin–Goltz syndrome
multiple endocrine adenoma syndrome (MENS), 44
    type III, 194
multiple hamartoma/ neoplasia syndrome   see Cowden's syndrome
multiple myeloma (myelomatosis), 36, 149

mumps, 36, 89
Munchausen's syndrome, 242, 324
Murray–Puretic–Drescher syndrome, 530
Mycobacterium spp., 100, 107, 108
mycoses, 111–24
  aspergillosis, 112
  blastomycoses, 38, 42, 112
  histoplasmosis, 30, 122
  mucormycosis, 36, 123
  see also candidosis
mycosis fungoides, 36, 151
myelodysplastic syndrome, 36, 230
myelomas
  localized, 157
  multiple, 36, 149
myelomatosis (multiple myeloma), 36–7, 149–50
myiasis, 127
myopathic facies, 533
myotonic dystrophy, 533
myxomas, 151

naevi, 11, 367, 534
  blue rubber-bleb, 495
  intramucosal, 534
  multiple basal cell *see* Gorlin–Goltz syndrome
  naevus unius lateris, 534
  of Ota, 367
  white sponge, 44, 547
Nager's syndrome, 544
nasopalatine duct cysts, 460
natal teeth, 298
neck swellings, 18
necrosis
  jaw, 587
  lingual, 263
  osteonecrosis, 61, 565
  osteoradionecrosis *see* osteomyelitis
necrotizing fasciitis, 423–4
necrotizing sialometaplasia, 36, 334
nefopam, 47
Nelson's syndrome, 183
neoplasms, 133–72
  drug-related, 565
  gastrointestinal, 381
  in liver transplantation, 389
  odontogenic, 454, 456, 461
  predisposition from prior irradiation, 585
  salivary, 158–62
  see also specific neoplasms
nerve damage, 577
nervous system, diseases of, 249–59
neuralgia
  migrainous, 10

trigeminal, 44
  idiopathic, 10
neuroblastomas, 152
neuroectodermal tumours (congenital epulis), 26, 153
neurofibromatosis, 38
  bilateral acoustic, 547
  generalized, 545–7
neuromas, 153
neutropenia, 230
  cyclic, 24, 231
'nicotine' staining of teeth, 312
Nikolsky's sign, 428
nitrazepam, 57
noma, 38
non-Hodgkin's lymphoma, 142
  drug-related, 565
  in HIV, 209
nonaccidental injury *see* child abuse syndrome; Munchausen's syndrome; self-mutilation
nonvital teeth, 299
Noonan's syndrome, 469
North American blastomycosis, 38, 112
nystatin, 48

occlusal line, 362
occlusion, traumatic, 329
  see also malocclusion
odontogenic abscesses, 301–4
odontogenic cysts/neoplasms, 453–64
odontogenic fibromyxoma, 461
odontogenic keratocyst, 461
odontogenic myxoma, 151
odontomes, 299–301
oedema, facial, 60
oestrogen replacement therapy, 400
oligodontia, 512
Olmsted's syndrome, 535
opalescent dentine, hereditary, 285
open bite, 296–7
oral dysaesthesia *see* burning mouth syndrome
oral focal mucinosis, 533
oral malodour (halitosis), 30, 270
  differential diagnosis, 7
  drug-related, 60
oral submucous fibrosis, 38, 367–8
orange staining of teeth, 311
orf, 38, 90
oroantral fistula, 577
orofacial granulomatosis, 38, 382, 550
  drug-induced, 565
orofaciodigital syndrome, 536

Osler–Rendu–Weber syndrome, 30, 264
osteitis
  alveolar (dry socket), 20, 470
  crani circumscripta, 479
  deformans (Paget's disease), 479–81
  syphilitic, 105
osteogenesis imperfecta, 28, 537
osteomas, 155
  in Gardner's syndrome, 521
osteomyelitis, 38, 476–7
  acute, 476–7
  chronic, 477
  maxillary, 477
osteonecrosis, 61, 565
osteopetrosis (Albers–Schönberg syndrome), 38, 467, 537
osteoradionecrosis *see* osteomyelitis
osteosarcoma, 38, 162, 163, 481
overjet, reverse, 296

pachyonychia congenita, 538
Paget's disease (osteitis deformans), 38, 479–81
pain
  differential diagnosis, 9–10
  drug-related, 61
  insensitivity, congenital, 252
pain dysfunction syndrome, 26
  of TMJ, 490
palate
  carcinoma of, 169–70
  lesions of, differential diagnosis, 17
papillary hyperplasia, 38, 368
papillitis, 89
  foliate, 28, 357
papillomas, 82
papillomatosis, 369
  in acanthosis nigricans, 381
Papillon–Lefèvre syndrome, 525, 526
paracetamol (acetaminophen), 46
paracoccidiodomycosis, 38
  see also South American blastomycosis
parkinsonism, 255
parotid duct calculi, 336
parotitis, recurrent, 40, 332–3
Parrot's furrows/nodes, 105
Parry–Romberg syndrome, 541
parvovirus infection (slapped cheek), 90
Patau's syndrome, 539
Paterson–Brown–Kelly syndrome, 233
peg-shaped teeth, 280
pemphigoid, 424–6
  bullous, 426

mucous membrane, 3, 36, 424–6
  ocular involvement, 425–6
  pemphigoid-like reactions, 61, 410
pemphigus, 38, 427–30
  benign (Hailey–Hailey disease), 430
  differential diagnosis, 3
  intra-epidermal IgA pustulosis, 430
  paraneoplastic, 430
  vegetans, 427, 428–30
    Neumann's *vs* Hallopeau type, 428–9
  vulgaris, 427
pemphigus-like reactions, 61–2
penicillins, 49–50
pentazocine, 47
peptic ulceration, 383
periadentitis mucosa necrotica recurrens, 343
perianal tags, 379
periapical abscesses, 301–4
  drainage, extraoral, 304
  facial swelling, 302–3, 304
periapical/radicular/dental cysts, 307
periarteritis (polyarteritis) nodosa, 40, 266
pericoronitis, 40, 325
perimyolysis, 240
periodontal/gingival disease, 317–30
periodontitis, 326–7
  accelerated (aggressive), 326
  acute apical, 40
  chronic, 326
  in HIV, 212
  juvenile, 326–7
  rapidly progressive, 326
periodontosis *see* periodontitis, juvenile
periostitis, proliferative, 477
peritonsillar abscesses, 273
perlèche *see* cheilitis, angular
pernicious anaemia, 185, 232
petechiae, 235
  in HIV, 217
  in SLE, 449
pethidine, 47
Peutz–Jeghers syndrome, 382, 540
pharyngitis, lymphonodular, 272
phenazocine, 47
phenoxymethyl penicillin (penicillin V), 49
phycomycosis *see* mucormycosis
Pierre Robin sequence syndrome, 540
pigmentation changes, 369
  chloasma, 400
  differential diagnosis, 10

gingival, 327
see also tattoos
pigmentation, racial, 540
pigmented lesions, benign, 11
pigmented purpuric
    stomatitis, 431
Pindborg tumour, 456
pink spot, 308
pinta, 108
plaque, dental, 320
plasmacytoma, 157
plasmacytosis, 233
pleomorphic salivary adenoma,
    40, 158–61, 338
Plummer–Vinson syndrome, 233
plunging ranula, 334
poisons, 557–9
Poland–Möbius syndrome, 255
polyarteritis (periarteritis)
    nodosa, 40, 266
polycythaemia rubra vera, 40, 234
polymyositis, 438
polyvinyl chloride
    acro-osteolysis, 488
porphyria, 312
prednisolone, 53, 54
pregnancy complications, 400–1
primary biliary cirrhosis, 389–90
primordial cysts, 461
procaine penicillin, 50
proliferative periostitis, 477
proliferative verrucous
    leukoplakia, 83
propanolol, 55
prurigo, actinic, 584
pseudoankylosis, 442
psoriasis, 431, 519
psychogenic conditions
    differential diagnosis, 19
    psychogenic oral disease,
        243–5
    see also mental disorders
pulp polyps, 292
pulpitis, 40
    hyperplastic, 292
purpura, 234
    differential diagnosis, 11
    localized oral, 3, 34, 235, 423
pyoderma gangrenosum, 384
pyogenic arthritis, 40
    of TMJ, 489
pyogenic granulomas, 40, 328,
    370, 400
pyostomatitis
    gangrenosum, 384
    vegetans, 40, 379, 384

quinsy, 273

radiation effects, 583–90
    radiation accidents, 589
    radiotherapy damage, 584–9

'rain-drop' hyperpigmentation,
    557
Ramsay Hunt syndrome, 81, 251
ranulas, 334
    see also mucoceles
Raynaud's phenomenon, 440, 443
recurrent aphthous stomatitis
    see aphthae
recurrent parotitis, 40, 332–3
red areas, differential diagnosis
    of, 11
Reiter's syndrome, 40, 101
renal failure, chronic, 394
renal transplantation, 395
Rendu–Osler–Weber syndrome,
    30, 264
residual cysts, 307
respiratory diseases, 269–74
retained primary teeth, 308
retained roots, 309
retention mucoceles, 334
rhabdomyosarcoma, 157
rheumatoid arthritis, 42, 440, 446
rickets, 42, 185
    vitamin D-resistant, 190
rifampicin, 53
Riga–Fedes disease, 372
Riley–Day syndrome, 247, 255–6
Romberg syndrome, 541
rubella (German measles), 28, 91
rubeola, 36, 87
Russell's sign, 240
Rutherfurd's syndrome, 530

saliva discolouration, 62
salivary gland disorders, 331–9
    differential diagnosis, 18
    drug-related, 62
    in HIV, 217
    neoplasms, 158–62
    salivary fistula, 336
    salivary tumour, mixed,
        158–61
    in Sjögren's syndrome, 446
    tumours, 338
sarcoidosis, 42, 127–9
sarcomas, 162–3
    rhabdomyosarcoma, 157
Schimke's syndrome, 194
scleroderma, 42, 442–5
    localized (morphoea), 445
scrofula, 108
scrotal tongue, 42
scurvy, 42, 185
seamstress' notch, 295
sedatives, 55
selective IgA deficiency, 201–2
self-mutilation/habit-induced
    lesions, 246–7
    cheek-chewing, 22, 348
    gingival, 240, 324
    labial, 348

lip chewing/biting (morsicatio
    buccarum), 36, 246, 348
lip licking, 247, 349
    tongue disorders, 246
    traumatic ulcers, 373
'shell teeth', 285
shingles (zoster) see herpes,
    zoster
sialadenitis
    acute bacterial, 20, 332–3, 447
    obstructive, 335–6
    recurrent, 332–3
sialadenosis (sialosis), 42,
    337, 388
sialolithiasis see calculus,
    salivary
sialometaplasia, necrotizing,
    36, 334
sialorrhoea (hypersalivation), 42
    differential diagnosis, 12
    drug-related, 60–1
sialosis (sialadenosis), 42,
    337, 388
sicca syndrome, 389–90
sickle cell disease, 226
simian crease, 509
simple bone cysts, 475
sinusitis, 42
    maxillary, 272
Sjögren's syndrome, 42, 445–7
    primary vs secondary, 446
    see also xerostomia
skin grafts, 575
skin/subcutaneous tissue
    diseases, 403–31
skip lesions, 378
slapped cheek see parvovirus
    infection
SLE see systemic lupus
    erythematosus
Smith–Lemu–Opitz
    syndrome, 541
smoker's palate, 370
'snow-capped' teeth, 278
South American blastomycosis,
    42, 112
    see also paracoccidiodomycosis
squamous cell carcinomas,
    165–70
    of alveolar ridge, 168
    of buccal mucosa, 169–70
    of gingiva, 167–8
    in HIV, 209
    of lip, 165
    of palate, 169–70
    of tongue, 166–7
Stafne bone cavity, 483
Staphylococcus aureus
    lymphadenitis, 44
Steinert's syndrome, 533
stem cell transplantation,
    haematopoietic, 222–4

Stevens–Johnson syndrome see
    erythema, multiforme
Still's syndrome, 440
stomatitis
    angular see cheilitis, angular
    chronic ulcerative, 422
    denture-induced, 24, 116–18
    geographic, 353
    geometric herpetic, 74
    migratory see erythema,
        migrans
    nicotina, 370, 566
    pigmented purpuric, 431
    recurrent aphthous (RAS) see
        aphthae
    vesicular, 66
streptococcal tonsilitis, 44
stroke, 44, 252
Sturge–Weber syndrome,
    542–3
subluxation of TMJ, 44, 489
submandibular duct calculi,
    335–6
sulfonamides, 50
sun damage, 584
'sunburst' ulcers, 423
superficial mucoceles, 334
supernumerary teeth, 291
Sutton's ulcers, 343
symblepharon, 425
syphilis, 102–6
    congenital, 105
    and HIV, 215
    and leukoplakia/glossitis, 362
    non-venereal, 108
    secondary, 103–4
    tertiary, 104–5
syphilitic osteitis, 105
systemic lupus erythematosus
    (SLE), 448–9
    nail involvement, 449

T-cell lymphoma, 142–3
'target' lesions, 410, 412
TASS syndrome, 183
taste disturbance, 62–3
    loss, 8, 588
tattoos, 371, 553
    amalgam, 11, 20, 327, 371,
        551–2
taurodontism, 310
teeth, disorders of see tooth
    disorders
telangiectasia
    differential diagnosis, 12
    hereditary haemorrhagic, 30,
        264, 525
    in primary biliary
        cirrhosis, 389
teletherapy, 584
temazepam, 57
temporal arteritis, 263

temporomandibular joint (TMJ)
  arthritides, 489
  dysfunction, 10
  pain-dysfunction syndrome, 490
  pyogenic arthritis, 489
  subluxation, 44, 489
teratomas, 311
tetracycline staining of teeth, 312–13
  detection, 313–14
tetracyclines, 50–1
tetralogy of Fallot, 543
thalidomide, 54
thioridazine, 55
thrombocytopenia, 73
thrush see candidosis, acute
thymoma, 122
thyroid, lingual, 543
TIE syndrome, 202
'tissue-paper' scarring, 108
'tobacco pouch' mouth, 442
tongue disorders
  carcinomas, 166–7, 254
  from chewing, 246
  cysts, 322
  differential diagnosis, 17
  discolouration, 559–60
  furred tongue, 357
  lingual arteritis, 263
  lingual haematoma, 364
  lingual hemihypertrophy, 365
  lingual laceration, 364
  lingual necrosis, 263
  lingual tonsils, inflammation of, 357
  traumatic ulcers, 372
tongue-tie (ankyloglossia), 492–3
tonsilitis, 44
tonsillitis, 273
tonsils, lingual, 357
tooth crowning, 570
tooth discolouration, 271, 559
  drug-related, 63, 559, 566
  extrinsic staining, 311–12
  fluorosis, 290

intrinsic staining, 312–14
tooth disorders, 273
  abrasion/abfraction, 276
  aesthetic damage, 295
  ankylosis, 279
  attrition, 281, 285, 303
  cusps, prominent, 307
  dental caries, 282–4, 314
  dilaceration, 286
  erosion, 240, 289, 388, 566
  fusion, 280
  in hypophosphataemia, 395
  impacted teeth, 294, 297
  localized damage, 295
  natal teeth, 298
  nonvital teeth, 299
  resorption
    external, 308
    internal (pink spot), 308
  shape anomalies, 280
  staining, extrinsic, 311
  tubercules, prominent, 307
tori, 44
  torus mandibularis, 483
  torus palatinus, 484
toxic epidermal necrolysis (TEN), 215, 434, 564
toxoplasmosis, 44, 129
tranexamic acid, 57
tranquilizers, 55
trauma to dentition, 578
Treacher Collins syndrome, 544
Treponema spp. 105, 108
triamcinolones, 53
trigeminal disorders
  neuralgia, 44, 256
  paraesthesia/hypoaesthesia, 63
  sensory loss, 257
  trismus, 12
tuberculosis, 44, 107–8
tuberculous cervical lymphadenitis, 108
tuberous sclerosis see Bournville–Pringle disease
Turner's tooth, 288
'twinning' of teeth, 299
tylosis, 383

ulcerative colitis, 384
ulcers/ulceration
  Bednar's, 373
  in Crohn's disease, 379
  differential diagnosis, 13
  drug-related, 63, 562
  eosinophilic, 351
  in HIV, 214–15
  in leukaemia, 138
  in SLE, 449
  'sunburst', 423
  Sutton's, 343
  traumatic, 327–8, 579
Urbach–Weithe disease, 192
urinogenital disorders, 390
uveitis, 346
uveparotid fever, 128
uvula
  absent, 492
  bifid (cleft), 494
uvulitis, 91

vaccinia, 92
vagal nerve palsy, 253
van der Woude's syndrome, 531, 545
vancomycin, 51
varicella (chickenpox) see herpes, varicella
varices, 266
verrucous hyperplasia, 373
verrucous leukoplakia, proliferative, 83
verrucous xanthoma, 374
vesicular stomatitis with exanthem, 66
Vincent's disease see gingivitis, acute necrotizing ulcerative
viral infections, 65–93
  glandular fever (infectious mononucleosis), 85–6
  hand foot and mouth disease, 30, 66
  herpangina, 30, 67
  in HIV, 204
  human papillomavirus infections, 30, 82–4

measles (rubeola), 87
mumps, 36, 89
orf, 38, 90
parvovirus infection (slapped cheek), 90
rubella (German measles), 28, 91
uvulitis, 91
vaccinia, 92
see also herpes
vitamin B deficiency, 184
vitamin C deficiency, 185
vitamin D deficiency, 185
vitiligo, 218, 434
von Recklinghausen's disease, 545–7
von Willebrand's disease, 236

warts, 82
warty dyskeratoma, 507
Wegener's granulomatosis, 267, 329
white lesions, 13
white sponge naevus, 44, 547
Wickham's striae, 419
Wiskott–Aldrich syndrome, 202

xanthoma, verrucous, 374
xerostomia (dry mouth), 26 338–9, 446
  after BMT, 222
  and caries, 284
  differential diagnosis, 5
  drug-related, 58–9, 563
  in HIV, 217
  radiation-induced, 586, 588
  see also Sjögren's syndrome

yaws, 108

Zimmermann–Laband syndrome, 529, 530
zinc deficiency, 180
zoster (shingles) see herpes, zoster
zygomycosis see mucormycosis

4th ed too expensive.
Selected alternate title.
1 checkout through 2011

DM 5/11/11